PRODUCTION OF BIOLOGICALS FROM ANIMAL CELLS IN CULTURE

PRODUCTION OF BIOLOGICALS FROM ANIMAL CELLS IN CULTURE

Editors

R. E. Spier

Department of Microbiology, University of Surrey,
Guildford, Surrey, UK

J. B. Griffiths

PHLS CAMR, Porton, Salisbury, Wilts, UK

B. Meignier

Institut Merieux, Marcy L'Étoile, Charbonnières, France

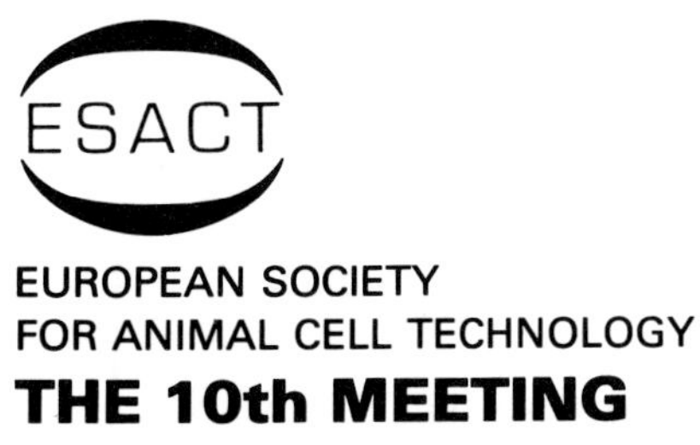

EUROPEAN SOCIETY
FOR ANIMAL CELL TECHNOLOGY
THE 10th MEETING

Butterworth–Heinemann Ltd
Halley Court, Jordan Hill, Oxford OX2 8EJ

 PART OF REED INTERNATIONAL P.L.C.

OXFORD LONDON GUILDFORD BOSTON MUNICH NEW DELHI
SINGAPORE SYDNEY TOKYO TORONTO WELLINGTON

First published 1991

© **Butterworth–Heinemann Ltd, 1991**

British Library Cataloguing in Publication Data

European Society for Animal Cell Technology.
   Meeting: 10th: 1990: Avignon, France
   Production of biologicals from animal cells in culture.
   1. Biological medicinal products. Production use of animal cells
   I. Title   II. Spier, R. E. (Raymond E.)
   III. Griffiths, J. B. (John Bryan). *1941–*   IV. Meignier, B.
   615.3

ISBN 0-7506-1103-0

Library of Congress Cataloging-in-Publication Data

European Society for Animal Cell Technology. General
   Meeting (10th: 1990: Avignon, France)
      Production of biologicals from animal cells in culture/
   editors, R. E. Spier, J. B. Griffiths, B. Meignier
         p.   cm.
      "European Society for Animal Cell Technology, the
   10th Meeting." Held in Avignon, France, 1990.
      Includes bibliographical references and index.
      ISBN 0-7506-1103-0
      1. Biologicals—Congresses.   2. Cell culture—
   Congresses.   3. Pharmaceutical biotechnology—
   Technique—Congresses.   I. Spier, R. (Raymond)
   II. Griffiths, J. B.   III. Meignier, B.   IV. Title.
   RS162.E88   1989
   615′.36—dc20

Printed and bound by Hartnolls Ltd, Bodmin, Cornwall

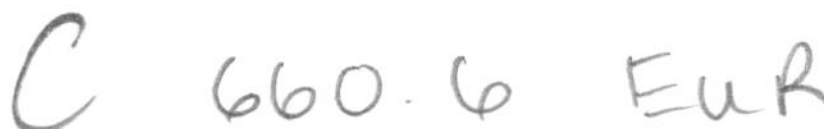

Organizing Committee

B. Meignier, *Meeting Secretary*

P. H. Archinard

J. M. Engasser

M. Koehl

B. Languet

J. Lupker

O. Merten

P. Trotemann

X. Pouradier-Duteil

Sponsors

The organizing committee acknowledges the financial support of:

AKZO
Alfa-Laval Centritech AB
Amicon
Applikon
B. Braun Sciencetec
B. D. Falcon
Biological Industries
BioMérieux
Bio/Technology
Bocknek Ltd
Butterworths
Cellon Sarl
Celltech Ltd
Charles River
Chemap Groupe Alfa-Laval
Comptoir Lyonnais de Verrerie
Cytolab
Diosynth
ECACC
Flobio
Gibco
Hyclone
IBF
Immuno-Chemical Products
Ingold France
Institut Jacques Boy

Institut Mérieux
Institut Pasteur Texcell
Intermed SA
Intervet
In Vitron Corporation
LH Fermentation Ltd
LSL Biolaffitte
MBR Bio Reactor AG
Medical and Veterinary Supplies Ltd
Microbiological Associates Ltd
Miles
Millipore
New Brunswick Scientific
NV Innogenetics
Organon
PAA-Labor-und Forschungs
Quality Biotech Ltd
Rhone-Merieux
Sera-Lab
SGI
Sigma Chimie
Sorebio
Verax Corporation

ESACT Executive Committee 1988–89

R. Spier	*Chairman*	University of Surrey, Guildford, UK
J. Stephenne	*Secretary/Treasurer*	Smith Kline Biologicals, Rixensart, Belgium
B. Meignier	*Meeting Secretary*	Institut Mérieux, Charbonnières, France
B. Griffiths		PHLS CAMR, Porton, UK
H. Katinger		Universität für Bodenkultur, Vienna, Austria
J. Lehmann		Universität Bielefeld, FRG
C. MacDonald		University of Strathclyde, Glasgow, UK
A. Mizrahi		Israel Institute for Biological Research, Ness Ziona, Israel

10th ESACT Meeting, Avignon, France

Session Officials

Chairmen

F. Horaud	D. G. Kilburn
M. Koehl	C. MacDonald
R. E. Spier	X. Pouradier Duteil
A. S. Lubiniecki	F. Wurm
S. Reuveny	J. Lehmann
P. Trotemann	T. Van Der Velden-de Groot
H. Katinger	B. Meignier
J. Lupker	G. F. Panina
O. Merten	B. Griffiths
E. J. Schlaeger	J. Stephenne
B. Montagnon	J. M. Engasser
J. Plana Duran	J. Litwin

Chairman's statement

At the conclusion of the 10th meeting of ESACT it is timely to look back at where we have come from and forward towards that to which we are impelled. We have met in nine countries over 15 years and attendance at meetings has risen from 75 to over 350. The next three meetings are likely to be first in the UK, followed by Germany and then Holland. The Dutch meeting could be a joint meeting with our Japanese sister society, JAACT. The subject too has undergone marked changes. From its twin, and very similar, foci of vaccines for foot-and-mouth disease and polio we have added monoclonal antibodies, recombinant proteins and recombinant vaccines. Cells too, are becoming serious products as such and there are many new proteins yet to be discovered.

Twenty years ago researchers who boasted green fingers were in demand, but the conceived costliness deterred many from entering the field and the need to operate free from contamination was also an inhibitory factor. Most such restrictions have now been overcome in the minds of those who increasingly turn to animal cells in culture as a means of achieving their contribution to commerce or society. Additionally, the view that animal cells are naked, fragile and defenceless blobs of amorphous protoplasm is gradually receding as more and more investigators discover how difficult it is to break the plasma membranes of healthy cells. Our new-found ability to design growth media for a wide variety of cells in different states of differentiation is also a pointer to a more varied and extensive future use of animal cells in culture.

There is little doubt that ESACT, by acting as a focus and a forum for the exchange of ideas, techniques and contacts, has been instrumental in increasing the rate of progress. Similar kinds of meeting are now regular occurrences under the auspices of the Federation of American Engineering Societies and the Japanese society referred to above. Mini-ESACTs are alive and well in Holland, Germany and the UK. This is clearly a process which is gathering momentum and from which this subject area can expect benefit.

There are yet new functions which fall to the parent society: ESACT has been very active in the formulation and promulgation of a T-project under the auspices of the European Community's BRIDGE program. Although the thrust of this project is biochemical, involving the understanding of the ways in which exogenous genes can be inserted and expressed in host animal cells, there is still a need for an equivalently sized project in the area of the bioprocess engineering of systems which can exploit, with the greatest efficiency, the capabilities of animal cells in culture. It is in this area that the commercial edge which controls success or failure is to be gained.

A second role for ESACT is its participation in scientific and technical meetings to determine ways in which the procedures used to ascertain the safety, efficacy, consistency and social benefit of product generating operations can be progressed. ESACT co-hosted one such meeting in Washington in the autumn of 1988 and is involved in the preparation of another in spring 1991. There is no doubt that much conjecture about conceptual hazards has given way to serious data on the properties of materials for which a licence is sought, but movements of this nature have not yet outrun their utility and further progress and rationalization can be expected.

ESACT is also active in setting up a repository of cells that can be used by the interested community for comparative studies of bioreactors or bioprocess technologies. Such studies are needed to enable differentiation between the myriad alternatives which are presented as potential systems for product generation. Readers may take these remarks as an invitation to send their donations to further this project to the ECACC cell bank at Porton UK. Professor Griffiths will implement it when sufficient funds have been raised.

The ingenuity of the genetic engineers abounds. Transgenic animals, transgenic crop plants and mini-, domaine- and chimeric-antibodies that can be produced in bacteria are with us. Claims are made that such systems could universally supersede the 'old hat' animal cell culture activities, but each such potential has to prove itself in generating and supporting a licensed, profit-making, commercial product. This eventuality seems some way off yet, and meanwhile the appropriately post-translationally modified materials made from animal cells in culture will in all likelihood hold sway.

Exciting times are ahead. Gauntlets have been thrown, prizes dangled and the field has been prepared for us to show our capabilities and ingenuity. I am sure that ESACT will continue to keep its members and participants in the forefront of this endeavour and retain its position as a force for progress in the years to come.

R. E. Spier
European Society for Animal Cell Technology Chairman, (ESACT)

Introduction

The 135 contributions to this volume constitute a state-of-the-art report on the field of animal cell biotechnology. They have been organized into sections reflecting the sequence of events that occur when generating a product from animal cells in culture. It is of interest to note that bioreactors still command intensive attention (some 32 (23%) of the papers), but downstream processing and regulatory aspects, including quality control and assurance activities, do not seem at this time to generate the science and technology which is to be presented in the public arena. This is strange, as much work is effected in these areas and although it may not be as glamorous as work with, say, cells or bioreactors, research in this area is just as vital for the progression of the field. Indeed it is *this* area of work, rather than the yield and properties, that is the prime determinant as to the success of a putative product. The design of cells and medium feature strongly and there is a proliferation of serum-free and/or low-protein media. Researchers are beginning to realise that many factors play a role in the system and that it is no longer necessary to keep media formulations secret for fear of commercial competition. Rather, use of a particular raw material or processing procedure is a more certain route to a commercial product than reliance on a particular recipe. Efforts are now in hand to derive and test models that account for the behaviour of cultures. Whether or not such models can be used to predict performance of cell systems that are not predicated in the model has yet to be determined. Nevertheless, methods are quoted here which enable adjustment of nutrient feed streams into perfusion bioreactors so as to increase productivities.

There were a number of issues raised from the papers and ensuing discussions which have been transcribed, edited and presented along with the paper which inspired them. For example, questions were raised as to the usefulness of the fingerprint method for cell characterization. It was adduced that gross differences between HeLa cells and BHK cells could be observed with reliable discrimination, but a HeLa cell and another human cell line (WI38) could *not* be differentiated. Indeed, it was brought out in discussion that it would not be possible to tell the difference between an engineered cell line and the original host cell using this technique, based as it is on enzymic hydrolysis of a section of the total genome. However, the system could be refined so as to determine differences based on changes of fewer nucleotides than at present. It is clear that such refining is awaited with interest, as methods for the clear and specific characterization of a cell substrate are of great value in the achievement and demonstration of consistency in any bioprocess based on animal cells.

In a similar vein, methods are needed for the characterization of the glycoforms of glycoproteins. Nutrient conditions and the state of the culture can affect changes in the particular glycoforms produced so that a rapid, reliable and inexpensive test would be of value in quality control. A rider to such work would be that it may be necessary to determine the state of the other post-translational modifications in addition to those involved in glycosylation.

Two enzymes surfaced as worthy of discussion. One was lactic dehydrogenase and its use as an indicator of cell lysis and, by inference, cell number. It would seem that whereas many investigators can use this system to good effect as they have a stable enzyme, others find that their enzyme activity is not stable, which could be a factor of the source of the enzyme, conditions in the medium, or the conditions of the assay. The other enzyme or enzyme system discussed is that involved in proteolysis. Here again, investigators differed in their experiences: some spoke of stable product proteins, while others could only explain the decrease in product protein as hydrolysis by secreted proteolytic enzymes. It would appear that such enzymes could be multifarious in nature, and that the nature of both the suspending medium and the cell type determine the nature and specificity of the particular protease secreted.

It is difficult to review the new developments in bioreactors. In some cases the action occurs peripherally to the bioreactor itself, in the removal of dead cells or in the separation of perfusate from the cell suspension. In other cases advances are reported in the instigation and exploitation of cell clumps. This latter propensity entails much in prospect, yet the control of these systems and understanding how cells perform under the conditions within these systems will provide a potentially fruitful experimental system. Membrane-based systems and different ways in which perfusion can be achieved are also highlighted topics and ways in which bioreactor systems can be optimized are reported.

Many investigators (and their managers/accountants) need to be sure that the bioreactor system that they are considering is the most effective for their needs, and the comparison of different bioreactors is an active area. Comparative studies should be carried out using a cell system whose performance is well characterized, under optimal conditions for that system; which could present problems as there is as yet no definition of the characteristics of an 'optimized performance'. An operational definition could be: 'the procedures which result in a situation where further modifications to the system do not further improve that system'. (The difficulty in such a definition is that, unknown to the investigator, there may exist a procedure that *could* make a dramatic improvement to one or other of the systems under test. It would therefore be unwise to compare systems where efforts to optimize each system individually had not been part of the programme.

The presentations in this volume represent the breadth and depth of the recent investigations to make the animal cell cultures used to generate commercial products more versatile, efficient and cost-effective. It is clear that we have a lot yet to learn. These papers and discussions highlight areas where problems have emerged and where progress needs to be made. This volume faithfully represents that situation and serves the dual purpose of transmitting information about the state of play as well as being the springboard for much new and exciting work.

R. E. Spier
J. B. Griffiths
B. Meignier

Editors

Contents

Section 3 Serum-free and protein-free media   131

Section 4 Cell physiology   205

Section 5   Gene expression in animal cell systems   285

Section 6.6 Bioreactors: comparative studies 517

Section 11 Regulatory issues 757

Hyclone Award Lecture

ANIMAL CELL CULTURE: THE PROBLEMS AND REWARDS

N B Finter
Wellcome Biotechnology Ltd, Beckenham, Kent BS3 3BS, England

It is an honour to receive this Award, which I accept
with great personal pleasure and on behalf of my colleagues
at Wellcome Biotechnology, too many to name individually,
who made possible the production of interferon from mass
culture of human lymphoblastoid cells.

Animal cell culture was an esoteric art practised by only
a few until the 1950's, when the urgent need for a vaccine
to combat poliomyelitis led to the use of primary monkey
kidney cells for growing the virus. These vaccines were very
successful, but the monkey cell substrate posed many
problems because contamination with wild simian viruses was
so frequent. One of these, SV40, was discovered for the
first time after a considerable amount of contaminated
vaccine had been released for use: epidemiological studies
have shown that, fortunately, the recipients do not appear
to have suffered any harm. Because of these problems, other
cells were considered as alternative substrates, including
the diploid human fibroblast cell strains. These are now the
preferred substrate, and after use for more 20 years, have
proved remarkably free from problems. Nevertheless, in spite
of their obvious advantages, there were at first some who
expressed grave concern about the safety of products made
from them, and this greatly delayed their general
acceptance, for example in the USA. Under such

circumstances, it seemed to many almost unthinkable that cells of transformed lines should even be considered as a source for a pharmaceutical product. Again, the urgent need to solve a problem led to innovation.

Foot-and -mouth disease (FMD)is a major scourge of cattle and pigs, and unless controlled, causes enormous economic losses. A vaccine with virus grown in primary bovine tongue epithelium collected from animals at slaughter, was developed, but much larger amounts of cheaper vaccine were badly needed. In 1964, workers in the Agricultural Research Council's laboratories at Pirbright in southern England found that FMD viruses replicated in monolayer cultures of the BHK 21 line of transformed baby hamster kidney cells. Later, it was shown that the viruses also grew in suspension cultures, and a process for making inactivated FMD virus vaccines from these was developed and scaled up in the adjoining Wellcome Foundation FMD virus laboratory. The vaccines proved innocuous in tests in cattle and pigs, and were introduced in routine use in 1966. They are now manufactured in plants in many parts of the world, and have been administered to many millions of animals.

In spite of this example, it was still generally considered that transformed cells should not be used to make a human pharmaceutical for fear that some virus or oncogenic factor derived from the cells might contaminate the product, causing serious disease in recipients, perhaps after a long interval. Indeed, many scientists believed that there were formal regulations in the USA that proscribed this possible route to manufacture. The need to make much larger amounts of interferons available for use in clinical trials led to this view being challenged.

Although from the time of their discovery in 1957, it seemed certain that interferons would have uses in medicine, it took many years to prove this. The main problem was to -make material for evaluation. For use in man, interferons must be derived from human cells, and thousands of millions of cells are needed to make sufficient for even a small clinical trial. In the first production system developed in Finland in 1966, human white blood cells were centrifuged from blood donated for transfusion purposes and induced to form interferon by treatment with a harmless mouse virus, Sendai. This process was applied in Finland to the cells from hundreds of thousands of donations, and provided almost all the material available for clinical trials until 1979, but even so, the amounts made were relatively very small. Furthermore, this process is labour-intensive and so costly, and only limited safety and quality controls can be applied to a product made from fresh human blood.

In 1959, the British Medical Research Council set up a Scientific Committee to develop interferons for medical use. After 12 years, the prospects for carrying out even limited clinical trials seemed so poor because of the supply situation, that the Committee was dissolved. Fortuitously at about that time, I and a number of scientists who had collaborated as members of this Scientific Committee while working in various other organisations, joined the staff of the Wellcome laboratories in Beckenham. In spite of the apparently dismal prospects, we remained convinced that

interferons would ultimately prove to be useful. What was a
needed was a new manufacturing route to provide plentiful
supplies of a safe and relatively inexpensive product.
Because there seemed no alternative way of obtaining the
requisite huge numbers of humam cells, we decided in 1974 to
explore the use of cells from some suitable transformed cell
line. The criteria were that the cells should be of human
origin, and able to grow well in suspension in large tanks
in some relatively simple medium and to yield large amounts
of interferon when induced with Sendai virus. We screened
nearly 100 cell lines, and selected from these the
lymphoblastoid cell line, Namalwa, derived from a Burkitt
tumour biopsy which best met our requirements.

In taking this decision to use this human cancer cell as
tkhe source of an intended medical product, we knew we were
challenging the accepted scientific wisdom of that time.
This was not done lightly, but against the background that
there was a medical need that could not apparently otherwise
be met. We felt sure that that by developing and applying a
rigorous purification procedure to the starting material, we
should be able to produce a safe and acceptable final
product, as for example, insulin is made from animal
pancreases collected from abattoirs.

A Master Bank of Namalwa cells was laid down in liquid
nitrogen, and used as the source of all cells for the
production area. When cells from this Bank and samples of
crude product were carefully tested, no infectious virus or
other contaminants were detected, and the latter only
occasionally contained very traces of nucleic acid derived

from lysed cells (most lymphoblastoid cells contain Ebstein

Barr virus; in Namalwa cells, the virus DNA genome is

present but no infectious virus is ever formed). Meanwhile,

Karl Fantes, the chemist in our team, had developed a

purification sequence involving a number of chemical and

physical procedures. These were chosen not only to yield a

highly pure product but also as likely to destroy or

eliminate any virus or other undesirable agent that might be

present in the starting material. As none had been found,

apart from traces of nucleic acid, we could not directly

evaluate the effects of our purification sequence.

Therefore, instead, we deliberately added various substances

as markers to the crude product and measured the residual

amounts after the successive stasges in purification.

Usually, only very small amounts were found even after the

first step; therefore, markers were also added to

intermediate products and their elimination followed. The

detailed results have been given elsewhere and will only be

briefly summarised here. We were able to show that no virus

of whatever size or type added to the crude material came

through the purification process, and bacteria, mycoplasmas

and other micro-organisms, and even the scrapie agent

similarly disappeared. With these data, we felt confident

that should some newly discovered virus be found in Namalwa

cells in the future, this would also be eliminated from the

product. The discovery since that time of various new human

viruses, including the T cell leukaemia viruses, even though

none have been detected in Namalwa cells, has shown ; the

wisdom of proving the general case in this way.. Similar

marker studies were carried out with highly radioactive
nucleic acid samples; these also vanished to levels below
the limits of detection. Nevertheless, every batch issued
for use is shown directly to be negative in a test able to
measure 10pg DNA per ml.

In 1975, some preliminary results of trials with
leucocyte interferon in bone cancer in Sweden became public;
these led to a surge of interest in interferons and a demand
for large amounts for detailed clinical evaluation in
patients with various forms of cancer. One consequence was
that the acceptability of the different sources of
interferon became the subject of debate, and it was soon
apparent that there was considerable sympathy with our view
that it might be possible to produce an acceptable product
from Namalwa cells. A second consequence of more immediate
benefit was that the U.S. National Institutes of Health made
arrangements to purchase leucocyte, fibroblast and
lymphoblastoid interferons. In consequence, we received a
contract initially to supply material for reagent use, and
later, to supply for clinical trial use. These
arrangements, which confirmed that there was a demand for
interferon derived from Namalwa cells was a considerable
encouragement to our team and to our management at a time
when costs were beginning to rise steeply.

By 1977, the complete process for making and purifying
lymphoblastoid interferon had been finalised, and with
valuable technological advice from colleagues in the
Wellcome FMD virus laboratory, my colleague, Gareth Ball,
was able to design the first of a number of successful

production plants for which he has been responsible. This first pilot plant with a single 1000 litre production vessel came into use towards the end of 1978 and under the capable control of Ken Pullen, made high quality product from the very first batch. With the fully tested final product, "Wellferon" and all the supporting data required, we approached the the Control Authorities in the UK and USA to seek permission to start clinical trials; these began in the UK in 1979, and in the USA, Canada and Japan in 1980 - 1981.

   Wikth rapidly increasing demands for clinical trial supplies, it was soon an urgent matter to manufacture on a larger scale. Fortunately there was an almost ready made solution in the shape of a large virus vaccines plant which had very recently been completed in North West Spain. This well- managed and equiped plant was relatively simply converted to make interferon, and it remained dedicated to this throughout the past 11 years, during which time, the scale of production has been progressively increased. Currently, crude interferon is made in batches of 10,000 litre batches, each yielding about as much interferon as all that was made from leucocytes in Finland in the years up to 1979.

   While we were developing our tissue culture process, big advances were taking place in recombinant DNA procedures. We collaborated with Professor Burke at the University of Warwick to try to obtain expression of an alpha interferon gene in *Escherchia coli*, but were beaten in the race to this goal by two other groups in 1980, who independently reported

9

their success. In view of this new route to the production
of interferon, which according to media reports of the time
would provide limitless and almost costless supplies, we
nsaturally considered carefully whether to go on with the
clincal development of Wellferon. We decided to continue for
two reasons. The first was that we had a considerable
headstart with our clinical trials; the second and more
important reason was that by then we knew our final product
was not only extremely pure but also contained at least 6
distinct alpha inteferons. Each of these subtypes was
unique in its chemical structure and biological properties,
perhaps reflecting some special role in the body. Thus it
seemed possible that our mixture would differ from any
single subtype made by recombinant DNA procedures in its
behaviour in the clinic, and perhaps have advantages under
at least some circumstances. We therefore continued and
expanded our programme, and in 1986, Wellferon was the first
interferon preparation to be approved by the responsible
United Kingdom government agency for routine use in
medicine, the indication being the treatment of hairy cell
leukaemia.

Three variants of the same interferon subtype, IFN- α_2,
made by recombinant DNA procedures, are now also in clinical
use. A proportion of the patients treated with these
recombinant interferons, in some studies as many as 20% or
more, develop antibodies which neutralise this interferon,
and in consequence no longer respond to the treatment.
Although the different interferons have not been directly
compared in the same trials, it seems that antibody

formation is very much less frequent with Wellferon.
Patients that develop antibodies to IFN- α_2 often respond
again when treated with a leukocyte or lymphoblastoid
interferon; in such patients, the levels of neutralising
antibody against interferon α_2 slowly fall to below the
threshold of detection(von Wussow, personal communication,
1990). These results strongly suggest that there is some
antigenic difference between recombinant and human cell
derived interferons. Wellferon contains at least 22
distinct alpha interferon subtypes, and three of these are
glycosylated including two which match IFN- α_2 in amino acid
composition. As products expressed in *Escherchia coli* are
not glycosylated, and as glycosylation can greatly modify
the antigenic behaviour of a protein, it is tempting to
speculate that this is the basis for the difference between
recombinant interferons and those derived from human cells.
With another cytokine, GM-CSF, Gribben and colleagues
recently showed that O-linked sugars present in a
recombinant version expressed in mammalian cells mask an
epitope that is exposed and antigenic in recombinant
products made in bacteria or yeast. Experiments are in
progress to see if the position is similar with IFN- α_2
(Brand, personal communication, 1990).

I have outlined the development of Wellferon at some
length because it established several important precedents.
Its example showed that cells of a transformed human line
can be used to make a product for use in man. It was the
first cytokine made from cultured cells to be prepared
routinely at more than 95% purity. It established the value

of using marker substances to validate the elimination of micro-organisms and nucleic acids from a product. It showed that animal cell culture on a scale up to at least 10,000 litres is not only possible but economically viable. These examples have contributed to and hastened the now general acceptance of animal cell cultures as the substrate for making therapeutic proteins. Often these are now obtained by expressing the gene concerned in some suitable mammalian cell, such as CHO hamster cells. Of course some proteins will be more cheaply or simply made in bacteria, yeast or insect cells, and no doubt in the future others will be better made by total chemical synthesis (though the closely coupled chemical machinery in a mammalian cell that makes proteins with the correct folding and glycosylation will be hard to reproduce in vitro). Thus with such future developments as serum-free media and techniques for growing cells to even higher densities, I am confident that animal cell culture will become even more widely appreciated and used as the natural way of making proteins for medical use.

Section 1
Cell lines and their characterization

THE ISOLATION OF IMMORTAL MURINE MACROPHAGE CELL LINES

Ute Kreuzburg and Caroline MacDonald

Department of Bioscience and Biotechnology, University of Strathclyde, The Todd Centre, Glasgow G4 0NR, Scotland.

ABSTRACT

Two stable cell lines have been isolated by transfecting mouse peritoneal macrophages with plasmid constructs containing sequences from the oncogenic DNA virus SV40. These cell lines have been assayed for macrophage markers: they express Fc receptors; will stain with neutral red; are able to phagocytose immunoglobulin-coated red cells and latex beads; are F4/80 positive; and have non-specific esterase, lysozyme, collagenase, prostaglandin E2, acid phosphatase, 5' nucleotidase and plasminogen activator activities. Comparisons have been made between activated and non-activated cells.

INTRODUCTION

Differentiated mammalian cell lines can be isolated by transforming primary cells with viral genes. A variety of viral genes have immortalising activity, but comparative studies by Gallimore et al (1) showed that sequences from the SV40 virus give the best results for human embryo retinoblasts. Plasmids containing SV40 early region sequences have been used to immortalise human (2) and rodent (3) cells. A plasmid containing the SV40 genome with a deletion at the origin of replication (ori⁻) transforms human fibroblasts more efficiently than derivatives containing a functional origin of replication (4). However, the properties of cell lines isolated in this way vary considerably (5).

We describe results obtained with mouse peritoneal macrophages immortalised by plasmid sequences introduced by calcium phosphate precipitation. These cell lines have been isolated by transformation using either a plasmid containing the entire SV40 genome except for a small deletion at the origin (pUK42), or with DNA in which only the early region of SV40 was present and which had a deletion at the origin of replication and a disruption in the small t antigen coding sequence (pUKEdt).

MATERIALS AND METHODS

Cell culture

Peritoneal macrophages were cultured in DMEM containing 10% fcs, penicillin (50 IU/ml), streptomycin (50ug/ml), gentamycin (100 ug/ml) all from Gibco, and 50 U/ml granulocyte macrophage colony stimulating factor (GM-CSF, Genzyme). Conditioned medium was prepared from mouse spleen cell cultures set up at 10^6 cells/ml in RPMI 1640 + 10% fcs and stimulated for 48 hours with 10ug/ml concanavalin A, and from 3T3 cultures grown in DMEM + 10% fcs. Medium was collected, centrifuged, filtered through 0.2um filters (Millipore), and stored at -70°C. The conditioned medium was diluted 1:1 with DMEM + 10% fcs before use.

Vectors and DNA transformation

Two plasmid constructs derived from the origin deleted SV40 vector p6-1, were used: one, pUK42, contained all of the SV40 sequences present in p6-1 ligated to pRSVneo, and the other pUKEdt, contained an additional disruption in the small t antigen coding sequence. One day prior to transfection, cells were subcultured using a rubber policeman for removal and reseeded at approx. 1×10^6 cells/25cm^2 flask. DNA was introduced into the cells by calcium phosphate precitation (6) using 15ug plasmid DNA and 5ug salmon sperm carrier DNA per 4ml culture. DNA was washed off the cells after 24 hours and fresh DMEM + 10% fcs 650ug/ml Geneticin (G418, Gibco) was added twice weekly.

RESULTS AND DISCUSSION

Stable cell lines were isolated as a result of transfecting GM-CSF stimulated macrophages with DNA from two different SV40-containing plasmid constructs. The Balb/42 line was obtained by transfection with pUK42 which contains origin-deleted SV40 ligated to the neo gene expressed from the RSV LTR; and Balb/Edt was obtained with pUKEdt which contains a disruption in the SV40 small t antigen coding sequence. The cells were grown in the presence of GM-CSF prior to transformation since cell division is required for integration of foreign DNA (7) but subsequently GM-CSF has not been required. The two cell lines isolated have been cultured continuously for a period of 8 months each, whereas the non-transfected controls survive for a maximum period of 2 months in DMEM. The Balb/42 line was passaged 44 times and the Balb/Edt 33 times during this time in culture. In contrast to the non-transfected macrophages the cell lines could be removed from the culture vessel by trypsinisation.

Both of the cell lines stained with antiserum against F4/80 and were positive for Fc receptors. Fc receptor-mediated phagocytosis of antibody coated red cells was observed after the cells were activated by 24 hour exposure to spleen cell-conditioned medium. In addition, both macrophage lines were able to phagocytose latex beads. Both lines stained by the enzyme marker non-specific esterase but neither was positive for peroxidase. Acid phosphatase activities were quantified: Balb/42 released 1.5 Sigma Units/mg protein and Balb/Edt 1.35 Sigma Units/mg. One Sigma Unit is defined as the enzyme activity which will liberate 1umol of pnitrophenol per hour under defined test conditions.

Plasminogen activator was secreted by both cell lines and
the levels secreted could be increased by activating the
cells by culturing in conditioned medium obtained either
from spleen cells or 3T3 cells. In contrast, 5'-
nucleotidase activity was high in non-activated cells and
extremely low in activated cells. Both cell lines secreted
2ug of lysozyme/mg cell protein using chicken egg white
lysozyme as standard. Cell lysates from Balb/42 contained
55ug collagenase per mg cell protein and Balb/Edt contained
86ug/mg using tadpole collagenase as standard.

Finally, the cells were assayed for prostaglandin E2
production. Low levels of PGE2 have been described in
culture medium by Tanigawa <u>et al</u> (8) and we detected 11pg/ml
PGE2 in samples of DMEM supplemented with 10% fcs. Culture
medium without cells was incubated at 37°C for 2 days and
the level of PGE2 detected as background was subtracted from
levels observed in the cell cultures. This gave values of
35ug of prostaglandin E2/mg cell protein secreted by Balb/42
and 12ug/mg for Balb/Edt.

ACKNOWLEDGEMENTS

This work was supported by grants from the E.C. Stimulation
Action Programme [no. ST2J-0321-C (TT)] and the University
of Strathclyde Research and Development Fund.

REFERENCES

1   Gallimore, P.H., Grand, R.G.A, and Byrd, P.J.
     <u>Anticancer Res</u>. 1986, <u>6</u>, 499

2   Mayne, L.V., Priestly, A., James, M.R. and Burke, J.F.
     <u>Exp. Cell Res</u>. 1986, <u>162</u>, 530

3   Scott, D.M., MacDonald, C., Brzeski, H. and Kinne, R.
     <u>Exp. Cell Res</u>. 1986, <u>166</u>, 391

4   Small, M.B., Gluzman, Y. and Ozer, H.L. <u>Nature</u> 1982,
     <u>296</u>, 671

5   MacDonald, C. <u>CRC Critical Reviews in Biotechnology</u>,
     in the press.

6   Gorman, C. in <u>DNA Cloning</u>, (Ed. Glover, D.M.), IRL
     Press, Oxford and Washington, D.C., 1985, p 143-190

7   Schwarzbaum, S., Halpern, R. and Diamond, B. <u>J.
     Immunol</u>., 1984, <u>132</u>, 1158

8   Tanigawa, T., Suzuki, T., Takayama, H. and Takagi, A.
     <u>Microbiol. Immunol</u>. 1982, <u>26</u>, 59

PROPAGATION OF HUMAN CD4-IMMUNOGLOBULIN PRODUCING CELL LINES

E.-J. Schlaeger and B. Schumpp
F. Hoffmann-La Roche Ltd., 4002 Basel, Switzerland

Abstract

Transfected mouse myeloma cells were used for the production of different CD4 chimaeric molecules based on immunoglobulin-expression systems described by A. Traunecker et.al. (1). The soluble CD4 proteins which neutralize human immunodeficiency virus type 1 were secreted into the cell culture supernatant. In a first step the cells were adapted to grow in serum-free medium. The metabolic activities including amino acid consumption or excretion were evaluated and the production of the recombinant CD4 receptors more precisely characterized. The initial results of studies of the CD4 production from lab to 60 l fermentor scale will be described and discussed.

Introduction

The gene region coding for the extracellular region of CD4 (more precisely, the gp120 binding domains 1 and 2) was inserted upstream of the HC (heavy chain) coding sequences of immunoglobulins (Ig) to generate chimaeric molecules (1,2). After transfection into mouse myeloma cells CD4-γ1 and CD4-γ3 chimaeric proteins were secreted as homodimers, whereas the CD4-μ product was processed as a homopentamer as expected. The recombinant proteins of these three chimaeric gene constructs were of interest to serve as potential therapeutic decoy attracting and neutralizing the HIV in the body before the virus infects healthy cells.

The use of mouse myeloma cells for expressing the recombinant CD4 antibody is based on four main rationales (3):
1. Myeloma cells are dedicated secretory cells, the malignant counterparts of immunoglobulin secreting plasma cells.

2. Myeloma cells have the machinery to correctly glycosylate heterologous
   proteins.
3. The genetic elements required for high Ig expression in myeloma cells are
   well characterized.
4. Myeloma cells are easy to handle. Cells grow well in suspension in
   protein-reduced media up to cell densities of 3-6 x 10^6 cells/ml.

The present work shows some preliminary results from our study with the
CD4-Ig secreting myeloma cell line J558L.

Materials and Methods

Medium:
DMEM, Ham F12 and IMDM were mixed together and supplemented with
insulin (5µg/ml), selenite (20 mM), ethanolamine (20 µM), human transferrin
(6µg/ml), Primatone RL (2,5 mg/ml), Pluronic F 68 (0,1 mg/ml) and 0 or 2 %
FCS.

Cells and cell culture:
Transfected and originally untransfected myeloma cells X63/0 and J558L
were obtained from A. Traunecker and K. Karjalainen and have been
described (1,2). Cells were routinely cultured in T-flasks and roller bottles.
Fermentation cultures were performed in 20 l or 75 l airlift fermentors
(Chemap).

Dialysis tubing growth system:
Dialysing tubings were prepared as desribed elsewhere (4).

Results and Discussions

In a first series of experiments we used mouse myeloma X63/0 to produce
CD4-Ig proteins. The untransfected cell line grew well under our conditions to
cell densities up to 5 x 10^6 cells/ml. However the transfected clones exhibited
poorer growth properties and respectively low product titers. To overcome
these serious problems the myeloma cell line J558L which constitutively
secretes Ig λ_1 light chain was used. The producing cells grew well and the

CD4 titers in the cell culture supernatant ranged from 10-80 µg/ml. The three chimaeric proteins of interest are listed in Table 1.

Table 1   Some properties of the CD4-Ig chimaeric molecules

Constructs	hCD4-hγ1	hCD4-hγ3	hCD4-hμ
CD4-regions	2	2	10
Heavy chain	IgG1 (Hi-C$_2$,C$_3$)	IgG3 (Hi-C$_2$,C$_3$)	IgM (C$_2$,C$_3$,C$_4$)
Structure	homodimer	homodimer	homopentamer
MW	~ 90 Kd	~ 90 Kd	~ 700 Kd
Selection	gpt	histidinol	gpt

The growth properties of the individual transfected cell clones were roughly similar in medium supplemented with 2 % FCS in the presence of mycophenolic acid and xanthine (gpt selection) as well as of histidinol. In Fig. 1 A,B growth curves of a CD4-γ3 producing subclone (BG2) in the presence as well as in the absence of fetal calf serum are shown.

In both cases the final cell titer reached 4-6 x 10^6 cells/ml. Additional feeding of the culture at about 2 x 10^6 cells/ml with a mixture of amino acids, glutamine, glucose and vitamins did not increase the cell density significantly but prolonged the high cell density state. As can be seen from the graph (Fig. 1 C,D) the CD4-γ3 production occured predominantly during the growth phase. Feeding did not increase significantly the CD4-γ3 titer. In the presence of FCS the product titer is slightly higher compared to the serum-free culture. Growth-linked synthesis was also observed with the CD4-γ1 and CD4-μ producing cells. In contrast, it is interesting to note that the accumulation of the light chain in the cell culture supernatant continued during the feeding period, as documented by SDS-PAGE in Fig. 2 A,B. This production property is exhibited by most antibody-producing mouse hybridomas in our laboratory.

Fig. 1 A,B: Comparison of growth of CD4-γ3 producing cells in medium supplemented with 2 % FCS (A) or without FCS (B). Cells were grown in roller bottles and feeding (F) occured daily from the day indicated by the arrow.

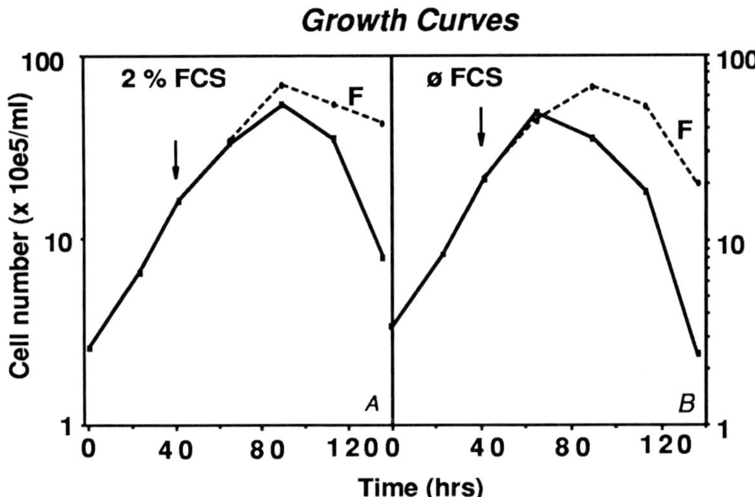

Growth Curves
Cell number (x 10e5/ml)
100
10
1
2 % FCS
ø FCS
F
F
A
B
0 40 80 120 0 40 80 120
Time (hrs)

Fig. 1 C,D: Comparison of CD4-γ3 productions from the cultures shown in Fig. 1 A,B (same symbols). CD4-γ3 concentrations during growth were quantified by a sandwich type ELISA test.

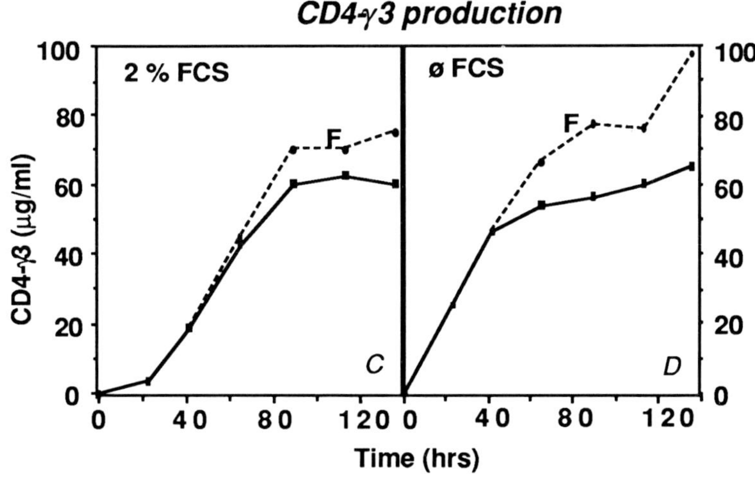

CD4-γ3 production
CD4-γ3 (µg/ml)
100
80
60
40
20
0
2 % FCS
ø FCS
F
F
C
D
0 40 80 120 0 40 80 120
Time (hrs)

The study of metabolic activity during growth (see Fig. 1 A,B) revealed that the final lactate and ammonia concentrations were higher in the serum-free culture (1,87 g/l, 4,2 mM) compared to the culture supplemented with serum (1,23 g/l, 2,76 mM). The ammonia concentration increased to 7-8 mM in the fed samples of both cultures whereas the lactate level remained at about 2 g/l (data not shown). Except for glutamine, which was almost totally consumed, all amino acids needed were only consumed in small quantities. In contrast the amino acids which were produced reached concentrations 3-5 times the original level (not shown).

Fig. 2: Electrophoretic analysis of culture supernatants (from Fig. 1) in a 10 % SDS-PAGE under non reduced conditions. Time course of CD4-γ3 production in:
(A) serum-free culture and (B) 2 % serum culture

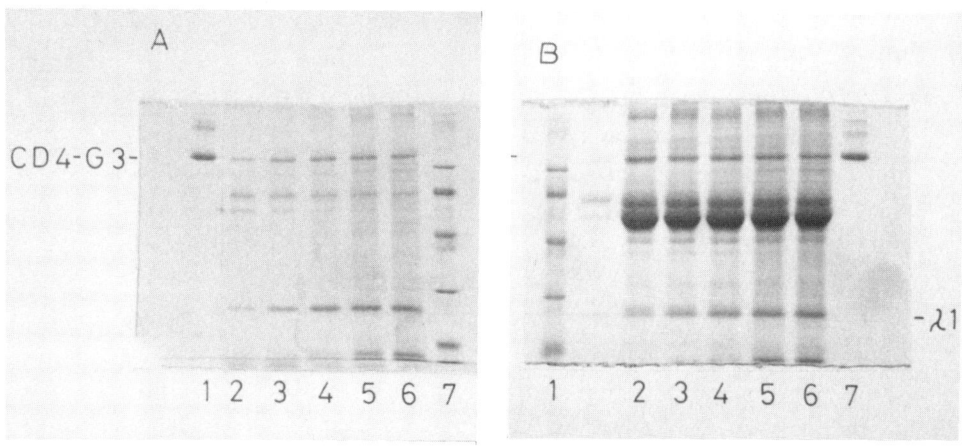

In order to overcome the limits of batch culture (low cell density) we have grown CD4-γ3 cells in non-toxic dialysis tubings which were incubated in roller bottles in excess of medium. This small "perfusion" system appeared to be a fast and simple culture approach to obtain high cell density up to 2-3 x 10^7 cells/ml. The result of the investigation is shown by a time course of CD4-γ3 production using SDS-PAGE (Fig. 3). As expected the increase of the CD4-γ3 molecules was related to the cell number during growth.

Fig. 3: CD4-γ3 production in dialysis tubings related to the cell number during growth analysed in a 10 % SDS-PAGE under non reduced conditions.

Lane 1:	low molecular weight marker proteins
Lanes 2 and 8:	purified CD4-γ3
Lanes 3-7:	1/2 diluted culture supernatants (as indicated on the gel)

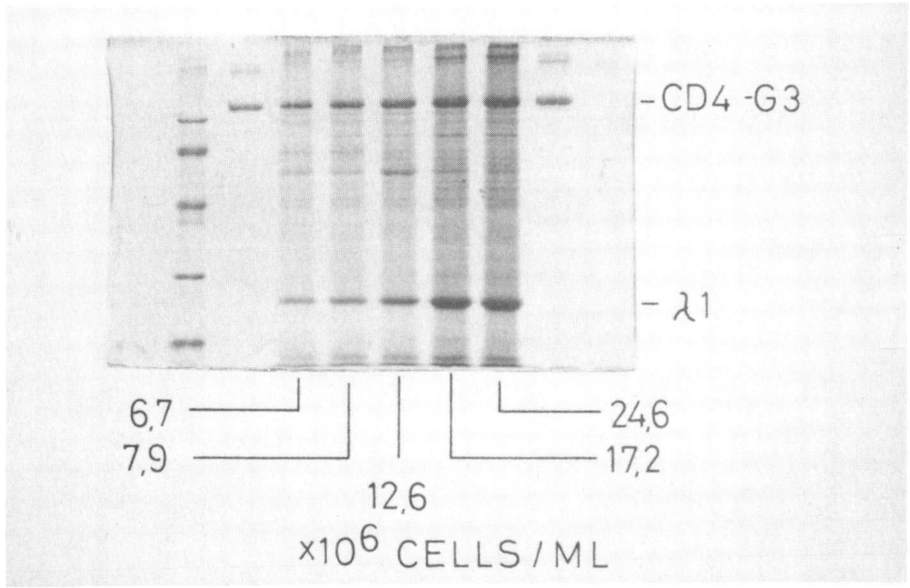

In the following 3 figures the production of the three recombinant proteins in airlift fermentors using a batch fermentation mode are shown (Fig. 4 A,B,C). The fermentation runs were performed without selection pressure. The growth properties as well as the yields of the CD4-Ig were similar to the results obtained in the laboratory study.

Fig. 4: Growth and production of three chimaeric proteins producing cell lines in airlift fermentors

A:	CD4-μ
B:	CD4-γ3
C:	CD4-γ1

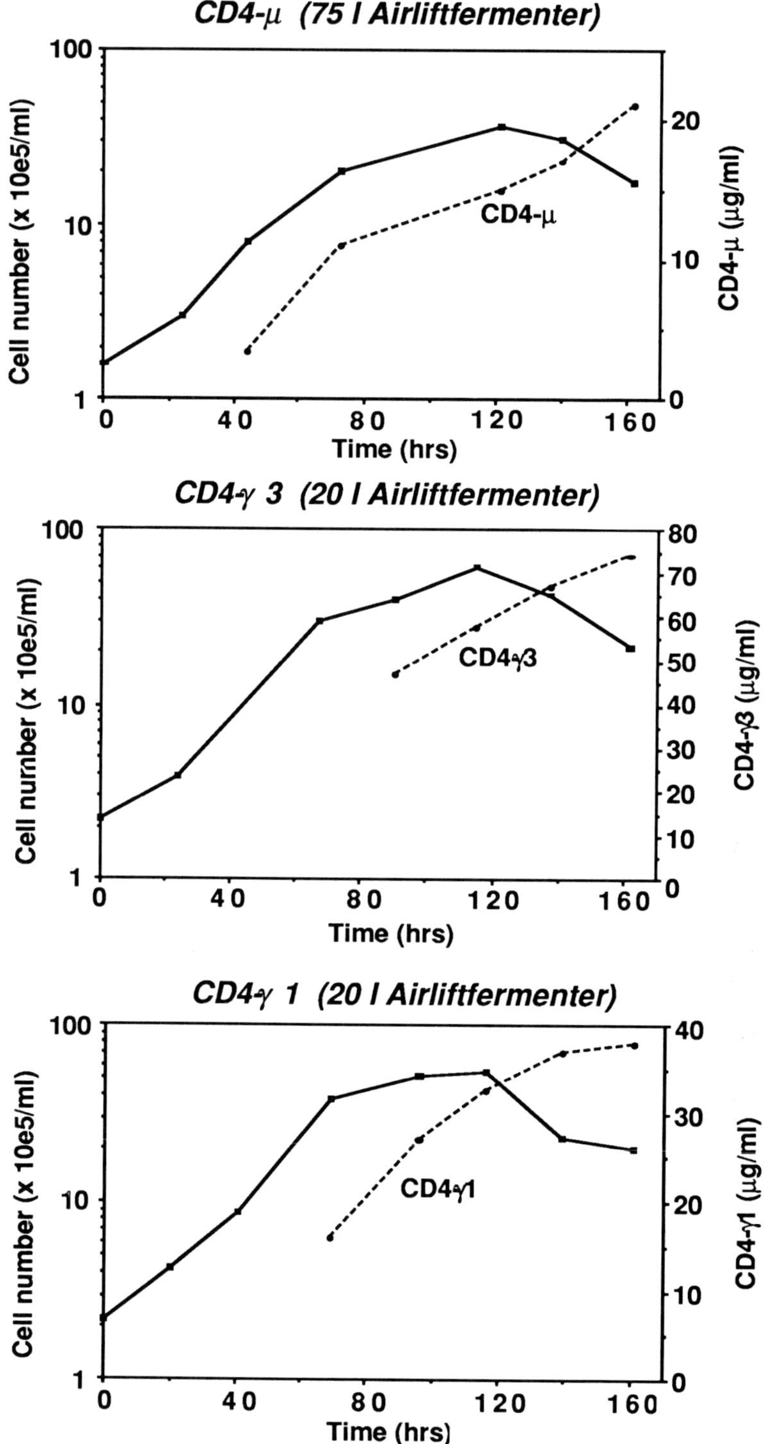

CD4-μ (75 l Airliftfermenter)
Cell number (x 10e5/ml)
CD4-μ (µg/ml)
CD4-μ
Time (hrs)
CD4-γ 3 (20 l Airliftfermenter)
Cell number (x 10e5/ml)
CD4-γ3 (µg/ml)
CD4-γ3
Time (hrs)
CD4-γ 1 (20 l Airliftfermenter)
Cell number (x 10e5/ml)
CD4-γ1 (µg/ml)
CD4-γ1
Time (hrs)

In conclusion we have shown that the myeloma cell line J558L appears to be a good producer of CD4-Ig chimaeric molecules. The proteins were stable during fermentation runs with the yields ranging from 20-25 µg/ml (CD4-µ) to 70-90 µg/ml (CD4-γ3). The subclones of transfected J558L grow well in protein-reduced medium without significant loss of productivity. The selection system using histidinol caused some problems in production stability, which were not observed if gpt selection pressure was used.

References

1.   Traunecker, A., Lüke, W. and Karjalainen, K.
     Soluble CD4 molecules neutralize human immunocleficiency virus type
     1. Nature 331, 84-86 (1988).

2.   Traunecker, A., Schneider, J., Kiefer, H. and Karjalainen, K.
     Highly efficient neutralization of HIV with recombinant CD4-
     immunoglobulin molecules. Nature 339, 68-70 (1989).

3.   Traunecker, A., Oliveri, F. and Karjalainen, K.
     Myeloma based expression system for production of large mammalian
     proteins. Submitted (1990).

4.   Schumpp, B. and Schlaeger, E.-J.
     Advances in animal cell biology and technology for bioprocesses,
     224-229, ESACT, The 9th Meeting. Butterworths & Co. (1989)

<u>**Paper of Schlaeger**</u>

Vournakis: Have you done any biological studies with the
             molecule, either <u>in vitro</u> or in animal models?

Schlaeger: These molecules are able to go to the placenta, and
             the half life was determined. This was a reason
             to link the CD4 molecule with the Ig molecule which
             increased the half life to several days.

Hentschel: The molecule you have constructed will clearly
             interact with the HIV gp120, but I cannot
             understand the rationale why this should be useful
             for HIV therapy. The disease is not fundamentally
             a virus killing cell type disease - this is only
             a trigger to a secondary disease which is more like
             an autoimmune or graft versus host disease.

Schlaeger: There is a hope that the infected cells themselves
             may be attacked by this type of molecule. Also
             free gp120 molecules bind to CD4 receptors of
             uninfected cells. Blood from an AIDS patient
             cultivated <u>in vitro</u> with these molecules showed
             that virus propagation was stopped.

Hentschel: I have no doubt this molecule will act as an anti-
             viral and prevent infectivity in culture in
             experiments such as you have described. The
             problem is that this is not the pathophysiology of
             the HIV disease, and it seems it is producing a
             form of autoimmune-like diseases, possibly through
             the interaction of gp120 with CD4. You may be
             mimicking that kind of situation with this
             molecule, especially if it has got Fc receptors.

Schlaeger: If there is a possibility of hitting the virus
             during birth as the molecule goes to the placenta,
             then its use would be appropriate at least in this
             specialist situation.

Wurm: At Genentech we are in clinical studies with CD4
             IgG, and we have shown that it kills infected
             cells. We have not yet seen any adverse effect in
             clinics. AIDS is very complex, there are many
             issues to be solved, and I am sure there will not
             be a single drug to cure the patient in a short
             time frame. I am hopeful that a combination
             therapy with several drugs, including AZT, will at
             least prolong life of patients and maybe prevent
             placenta transfer.

Eberhar: Clinical studies have been going on with Biogen
           soluble CD4 for some time and are now entering
           phase II. There have been no signs of adverse
           effects of this molecule.

Hofmann: Has the possibility of a severe immune response in
           patients been noticed?

Wurm: The purpose of doing phase I studies is to
           investigate that question. However the data are
           not available yet.

CHARACTERISATION OF CELL BANKS BY DNA FINGERPRINTING

Stacey, G.N., Lanham, S., Booth, S.J. and Bolton B.J.

European Collection of Animal Cell Cultures, PHLS Centre for Applied
Microbiology and Research, Porton Down, Salisbury, Wiltshire, SP4
0JG, UK.

INTRODUCTION

DNA fingerprints originate from the repetitive DNA called minisatellite
DNA which occurs throughout the human genome. When the genome is
fragmented by a restriction enzyme such as Hinf1 a pattern of
minisatellite bearing fragments is produced that is unique to each
individual. The multilocous method of fingerprinting developed by
Alec Jeffreys has been demonstrated to have great potential in the
investigation of cell lines from a wide range of species[1-2].
The Jeffreys probes 33.6 and 33.15 have been used to analyse cell
lines at the European Collection of Animal Cell Cultures (ECACC)
where DNA fingerprinting has been used in the quality control of cell
stocks. In addition the stability of DNA fingerprints was analysed
in cell lines subjected to some of the common variables in animal
cell tissue culture.

MATERIALS AND METHODS

All methods were carried out according to ICI-Cellmark Diagnostics
(UK) protocols under licence from ICI. The methods and DNA probes
of Jeffreys et al are described in references 3 and 4. DNA probes
33.6 and 33.15 were obtained through ICI-Cellmark Diagnostics (UK)
and were produced according to "Good Manufacturing Procedures". Samples
from cell lines comprised approximately 10^7 cells which had been washed
twice in phosphated buffered saline and stored as frozen pellets over
liquid nitrogen.

RESULTS

DNA fingerprints were produced from samples of master and extended
cell stocks of six lines (K562, MOLT4, 3T3, HelaB, HL60 and P3X63)
deposited at the ECACC. The fingerprint profiles were identical for
all lines studied with probes 33.6 (all six lines) and 33.15 (K562
and MOLT4) and an example is shown in Figure 1a).
The influence of culture conditions and growth phase on fingerprints
were investigated in a number of situations. Identical DNA fingerprints
with probe 33.6 were produced for samples of the B lymphoblastoid
cell line JHAF which had been split and cultured separately with 10%
foetal calf serum (Gibco-BRL) and 10% donor calf serum (TCS). Similarly
probes 33.6 and 33.15 showed no difference in fingerprints from samples
of a hybridoma cultured with a 10% foetal calf serum supplement and
(Gibco-BRL) a serum free medium.
Mixtures of cell lines were readily detected by DNA fingerprinting
as demonstrated with probe 33.6 for samples from B lymphoblastoid
lines KAS011 and BM15 as shown in Figure 1b. Dilution experiments
are under way to determine the level of cross contamination that can
be detected. The DNA fingerprint of the vero cell line infected with

<u>Mycoplasma orale</u> was found to have the same band pattern with
33.6 as the uninfected control(See Figure 1c). However, two bands
showed reduced intensity in the infected sample.

CONCLUSIONS

DNA fingerprinting has given increased confidence in the genetic
stability and purity of cell stocks produced from the master cell
bank at the ECACC. Other investigations indicate that a cell
lines fingerprint is independent of culture conditions. Mycoplasma
infection did not change the fingerprint pattern of the vero cell
line. However, the decreased intensity of two bands may indicate
chromosomal losses. The effect of long term infection and eradication
has yet to be assessed.
In the future it is intended to produce a directory of representative
DNA fingerprint profiles from the ECACC. This could act as a central
point of reference for the authentification of cell lines. Another
important aspect in future work will be the production of species
specific probes to widen the species range that can be tested and
simplify the interpretation of DNA fingerprint data.
Experience with multilocous DNA fingerprinting at the ECACC indicates
that this technique will become a vital component in cell banking
quality assurance.

REFERENCES

1 Thacker, J., Webb, M.B.T. and Debenham, P.G. Fingerprinting
   cell lines: use of human hypervariable DNA probes to characterise
   mammalian cell cultures. <u>Somatic Cell and Molecular Genetics</u>
   1988, <u>14</u>, 519-25.

2 van Helden, P.D., Wiid, I.J.F., Albrecht, C.F. et al.
   Crosscontamination of human esophageal squamous carcinoma cell
   lines detected by DNA fingerprint analysis. <u>Cancer Research</u>
   1988, <u>48</u>, 5660-2.

3 Jeffrey, A.J., Wilson, V. and Thein, S.L. Hypervariable
   'Minisatellite' regions in human DNA. <u>Nature</u> 1985, <u>314</u>, 67-
   73.

4 Jeffreys, A.J., Wilson, V. and Thein, S.L. Individual specific
   'fingerprints' of human DNA. <u>Nature</u> 1985, <u>316</u>, 76-79.

Figure 1. DNA Fingerprints with Probe 33.6

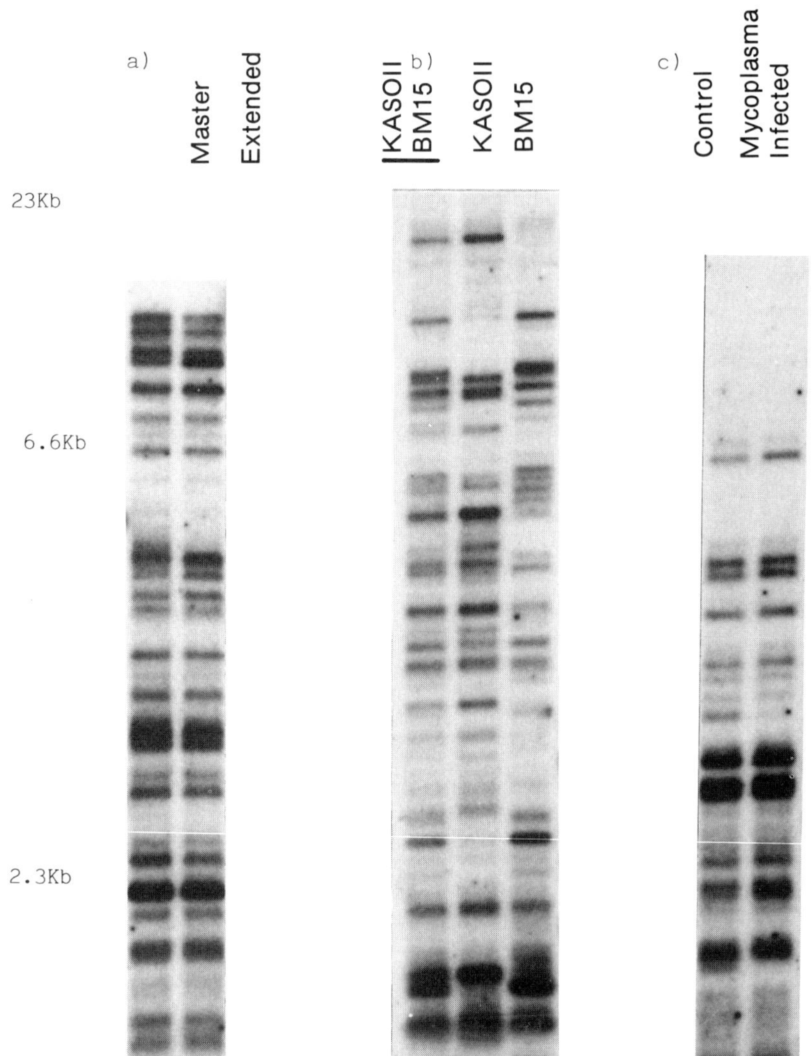

a)
Master
Extended
b)
KASOII
BM15
KASOII
BM15
c)
Control
Mycoplasma
Infected
23Kb
6.6Kb
2.3Kb

Paper of Stacey:

Spier: Would if not be possible to effect a densitometric scan of the gels and then by computer processing of the data generate an intensity corrected profile. You could calculate ratios of intensities between those bands which would cater for loading differences. This would enable more objective comparisons.

Stacey: A lot of work has been done on scanning of DNA fingerprints to produce better bases. (Cellmark, Diagnostic have investigated this) but we are looking for the presence or absence of bands not just the intensity. We may be able to use the most intense bands as a screen to identify the cell line. The technology for doing densitometry of radioautographs of this type is still at its early stages.

Horaud: Do you have a problem in terms of the reproducibility of your results due to restriction enzyme variations causing splitting into differing fragments.

Stacey: With human cell lines you can assess the activity of the restriction enzymes quite effectively. We can use a probe to look for a particular restriction site in such cell lines. But normally we work with an excess of restriction enzyme to overcome the effects of any partial digestion.

Kleuser: Do you think the method can be used to monitor the stability of a cell line during a production run? Or is it a method limited to cell line identification which can detect cross contamination.

Stacey: Yes: It has been used for such a situation where minor genetic variations in the cell line can be studied.

Kleuser: So what do we do with the results if we see a change in the pattern having excluded a cross contamination. Do you not get the same problems that you get from karyotyping. We know we get changes in karyotype but I would not throw away a cell line that is not stable in karyotyping but where the product is OK.

Stacey: If there was a genetic variation you might see a one or two band difference on the fingerprint; whereas with cross contamination you would see something very different.

Horaud: This technique is valuable when it comes to examining cell identity. I am not sure that tells us everything about the cell. It is well known that cells having different phenotypes in terms of microscopic appearance, EB, Hep2 cells and HeLa cells, are the same

cell but they are morphologically different and they
have the same fingerprint. So such a test should be a
component of the package but should not be considered
as a unique measure but it is still better than
karyology and isoenzyme analysis which gives little
information.

Hoppe:

Many of us work with the same host cell but we
transfect into the host cell a variety of different
vectors. Is the technique sensitive enough to do the
identity of the cells at the end of the run? Can you
determine if you have contamination by the same host
cell but with a different vector in it?

Stacey:

One of the problems is that the sensitivity of the test
may vary with the cell type. We are presently trying
to establish what those variations in sensitivity are.
At the present we expect to be able to detect 5-10%
contamination. If the contaminant level decreases in
the process it is of little significance ultimately.

Montagnon:

We have started to use DNA fingerprinting to
characterise the VERO cell line using 3 different
enzymes I3, pru 2 and tech 1 and using different probes
from the HLA Class I we were able to detect the
stability of the different levels of the master and
working cell banks up to passage level of 200. The
stability of the cell line was well established by this
technique and it was possible to check the identity of
our VERO cell line in comparison with other sources of
the VERO cell line. Eg, one cell line described as
VERO from Japan had a different pattern. I think the
sensitivity of the test will detect a 1-2%
contamination by other cell lines.

Horaud:

Is your VERO cell line called WHO-VERO cell.

Montagnon:

Our VERO cell started from one ATCC cell ampoule
received in 1979 and later we produced cells for the
WHO cell bank at passage 134. The cell came from the
ATCC at passage 125.

Horaud:

It is important for all to realise that at the European
Cell Bank at Porton, there is available VERO cells that
were established under WHO supervision and those cells
were extensively characterised for their viral
contaminants and sequences. Using hybridization and
PCR techniques we failed to find viral sequences for
SIV or B Herpes Virus and Sinomalgus. This is a useful
source of cells for production purposes.

Gannon:

DNA fingerprinting is a good way to detect the
difference between different cell lines however the
method will not detect subtile differences and a few

instances genetic differences were not detected. What
you observe in your bonding patterns can be attributed
to 50 base pair differences and quite obviously there
is plenty of room for point mutations and deletions and
insertions which would lead to genetic differences
which would not be detected by these fingerprints. The
other point where you have two cell lines of common
origin but with different inserts at different loci in
the chromosome, they will not be detected either. This
puts some obvious limitations to the usefulness of the
DNA fingerprinting techniques.

EVALUATING THE SAFETY OF MURINE AND HUMAN HYBRIDOMAS : NEW
PROBLEMS AND NEW TECHNIQUES

David Onions[1] and Gillian Lees[2]

[1]LRF Virus Centre, University of Glasgow, G61 1QH
[2]Quality Biotech, 6.04 Kelvin Campus, West of Scotland Science
Park, Glasgow G20 0SP Scotland.

ABSTRACT AND INTRODUCTION

The retroviruses and herpesviruses pose a particular problem in
safety evaluation for several reasons: Some retroviruses, the
endogenous viruses, are inherited through the germ line, whereas
exogenous retroviruses and herpesviruses may remain as latent
infections within cells. Both groups of viruses are associated
with oncogenic and systemic disease.

SCREENING FOR MURINE RETROVIRUSES

Murine cells may contain several endogenous retrovirus families,
ecotropic viruses that infect murine and rat cells and
xenotropic viruses that infect non-murine cells including human
cells. Polytropic (MCF) viruses are recombinant viruses between
ecotropic viruses and xenotropic-like sequences. These viruses
infect murine and other cells and are the proximal cause of
retrovirus induced leukaemia in mice. These viruses can be
detected by electron microscopy, reverse transcriptase and
infectivity assays. It is important to understand that each
assay yields different information. Not all viruses detected by
EM are infectious and the ratio of defective, non-infectious
viruses to infectious virus varies from cell line to cell line.
When conducting infectivity assays, direct assays like the
direct S+L- assay for xenotropic virus are less sensitive than
extended assays which in turn are less sensitive than co-culture
assays. Using each assay provides a picture of the infectious
virus levels.

The stage of harvesting the supernatant for analysis also
profoundly affects the detection of retroviruses. They are only
released from mitotically active cells as shown in the pattern
of type-C retrovirus released from the T3 cell line.

LABORATORY 1

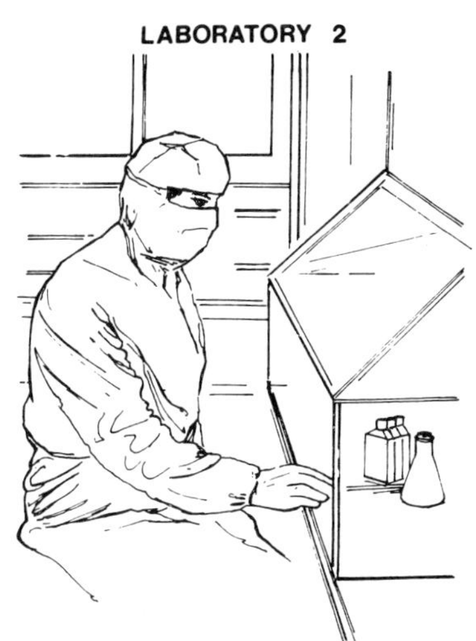

Reagent Aliquots

in sterile packs

PCR supplies including Plasticware & reagents
- Reagents prepared and aliquoted
- No samples or controls handled
- Separate personnel from other labs.

LABORATORY 2

- Samples added to pre-prepared reagents
- Protective clothing
- Class II hood
- Sentinel controls
- Positive displacement pipettes
- Gloves changed between samples

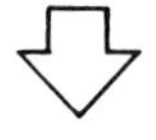

LABORATORY 4

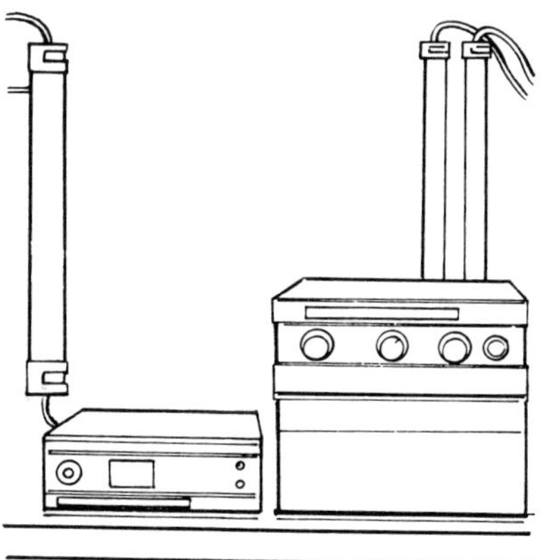

- Run samples in PCR Block
- Electrophoresis
- Detection by 32p- Probe

LABORATORY 3

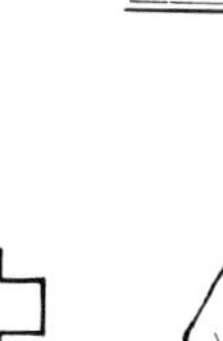
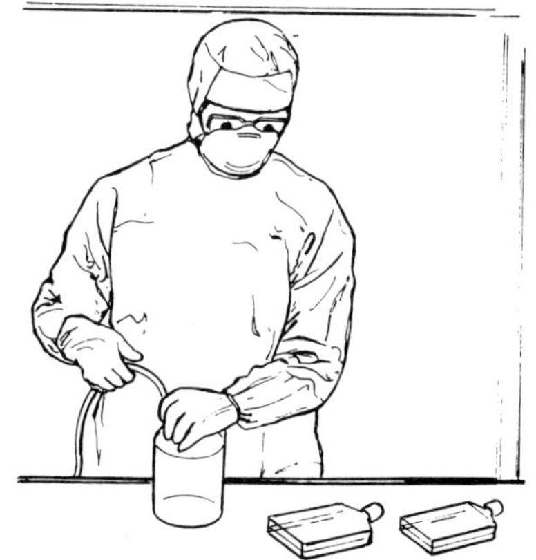

- Positive control added
- Separate dedicated pipettes used
- Added in containment hood

<u>Detection of C-Type Retrovirus in T3 Cell Line</u>

Days after Passing Cells	ffu/ml Direct S+L- Assay	Extended	RT Assay
0.5	–	+	–
1.0	76	+	–
2.0	8.9×10^2	+	+
3.0	3.2×10^3	+	+
4.0	6.4×10^2	+	+
5.0	1.35×10^2	+	+[a]

[a] Build of cellular DNA polymerases in static culture led to an equivocal results in reverse transcriptase assay.

<u>HUMAN RETROVIRUSES</u>

The human oncogenic and immunosuppressive retroviruses HTLV-1, HTLV-2, HIV-1 and HIV-2 are all exogenous and therefore screening can be initiated by detecting the presence of the proviruses in cells by Southern hybridisation or PCR techniques. However, the recent description of a variant of HTLV not detected at high stringency by HTLV-1 indicates that it is important to include culture techniques for human retroviruses (1). For the HTLV group syncitium formation on HOS cells is usually more sensitive than co-cultivation technique with cord blood lymphocytes (2).

<u>HERPESVIRUS SCREENING</u>

Where EBV is used it is essential to demonstrate the stability of the latent state. This can be tested by inducing the cells with phorbol esters and assaying for the induction of viral capsid antigen. A proportion of VCA positive cells will proceed to the full lytic cycle and the production of infectious virus, which can be detected by co-culture with cord blood cells.

Two new herpesviruses require assay. We have recently shown that HHV-6 is present in some human lymphomas and can be detected by PCR in a small proportion of peripheral blood mononuclear cells of most individuals (3,4). Similarly a new rodent gamma-herpes virus has recently been characterised. Gamma-herpesviruses include the lymphomogenic viruses like EBV and murine hybridomas should be screened for this class of virus.

<u>PCR BASED TECHNIQUES</u>

We have developed PCR based techniques for final product for the human and animal herpesviruses and retroviruses described above. PCR should only be conducted in a facility with a validated system for controlling contamination. Our procedure for conducting PCR involves 4 separate laboratories as outlined in

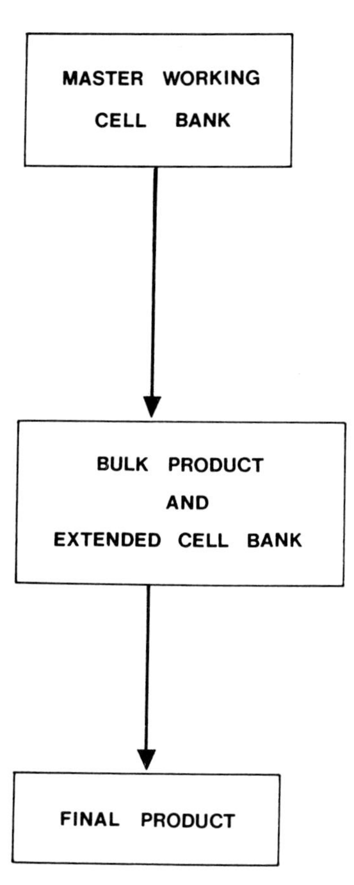

1   Direct xc and S+L– assay   ± Induction
2. Extended xc and S+L– assay   ± Induction
3. Co-cultivation with human cells if 1 or 2 positive
4. Reverse Transcriptase
5. EM Level 1
6. Murine gamma herpesvirus

1. Direct xc and S+L–
2. Reverse Transcriptase
3. Murine gamma herpesvirus
4. Extended or co-cultivate if 1 or 2 positive

1. Extended xc and S+L– assay
2. PCR detection for virion RNA

Similar assays for CHO cells although CHO c-type virus does not appear to infect a wide range of cell types including :–

xc	–	Rat
NIH 3T3	–	Mouse
MRC-5	–	Human
HeLa	–	Human
J/Jhan	–	Human

37

the accompanying diagram.   PCR is of great value for final
product testing but it will not replace infectivity assays which
may detect variant viruses.

SUMMARY

Outlined in the diagrams below are testing systems applicable to
murine and human hybridomas.

REFERENCES

1.   Manzari V, Gismandi A, Barillari G, Morrones _et al_. A new
     human   retrovirus   isolated   in   Tac   negative   T-cell
     Lymphoma/Leukaemia. _Science_ 1987, _238_, 1581-1583

2.   Clapham P, Nagy K, Cheingsong-Popov R. and Weiss RA.
     Productive infection and cell free transmission of human T-
     cell leukaemia virus in a non-lymphoid cell line.   _Science_
     1983, _222_, 1125-1127

3.   Jarrett RF, Gledhill S, Qureshi F, Crae SH, Madhok R, Brown
     I, Evans I, Krajewski A, O'Brien CJ, Cartwright R, Venables
     P. and Onions D. Identification of human herpesvirus-6
     specific DNA sequences in two patients with Non-Hodgkin's
     Lymphoma. _Leukemia_ 1988, _2_, 496-502

4.   Jarrett RF, Clark D, Josephs J. and Onions D. Detection of
     human herpes virus-6 in saliva and peripheral blood. _Lancet_
     In press.

DEFECTIVE ENDOGENOUS RETROVIRUSLIKE PARTICLES OF CHINESE HAMSTER OVARY CELLS

Kevin P. Anderson*, Mari-Anne L. Low*, Yolanda S. Lie*, Richard Lazar*, Gilbert Keller+, Marshall Dinowitz*.

Departments of Medicinal and Analytical Chemistry*, and Safety Evaluation+, Genentech, Inc., 460 Point San Bruno Blvd, South San Francisco, CA 94080, U.S.A.

ABSTRACT

The presence of budding C-type and intracytoplasmic A-type particles in Chinese hamster ovary (CHO) cells is well documented. However, extensive screening has failed to detect any evidence of infectivity. We have used a high-capacity, continuous-flow, ultracentrifuge rotor to concentrate extracellular particles from culture fluid of recombinant CHO cells for molecular characterization. Equilibrium sucrose gradient sedimentation of particle preparations results in co-fractionation of reverse transcriptase activity and mammalian C-type retrovirus core proteins at a density characteristic of retrovirus particles. Electron microscope examination of gradient fractions at this density revealed the presence of particles with morphology and size similar to other characterized retroviruses. Several cDNA clones of particle RNA homologous to the endonuclease region of Moloney murine leukemia virus have been isolated and sequenced. None exhibit open reading frames capable of encoding an intact endonuclease, providing one possible explanation for the non-infectious nature of the observed particles. The presence of conserved C-type provirus sequences in the DNA of all CHO cell lines examined, as well as in Chinese hamster liver DNA, suggests that the observed particles are the products of endogenous retroviruslike elements present in the germline of Chinese hamsters.

Keywords: CHO cells, C-type particles, intracisternal A-particles, endogenous retrovirus, endonuclease, reverse transcriptase, core protein, cDNA, continuous-flow ultracentrifugation, sucrose gradients.

INTRODUCTION

All CHO cell lines exhibit low levels of retrovirus-like particles when thin-sections of cells are viewed by transmission electron microscopy. Two types of particles are consistently observed: Intracytoplasmic A-type particles frequently associated with centrioles, and budding C-type particles[1-5]. Infection or transmission to other cells has never been detected despite extensive screening[2,3,6]. Because of the low numbers of retroviruslike particles present in CHO cells, characterization has been difficult. We have used a high-capacity, continuous-flow, ultracentrifuge rotor to concentrate extracellular particles from large volumes of culture fluid of a recombinant CHO cell line. Sufficient quantities of particles were obtained for detailed molecular characterization.

MATERIALS AND METHODS

Concentration of particles from extracellular fluid of CHO cells. A recombinant CHO cell line derived from the dihydrofolate reductase deficient (dhfr-) CHO-DUXB11 line[7] was used as the source of extacellular fluid for particle concentration. Clarified cell culture fluid (20-30 L) was passed through a high-capacity, continuous flow ultracentrifuge rotor (Beckman model CF32) at approximately 100,000xg. Pelleted material was harvested and recentrifuged in a Beckman Ti45 rotor. The final pellet was resuspended in 4-5 ml of 10 mM Tris-HCl (pH7.5), 150 mM NaCl (TN) and stored at -80°C.

Sucrose gradient fractionation. For purification of particles, concentrated culture fluid was adjusted to 50% sucrose, and overlayed with equal volumes of 40%, 30%, and 20% sucrose in TN. After sedimentation to equilibrium, reverse transcriptase (RT) containing peak fractions were pooled, dialyzed and spun again through a linear 10-60% continuous sucrose gradient. For some analytical experiments fractionation was performed using a single 10-60% continuous sucrose gradient.

Reverse transcriptase (RT) assays. Incorporation of [^{3}H]-TTP into DNA after a 60 min incubation in the presence of poly(rA):oligo(dT) as template and Mn^{++} as divalent cation was monitored by counting radioactivity bound to DE81 filters after thorough rinsing in 1X SSC.

Western blot analysis. Samples were fractionated on reducing SDS-polyacrylamide gels and transferred electrophoretically to Immobilon filters (Pharmacia). Primary antisera was goat anti-feline leukemia virus p27 (NCI repository, Microbiological Associates). Secondary antibody was donkey anti-goat IgG coupled to horseradish peroxidase. The resulting signal was developed using 4-chloro, 1-napthol.

Electron microscopy. After dialysis, samples of gradient fractions were spotted onto grids. Particles were visualized in a transmission electron microscope following negative staining with uranyl acetate.

Isolation and characterization of nucleic acids. Nucleic acids were extracted from sucrose gradient fractions by phenol/chloroform extraction. Samples were applied to membranes (Genescreen plus; NEN Research Products) using a slot-blot manifold (Schleicher and Schuell mini-fold II). Hybridizations were performed in 50% formamide (high stringency) or 25% formamide (low stringency) at 42°C. Cloned probe for the endogenous, polytropic murine leukemia virus (MLV) isolate, MX27[8], was provided by J. Coffin and J. Stoye. Probes for endogenous CHO intracisternal A-particle sequences have been described elsewhere[9]. C-type clones were isolated from a randomly primed cDNA library of particle RNA in λgt10. Low stringency hybridization using MLV probe allowed identification of plaques of interest. DNA sequencing was performed using the dideoxy chain termination method on subcloned single-stranded template[10]. Standard procedures were used for preparation and hybridization of genomic DNA blots[11].

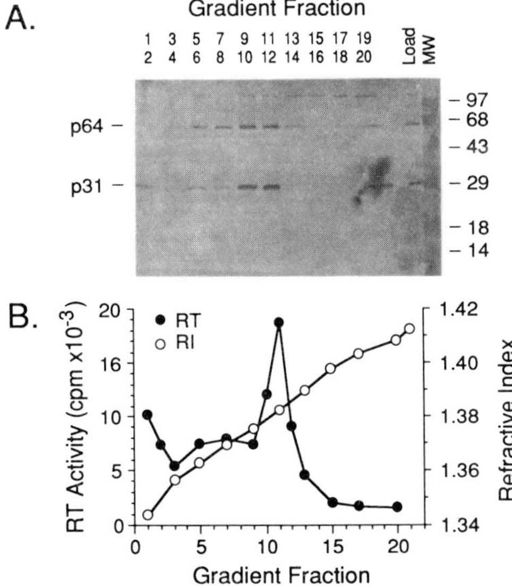

Figure 1. Cofractionation of RT activity and C-type retrovirus proteins on sucrose gradients. Concentrated culture fluid from CHO cells was fractionated on a sucrose gradient and fractions were tested for the presence of RT activity and C-type retrovirus core polypeptides. Fraction 1 represents the top of the gradient. (A) Western blot analysis of pooled samples of 2 fractions each using anti-FeLV p27 sera. The p31 band represents the major core protein and the p64 band represents unprocessed gag precursor. (B) Closed circles represent RT activity of fractions from the same sucrose gradient analyzed in A. Open circles represent refractive index of fractions.

RESULTS

Co-fractionation of reverse transcriptase (RT) activity, C-type core polypeptides, and retroviruslike particles. Concentrated culture fluid from CHO cells was fractionated on a 10-60% sucrose gradient, and fractions were tested for RT activity. A peak of RT activity banded at a density characteristic of retrovirus particles (1.12-1.14 g/cc; Fig. 1B). Preference of activity for poly(rA):oligo(dT) over poly(dA):oligo(dT) as template, and for Mn^{++} over Mg^{++} as divalent cation was verified in a seperate experiment (not shown).

Reverse transcriptase activity with a preference for Mn^{++} is characteristic of mammalian C-type retroviruses. Samples of gradient fractions were tested for the presence of C-type related core polypeptides by western blot analysis using antisera to purified feline leukemia virus p27 protein. As shown in Fig. 1A, a 31 kd core polypeptide (p31) as well as a 64 kd gag polyprotein precursor (p64) are most abundant in fractions exhibiting the highest levels of RT activity.

Electron microsopic examination of RT containing fractions following negative staining allowed visualization of pleiomorphic particles compar-able in size and morphology to characterized C-type retroviruses (not shown).

Nucleic acid content of purified C-type particles. RT containing fractions obtained after a single sucrose gradient fractionation contained significant amounts of contaminating cellular DNA and were not suitable for evaluating nucleic acid content of particles. Therefore, a double-gradient protocol was devised for purification of extracellular particles (Materials and Methods). Pools of 4 fractions each from the second sucrose gradient were

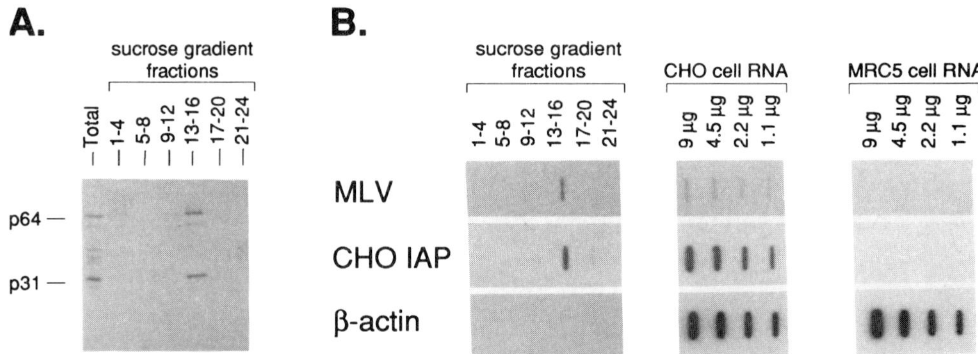

Figure 2. Retrovirus related nucleic acids in purified particles of CHO cells. Pools of 4 fractions each from the second gradient of a double-gradient particle purification were evaluated for the presence of C-type capsid proteins and retrovirus nucleic acid sequences. (A) Western blot analysis using anti-FeLV p27 sera. (B) Nucleic acids were extracted from samples of each pool, applied to membranes and hybridized to the indicated probes. Cytoplasmic RNAs from CHO cells and MRC5 cells (human diploid fibroblasts) were used as controls.

combined and tested for the presence of C-type structural proteins and retrovirus homologous nucleic acid sequences. Only the pool containing fractions with RT activity (fractions 13-16) exhibited substantial p31 and p64 levels indicating the presence of C-type particles (Fig. 2A). Nucleic acids hybridizing to a murine leukemia virus (MLV) probe were detected in this same pool using low stringency hybridization conditions (Fig. 2B). Nucleic acids from RT-containing, p31-positive fractions also hybridized to probe for family II CHO cell intracisternal A-particle (IAP) sequences[9]. Nucleic acids with homology to a major cellular mRNA (β-actin) were not detected in any gradient fractions. Elimination of the hybridization signal by treatment of nucleic acids prior to blotting with alkali or RNAse, but not DNAse, confirmed that hybridization was to RNA and not DNA.

Characterization of particle cDNA sequences homologous to MLV. Eleven cDNA clones of purified particle RNA which hybridized to MLV probe were isolated and characterized. Of three clones which were sequenced, all showed homology to the endonuclease domain of MLV (Fig. 3), but none contained uninterrupted translational reading frames. The largest clone (pCHOC.ML10, 949 bp) exhibited 73% nucleotide identity with the published sequence of Moloney MLV[12]. This sequence contained multiple interruptions of potential coding sequences in all 3 reading frames.

Presence of homolgous DNA sequences in the Chinese hamster genome. Southern blot analysis of Chinese hamster DNA using the pCHOC. ML10 clone as probe revealed that conserved, homologous sequences were present at approximately 100 copies per genome in DNA of both parental and recombinant CHO cell lines, as well as DNA from Chinese hamster liver (data not shown).

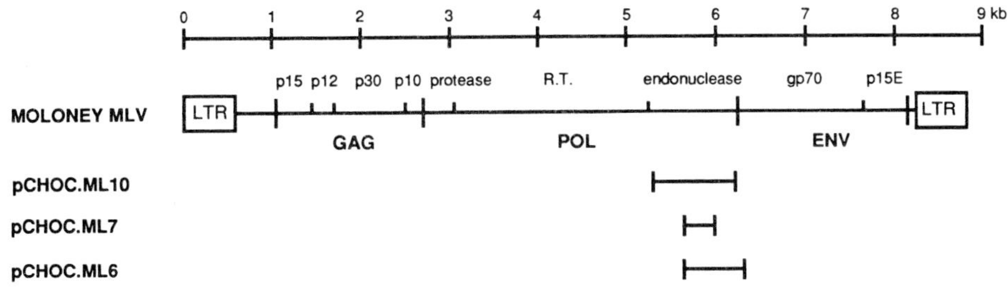

Figure 3. Nucleotide homology of particle cDNA clones to Moloney MLV genome. Regions of nucleotide homology with the Moloney MLV genome are shown for 3 partial cDNA clones, representing RNA from purified extracellular particles of CHO cells. All 3 clones exhibited greater than 70% nucleotide identity with the Moloney MLV sequence over the indicated regions.

DISCUSSION

Particles morphologically similar to retroviruses have previously been observed in CHO cells, but further characterization has not been reported. High-capacity, flow-through, ultracentrifugation of large volumes of culture fluid has facilitated purification and biochemical characterization of these particles. The extracellular particles are similar to those of characterized mammalian C-type retroviruses not only morphologically, but also by a number of biochemical criteria. They band in a sucrose gradient at an appropriate density, and exhibit RT activity with a preference for Mn^{++}. Polypeptides of the particles are immunologically related to those of mammalian C-type retroviruses, and RNA from purified particles is partially homologous to murine C-type retrovirus genomes.

Purified extracellular particles also contain RNA sequences homologous to endogenous intracisternal A-particle (IAP) sequences of CHO cells[9]. Current information does not allow differentiation between the presence of 2 types of particles with similar buoyant densities, or a single type of particle which encapsidates two different RNAs.

Characterization of cDNA sequences representing purified particle RNA revealed significant homology to the conserved endonuclease region of the MLV genome. However, none of the 3 sequenced clones contained open reading frames. Since the retrovirus endonuclease is required for retrovirus integration, these findings provide one possible explanation for the non-infectious nature of particles observed in CHO cells.

The presence of multiple, conserved C-type provirus sequences in the DNA of both parental and recombinant CHO cell lines, as well as in Chinese hamster liver DNA, implies that the observed particles are the products of endogenous retroviruslike elements present in the germline of Chinese hamsters.

ACKNOWLEDGEMENTS

We thank R. Arathoon, J. Obijeski, M. Wiebe, and F. Wurm for suggestions and encouragement, and T. Nguyen, E. Chen, and E. Penuel for determining DNA sequence. J. Coffin and J. Stoye provided cloned MX27 murine leukemia virus probe, and K. Lueders provided Chinese hamster liver DNA.

REFERENCES

1. Heine, U. I., B. Kramarsky, E. Wendel, and R. G. Suskind. 1979. Enhanced proliferation of endogenous virus in Chinese hamster cells associated with microtubules and the mitotic apparatus of the host cell. J. Gen. Virol. 44:45-55.

2. Lubiniecki, A. S., M. Dinowitz, E. Nelson, M. Wiebe, L. May, J. Ogez, and S. Builder. 1989. Endogenous retroviruses of continuous cell lines. Develop. Biol. Standard. 70:187-191.

3. Lubiniecki, A. S. and L. H. May. 1985. Cell bank characterization for recombinant DNA mammalian cell lines. Develop. Biol. Standard. 60:141-146.

4. Manley, K. F., J. F. Givens, R. L. Tuber, and R. F. Zeigel. 1978. Characterization of virus-like particles released from the hamster cell line CHO-K1 after treatment with 5-bromodeoxyuridine. J. Gen. Virol. 39:505-517.

5. Tihon, C. and M. Green. 1973. Cyclic AMP amplified replication of RNA tumor virus-like particles in Chinese hamster ovary cells. Nature New Biol. 244:227-231.

6. Hojman, F., R. Emanoil-Ravier, J. Lesser, and J. Peries. 1989. Biological and molecular characterization of an endogenous retrovirus present in CHO/HBs-A Chinese hamster cell line. Develop. Biol. Standard. 70:195-202.

7. Simonsen, C. C. and A. D. Levinson. 1983. Isolation and expression of an altered mouse dihydrofolate reductase cDNA. Proc. Natl. Acad. Sci. USA 80:2495-2499.

8. Stoye, J. P. and J. M. Coffin. 1987. The four classes of endogenous murine leukemia virus: structural relationships and potential for recombination. J. Virol. 61:2659-2669.

9. Anderson, K. P., Y. S. Lie, M. L. Low, S. R. Williams, E. H. Fennie, T. P. Nguyen, and F. M. Wurm. 1990. Presence and transcription of intracisternal A-particle related sequences in CHO cells. J. Virol. 64: 2021-2032.

10. Sanger, F., S. Nicklen, and A.R. Coulson. 1977. DNA sequencing with chain-terminating inhibitors. Proc. Natl. Acad. Sci. U.S.A. 74:3463-3467.

11. Maniatis, T., E. F. Fritch, and J. Sambrook. 1982. Molecular cloning: a laboratory manual. Cold Spring Harbor Laboratory, Cold Spring Harbor, N.Y.

12. Shinnick, T. M., R.A. Lerner, and J. G. Sutcliffe. 1981. Nucleotide sequence of Moloney murine leukemia virus. Nature 293: 543-548.

<u>**Paper of Anderson**</u>

Brown: Can we assume that these particles found their way in through cell lysis?

Anderson: The particles are present in the supernatant of cells and we do not know the mechanism of their release although when you look at thin sections of cells you can visualise budding C-type viruses so they don't have to be released from lysed cells.

Onions: In work we published in Nature two years ago we found a virus which had many of the characteristics you described it was predominantly a defective virus. It has defects in both endonuclease and in pol. If you look at the culture of these after one passage there is replication competent virus there which is generated by recombination from 2 defectives. So we have to be cautious with such data in situations where we have apparently replication in competent viruses emerging. This is reinforced with HIV where we have transdominant mutants which also are effective in suppressing replication competent virus.

Anderson: This is why we intend to continue our process validation studies and testing to ensure removal of these particles.

REFERENCE CELL LINES

R Bliem and JB Griffiths

Bristol Myers Squibb, Syracuse, USA, and *PHLS CAMR, Porton, Wiltshire SP4 0JG, UK.

BACKGROUND

The need for Reference Cell Lines to impart a higher level of standardisation to Animal Cell Technology is now well understood and documented (1, 2). The aim has been to get agreement on the 3 most useful cell lines and then to get funding to set up fully authenticated cell banks at the major international cell culture collections.

The standardisation is needed so that alternative bioreactors, media, processes and techniques can be usefully compared and a quantitative evaluation of the systems' productivity made. To do this we need authenticated and characterised cell cultures, a common source of reference cell lines, and a universally accepted system of units of measurement.

Since this need was voiced at the ESACT meeting in Belgium (September 1988) questionnaires have been sent to ESACT members, to scientists responding to the Bio/Technology Article (1) and to the participants of the Cell Engineering II Meeting (Santa Barbara, USA). There has been considerable support and comment on the subject such that the following proposal is now being made.

PROPOSAL

The need has been clearly demonstrated from the responses to the questionnaire and we will now seek funding to establish a minimum of 3 reference cell lines. Many cell lines have been proposed for this purpose but the consensus opinion is that the following should be chosen:

1 Recombinant CHO (with an easily assayed product eg antibody).

2 Mouse hybridoma

3 Vero, BHK or Sf-9 (if resources permit only 1 of these to be chosen then additional feedback is needed for selection)

Other cell lines that have been suggested include Sf-9, Myeloma (Sp2/0), HeLa, MDCK, MRC-5, and 3T3.

ACTION

1 Further comment will be welcomed on the selection of the
  third choice of cell line.   Ideally it should be an
  anchorage dependent cell and possibly Vero may be the best
  choice.

2 Industrial sponsorship and Governmental support will be
  sought to raise initially $10-15,000 to establish 3 fully
  characterised reference cell lines at recognised culture
  collections (ATCC, ECACC, Riken). Hopefully this will be
  extended to 5 cell lines in due course. An efficient way
  of proceeding will be if each of these cell banks can get
  sponsorship funding from their own geographical region to
  set up one of the 3 chosen cell lines.

REFERENCES

1 Bliem, R. and Griffiths, J.B. (1989) Bio/Technology 7, 759

2 Griffiths, J.B. (1990). Cytotechnology 3, 1.

A EUROPEAN DATABASE FOR ANIMAL CELL LINES

A Doyle*, J B Griffiths+ and C Caulcott**.

*European Collection of Animal Cell Cultures, PHLS Centre of Applied
Microbiology and Research, Porton Down, Salisbury, Wiltshire, SP4 OJG,
UK.
+Animal Cell Technology, PHLS Centre of Applied Microbiology and Research
Porton Down, Salisbury, Wiltshire, SP4 OJG, UK.
**Bioscience 1, ICI Pharmaceuticals, Mereside, Alderley Park,
Macclesfield, Cheshire, SK10 4TG, UK.

ABSTRACT

A workshop jointly organised by ECACC, ESACT and ETCS to discuss a
proposed European Database for Animal Cell Lines was held at Graz,
Austria in September 1989. There was overwhelming agreement on a need
for such a resource for animal cell technologists as current databases
are either regional or too specialised. There are an enormous number
of cell lines produced in scientific centres throughout Europe for
which presently no system exists for learning of their existence.
This has led to the establishment of a working party with representation
from major interest groups to develop this project further. Existing
databases such as the IST/Interlab, Genoa and Hybridoma Databank, Nice
are collaborating with the project and are forming the basis of an
agreed consensus data format. The aim is to retain compatability with
the existing projects. Important criteria for the database are that it
should be readily available to the end user in a confidential and
user-friendly format. The immediate goal is to produce a PC version of
the database to enable as wide a number of users as possible. A number
of suitable programs exist but it is likely that ORACLE is the most
appropriate. Once established in a final agreed format, the system
will be promoted via regional coordination centres using training
courses and workshops to allow for easy installation in all
laboratories handling cell lines and needing an in-house database.
Copies of the non-confidential part of the data set can then be
submitted by these laboratories to a collating centre to form the
database which will enable much more efficient usage of cell line
resources with open access to contributing groups. An application has
been made to the EEC DG XII for grant funding under the "BRIDGE"
programme to support the setting up of the database with the aim of the
project becoming self financing in the long-term.

CELL LINE DATA BASE: AN ON-LINE DATA BANK WHERE INDUSTRY
MEETS RESEARCHERS

Ottavia Aresu, Beatrice Iannotta, Barbara Parodi, Paolo
Romano, Tiziana Ruzzon

Servizio Tecnologie Biomediche, Istituto Nazionale per la
Ricerca sul Cancro, Viale Benedetto XV, 10, Genova, Italy

ABSTRACT

The Interlab Project, meant to create data banks, to provide
services of biomedical interest and to develop a communication network, collaborates with European institutions for
the creation of a European Data Base for Animal Cell Lines.

INTRODUCTION

The swift development of biotechnology has led in the last
years to an enormous yield of data, and it becomes very important for researchers to gain rapid access to updated,
reliable and comprehensive information. The same need is
felt by industry scientists, for which data accuracy is essential. For animal cell lines in particular the need is
felt for a user-friendly European data bank. A centralised
data base, providing an adequate quality control, should be
set up in order to make the whole data internationally
available. Local versions, sharing the same structure,
should be installed on PC for the management of local
collections and periodical uploadings.
The Interlab Project foresees the creation of centralized
data banks and additional services of biomedical interest,
as well as the development of a communication network among
Italian and European Research Institutes. At present, the
following data bases are being developed: B Line Data Base
(BLDB), Molecular Probe Data Base (MPDB) and Cell Line Data
Base (CLDB).
BLDB is the first of a series of data bases designed to give
specific information on particular clusters of lines. Information on a large number of HLA typed B lymphoblastoid cell
lines is given, including complete HLA typing and com-
plotyping, ethnics, family trees, genetic disease status,
and the possibility of performing very specific searches.
MPDB is designed to collect and make information on oligonucleotides available on-line; sequence data on oligos of up
to 100 nucleotides will be stored. The following information
is included: identification (name, nucleotide sequence,
aminoacid sequence, catalogue codes, ...), target gene
(name, EMBL/GENBANK sequence access number, allelic variants

recognized, ...), technical data (melting temperature, NaCl
molarity, G+C, advices, ...), origin data (originating
laboratory, bibliography, ...) and applications.

TECHNICAL DESCRIPTION

Data bases have been developed by means of the relational
data base management system Oracle, that is available on a
wide range of computers (from personals to mainframes) and
utilizes the standard query language SQL (Structured Query
Language). Unix has been as well adopted. These choices
ensure good modularity and portability to the system.
A particular care has been devoted to the user interface;
every principal function, which can be fulfilled simply following a series of menus, has been built with easy to understand windows, fitted up with help "on-line". The relational
nature of the data bases, combined with the intensive use of
reference tables instead of textual description, makes the
carrying out of searches very simple and accurate.
Remote access to data bases, which are currently located at
the National Cancer Institute in Genoa, can be achieved by
means of a modem equipped Personal Computer.

CELL LINE DATA BASE

CLDB is based on a central nucleus of information corresponding to the cell line basic data set, and containing the
following items: identification (name, catalogue codes, ..),
origin (species, tissue, ...), specific functions, preserva-
tion and culture characteristics, retrieval sources (references, availability, ...). At present, 390 cell lines are
described, about 70% of which being "original lines", not
present in other catalogues. Data on more than 200 further
cell lines are ready to be inserted in CLDB.
Data collection is being carried out in cooperation with the
Italian National Research Council Project "Biotecnologie e
Biostrumentazione", with the Associazione Italiana Colture
Cellulari and the Scuola Superiore di Oncologia e Scienze
Biomediche. Moreover, at an international level, close col-
laborations have been established with the European node of
Hybridoma Data Bank, the European Collection of Animal Cell
Cultures and the Microbial Strain Data Network.
So far developed applications give the user the opportunity
of performing searches on the basis of the following features: name and catalogues code ("query by name"), species,
strain, tissue, tumor ("query by origin"), specific function, application ("query by function"). Mnemonic codes can
be used to define the corresponding item. Furthermore, <%>
and < _ > keys can be used as substitutes of characters.
In fig. 1 the result of a query by origin restricted to tum-
or cell lines from mammary gland is shown.
A catalogue will be produced, in volume or floppy disk; an
example of line description is given in fig. 2.

Fig. 1 Query by origin

```
--------------------------------------------------------------------
INTERLAB PROJECT          === QUERY BY ORIGIN ===           CLDBV v 1.0
                       ( results ordered by name )

Name  MCF7_______________________________
Species   HU Human___________________ Tissue MNGL_ Mammary gland__________
Strain CAUCA Caucasian_____________ Tumor CA___ Carcinoma_______________

Name  MDA-MB-157__________________
Species   HU Human___________________ Tissue MNGL_ Mammary gland__________
Strain BLACK Black_________________ Tumor CA___ Carcinoma_______________

Name  META-1___________________
Species   MS Mouse__________________ Tissue MNGL_ Mammary gland__________
Strain BALBC BALB/c________________ Tumor CA___ Carcinoma_______________

Name  META-10__________________
Species   MS Mouse__________________ Tissue MNGL_ Mammary gland__________
Strain BALBC BALB/c________________ Tumor CA___ Carcinoma_______________
--------------------------------------------------------------------
 ^ v  Char Mode: Replace  Page 5                        Count:  17
```

Fig. 2 Line description for the catalogue

H4-II-E-C3   (Liver, Rat)
ATCC CRL 1600   ECACC 85061112
Monoclonal established culture, grown as monolayer
Epithelial-like morphology
Species: Rat male   Strain: AxC
Tissue/organ: Liver   Tumor: Hepatoma
Derived from: Reuber-H-35 hepatoma
Transformed by: N-2 fluorenyldiacetamide
Tumorigenic in syngeneic animals
Endogenous viruses: Type C viruses
Specific function: Plasma protein secretion
Applications: Factor   sensitivity   *   Somatic   cell
hybridization * Gene expression * Enzymatic studies
Data received from:
- PAGPG   Facolta' Medicina e Chirurgia   Perugia
  C: SWIM01 F: CMGL01   Tyrosine aminotransferase positive
Bibliography: N.C.I. Monogr. 1964, 13:229

ACKNOWLEDGEMENTS

The project is partly supported by the Italian Ministry for University and Scientific and Technological Research.

REFERENCES

1 Maschio, C., Parodi, B., Romano, P. and Ruzzon, T. Interlab Project: a cell line data base. _Proceedings of the 5th European Edition of the Oak Ridge Conference on "Advanced Technology for the Clinical laboratory and Biotechnology"_, Milan, November 23-25, 1989

2 Aresu, O. et al. A data base for HLA typed B lymphoblastoid cell lines. _Proceedings of the European Histocompatibility Conference_, Strasbourg, March 21-23, 1990

ADHESION AND MOTILITY OF EMBRYONIC AND CANCER CELLS

J.P. Thiery, J.L. Duband, S. Dufour, B. Boyer, G.C. Tucker, A.M. Valles, J. Gavrilovic, G. Moens and J. Jouanneau
CNRS-ENS, Laboratoire de Physiopathologie du Développement, 46 rue d'Ulm, 8ème étge, 75230 Paris Cedex 05, France.

Cell-cell and cell-extracellular matrix adhesion mechanisms play a key role in morphogenesis and in cancer invasion and metastasis. We have analysed in detail the program of expression of several adhesion molecules in epithelial-mesenchymal cell interconversion and in migratory events in the neural crest. The pattern of expression and modulations of the cell adhesion molecules (CAMs) and the substrate adhesion molecules (SAMs) correlate with the different morphogenetic steps in the neural crest. During migration crest cells do not express functional CAMs but interact specifically with fibronectins in the extracellular matrix. Several distinct cell binding domains on the fibronectin molecules have been mapped and their relative contribution to adhesion, spreadind and motility will be described. A rat bladder carcinoma has been used as a model system to study early events in the dissociation and the acquisition of motility and invasive properties of carcinoma. This epithelial cell line undergoes a conversion to a migratory fibroblast-like state in response to different collagen types but not to fibronectins or laminin. A similar conversion is obtained when acidic FGF is added to the culture medium. This multifunctional growth factor induces a rapid internalization of desmosomes, and a progressive disappearance of cytokeratins which are replaced by vimentin intermediate filaments. Acidic FGF also triggers cell motility. On collagen substrates, the speed of locomotion is enhanced in the presence of acidic FGF and under these conditions the bladder carcinoma cells readily invade 3D collagen gels. Thus this model systems may offer a unique opportunity to evaluate the role of the different adhesion modes and soluble factors in the dispersion of carcinoma cells.

Spier:

There are these connections between the fibronectins and the cytoskeleton but we also know that the way the cell interacts with its surface controls the way the cell differentiates. So interactions occur between the site of attachment and the expression of the gene. Could you tell us what your thinking is as to how that connection is made.

Thiery:

Our knowledge is still extremely primitive because people are still involved in unravelling the secondary messengers involved in these interactions. In the case of our bladder carcinoma, if you treat the cell with growth factors you change the adhesive properties so the cells become fibroblastic, the cell then changes its properties; it starts to make vimentin instead of cytokeratins. The cell is a rich source of collagenase type IV. The genes for this latter material are induced to function within 2 hours after the loss of cell adhesion. Whether these gene activities are linked is a major question. How you link morphogenesis and differentiation could involve the homoeobox and master genes with programmes and subprogrammes of genetic expression. My prejudice indicates that by simply changing the adhesive state of the cell you can get that cell to produce any biochemical of choice.

Spier:

We have the relationship between the cytoskeleton and the substratum.

Thiery:

This is a mechano-chemical link

Spier:

How do we get to the genes

Thiery:

No one knows the secondary messengers which go to the nucleus

Spier:

Are there phosphorylated proteins involved.

Thiery:

Oh yes, too many. If you do a 2D-gel with acidic SDS within two minutes you can detect 200 spots. This would take 15 post-docs 18 years to unravel. If you activate a molecule on the surface of a T-cell you induce the production of a cell adhesive molecule which was not previously detectable. You must not have your adhesion molecule active all the time or you would have strokes etc.

Pouradier:

May I have your opinion about the therapeutic potential of the RGD molecule as marketed by Tebens and others.

Thiery:

A lot of excitement was generated by an experiment

showing an inhibition of metastatic development in the lung. The RGD peptides per se have a half life in the blood of 8 minutes. So you would have to design either cyclic peptides or peptide analogues. Such a peptide now exists which has a half life of one day. Some of them are being used but not to treat metastasis because we do not know when such metastasis occur. So they are used in different combinations for leg venous ulcers. This can cure people when the peptides are combined to beads. The second kind of reagent which will be used which will be much better than tissue plasminogen activator for the metastasis is the anti-integrin antibodies. These can be injected i.v. and dissolve platelet aggregates very rapidly without any side effects, where with tPA you get immediate reoccurrences of the thrombosis and platelet aggregation. So this will be a marketed product in the near future. So anti-adhesive components will be used to counteract some diseases while adhesive components (mini fibronectins) or others will be used for tissue repair.

IMMORTALIZATION OF CELLS WITH ONCOGENES

Jacques SAMARUT,
Laboratoire de Biologie Cellulaire et Moléculaire, Ecole Normale
Supérieure de Lyon, 46 allée d'Italie, 69364 Lyon cedex 07,
France

Spontaneous immortalization of vertebrate cells is an extremely
rare event and its frequency of occurence varies according to
animal species. Immortalization and establishment into cell lines
can be induced by transferring oncogenes into primary cells.
Several parameters should be considered to establish cells into
permanent cell lines with oncogenes : first the nature of the
oncogene, second the route of introducing the oncogene into
cells, third the strategy of expression of the oncogene in the
targeted cells. Two kinds of oncogenes can be used.
Oncogenes like the E1A gene of the human adenovirus, the
large T of SV40 or Polyoma Virus, E7 of Human Papilloma Virus
induce immortalization of several kinds of cells, mostly epithelial
cells, without over neoplastic transformation. These oncognes
induce permanent replication of the cells by inactivating cellular
proteins like the p53 and Rb proteins which are involved in
negative feedback control of cell proliferation (anti oncogenes).
However these oncogenes are poorly efficient in immortalizing
some kinds of cells like hemopoietic cells. In this case,
transforming oncogenes which block the differentiation at
specific differentiation stages can be used. Cells immortalized
through this way are generally tumorigenic.
DNA transfection is the usual way of transferring oncogenes into
cells. However this technique can be used only on cells in
culture and is poorly efficient on hemopoietic cells. Recombinant
retroviruses are efficient vectors to introduce immortalizing
oncogenes into most kinds of cells and can be used for in vivo
infection. The recent development of transgenic animals has
made it possible to construct animal species which harbor
specific oncogenic sequences in all tissues. In this case the
immortalization of specific cell lineages requires targeting the
expression of the oncogene with tissue specific promoters.
Transformation of normal cells into immortal cells requires
multiple genetic events most of which are still unknown. Forced
expression of an exogenous oncogene might represent only
one initial event in this process.
As a matter of fact, the procedures for immortalizing specific
cells are still empirical. The in vivo approach is promising since
the cells are maintained in their proper environment and then
can fully develop their proliferation potential allowing then the
emergence of rare immortalized cells.

Brown: It seems obvious that people would have tried anti-sera technology to reduce retinoblastoma (RB); has that been done?

Samarut: I have not seen anything published although I know of people who have tried it without success.

Horaud: There was a lot of work done on immortalised human fibroblasts using SV40 (Girard). Are the oncogenes you have described a useful way of establishing immortalised human cell lines. I would prefer to have B-cells immortalised by an oncogene than the full EB virus genome.

Samarut: Many human cells have been immortalised by oncogenes. Epithelial cells, Keratinocytes . Many cells have been so established. People do have difficulty immortalising B-cells using parts of the EB genome as it is possible there is more than one transcription unit involved. You need the HPV to obtain immortalisation of Keratinocytes.

Muller: You said that immortalisation is one step towards tumorigenic transformation. Barnes and Sato used a serum-free medium to grow mouse fibroblasts and they bye-passed senescence with such cells and did not show chromosomal rearrangements; you can get immortalisation without using oncogenes therefore.

Samarut: In whole organisms some cells might be regarded as immortal such as the hematopoietic stem cells, but there is a difference between in vivo and in vitro situations. It is impossible to keep the hemopoeitic cells in culture in the way they continue to proliferate in the body; there is something inappropriate in the medium. But with mouse embryonic stem cells from early embryos (the blastocysts) at which stage all the cells are totipotent. These cells can now be maintained with their totipotent feature in vitro, and these cells are not tumorigenic. So if we can provide the right growth factors, etc we should be able to maintain in vitro cells with self renewal capability in vivo.

Miller: I am against the use of transgenic animals as are many others. I am also against the use of retroviruses because it is not a good system as you cannot control the site of virus integration. Anderson at the NIH has tried to use it to cure human disease, I think this is a wrong approach.

Freshney: Jim Smith in the USA has described 4 complementation groups of dominant acting genes which he calls senescence genes. Clearly within that complex there are genes which not only regulate growth but which control the number of times a cell can go through a replication cycle. Do you see a difference between these two gene types.

Samarut: Senescence is a complicated phenomenon; a reason for senescence is a degradation of the DNA and a failure of the repair mechanisms.

Freshney: But that would be a recessive gene; I asked about dominant acting genes as shown by hybridization experiments.

Samarut: I cannot say.

Katinger: Many people use cell fusion for immortalization, you did not mention this.

Samarut: I focused on a controlled way of introducing specific sequences.

Katinger: You would not recommend fusion?

Samarut: No, it has been very useful but people would be happier if they could achieve the same results by transfecting one or two genes.

Katinger: What about microinjection.

Samarut: It would be a useful way of introducing genes into cell; this technique is very difficult for non-adherent cells.

             If we want to target cells for immortalization it is useful to go for the cells which are early on in their differentiation pathway.

Hentschel: The problem of immortalizing human B-cells is that there is a loss of the phenotype after a while. Do the example of other differentiated cell types which have been immortalized also loose that phenotypic characteristics.

Samarut: It depends of the cells. But even in early passages the immortalized cells do not express the fully differentiated phenotype although some of genes of the differentiated phenotype are expressed in immortalized Keratinocytes.

Section 2
Nutrient media with special supplements

LIPID METABOLISM OF ANIMAL CELLS IN CULTURE - A REVIEW

Georg Schmid

Central Research Laboratories, ZFE/MB, Bld. 66/302, F. Hoffmann-La Roche AG, CH-4002 Basle, Switzerland

ABSTRACT

The fatty acid composition of mammalian cells with respect to cellular storage lipids and membrane phospholipids reflects that of lipids present in the culture medium. Modification of membrane phospholipid fatty acyl groups leads to differences in cell function (membrane enzyme activity and transport properties). The specific growth rate μ of cultured cells may likewise be affected by different concentrations and combinations of exogenous lipids. Thus, lipidic supplements for large-scale cell culture media used in the production of monoclonal antibodies and recombinant protein products should be more closely evaluated for their potential impact on cell growth, product formation, and metabolism.

BACKGROUND

A number of extensive review articles (1-5) provide an excellent overview on the current knowledge of fatty acid, glyceride, and phospholipid metabolism of cultured cells in the biochemical literature.

Essentially all cells examined have been found to readily take up any exogenous lipids contained in the culture medium. Lipids may be present in the medium as components of added serum or they can be supplemented in the form of isolated plasma lipoprotein fractions, free fatty acids complexed to serum albumin or fatty acid/phospholipid microemulsions. Incorporated lipids are utilized within the cell, either as a source of energy or as building blocks for cell growth. When adequate supplies of lipids are available in the medium de novo synthesis is inhibited. In spite of this the cells accumulate excessive triglycerides and cholesterol esters in the form of cytoplasmic inclusions when they are exposed to an overabundance of lipids. The fatty acid composition of cellular storage lipids as well as of membrane phospholipids resembles that of lipids present in the medium. Modification of membrane phospholipid fatty acyl groups was shown to lead to differences in cell function (transport properties and membrane enzyme activity). The specific growth rate of cultured cells was found to be profoundly affected by different combinations and concentrations of fatty acids.

Research activities towards the development of serum-free and/or protein-free cell culture media have long recognized the potential growth promoting effects of exogenous fatty acids, phospholipids, or lipoprotein fractions. Thus, lipids are included in most serum-free medium formulations (6-11). However, there is very limited or no quantitative data available on the utilization of (or limitations in) exogenous lipid supplements. Their potential influence on cell growth, product formation, and metabolism of recombinant cell lines and hybridoma cells relevant to the biotechnological industry still has to be explored.

UTILIZATION OF EXTRACELLULAR LIPIDS

All cells tested so far can utilize exogenous lipids from the culture medium. The medium may be supplemented with serum, free fatty acids bound to a carrier protein, plasma lipoprotein fractions, or fatty acid/phospholipid/cholesterol microemulsions (3,4,6,7,16). Incorporated lipids are used either as a source of energy or as builing blocks for synthesis of complex lipid esters. Mammalian cells in culture seem to have a virtually unlimited capacity to incorporate exogenous fatty acids (1,3,4). Rosenthal (20) observed that higher exogenous free fatty acid concentrations resulted in increased incorporation of both oleic and linoleic acids by human skin fibroblasts. Schmid et al. (27) calculated higher metabolic quotients (incorporation rates) with higher initial free fatty acid concentrations for recombinant BHK cells in low-serum medium. With no apparent regulatory mechanism to limit fatty acid uptake excess fatty acyl groups are eventually stored as cytoplasmic inclusions that are composed mostly of triglycerides (21,22,17).

TURNOVER AND MODIFICATIONS OF CELL LIPID COMPOSITION

Lipids of mammalian cells in culture are in a dynamic state of rapid turnover (3,4). Depending on culture conditions (i.e., exponential growth phase or onset of density inhibition) and external free fatty acid supply this turnover will include exchange of cellular acyl groups (from membrane phospholipid and triglyceride pools) with free fatty acids bound to albumin and/or other proteins present in the culture medium. The composition of cellular storage lipids, such as triglycerides and cholesterol esters, and also of membrane phospholipids does reflect the composition of lipids contained in the medium (14,23,25,12,20,27).

INFLUENCE OF LIPIDIC SUPPLEMENTS ON CELL GROWTH RATES

It is now well established that a number of mammalian cells can be grown in the complete absence of polyunsaturated (linoleic) fatty acids without any apparent alterations in cell morphology or energy metabolism (3,4,6,11,29). However, low concentrations of exogenous unsaturated fatty acids often promote cell growth and/or differentiated function in normal as well as transformed cells (3,4). For example, growth stimulation was found to be a function of different combinations and concentrations of free fatty acids bound to albumin or β-lactoglobulin (as assessed by monitoring tritiated thymidine incorporation into DNA) for Con A-stimulated lymphocytes (24). Rintoul et al. (18) reported that except for the saturated fatty acids stearate and palmitate all fatty acids tested (linoleic, oleic, and elaidic) supported the growth of CHO K1 cells equally well. Hatzfeld et al. (15) observed a strong additive effect of saturated and unsaturated free fatty acids bound to bovine albumin with various cells of the human hematopoietic and immune systems (U937, K562, HL-60, Jurkat, Raji). Similar synergistic effects have been communicated by other authors (3,4,26,13,19). Doi et al. (13) demonstrated a good correlation between the unsaturated fatty acid content of membrane phospholipids and cell growth. When incorporated saturated fatty acids reduced the percentage of unsaturated fatty acids in membrane phospholipids to less than 50%, severe inhibition of cell growth was found.

POTENTIAL IMPACT ON LARGE-SCALE MAMMALIAN CELL CULTURE

Schmid et al. (27) reported on the effects of free fatty acids and phospholipids on growth of and product formation by recombinant BHK and CHO cell lines that produce human antithrombin III. The specific growth rate of adherent rBHK cells cultured in medium containing 0.1% fetal bovine serum and additional supplements was found to be unaffected by different combinations and concentrations of free fatty acids. Interestingly, antithrombin III formation, however, was a function of free fatty acid combinations and concentrations. Palsson and coworkers (28) communicated some preliminary results on the influence of free fatty acids on specific growth rates, metabolism, and cell composition of a murine hybridoma cell line. They studied the effects of added linoleic and linolenic acids at concentrations of 0–15 μg/mL on cell growth and death rates in stationary and spinner cultures using RPMI medium supplemented with 1% FBS.

REFERENCES

1 Howard, B. V., and Howard, W. J. Lipid Metabolism in Cultured Cells. _Adv. Lipid Res._ 1974, _12_, 51

2 Spector, A. A. Fatty Acid, Glyceride, and Phospholipid Metabolism. In: _Growth, Nutrition, and Metabolism of Cells in Culture_, Vol. 1 (Eds. Rothblat, G. H. and Cristofalo, V. J.) Academic Press, New York, 1972, pp 257–296

3 Rosenthal, M. D. Fatty Acid Metabolism of Isolated Mammalian Cells. _Prog. Lipid Res._ 1987, _26_, 87

4 Spector, A. A., Mathur, S. N., Kaduce, T. L., Hyman, B. T. Lipid Nutrition and Metabolism of Cultured Mammalian Cells. _Prog. Lipid Res._ 1981, _19_, 155

5 Cornwell, D. G., and Morisaki, N. Fatty Acid Paradoxes in the Control of Cell Proliferation: Prostaglandins, Lipid Peroxides, and Cooxidation Reactions. In: _Free Radicals in Biology_, Vol. VI (Ed. Pryor, W. A.) Academic Press, New York, 1984, pp 95–137

6 Barnes D., and Sato, G. H. Methods for Growth of Cultured Cells in Serum–Free Medium. _Anal. Biochem._ 1980, _102_, 255

7 Bettger, W. J., and Ham, R. G. The Nutrient Requirements of Cultured Mammalian Cells. Adv. Nutr. Res. 1982, _4_, 249

8 Higuchi, K. Cultivation of Animal Cells in Chemically Defined Media: A Review. Adv. Appl. Microbiol. 1973, _16_, 111

9 Bjaere, U. Serum–Free Cultivation of Lymphoid Cells. In: _Advances in Biochemical Engineering/Biotechnology_, Vol. 34 (Ed. A. Fiechter) Springer–Verlag, Berlin, 1987, pp 95–109

10 Glassy, M. C., Tharakan, J. P., and Chau, P. C. Serum–Free Media in Hybridoma Culture and Monoclonal Antibody Production. _Biotechnol. Bioeng._ 1988, _32_, 1015

11 Barnes, D., and Sato, G. H. Serum–Free Cell Culture: A Unifying Approach. _Cell_ 1980, _22_, 649

12 Daniel, L. W., Kucera, L. S., and Waite, M. Metabolism of Fatty Acids by Cultured Tumor Cells and Their Diploid Precurser Fibroblasts. _J. Biol. Chem._ 1980, _255_, 5697

13 Doi, O., Doi, F., Schroeder, F., Alberts, A. W., and Vagelos, P. R. Manipulation of Fatty Acid Composition of Membrane Phospholipid and its Effects on Cell Growth in Mouse LM Cells. _Biochim. Biophys. Acta_ 1978, _509_, 239

14 Gallaher, R. W., and Blough, H. A. Effects of Density–Dependent Inhibition of Growth on Phospholipid Metabolism in Monolayer Cultures of Animal Cells. _Arch. Biochem. Biophys._ 1976, _173_, 739

15 Hatzfeld, J., Hatzfeld, A., Maigne, J., Sasportes, M., Willis, R., and
McClure, D. B. Specific Roles of Lipids, Transferrin, and Insulin in Defined
Media for Cells of the Human Hematopoietic and Immune System. In: Growth of
Cells in Hormonally Defined Media, Book A (Eds. Sato, G. H., Pardee, A. A.,
and Sirbasku, D. A.) Cold Spring Harbor Press, 1982, pp 703–710
16 Iscove, N. N., and Melchers, F. Complete Replacement of Serum by Albumin,
Transferrin, and Soy Bean Lipid in Cultures of Lipopolysaccharide-Reactive
B Lymphocytes. J. Exp. Med. 1978, 147, 923
17 MacKenzie, C. G., MacKenzie, J. B., and Reiss, O. K. Increase in Cell Lipid
and Cytoplasmic Particles in Mammalian Cells Cultured at Reduced pH.
J. Lipid Res. 1967, 8, 642
18 Rintoul, D. A., Sklar, L. A., and Simoni, R. D. Membrane Lipid Modification
of Chinese Hamster Ovary Cells. J. Biol. Chem. 1978, 253, 7447
19 Rockwell, G. A., Sato, G. H., and McClure, D. B. The Growth Requirements of
SV40 Virus Transformed Balb/c-3T3 Cells in Serum-Free Monolayer Culture.
J. Cell Physiol. 1980, 103, 323
20 Rosenthal, M. D. Selectivity in Incorporation, Utilization, and Retention of
Oleic and Linoleic Acids by Human Skin Fibroblasts. Lipids 1980, 15, 838
21 Rothblat, G. H., Rosen, J. M., Insull, Jr., W., Yau, A. O., and Small, D. M.
Production of Cholesterol Ester-Rich, Anisotropic Inclusions by Mammalian
Cells in Culture. Exp. Mol. Path. 1977, 26, 318
22 Schneeberger, E. E., Lynch, R. D., and Geyer, R. P. Formation and Disappearance of Triglyceride Droplets in Strain L Fibroblasts. Exp. Cell Res. 1971,
69, 193
23 Spector, A. A., and Steinberg, D. Turnover and Utilization of Esterified
Fatty Acids in Ehrlich Ascites Tumor Cells. J. Biol. Chem. 1967, 242, 3057
24 Spieker-Polet, H., and Polet, H. Requirement of a Combination of a Saturated
and an Unsaturated Free Fatty Acid and a Fatty Acid Carrier Protein for
In Vitro Growth of Lymphocytes. J. Immunol. 1981, 126, 949
25 Tsai, P.-Y., and Geyer, R. P. Effect of Exogenous Fatty Acids on the
Retention of Phospholipid Acyl Groups by Mouse L Fibroblasts. Biochim.
Biophys. Acta 1978, 528, 344
26 Yamane, I. Development and Application of a Serum-Free Culture Medium for
Primary Culture. In: Nutritional Requirements of Cultured Cells (Ed.
Katsura, H.) Japan Scientific Societies Press, Tokyo, 1978, pp 1–21
27 Schmid, G., Zilg, H., Eberhard, U., and Johannsen, R. Effect of Free Fatty
Acids and Phospholipids on Growth of and Product Formation by Recombinant
Baby Hamster Kidney Cells (rBHK) and Chinese Hamster Ovary Cells (rCHO) Cells
in Culture. J. Biotechnol. 1990, in press
28 Savinell, J. M., Lee, G. M., and Palsson, B. O. The Effects of Fatty Acids on
Hybridoma Growth, Metabolism, and Cell Composition. 198th ACS National
Meeting, Miami Beach, FL, 1989, paper no. 113
29 Katsuta, H., and Takaoka, T. Protein- and Lipid-Free Synthetic Media for the
Cultivation of Mammalian Cells in Tissue Culture. In: Nutritional Require-
ments of Cultured Cells (Ed. Katsura, H.) Japan Scientific Societies Press,
Tokyo, 1978, pp 257–275

<u>**Paper of Schmidt**</u>

Griffiths: The yields of ammonia to glutamine showed a gradual change but you were explaining it in terms of a change in pathway. If so, wouldn't you expect a switch rather than a gradual change?

Schmidt: It is only a suggestion, I cannot prove it.

Griffiths: The work of the Surrey, and other, groups show triphasic metabolic patterns with sudden death changes so I wondered if we could expect pathway switches with only gradual changes.

Schmidt: We never saw this sort of behaviour with all our studies at Berkeley, but that does not mean that different cells aren't different.

Caulcott: What do you think the limiting nutrient was in your system?

Schmidt: It can never be called a chemostat culture because we have several limiting nutrients. At dilution rates of 0.7 and below, glucose, glutamine, methionine and tryptophan are limiting.

Caulcott: Doesn't that invalidate some of your calculations as they are based on 'classical microbial' culture work with a single limiting nutrient, and everything else in excess? For example, I am not convinced that you would ever return to having a zero growth rate.

Schmidt: The mathematical balances of calculations still hold but the linear graphs for amino acid consumption and production rates are tentative. They hold over the expected growth rate but not to zero growth rate.

Bushell: But aren't they based on a simple Monod relationship which requires a single limiting nutrient?

Schmidt: The equations I presented are valid at any time.

Griffiths: With continuous flow culture of animal cells it does not entirely follow the microbial system, but there is a window of growth rates where it does follow, but not at or near zero growth rate.

Paper of Schmidt

Gerbert: Do you know of any lipids that can be added to cell culture media that will affect glycoproteins coming out of the ER?

Schmidt: I am not aware of any. The secretion of human anti-thrombin III is increased by different concentrations and combinations of fatty acids in the medium.

LIPOPROTEIN REQUIREMENTS OF CULTURED MAMMALIAN CELLS.

Guy Hewlett

Bayer AG, Institute for Virology, Wuppertal, Germany

ABSTRACT

Lipids are usually found in association with carrier proteins, the lipoproteins. Using the aqueous preparation of lipoprotein Ex-Cyte(R) as a source of cholesterol and fatty acids, we have found that different cell lines have their own particular requirement for Ex-Cyte and that the presence of albumin and selenous acid in the medium can enhance the effect of Ex-Cyte.

KEYWORDS: lipoprotein, lipid, fatty acid, serum-free, selenium, albumin, fibroblast, hybridoma, myeloma, keratinocyte.

INTRODUCTION

Many cultured cells require a source of fatty acids in the medium. Lipids and fatty acids, in a free state or bound to carriers like albumin or lipoproteins, act as precursors for prostaglandin synthesis, represent an alternative energy source and are major components of the cell membrane. Until recently, one of the major problems in serum-free culture was that of supplying a satisfactory source of preformed lipids to the cells. We have carried out extensive studies on the water-soluble mammalian lipid preparations known as Ex-Cyte(R), which contain a range of fatty acids, lipids and lipoproteins normally found in plasma, and their effects on serum-free culture of a variety of cell types.

MATERIALS AND METHODS

The cells described in the Results section were grown in a low-serum medium (see Results) or in a serum-free medium consisting of a 50/50 mix of Dulbecco's modification of Eagle's medium (DME) and Ham's nutrient solution F12 (F12) with the addition of bovine insulin (10 mg/l), transferrin (10 mg/l), Ex-Cyte lipoprotein/lipid (see Results), albumin (200 mg/l), and selenium (100 nmol/l). Basal medium was obtained from Gibco/BRL (Eggenstein, FRG) and selenous acid from Aldrich (Heidenheim, FRG). The remaining components were all supplied by Bayer Diagnostic GmbH (München, FRG).

RESULTS AND DISCUSSION

In Table 1 the production of Interleukin 1 (IL-1) by the A431
human keratinocyte line is depicted as a function of basal
medium supplemented with bovine serum albumin (BSA) alone or
Ex-Cyte V, a mixture of BSA and bovine lipids. The lipoprotein
preparation clearly improves the yield of IL-1 in the serum-
free medium:

| Medium | Day of harvest | | | |
Supplement	3	4	5	6
BSA	10.6	9.5	9.4	9.4
BSA + Ex-Cyte	10.8	12.3	14.4	14.8

Table 1: Ex-Cyte (30 ug cholesterol/ml) increases the
production of IL-1 by A431 cells in serum-free medium. Data
represent mean levels of IL-1 in the supernatants in U/ml.

We have also found that Ex-Cyte lipids and albumin together
stimulate the growth of L929 mouse fibroblast cells in serum-
free medium (figure 1):

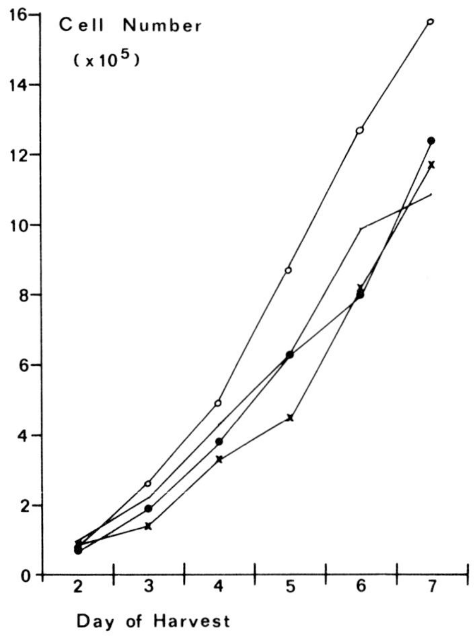

Figure 1: Ex-Cyte (30
ug cholesterol/ml) and
Fraction V BSA act
synergistically on the
growth of L929 cells in
serum-free medium:
X---X: basal medium;
•----•: + BSA
●---●: + Ex-Cyte;
o---o: + BSA + Ex-Cyte

Some cells require lipoprotein/lipids when serum is reduced to
low levels. Table 2 shows the positive effect of Ex-Cyte on

the yield of 3T3 cells in basal medium containing only 0.5 %
FCS:

Medium Supplement	6 day cell yield $(x\ 10^5)$	Viability (%)
0.5% FCS	5.6	17
0.5% FCS + Ex-Cyte	8.0	4

Table 2: Ex-Cyte (30 ug cholesterol/ml) improves the yield and
also the survival of 3T3 cells in low serum medium.

P3X63Ag8.653 (X63) myeloma has an optimum level of Ex-Cyte at
100 ug cholesterol/ml in low-serum medium but under serum-free
conditions, the optimal level of Ex-Cyte was found to be 30 ug
cholesterol/ml (data not shown). Similar results were found
for the hybridoma AHT 107 in serum-free medium. Previously
reported studies with AHT 107 showed that a serum-free medium
supplemented with Ex-Cyte lipoprotein (30 ug cholesterol/ml)
induce a more sustained period of antibody production at a
higher level than in the serum-containing control medium (1).

Finally we have found that in the case of HeLa cells, the
response to Ex-Cyte is improved when selenium is also included
in the medium (table 3):

Cell Type	Medium	Selenium	Growth
Hela	0.5% FCS + Ex-Cyte	+	+++++
..	0.5% FCS + Ex-Cyte	-	+
..	0.5% FCS	+	-

Table 3: Selenium stimulates the growth of HeLa cells in low-
serum medium supplemented with Ex-Cyte (30 ug cholesteron(ml).

CONCLUSION

Our studies show that each cell line has its own requirements
for lipoprotein as supplied in the form of Ex-Cyte and that
the presence of low amounts of serum in the medium can alter
those requirements. In many cases, a serum-free medium has to
be supplemented with selenium and albumin for Ex-Cyte to exert
its positive effects on growth rate, cell survival and the
synthesis/release of cytokines and monoclonal antibodies.

REFERENCE

1. Hewlett, G., Duvinski, M.S. and Montalto, J.G. Pentex Ex-
Cyte growth enhancement media supplement as a lipoprotein
additive for mammalian cell culture. Miles Science J. 1989,
11, 9-14

EFFECT OF NUTRIENTS AND WASTE METABOLITES ON GROWTH, METABOLISM AND PROTEIN SYNTHESIS IN HYBRIDOMA

Mohamed Al-Rubeai and A N Emery

Centre for Biochemical Engineering, School of Chemical Engineering
University of Birmingham, Birmingham B15 2TT, UK

ABSTRACT:
Several different metabolic events in murine hybridoma cells are affected by both nutrient depletion and waste metabolites. The incorporation of [^{3}H] thymidine into DNA and [^{35}S] methionine into protein and the reduction of MTT salt by active mitochondria are highly affected by the depletion of both glucose and glutamine. Serum depletion results in a 20% inhibition of thymidine incorporation; MTT reduction is also inhibited by 25%, whereas methionine incorporation is unaffected. Lactic acid and ammonia additions result in 79%, 75% and 57% inhibition of thymidine and methionine incorporation and MTT reduction respectively.

KEYWORDS :
Hybridoma; cell culture; DNA synthesis; protein synthesis; metabolic activity.

INTRODUCTION:
We have reported (1,2,3) that Ig production in murine hybridomas is maximal in the G1 and S phases and also that the total Ig accumulated can be increased if cells are arrested and maintained in late G1/S phases. Higher specific antibody production (QA) is also found when the viability is decreased (3) and such an observation is reasonably explained and justified (3) as due to the passive release of accumulated intracellular antibody during cell death and lysis. While reports of increased antibody production in serum-free medium (4) and when cells are subjected to stress (5) suggest that the synthesis of the targeted product may be influenced by physiological conditions, it may be postulated that such apparent changes in specific productivity result primarily from variations in the population viability and proliferation rate.

In this present study, we investigated the effects of nutrient depletion and accumulation of toxic metabolites on the rate of protein and DNA synthesis. While similar studies have been widely reported, most have neglected the importance of the relationship between growth and death and protein synthesis, and "secretion".

MATERIALS AND METHODS
TB/C3 murine hybridomas producing antibodies against human IgG were maintained in RPMI1640 medium supplemented with 5% of either foetal or newborn calf serum. Cells were resuspended into glucose and glutamine-free RPMI in 5ml aliquots at 5×5^5 ml^{-1}. Various concentrations of foetal calf-serum, glucose, glutamine, lactic acid and ammonia were added to each tube and incubated for 3hr at 37°C. Either 1 μCi/ml of [^{3}H] thymidine or 3 μCi ml^{-1} [^{35}S] methionine or 10 μl of MTT (to 0.1 ml culture medium in a microtitre plate) was added to each set and reincubated for 1 hr in the case of [^{3}H] thymidine or 3 hr for the others. Incorporation of the labelled thymidine and methionine was determined by TCA precipitation and scintillation counting. MTT formazan precipitates

were dissolved and measured at OD 540nm.   Labelling and staining procedures were as described in (3).

RESULTS AND DISCUSSION :
The results presented in Fig. 1 show that protein and DNA synthesis and metabolic activity were affected to various degrees by nutrient limitation and product concentrations.   Serum depletion reduces both thymidine incorporation (by 20% at zero serum concentration) and MTT reduction (by 25%) but methionine incorporation is completely unaffected, at least over the timescale examined.   Glucose deprivation has insignificant effects on methionine incorporation and MTT reduction, but does reduce thymidine incorporation by 20%, the rate of nucleotide synthesis apparently limited by the absence of glucose.   Deprivation of glutamine reduces methiomine incorporation drastically (>90%), and reduces thymidine incorporation by 50% but MTT reduction is barely affected.

Addition of lactic acid (15mM) and ammonia (2mM) both separately andtogether results in reduced synthesis and metabolic activity.   The individual effects appear to be directly additive so that the thymidine and methiomine incorporation and MTT reduction are reduced to 79%, 75% and 57% respectively of the control values.   Lactic acid has the greater effect on metabolic activity.   Ammonium lactate does not show a particular cytotoxic effect.   The clear implication is that while serum and glucose affect cell proliferation by some reduction of DNA synthesis and energy metabolism, protein synthesis is only affected, and then critically by deprivation of glutamine.   Most batch growth curves in standard media show that glutamine is completely consumed at the same time as the maximum cell number is achieved.   Clearly glutamine is essential as a component for protein accumulation and biomass increase as well as for energy metabolism.

In asynchronous batch culture DNA and protein synthetic activity peak during the early exponential phase and decline rapidly during mid and late exponential and death phases (3).   Metabolic activity however peaks up to 20 hrs after the peak in DNA synthesis and declines similarly during the death phase.   It is not unreasonable to presume that the shutdown of protein synthesis is reflected also in MAb synthesis.   This would suggest that MAb synthesis declines rapidly as the viable cell numbers decline. Therefore the observed increase in specific antibody production in the death phase can only arise through the release of stored product from lysing cells.

REFERENCES
1 Al-Rubeai, M., Rookes, S. and Emery, A.N., 1989.   In: Advances in Animal Cell Biology and Technology for Bioprocesses.   Eds. Spier, R.E. et al, pp 241-245, Butterworths, London.

2 Al-Rubeai, M. and Emery, A.N., 1989.   Proceedings of 37th Ann. Meet. Eur. Tissue Culture Soc., Austria.

3 Al-Rubeai, M. and Emery, A.N., 1990.   J. Biotechnology (in press).

4 Glassy, M.C., Tharakan, J.P. and Chau, P.C., 1988.   Biotechnol. Bioeng. 32, 1015-1028

5 Miller, W.M., Blanch, H.W. and Wilke, C.R., 1988.   Biotechnol. Bioeng. 32, 947-965.

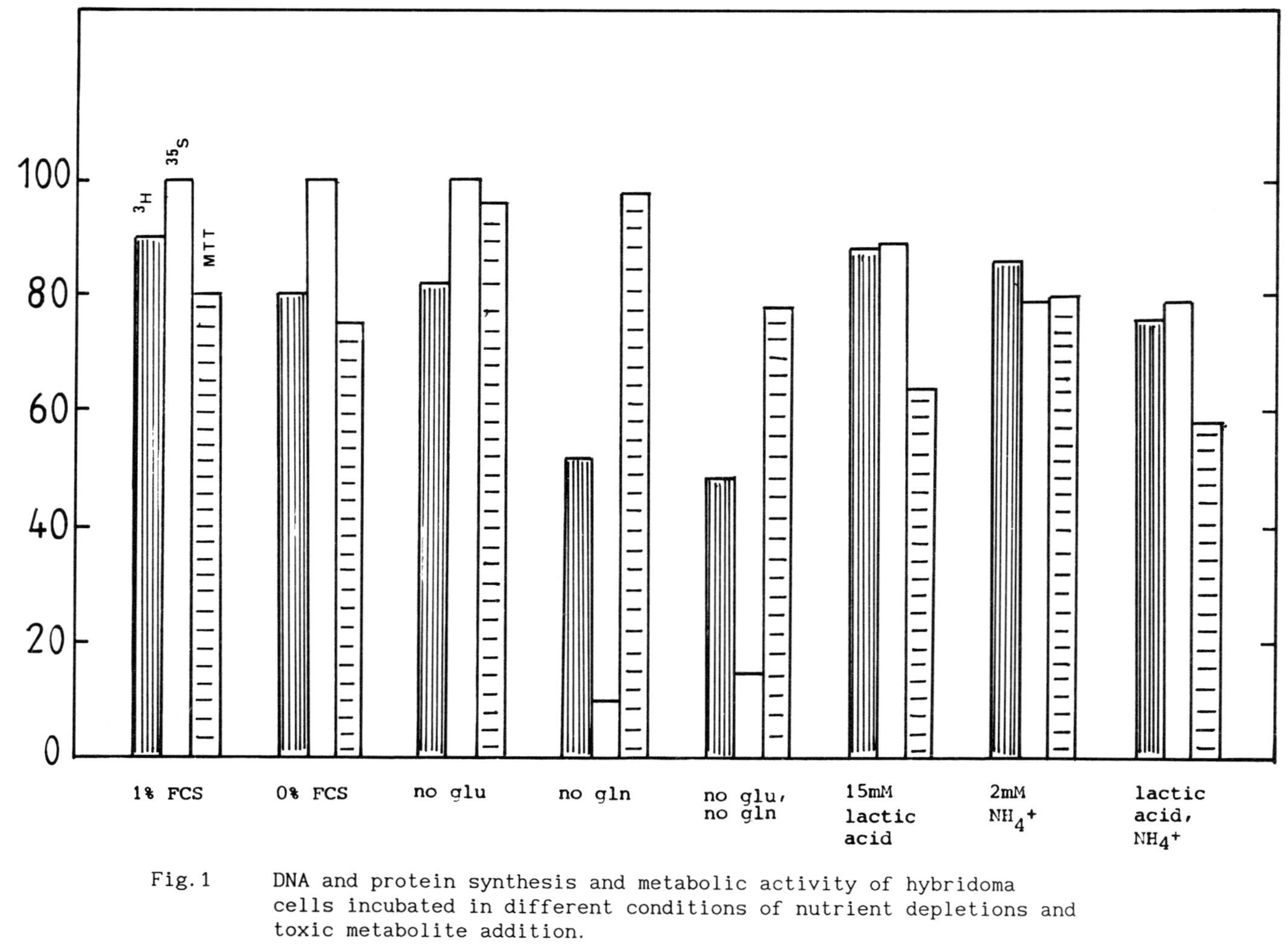

Fig. 1   DNA and protein synthesis and metabolic activity of hybridoma cells incubated in different conditions of nutrient depletions and toxic metabolite addition.

72

HYBRIDOMA GROWTH, METABOLISM, AND PRODUCT FORMATION IN HEPES-BUFFERED MEDIUM:
EFFECT OF PASSAGE NUMBER AND pH

Georg Schmid[#], Harvey W. Blanch, and Charles R. Wilke

Department of Chemical Engineering, University of California, Berkeley, CA
94720, USA. [#]Present address: Central Research Laboratories, ZFE/MB,
F. Hoffmann-La Roche AG, CH-4002 Basle, Switzerland

ABSTRACT

The effects of passage number and pH on hybridoma growth, metabolism, and antibody formation in small-scale HEPES-buffered cultures were evaluated. Prolonged
serial propagation resulted in much reduced final MAB concentrations due to the
lack of a growth phase during which cells produced significant amounts of MAB at
low specific growth rates μ. Maintaining the pH at 7.2 resulted in a reduction
of the maximum MAB and viable cell concentrations as well as increased specific
nutrient consumption rates. When the pH was allowed to fall to 6.7 there was MAB
production and growth after glutamine was exhausted using branched-chain amino
acids as substrates. Y'[lac/gluc] increased from 1.3 at pH 6.7 to 1.5 at pH 7.2.

INTRODUCTION

In preliminary experiments Miller (1,2) found that AB2-143.2 cells maintained in
HEPES-buffered DME medium reached significantly lower viable cell concentrations
but continued to grow at a reduced growth rate μ for several days compared to
cells cultivated in bicarbonate-buffered medium. In this paper we present more
detailed results on growth, metabolism, and product formation of this cell line
in HEPES-buffered medium as function of passage number and pH.

MATERIALS AND METHODS

A mouse hybridoma line AB2-143.2 (3) was grown in Dulbecco's Modified Eagle's
medium supplemented with 10% fetal bovine serum, MEM nonessential amino acids,
and pyruvate. Buffering capacity was provided by 25 mM HEPES (N-2-Hydroxyethyl-
piperazine-N'-2-ethanesulfonic acid) sodium salt (4). pH adjustments were made
twice daily (from day three onwards) with 0.5 N NaOH so as to keep the pH-value
at 7.1-7.2, whereas the pH decreased from an initial value of 7.2 to pH 6.6-6.7
in the control experiments.
Viable and nonviable cells were estimated by hemacytometer counting (trypan blue
staining). Glucose and lactate were determined by enzymatic assays; ammonia was
measured with an ion-selective electrode. Fluorescent amino acid derivatives
were separated by reverse phase HPLC and antibody concentrations quantitated by
high pressure Protein A affinity chromatography.
Details on the hybridoma cell line, medium composition, and growth conditions as
well as the assay procedures for metabolite and product concentrations are given
elsewhere (5).

RESULTS AND DISCUSSION

As a function of passage number
(1) the maximum cell concentration and total cell yield per mL of medium [i.e.,
area under concentration-time plot $(=\int n_v dt]$ increased considerably (cell yield

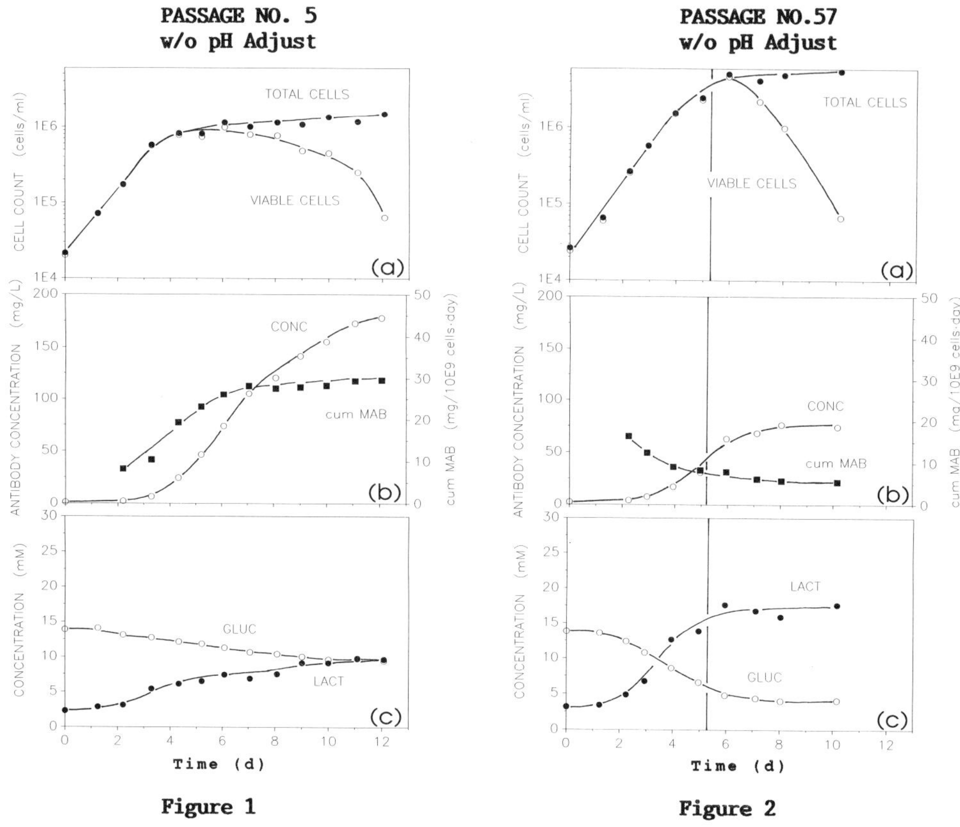

Figure 1   **Figure 2**

tripled). **(2)** At the same time final MAB concentrations decreased from 180 µg/mL to 90 µg/mL (after 3 months of serial propagation) and 75 µg/mL (after 10 months = 57th passage). The cumulative antibody production rates decreased from 30 to 6 mg/10E9 cells·d. **(3)** The apparent yield coefficients Y′[lac/gluc] declined from 1.80 to 1.50 and 1.32, whereas the apparent yield coefficients Y′[NH4+/GLN] were constant at ≃1. **(4)** The maximum specific growth rate μ_{max} was 1.10±0.05 d^{-1} for all experiments. For unknown reasons – after prolonged propagation in the HEPES-buffered DME medium – AB2-143.2 cells were able to grow at μ_{max} to higher viable cell densities, but there was no growth phase during which cells produced significant amounts of antibody at low µ (data not shown).

As a function of pH
(1) the cell metabolism was influenced so that the specific glucose and amino acid consumption rates were reduced at pH 6.7. After glutamine was exhausted there was additional growth and antibody production at low growth rates µ using branched-chain aliphatic amino acids (data not shown). **(2)** If the pH value was maintained at 7.2 the glucose metabolic quotient was much elevated and glucose and glutamine became limiting substrates simultaneously. Growth and antibody production ceased as there was no more glucose available for biosynthesis. The maximum antibody concentration was reduced by ≃40%. **(3)** The apparent molar yield coefficients Y′[lac/gluc] increased from 1.32 at pH 6.7 to 1.50 at pH 7.2. This indicates that glucose is used more efficiently at low pH values.

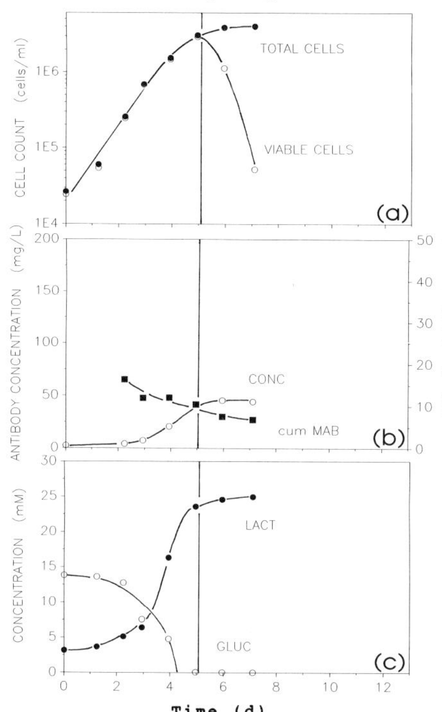

Figure 3

Growth of murine hybridoma cell line AB2-143.2 in HEPES-buffered DME medium

Figure 1: Passage No.05 w/o pH adjust

Figure 2: Passage No.57 w/o pH adjust

Figure 3: Passage No.57 w/ pH adjust

(a) viable and total cell counts vs time.
(b) MAB concentration and cumulative antibody production rate vs time.
(c) glucose and lactate concentrations vs time.

Culture conditions: AB2-143.2 cells were grown in DME medium supplemented with 10% serum in 200 mL polystyrene bottles placed on a shaker ($\approx$70 rpm) and equilibrated with 1% CO_2 in air in a 37°C incubator. Initial cell concentrations were $\approx 2 \cdot 10E4$ cells/mL.

Passage	n_v^{max} (vc/mL)	$\int n_v dt$ (vc d)	c_{MAB}^{max} (µg/mL)	cumMAB (mg/10E9 vc d)	$Y'_{(lac/gluc)}$ (mol/mol)	$Y'_{(NH4^+/GLN)}$ (mol/mol)
No 5 w/o pH Adjust	$0.9 \cdot 10^6$	$5.3 \cdot 10^6$	180	30	1.80	$\approx$1
No57 w/o pH Adjust	$4.8 \cdot 10^6$	$13.8 \cdot 10^6$	75	6	1.32	$\approx$1
No57 w/ pH Adjust	$3.0 \cdot 10^6$	$6.5 \cdot 10^6$	45	7	1.50	$\approx$1

Table 1   Selected parameters as function of passage number and pH

ACKNOWLEDGEMENTS
G. S. was supported by a postdoctoral fellowship from the Deutscher Akademischer Austauschdienst (DAAD).

REFERENCES
1 Miller, W. M., Blanch, H. W., Wilke, C. R. Biotechnol. Bioeng. 1988, 32, 947
2 Miller, W. M. Ph.D. Thesis 1987, University of California, Berkeley, CA
3 Hornbeck, P. V., and Lewis, G. K. J. Exp. Med. 1985, 161, 53
4 Shipman, Jr., C. PSEBM 1969, 130, 305
5 Schmid, G., Blanch, H. W., and Wilke, C. R. Biotech. Lett. 1990, in press

A SCREENING EXPERIMENT OF MEDIA SUPPLEMENTS ON CHO CELLS.

Carol Gebert, Peter P. Gray
Dept of Biotechnology, University of New South Wales, Sydney, Australia.

KEYWORDS: serum free, media supplement, CHO cells, beta actin

INTRODUCTION:

Optimisation of protein production in animal cell culture requires the testing of many potential media components. Since many components can act synergistically, a screening experiment should be designed where all factors are tested simultaneously, allowing for the calculation of two or more factor effects as well as single factor effects. This can involve much effort, but experiments can be designed which minimise the number of trials required.
Here, 15 different media supplements were tested in only 32 trials in a fractional factorial experimental design, to study induction of the beta actin promoter, used in a construct to drive Follicle Stimulating Hormone expression in CHO cells.
In serum free media, the protein expression levels dropped to a third of those observed in serum containing media. The screening experiment was performed to determine which factor/s can increase heterologous protein expression.

EXPERIMENTAL DESIGN:

A special design[1] for a fractional factorial experiments was used to keep single factor effects and certain two factor interactions mathematically clear of each other
The two factor interactions thought likely from table 1 to have significant interactions were AB, AC, BC, CD, EF, EG, FG, HI, BK, BD, GH, AN, EH, JL, FH. This gave a total of 30 effects to be calculated. The experiment was run in 32 trials, allowing calculation of 31 effects, which were in triplicate and randomized order. The results were analysed with Yates' theorem, which gives a relative significance to each factor. Only factors giving obviously large effects were taken to be significant. Numbers close to zero were taken to be zero.

MATERIALS AND METHODS:

CHO cells expressing FSH were provided by Pacific Biotechnology, Sydney. 24 well plates were inoculated with 10^5 cells/mL Coons/DMEM media with 10% FCS. At confluence, the media was replaced with 0.5mL serum free media containing the supplements valid for the various trials. The cells were incubated 4 days, with media replaced on day 2. Cell counts were done on day 2 and 4. Conditioned media was assayed for FSH by RIA.
After determination of the major factors, these were tested simultaneously on cells in spinner flasks against a flask with no supplements. The cells were grown to confluence on cytodex 2 microcarriers, incubated for five days, with a serum free media change every day.

MEDIA SUPPLEMENTS: table 1   These fell into 4 categories.

1.	Growth factors		2.	hormones	
A.	HB CHO[a]	as directed	E.	estradiol[c]	2.7 ng/mL
B.	IGF-1[b]	50 ng/mL	F.	progesterone[c]	3.1 ug/mL
C	EGF[c]	10 ng/mL	G.	testosterone[e]	2.9 ug/mL
D.	ECGF[d]	10 ng/mL	H.	LH[c]	50 ng/mL
			I.	LHRH[c]	11.8 ng/mL
3.	stimulators of cellular pathways,		4.	miscellaneous	
J.	forskolin[f]	103 ug/mL	N.	ribose[f]	1 mg/mL
	IBMX[g]	11 ug/mL		albumin[f]	1 mg/mL
K	A23187[f]	260 ng/mL	O.	Na butyrate[f]	110 ug/mL
L.	phorbol dibutyrate[g]	42 ug/mL			
M.	vasopressin[g]	11 ng/mL			

sources: a. gift from Cytosystems, agent for Hana Biologicals. b. gift from Div. Nutrition, CSIRO, Adelaide. c. gift from Garvan Institute. d. gift from Centre for Immunology, St Vincent's Hospital. e. gift from Dept of Biochemistry, UNSW. f. Sigma. g. Calbiochem. All from Sydney, unless otherwise indicated.

RESULTS AND DISCUSSION:

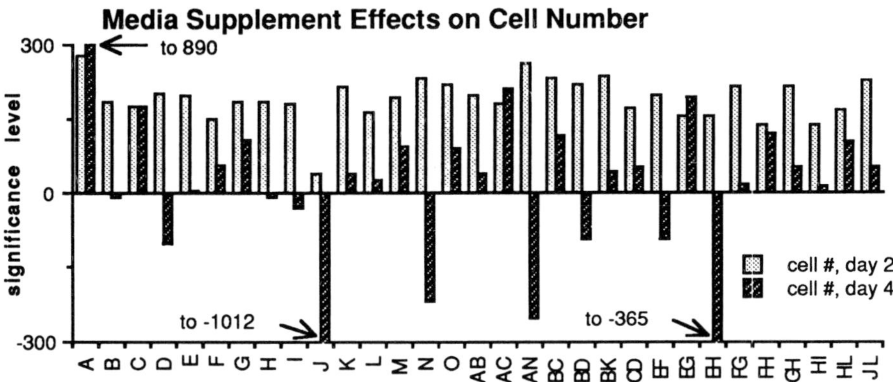

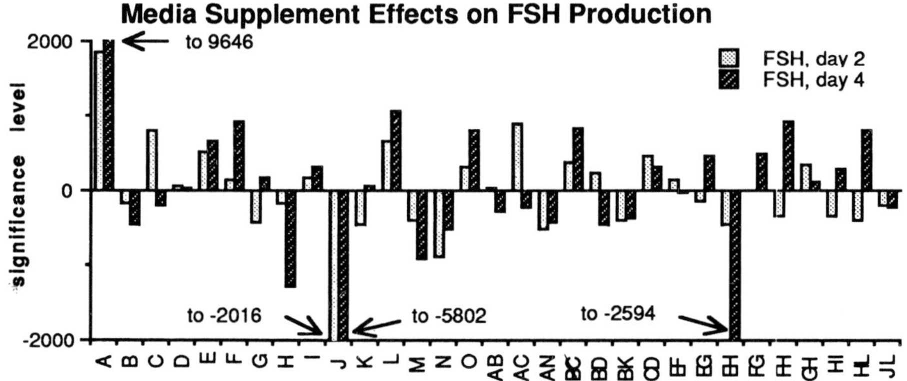

Cell numbers	
day 2:	All factors of similar significance value
day 4:	positive: HB CHO, EGF, testosterone, vasopressin, Na butyrate negative: forskolin-IBMX, ribose-albumin, ECGF

FSH production	
day 2:	positive: HB CHO, EGF, phorbol dibutyrate, estradiol, Na butyrate negative: forskolin-IBMX, ribose-albumin, testosterone
day 4:	positive: HB CHO, phorbol dibutyrate, progesterone, Na butyrate, estradiol negative: forskolin-IBMX, LH, vasopressin, ribose-albumin

1. The strong negative effect of forskolin-IBMX may have been partly due to 0.1% DMSO necessary to solubulise the forskolin.

2. EGF and HB CHO/EGF's positive effect on FSH production on day 2 is reduced to zero on day 4 despite a positive effect on both days for cell number, perhaps due to downgrading of some cellular signal.

3. Important interactions: LH/estradiol, HB CHO/ribose-albumin, HB CHO/EGF, estradiol/testosterone, LH/progesterone and IGF-1/EGF.

4. Trials indicated specific productivites up to levels observed in 10% FCS.

5. The effect HL, the spare effect from the design, could have also been IN, FM or CG, but HL is most likely considering the effects of H and L.

6. When HB CHO supplement, EGF, estradiol, progesterone, testosterone, LHRH and Na butyrate were added simultaneously to cells in a spinner flask, specific productivities comparable to serum containing levels were maintained for five days, against one third this level in the control spinner without supplements.

CONCLUSION:

1. Identification of important factors and important interactions can be done in compact experiments to save effort in screening many potential media supplements.

2. Stimulation of the beta actin promoter, resulting in expression of FSH can be increased three fold by a combination of media supplements, as identified with a special experimental design.

ACKNOWLEDGEMENTS:

Help was provided by Dr D. Street, UNSW for statistical design., Dr M. Stuart, Garvan Inst, and Dr C Morris, UNSW, for factor choice, R. DeKroon and M. Albrecht for performing the FSH radio-immuno assays. Support was given by the Generic Technology component of the Industry Research and Development Act, 1986.

REFERENCES:

1. Franklin, M.F., Bailey, R.A. Selection of Defining Contrasts and Confounded Effects in Two-level Experiments. Appl. Statist. 1977, 8(1), 321-6.

ENERGETICS OF GLUTAMINOLYSIS - A THEORETICAL EVALUATION

Lena Häggström

Department of Biochemistry and Biotechnology, Royal Institute of Technology, S-100 44 Stockholm, Sweden

ABSTRACT

From a general metabolic network describing glutaminolysis, eight individual metabolic pathways have been identified. They all originate from glutamine but end in different combinations of the products CO_2, NH_4^+, alanine, aspartate, and lactate. From the stoichiometry of the individual pathways the ratio of ATP/glutamine and ATP/NH_4^+ could be calculated. It was found that complete oxidation of glutamine to CO_2 and water was most favourable in both respects. The other metabolic routes were far less efficient in terms of energy production and the ATP/NH_4^+ ratio was lower. Two pathways were inferior in respect to the ATP/NH_4^+ ratio.

Glutaminolysis, glutamine, metabolic pathways, energetics, stoichiometry, ATP

INTRODUCTION

The energy metabolism of glutamine in cultured animal cells is named glutaminolysis. A general metabolic scheme of glutaminolysis, based on known enzymatic steps and their localisation in the mitochondrion and/or the cytosol, shows that glutaminolysis is not a unit pathway but composed of several alternative paths with common parts. Individual pathways leading to various end products can be described and stoichiometrically defined, enabling the calculation of released ammonia and produced energy.

RESULTS

A general metabolic network of glutaminolysis was based on the scheme proposed by McKeehan (1). Individual pathways are described briefly below and summarised in Table 1. Energy yields have been calculated on basis of the generation of energy equivalent to 3 ATP / NADH and 2 ATP / FADH. GTP was considered equal to ATP.

1. Complete oxidation of 1 mole of glutamine to CO_2 and water within the mitochondrion results in the production of 2 moles NH_4^+ and energy equivalent to 27 moles ATP. The ATP/ NH_4^+ ratio becomes 13.5. This pathway requires the participation of the enzymes glutaminase, glutamate dehydrogenase and malic enzyme in addition to the usual TCA enzymes. Since it is not possible to determine

"

which of the mitochondrial isoenzymes of malic enzyme (NADP or NAD requiring) that is active energy yields have been calculated for both alternatives (Table 1). It should be noted that acquisition of NADPH instead of NADH might be a good alternative since the cost for synthesis of one NADPH corresponds to 4 ATP (2).

2) Another possible pathway, also completely located in mitochondria, leads to partial oxidation of glutamine with alanine as an end product in addition to NH_4^+ and CO_2. The necessary enzymes are glutaminase, glutamate-pyruvate transaminase, TCA-enzymes from α-ketoglutarate to malate, and malic enzyme. Although only 1 mole NH_4^+ is released per glutamine the ATP/NH_4^+ ratio is only 9.

3) This path way is similar to 2) except for the transaminase being located in the cytosol. Glutamate used in the transaminase reaction is derived from glutamine deamidated in biosynthesis and not by glutaminase. This is a very interesting metabolic route since no ammonia is liberated at all but it is doubtful if it can contribute significantly to the overall generation of energy due to shortage of glutamate generated as proposed.

4) As 3) i.e. transaminase in cytosol but glutamate is exported from mitochondrion. The formed α-ketoglutarate returns to mitochondrion. The energy yield equals 2).

5) In this pathway aspartate, ammonia and CO_2 are the end products. The participating enzymes are glutaminase, glutamate-oxaloacetate transaminase and TCA-enzymes from α-ketoglutarate to oxaloacetate, all of them in mitochondria.

6) Glutamine can also be oxidised to lactate. Glutamine is first oxidised to malate, CO_2 and 2 NH_4^+/glutamine. Malate is further oxidised to pyruvate by malic enzyme either in the mitochondrion or in the cytosol. Cytosolic pyruvate is reduced to lactate with lactate dehydrogenase using NADH. These NADH cannot be provided by cytosolic malic enzyme which is NADP dependent nor by glycolysis since glycolytically derived NADH are consumed for production of glucose derived lactate. If there are excess reducing power in the cytosol from unrelated reactions e.g. bio- synthesis of serin the energy calculation becomes as in 8). Otherwise NADH has to be produced from malate that is oxidised in the cytosol to oxaloacetate and NADH with malate dehydrogenase. The so formed oxaloacetate can not return to the mitochondrion but is transformed to aspartate by cytosolic glutamate-oxaloacetate transaminase.Glutamate used in this reaction is derived from glutamine used in biosynthesis. Thus, the complete sequence of reactions requires 2 moles of glutamine, one ending up as lactate and the other as aspartate.

7) This way is similar to 6) but glutamate used in the transaminase reaction is exported from mitochondrion and formed α-ketoglutarate returned to it. Thus the production of NH_4^+ increases and the ATP/NH_4^+ ratio decreases compared to 6).

8) In this last pathway of glutamine oxidation lactate, NH_4^+ and CO_2 are the end products. Glutamine is metabolised to cytosolic oxaloacetate and NADH as in 6)

and 7). Oxaloacetate can be converted to phosphoenolpyruvate (PEP) by PEP - carboxy- kinase, an enzyme normally participating in gluconeogenesis. PEP can in turn be converted to pyruvate (by pyruvate kinase) which finally is reduced to lactate. The significance of this pathway is doubtful since i) for thermodynamical reasons the oxaloacetate to PEP reaction can only occur at low PEP concentrations (i.e. when glucose is exhausted from the medium), and ii) if this reaction is triggered it means that gluconeogenesis is turned on.

Endproducts	ATP/glutamine	ATP/NH_4^+
1) $5 CO_2 + 2 NH_4^+$	27 (24+NADPH)	13.5
2) $Ala + 2 CO_2 + NH_4^+$	9 (6+NADPH)	9
3) $Ala + 2 CO_2$	9 (6+NADPH)	∞
4) $Ala + 2 CO_2 + NH_4^+$	9 (6+NADPH)	9
5) $Asp + CO_2 + NH_4^+$	9	9
6) $Asp + 3 CO_2 + 2 NH_4^+ + HLac/2 Gln$	9 (7.5+0.5NADPH)	9
7) $Asp + 3 CO_2 + 3 NH_4^+ + HLac/2 Gln$	9 (7.5+0.5NADPH)	6
8) $HLac + 2 CO_2 + 2 NH_4^+$	9	4.5

Table 1. Energy yields in various individual pathways of glutaminolysis. Numbers in front of rows refer to the descriptions of the pathways in the text. Data in parenthesis refer to the alternative where malic enzyme uses NADPH as cofactor.

DISCUSSION

Complete oxidation of glutamine to CO_2 and water gives, as expected, the highest ATP/glutamine ratio. In practise, it is also the most favourable pathway in terms of the ATP/NH_4^+ ratio since the route with alanine and CO_2 as the only end products is of less significance for energy production. All other pathways identified here give a much lower ATP/glutamine ratio. Pathways 7) and 8) are least favourable with respect to the ATP/NH_4^+ ratio. Results obtained from theoretical evaluations like these are important for developing strategies for metabolic control of cultured cells in order to decrease the production of toxic metabolites.

REFERENCES

1 McKeehan, W.L. Glutaminolysis in animal cells. In: Carbohydrate metabolism in cultured cells (Ed) M.J. Morgan, Plenum Press, New York, 1986, chap. 4
2 Atkinson, D.E. Cellular energy metabolism and its regulation Academic Press, New York, 1977, pp 42-45
3 Glacken, M.W. Catabolic control of mammalian cell culture. Bio/technology, 1988, 6, 1041

DEGRADING EFFECT OF LIGHT ON CELL CULTURE MEDIA

Hans Ingolf Nielsen[1] and Kjell Bertheussen[2]

[1]Medi-Cult a/s, Kanalholmen 12, DK-2650 Hvidovre, Denmark, and
[2]Dept. of Clinical Medicine, University of Tromsø, Norway.

ABSTRACT

The effect of light on the protein-free RPMI-SR3 medium and
RPMI 1640 with 10% horse serum was studied using the growth
rate of the 1E6 murine hybridoma cell line as a parameter.
Storage in the dark at room temperature has no effect on the
medium the first 2 - 3 days, but then the growth inhibition
rises to 15% at day 6 for the serum-free medium. In sunlight
the growth inhibition has reached 90% in 1 hour. A similar
level is reached in artificial light after 3 days, and in stray
daylight and UV-C-light after 4 - 5 days. It is worth noticing
that the medium with serum have a similar light sensitivity as
the serum-free medium.
Keywords: Cell culture, Serum-free media, Culture media,
Degradation, Light, Light sensitivity.

INTRODUCTION

It is a well known fact that light has a degrading effect on
cell culture media, but in the daily routine this fact is
frequently neglected. In the authors' laboratories, cells are
largely cultivated in media which are not only serum-free, but
to a high degree also protein-free. This system is obviously
very sensitive, since there are no proteins present to bind and
neutralize toxins. Light degradation of media components are
therefore likely to be particularly important under such
circumstances.

MATERIALS AND METHODS

Samples of the practically protein-free medium RPMI-SR3 (0.5
mg/ml insulin is the only peptide present) (Medi-Cult a/s,
Denmark) in clear polystyrene bottles were placed:
1) exposed to sunlight in a laboratory window
2) in stray daylight behind a glass door in a lab closet
3) continuously exposed to artificial light (Luxo 11W fluorescent tube)
4) continuously exposed to UV-C-light in a laminar air flow
   hood
5) wrapped in aluminium foil at room temperature.
As a control the same batch of medium was stored in the dark
at 5°C for a similar periode of time. As a serum-containing
control, RPMI 1640 with 10% horse serum was exposed to light
as described above.

The media were exposed for various lenghts of time, and then
used for culture of the sensitive, but rapidly growing 1E6

murine hybridoma cell line, also used in the Medi-Cult® Hybritest (1,2,3).

The cells were seeded at a density of 10^4 cells per ml in 24-well plates, incubated at 37°C in 5% CO_2, and counted after 4 days. The percentage growth inhibition was then calculated relative to control cultures.

RESULTS AND DISCUSSION

Figures 1 - 2 show the growth inhibition as a function of the exposure time to the various types of light of RPMI-SR3 (filled symbols) and RPMI 1640 (open symbols).

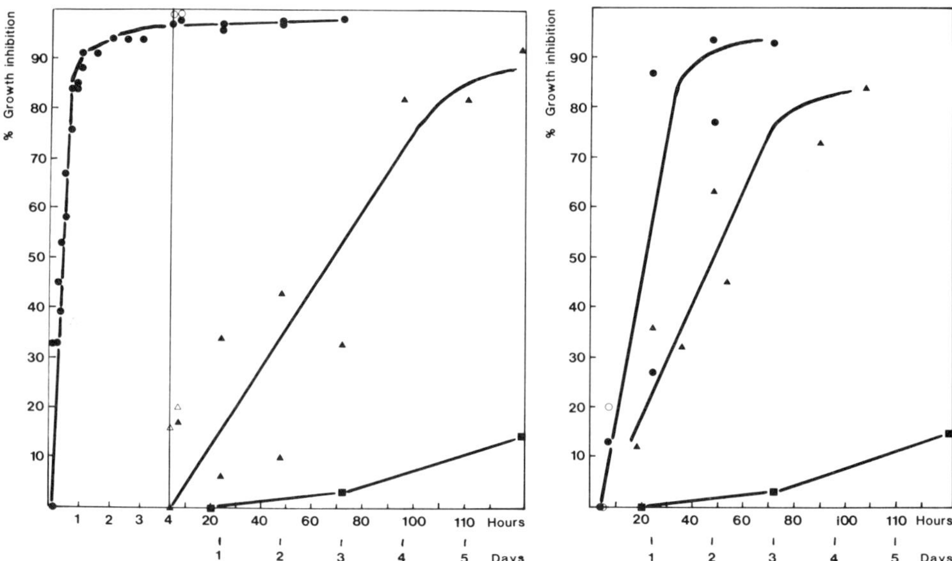

Figure 1. Effect of light.
● sunlight; ▲ stray daylight;
■ darkness, 20°C.

Figure 2. Effect of light.
● artificial light; ▲ UV-light; ■ darkness, 20°C.

Storage in the dark at room temperature has no effect on the medium the first 2 - 3 days, but then growth inhibition slowly rises to 15% at day 6 for the serum-free medium. This just shows the normal degradation of media with time, and is why ready-made media should be used within relatively few weeks, if one wants an optimal cell growth.

The reaction to sunlight is dramatical. Within one hour the growth inhibition has reached 90% for the serum-free medium. And somewhat surprising: This seems to be the case for serum-containing medium, as well. A similar level is reached in artificial light after 3 days, and in stray daylight and UV-C-light after 4 - 5 days. It should be noticed that the illumination was continuous for artificial light and UV-C-light, while daylight obviously was on only during the day. The reason, why UV-C-light did not have a stronger effect, is probably that it does not efficiently penetrate plastic or water.

A couple of things should be noticed here:
1) The very rapid degradation of media by light, especially sunlight, and
2) the fact that serum-containing medium seems to be as light sensitive as the serum-free medium.
This latter fact is especially surprising, since the serum-containing medium contains toxin-neutralizing proteins, and at the same time does not contain two of the potentially light sensitive components - HEPES and one of the components of the SSR3 Synthetic Serum Replacement.

Further experimentation is now needed to determine the harmful wavelengths and the nature of the degradation.

ACKNOWLEDGEMENTS

The skilful assistance of Anna-Lise Poulsen and Susanne Rasmussen is gratefully acknowledged.

REFERENCES

1. Bertheussen, K., N.Holst, F.Forsdahl and K.E.Høie. A new cell culture assay for quality control in IVF. <u>Human Reproduction</u>, 1989, <u>4</u>, 531-535.
2. Nielsen, H.I. and K.Bertheussen. The Medi-Cult® Hybritest for *in vitro* toxicology and quality control. <u>ATLA</u>, 1990, <u>17</u>, 199-202.
3. Nielsen, H.I. and K.Bertheussen. The Medi-Cult® Hybritest - a new test for *in vitro* toxicology. <u>This volume</u>.

CULTURE OF HYBRIDOMA IN DIALYSED MEDIA

C. MAZARS, L. POUGET ***, B. PINGEON **, S. PROVENCHERE * ET P. HENNO ***.

* Centre National de Transfusion Sanguine - B.P. 100 - 91943
Les Ulis Cédex

** Diagnostic Pasteur - 3, Bd Poincaré - 92430 Marnes La Coquette

* * * Biosys S.A. - 21, Quai du Clos des Roses - 60200 Compiègne

ABSTRACT

Hybridoma cells were cultivated in RPMI 1640 medium supplemented with a serum substitute, primatone and pluronic F68. After 52 hours of batch culture, the cells die rapidly. This observation was attributed to either the exhaustion of nutrients in the culture medium or to the release of toxic compounds by the cells.

The "exhaustion" hypothesis was ruled out by supplementing the medium with glutamine, glucose and amino acids, but no improvement in cell viability at 52 h was observed. As regards toxicity, neither the addition of ammonium salts, of lactate at concentrations similar to those found in 52 h batch cultures decreased cell viability.

On the contrary, dialysis of the 52 h and 72 h culture medium against complete medium (cut off 10 000 d) permetted normal growth. In an attempt to scale up this dialysis procedure, a hollow fiber dialysis system (ENKA) was connected to a 2 liters fermentor (Biolafitte).

The described cultivation process allows to increase the concentration of living cells as well as concentration of immunogloblulins.

Key words : Hybridoma, dialysis cartridge, conditioned medium.

INTRODUCTION

One of the problems remaining in monoclonal antibody production is the evolution of medium constituents during culture (1). Some authors (2,3) have reported the results of different studies related to the evolution of energetic substrates and amino acids (4) during culture of an hybridoma cell line.

The typical growth pattern of a hybridoma batch culture shows a rapid decrease in the concentration of living cell after the growth phase .

In this report, we present first the results of a study of the growth and antibody production by murine hybridoma cell line cultivated in 72 hour conditioned medium dialysed against fresh medium and secondly the production of monoclonal antibodies in a fermentor connected to a dialysis cartridge.

MATERIAL AND METHODS

Hybridoma cell line : A mouse x mouse hybridoma cell line producing IgM was used. The cells were cultivated in RPMI 1640 (Flow) supplemented with primatone RL (Sheffield) ; Pluronic F 68 (Serva) and FCS (Biosys) in Roller bottle (Falcon). Every two days, the cultures were split in a ratio of 1/5.

Fermentor cultivation : The cells were cultivated in a 2 l biolafitte reactor equiped with a 10 μm spin filter. Generally, the fermentors were running using the following conditions (pH 7,1, Temperature 37°C, pO2 20 % air saturation and stirring 20 to 30 rpm). The initial cells concentration was 10^5 cel./ml. To dialyse the medium during culture, a dialysis cartridge (ENKA) with a cut off of 10 000 daltons has been connected to the fermentor.

Assays :   Cells were counted in a hemacytometer by the trypan blue exclusion method. Immunoglobulin assays were performed as described elsewhere (5).

RESULTS AND DISCUSSION

1. <u>Preliminary results</u> :

The cell culture (fig.1) has been performed in roller bottles on different media :

- fresh medium
- 72 hour cultured supernatant
- 72 hour cultured medium dialysed against complete medium.
  Two membranes have been used : 6-8 000 d. and 12-14 000 d.

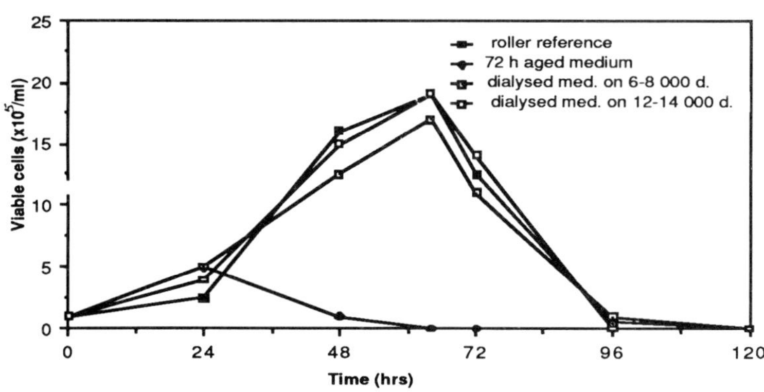

Fig.1 : Profile of growth in different media

From the results presented in figure 1, it is apparent that :
- A 72 hour aged medium can support a very poor growth of cells.
- When the 72 hour aged medium were dialysed, cell growth is comparable to that in fresh medium.

These results suggest that the dialysis step has brought about either the remplacement of an exhausted nutrient or the elimination of toxic compounds. According to the cut-offs which have been studied, MW of implied molecules would be less than 6 000 daltons.

Average productivities calculated after 120 hours culture are represented in table 1.

MEDIUM	FRESH MEDIA	72 h CULTURED MEDIA	DIALYSED MED
µg IgM/10^5 Cel. x d.	0,8	1,8	0,75

Table 1 : Average Specific productivities in different media

It seems that a 72 hour aged medium contains molecules with a MW lower than 6 000-8 000 daltons which stop cellular growth and stimulate IgM secretion. Molecules with a MW up to 12 000-14 000 daltons stimulate cellular growth.

2. Culture in a fermentor connected to a dialysis cartridge

Hollow fiber dialysis module connected to a 2 l fermentor as depicted in fig. 2 were used for cultivating hybridoma cells. 48 h after inoculation, the following conditions were used :

- flow rate of pump 1   0,2   - 1,5 l/h
- flow rate of pump 2   0,05 - 0,2 l/h

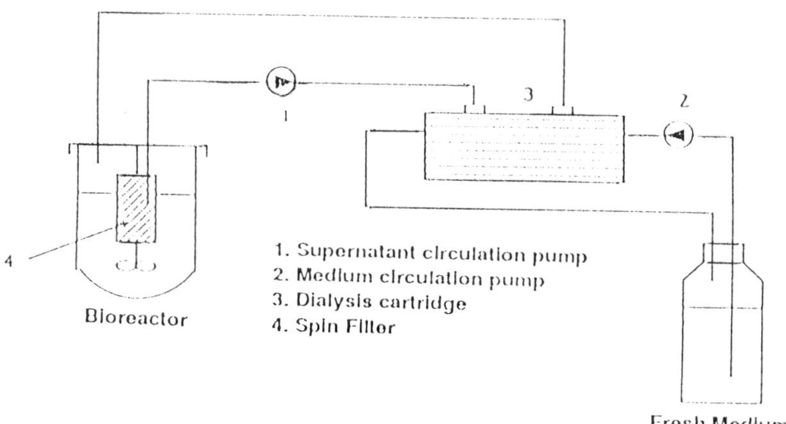

Fig. 2 : Schema of dialysis system

Growth and secretion are represented in fig. 3, and compared with a standard pattern obtained in a classical batch system. After 52 hours of culture, no decrease of growth is observed. 36.10^5 cel./ml are obtained after 128 hours. The IgM concentration reached 70 µg/ml after 150 hours. Compared to the results shown in fig. 1, dialysis carried out continuously during the growth phase enables us to regenerate or to deplete the medium of toxic substances and thereby reach higher concentration of living cells $(36.10^5$ versus $17.10)$.

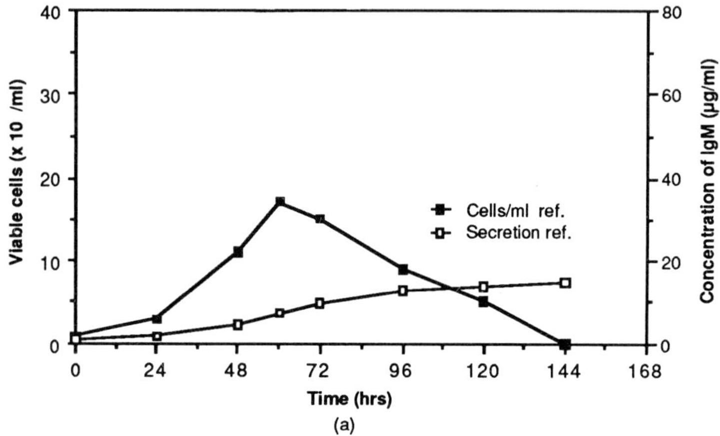

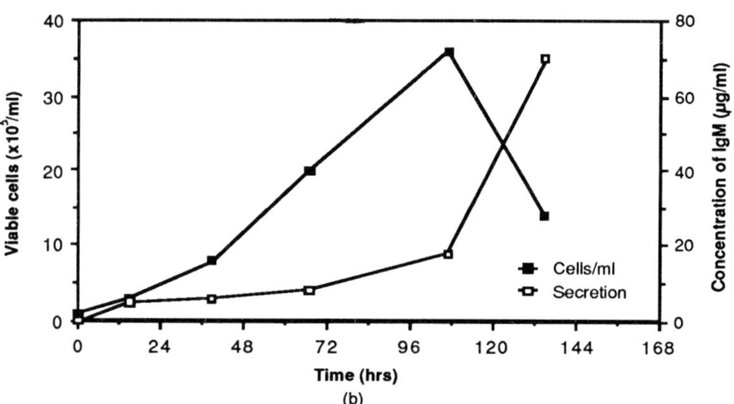

Fig. 3 : Profile of growth and Secretion
(a) Classical batch system
(b) Dialysis system

CONCLUSION

Dialysis led continuously during the growth phase enable to regenerate or epurate the media. Productivity was also improved compared to that obtained with a classical system. The isolation and characterisation of cells secreted factors capable of modulating growth and antibody secretion are currently being pursued.

REFERENCES

1. DODGE and Col. W.S. Enzyme Microbiol technol. 1987, 9, 607

2. LYAN and Col. Biotechnol. letters, 1987, 8, 535

3. ZIELKE and Col. in HAUSSINGER D, SIED H. (eds) 1984
   SPRINGER - VERLAG, 247

4. ADAM SON SR. et Col. in
    SEAVER SS (Ed. Commercial Production of monoclonal antibodies), 1987, Marcel DEKKER   17.

5. PRUSLIN and Col, 1986, 3 immunol. Meth., 94, 99.

EVALUATION OF FETAL BOVINE SERUM SUBSTITUTES ON CELL GROWTH AND
RECOMBINANT PROTEIN PRODUCTION

Luciano Ramos, Melvin S. Oka, and Amy A. Murnane
SmithKline Beecham, King of Prussia, PA   19406

ABSTRACT

This study describes the evaluation of a fetal bovine substitute
(FBSS; Alliance Pharmaceuticals) for use in mammalian cell culture.
These supplements are prepared from adult bovine blood by a proprietary
method. Cell lines secreting recombinant tissue plasminogen activator or
a recombinant form of T4 receptor (sT4) were used in these studies.
Spinner flasks were seeded with cells in either 5% (V/V) fetal bovine
serum supplemented medium or medium containing 1%(V/V) supplement "E" and
a concentration of the FBSS under evaluation. Cell counts and recombinant
product titers were determined daily. One of the FBSS identified as CGA-6
was found to be potentially useful as a FBS substitute.

INTRODUCTION

The recent surge in developing large-scale production processes for
recombinant products secreted from cultured cells provides the impetus
for evaluating the nutritional requirements of cells grown in this
manner. In the past, cells have been grown in basal medium supplemented
with Fetal Bovine Serum (FBS). FBS contains many components, including
trace elements and growth factors responsible for maintaining cellular
growth and viability (1,2). Although it has been highly successful in
enhancing the growth of many different cell lines, it has its
disadvantages. Drawbacks, including cost, availability, lot-to-lot
variability, and ease of product purification, are magnified when the
use of FBS for large-scale production of recombinant products is
critically evaluated. Therefore, the search for a substitute for FBS,
be it chemically defined or otherwise, continues.

CRITERIA FOR CHOOSING FETAL BOVINE SERUM-SUBSTITUTES

1. **ECONOMY:** The cost of the FBSS must be lower than the cost for
    FBS.
2. **CELL GROWTH:** This substitute would have to be similar to FBS in
    its growth promoting activity.
3. **PRODUCTION:** This material must contain the necessary components
    required to produce a comparable amount of product (if not
    more) per unit of FBS.
4. **PURIFICATION:** Ideally the substitute would present fewer
    difficulties than FBS in product purification.
5. **ADAPTATION:** The cells must be able to adapt readily to this
    serum substitute without alterations in productivity, culture
    doubling time, and cellular characteristics.

MATERIALS AND METHODS

The cell lines producing recombinant proteins (either tissue
plasminogen activator (tPA), or soluble T4 (CD4)) were developed by the
SK&F Molecular Genetics group, and transferred to the Animal Cell
Culture group. These cells were maintained as suspension cell lines in
basal medium supplemented with 5% FBS (Hazleton # 12-103) and 100nM
methotrexate (Sigma # A-6770) in a humidified atmosphere of 5% CO_2, 95%
air. Spinner flasks (125 ml) were seeded with 5.0x10e5 cells/ml in

either serum-containing medium (control), or medium containing 1%
supplement "E"(Otisville) and a concentration of the FBSS recommended
by the supplier (Table I). Cell counts were collected each day from the
spinner flasks, and trypan blue dye exclusion assays were performed to
assess cellular viability. Samples taken on day 4 post seeding were
centrifuged at 1200 rpm for 5 minutes and the resulting supernatants
were analyzed for recombinant protein production.

TABLE I

SERUM SUBSTITUTE	CONCENTRATION TESTED
CGA-A	2%
CGA-B	2%
CGA-1A	9%
CGA-2	2%
CGA-3	2%
CGA-4	3%
CGA-6	3%

RESULTS

Two independent sets of studies were performed to assess the utility
of the serum substitutes for the cell cultures. Each set of data
represents an average of two experiments. The cell viability in each of
these experiments ranged between 90-98%. In both studies, the growth of
cells cultured in medium supplemented with FBSS and their ability to
synthesize the recombinant protein was compared to control cells grown in
medium supplemented with 5% FBS.

In the first study, CGA-A, CGA-B, and CGA-1A were initially evaluated
for growth promoting activity of the tPA-producing cells. As indicated in
Figure 1A, cells grown in CGA-A showed similar growth to that of control
cells. Cultures grown in CGA-B yielded slightly decreased growth; CGA-1A
did not support the growth of these cells. The effect of the substitutes
on tPA production is shown in Figure 1B. Samples were analyzed on day 4
post seeding. From previous experiments (data not shown), cell culture
viability and corresponding recombinant protein levels reach a maximum day
4 in culture. When compared to the control culture, only CGA-B was able
to maintain similar production levels of the recombinant protein.
Therefore, the FBSS CGA-B partially fulfilled criteria described in the
introduction.

In the second study, a similar set of experiments were conducted to
evaluate four additional FBSS. The FBSS used in the experiments were CGA-
2, CGA-3, CGA-4, and CGA-6. Although none of these FBSS yielded the growth
observed with the control cells, CGA-6, CGA-4, and CGA-2 showed 83%, 74%,
and 79% of the total cell number attained with FBS respectively (Figure
2A). Production of the recombinant product in various day 4 culture media
is illustrated in Figure 2B. Concentrations of the recombinant protein in
media from both CGA-6 and CGA-3 supplemented cultures were comparable to
those levels observed from cells maintained in 5% FBS.

Similar studies were conducted for the CD4-producing cell line. Cells
were grown in Alpha(-)MEM medium supplemented with either 5% FBS (control),
CGA-A, CGA-B, or CGA-1A. As shown in Figures 3A & 4A, comparable growth
was observed with serum-containing, or CGA-A-containing media, whereas
media supplemented with CGA-1A did not support cell growth. Production of
CD4 appeared highest in serum and CGA-B-containing medium (Figures 3B &
4B).

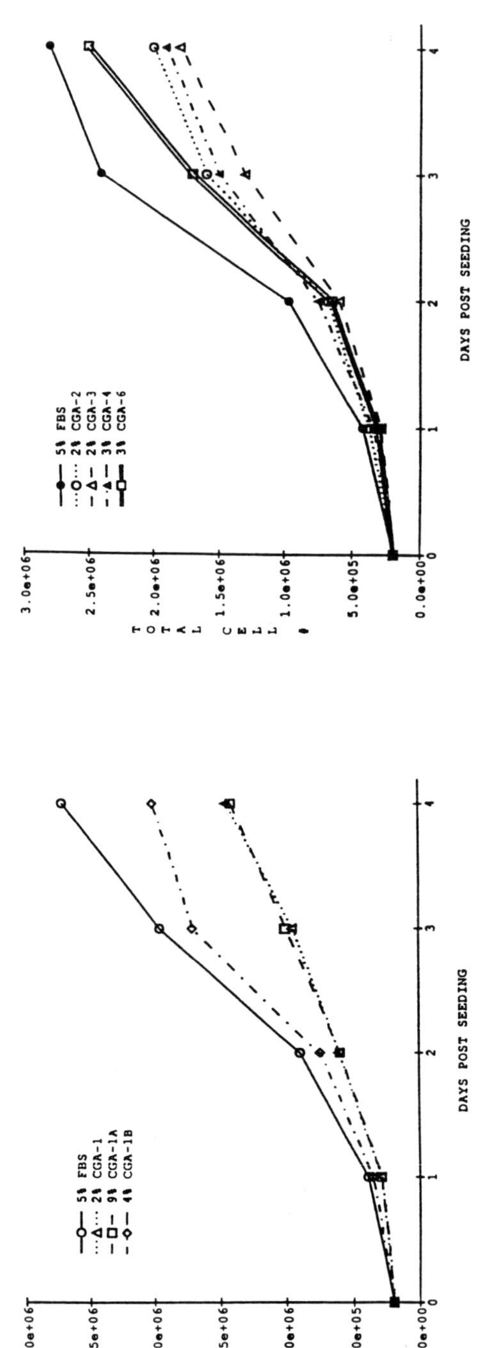

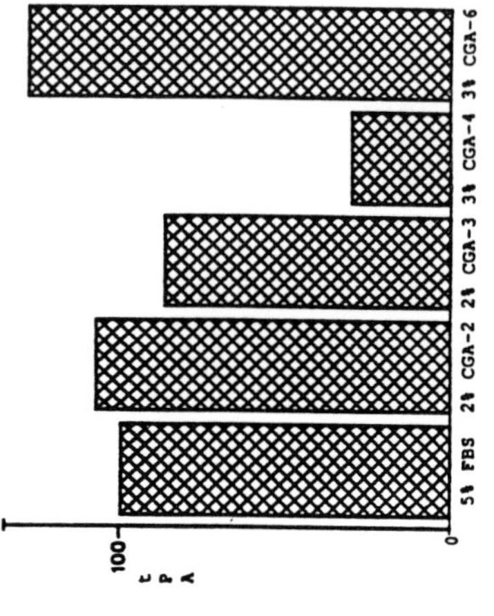

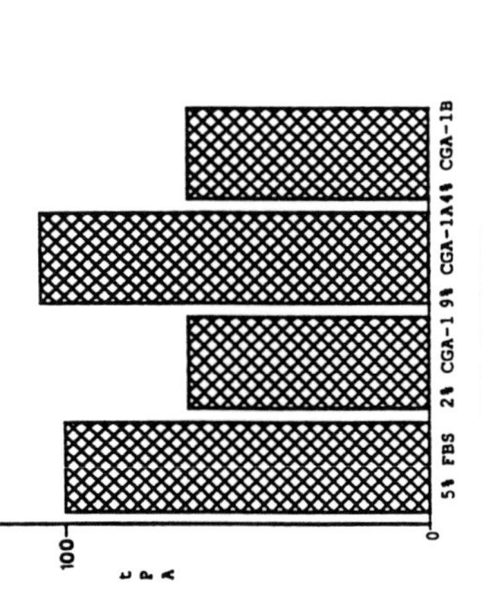

FIGURE2:
(a). Cells grown in Alpha(+)MEM for 4 days in medium supplemented with 5% FBS or CGA (a serum substitute).
(b). Production of tPA was assayed on day 4 (post seeding).

FIGURE1:
(a). Cells grown in Alpha(+)MEM for 4 days in medium supplemented with 5% FBS or CGA (a serum substitute).
(b). Production of tPA was assayed on day 4 (post seeding).

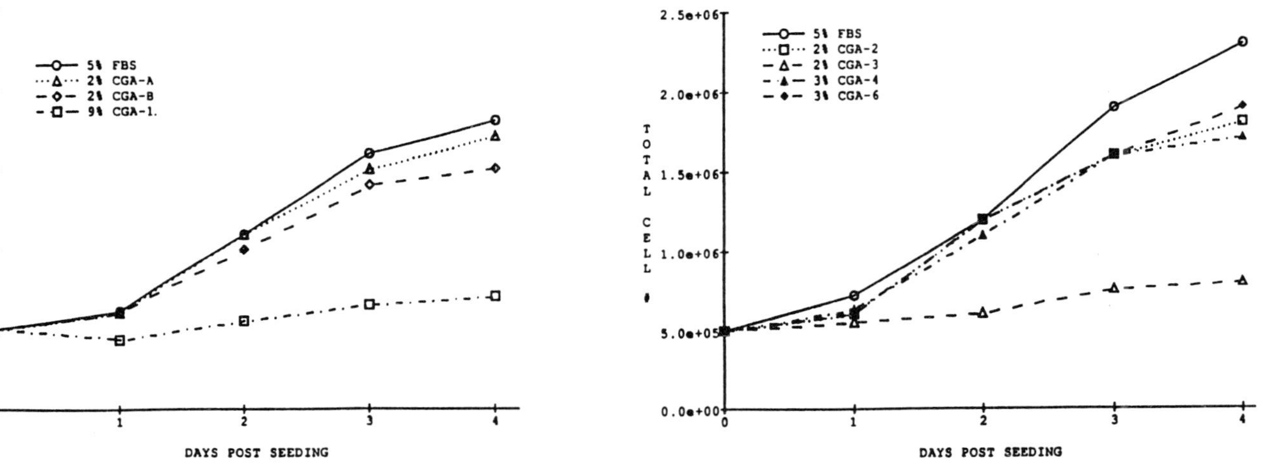

FIGURE 3:
(a). The recombinant cells were grown in Alpha(-)MEM medium supplemented with either 5% FBS or a serum substitute (CGA). (b). Samples collected on day 4 (post seeding) were evaluated for CD4 production.

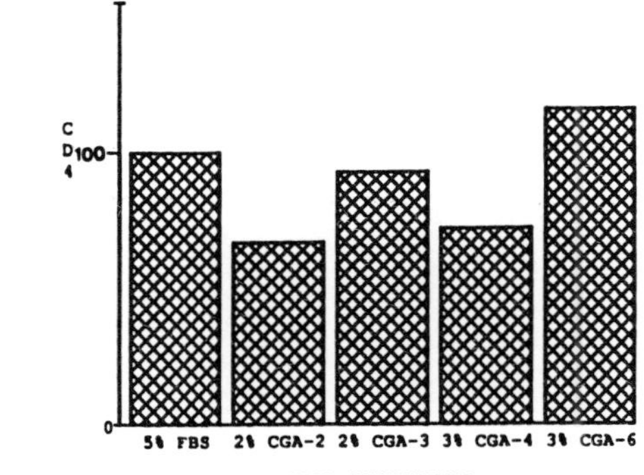

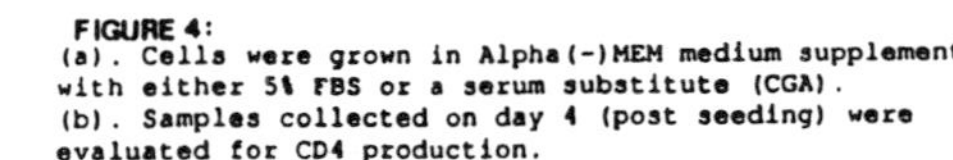

FIGURE 4:
(a). Cells were grown in Alpha(-)MEM medium supplemented with either 5% FBS or a serum substitute (CGA). (b). Samples collected on day 4 (post seeding) were evaluated for CD4 production.

DISCUSSION

The selection of a FBSS was based on the criteria described in the introduction. The best candidate partially suited to these criteria described in this study was CGA-6. The ability of the cells to adapt readily to a chosen serum substitute eliminates the time required to wean cells from one media to another. In this study, cells grown in 5% FBS could be directly transferred to medium supplemented with CGA-6 without any lag in growth, thereby eliminating the time required for adaptation. Another criteria required of the selected substitute was that it support cell growth and maintain levels of production observed in the control culture. Cells grown in CGA-6 were able to sustain cell growth at approximately 1.9×10^6 cells/ml, and secrete levels of the recombinant product day 4 in culture comparable to control. An economic advantage of using CGA-6 relates to its cost relative to that of serum. Alliance maintains that their FBSS are much less expensive than that of FBS because of the lower concentrations used. This coupled with the long term stable supply of adult bovine serum further supports the use of this as an alternative to FBS. The ease of purification of recombinant products secreted from cells grown in this substitute is yet to be determined. A preliminary investigation reveals increased protein content in CGA-6 as compared to 5% FBS (data not shown). Whether purification schemes can be devised to isolate these products without contaminating serum proteins awaits further investigation. We have demonstrated that CGA-6 can be directly substituted for FBS for the above cell line tested. The use of this substitute eases the economic and availability constraints FBS imposes. Indeed, this report reveals that FBSS may play an important role as an alternative to FBS.

REFERENCES

1.   HyClone Laboratories. Art to Science 1989, $\underline{7}$(2), 1-3.

2.   HyClone Laboratories. Biochemical Assay: Defined Fetal Bovine Serum. (product information sheet). 1989.

CELL GROWTH ACTIVATORS (CGA) AND CELL FUNCTION MODULATORS
(CFM) OF BLOOD: EFFECT ON CELL REPLICATION AND PROTEIN
EXPRESSION

S.K. Dinka, P. Dehazya, J.S. Dinka, P. Gariepy, E. Szekely,
P. Barber

Alliance Pharmaceutical Corp., Otisville, NY 10963, USA

ABSTRACT

Using the growth of certain recombinant and hybridoma cells
and their protein expressions (product yield) as criteria, a
large scale blood fractionation process was developed. This
resulted in formulation of CGA as a replacement for fetal
bovine serum (FBS). By further fractionation several fractions were identified where CGA and/or CFM activity was
highest. The fraction showing the highest activity for a wide
range of anchorage dependent cells would appear to be
     a family of similar proteins that have varying CGA-CFM
activity for specific cells. Further characterization of
these proteins is currently proceeding.

During this work it was found that the use of CGA did not
require adaptation of cells and that the optimal combination
of CGA-CFM and basal medium had to be established separately
for good cell growth and product yield. The level of product
yield or virus replication did not correlate with the level of
cell growth in this system. Moderate levels of cell growth
were frequently associated with high product yields. Thus;
cell growth rate cannot be considered an indicator of product
yield.

Keywords: cell culture, cell growth, growth factor, serum
            free medium, protein expression, virus replication,
            product yield, cell function modulator, blood
            protein fractionation.

INTRODUCTION

With the work of Carrel at the beginning of this century the
study of cell growth in culture (1) and the analytical approach to isolate the growth factors from blood (2) was
started. The analytical approach was abandoned by the end of
the 1970's because of the complexities of blood. The synthetic approach formulated by David Barnes and Gordon Sato in
their "Unifying Approach" (3) replaced serum in cell cultures
by combinations of hormones, nutrients, binding proteins and
attachment factors. This approach presently dominates the
field.

In addition to obtaining a practical serum replacement, the
guiding principle was that native biological cell modulator

molecules have to be isolated from blood to help understand
"in vivo" cell regulation. The study of these molecules
would reveal how they are produced by cells, their interactions with cells, tissues and the intact organism. These
factors could also be considered as indicators of physiological and/or pathological states and aging.

MATERIALS AND METHODS

The plasma fractionation process utilized different physico-
chemical principles in sequence. The fractionation steps
were based on the growth of different cell types and product
yield of certain recombinant and hybridoma cells. Primary
chick embryo and established anchorage dependent epithelial-
like (normal, recombinant and tumor), fibroblast-like, (human,
diploid, monkey) and suspension (human) T, (murine) myeloma
and hybridoma cells were used in the evaluation.

Anchorage dependent cells were seeded at densities ranging
from 25,000 to 50,000 while suspension cells were seeded at
100,000 viable cells/ml. Plates and flasks were seeded as
follows:

      o   24 multi-well plates - 1.0 ml per well
      o   25 cm^2 flasks - 6.0 ml
      o   75 cm^2 flasks - 25.0 ml
      o 150 cm^2 flasks - 40.0 ml

in the appropriate medium. After proper incubation at $36^{O}C$,
with 5% CO_2, the media were analyzed for product. The cells
were counted (anchorage dependent cells after removal by
trypsin) after staining with trypan blue and the cell growth
was expressed as viable cell number.

Enhancer (E) preparation is obtained from erythrocytes. Alone
it has little or no effect for most of the cells used. With
CGA-CFM it can markedly increase the cell growth and/or
product yield of specific cells.

Effect of CGA-III: S 37-2-Q: 1, 5 and 8 Fractions

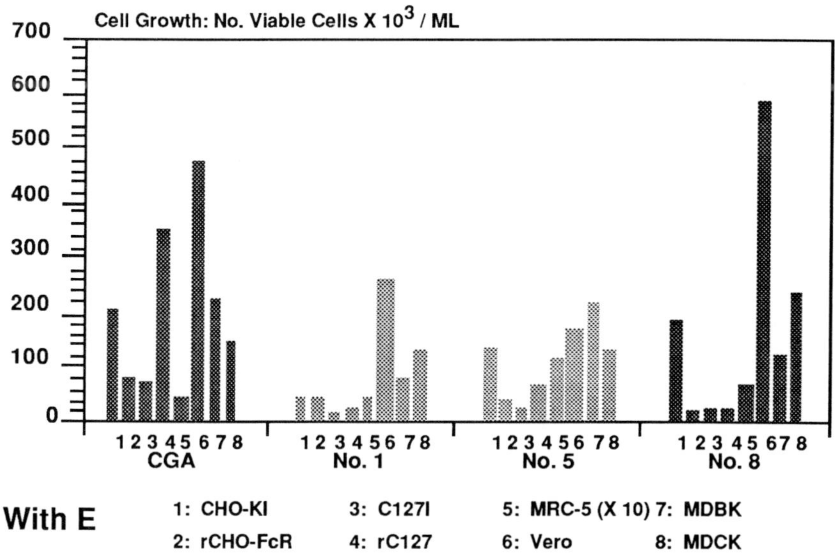

Fig. 1 shows the effect of fractions selected for activity on anchorage dependent cells. These fractions were used with the cells indicated. When compared to the starting CGA preparation, all three of the fractions have growth promoting activity for all the cells indicated, but the level of these activities varies greatly for specific cells in the different fractions.

Effect of CGA-III: S: 37-2-Q: 4 and 5 Fr on rC127 Cells

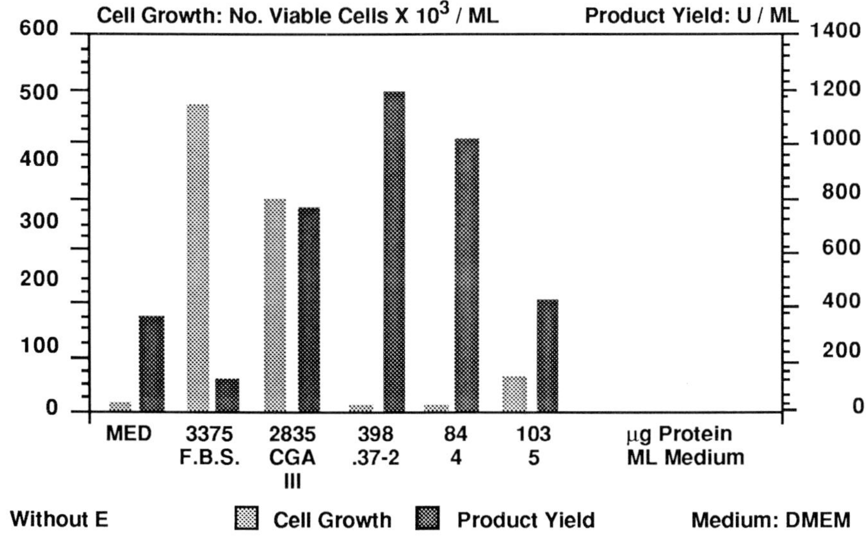

In Fig. 2, Fractions 4 and 5 of this group were tested with
rC127 cells. These fractions supported a higher level of
recombinant protein production than 10% FBS. Cell growth
with Fraction 5 was approximately ten times lower than with
FBS and with Fraction 4, cell growth was similar to that of
medium alone.

The experimental data seem to indicate that these fractions
represent proteins having similar physico-chemical characteristics with varying cell specific CGA-CFM activities.

In the work with CGA it was realized that the right combination of basal medium and CGA has to be established for good
cell growth and product yield. (Fig. 3). This applies not
only for different cells but also for recombinant or
hybridoma cells derived from the same parental cell.

Effect of Cell Growth Activators and Media on the Growth of CHO-KI and Recombinant CHO-FcR and CHO Cells

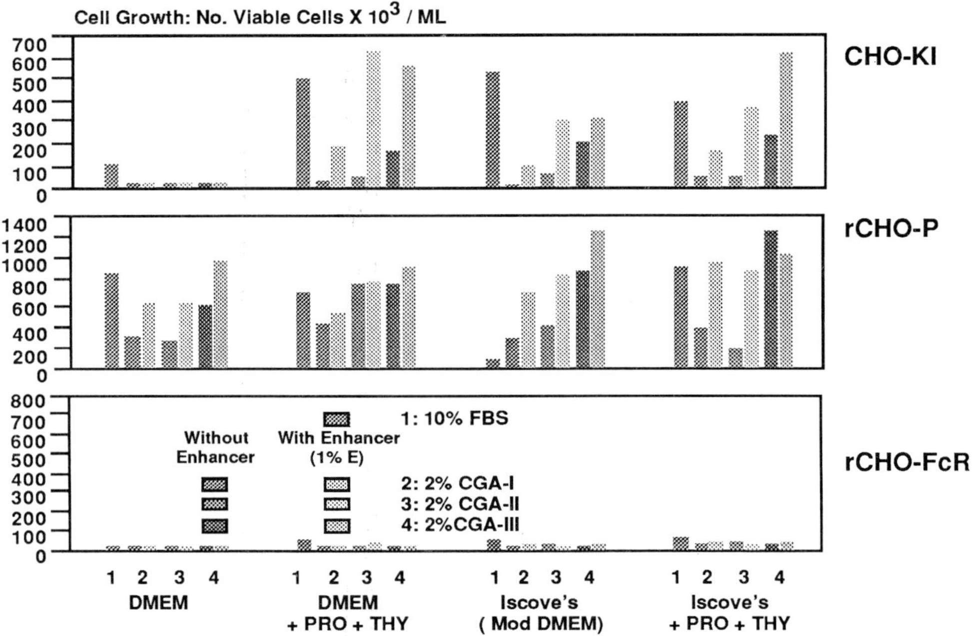

In Fig. 3 CHO-Kl and two recombinant CHO cells were seeded in different media with different CGA and FBS. Only Dulbecco's Modified MEM (DMEM), Iscove's Modified DMEM, the addition on proline and thymidine to these media are shown in the figure. In these media either 10% FBS, 2% CGA-I, CGA-II or CGA-III were used. The results indicate that:

1. The three cells showed very different growth rates under similar conditions.

2. The medium providing best cell growth was dependent on the CGA used.

3. The best medium-CGA combination for optimum cell growth varies from cell to cell.

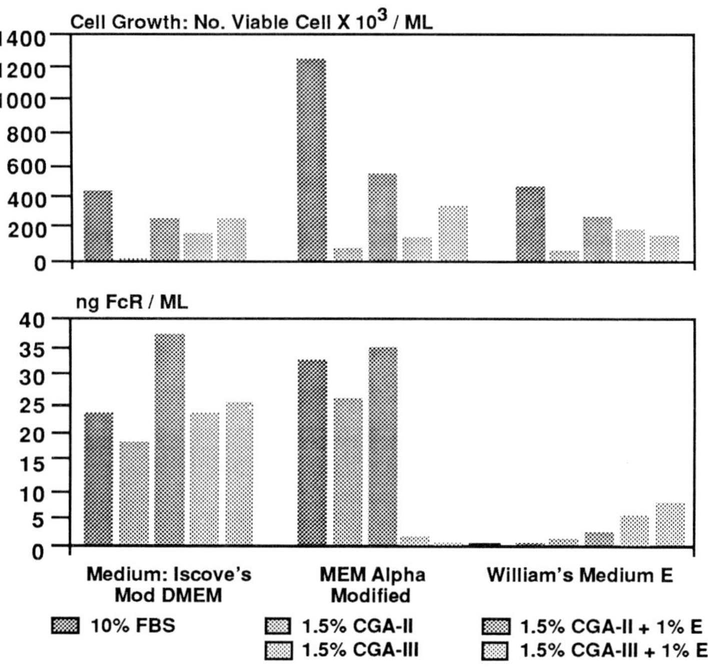

To examine the effect of CGA and medium combination on product yield (Fig. 4), rCHO-FcR cells were seeded in different media containing either FBS, CGA-II or CGA-III with and without E. Iscove's Mod. DMEM was the best with FBS, CGA-II, and CGA-III. MEM Alpha was good only for FBS and CGA-II. William's Medium was very poor for all. As with cell growth, the optimum protein expression depends also on the right medium - CGA-CFM combination. Relatively low cell growth can provide equal or higher product yield as FBS with very good cell growth.

Effect of Cell Growth Activator and 10μM Methotrexate on Growth and Recombinant FcR Expression of Serially Subcultured rCHO-FcR Cells

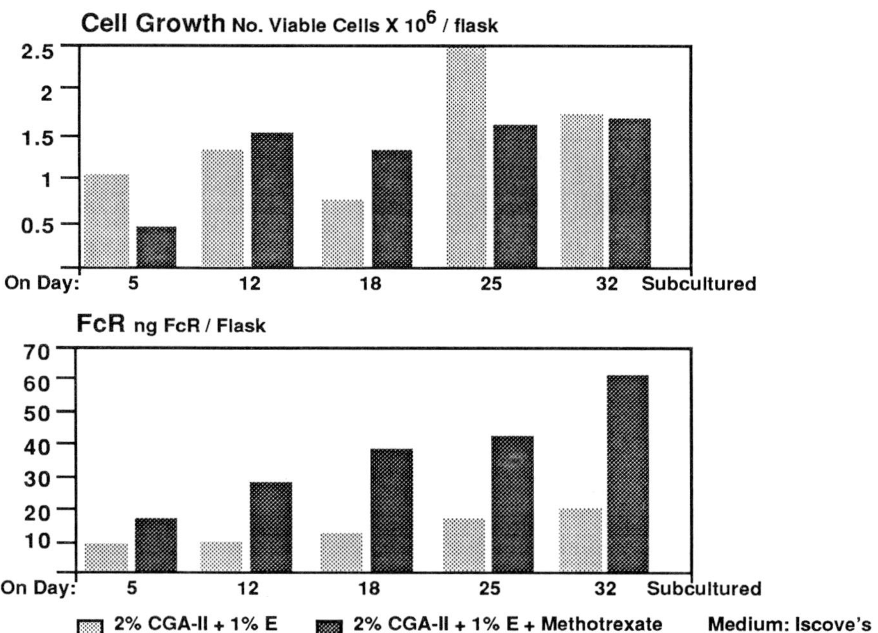

(Fig. 5) To examine how the cell growth and recombinant protein expression is maintained with CGA-CFM and the effect of methotrexate on these cells, 300,000 viable rCHO-FcR cells were seeded in Iscove's Mod. DMEM medium containing 2% CGA-II + 1% E with and without 10 μM. methotrexate into 25 cm^2 flasks. The media was tested for product yield on the indicated day, cells were counted and new subcultures were seeded at the same cell density. The results indicate that by establishing an optimum medium - CGA-CFM combination, a high level of recombinant FcR expression can be maintained. Product yield gradually increased in this experiment while cell growth remained at the same level. This is consistent with gene amplification by methotrexate.

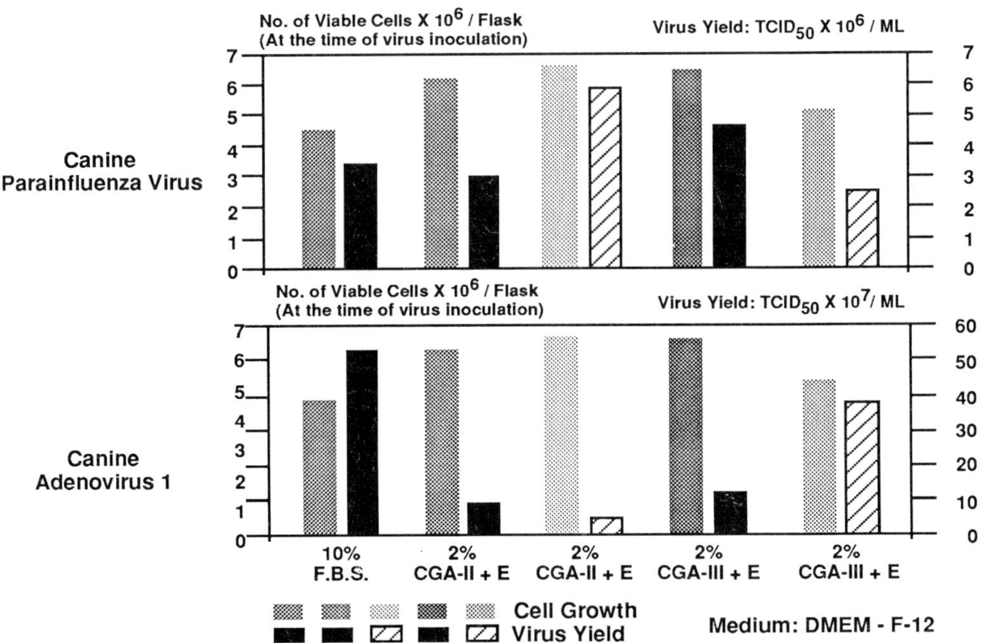

CGA has been shown to work well with other recombinant cells.
Significantly higher recombinant protein expression was obtained with another *rCHO* and *rC127* cells than with FBS. The
same basic observations apply for hybridoma cells and cells
infected with viruses. Using viruses as shown in Fig. 6,
300,000 viable MDCK cells were seeded per 25 cm^2 flask. At
the time of virus inoculation some flasks were used for cell
counting. The remaining flasks were divided into two groups.
One was inoculated with canine parainfluenza virus, the other
with canine adenovirus 1. The data indicate that the virus
yield was CGA-and E-dependent, with significantly higher
parainfluenza virus yield obtained with 2% CGA-II + 1% E than
with 10% FBS.

The results show also that different viruses can have significantly different CGA requirements for optimum virus
replication, as shown with CGA-II versus CGA-III in the test
using canine parainfluenza and adenovirus 1. The CGA-II + E
provided the highest parainfluenza virus titer whereas it
gave the lowest titer with adenovirus 1. With adenovirus 1
the CGA-III + E gave the highest titer which had given the
lowest parainfluenza virus titer for the same cells.

CONCLUSION

A large scale blood fractionation process yielded several
fractions with CGA and/or CFM activities. In the fraction
with the highest levels of CGA-CFM activities for anchorage
dependent cells; the activities seem to be associated with
similar proteins having varying CGA-CFM activity for specific
cells.

The right combination of basal medium, CGA-CFM has to be established for both good cell growth and for product or virus
yield. Different viruses may have different CGA requirements
in the same cell to obtain higher virus yield. The level of
product expression or virus yield did not correlate with the
level of cell growth in this system.

ACKNOWLEDGEMENTS

Special appreciation to Michelena Allen, Debra Cabe, Virginia
Russo, Louise Slaughter and Raymond Leidich for technical
assistance, to Christina Cameron for the computer graphic
work and Annette Vellake for the typing.

REFERENCES

1. Carrel, A. On the permanent life of the tissue outside
    of the organism. J. Exp. Med. 1912, 15, 516-528.

2. Carrel, A. and Ebeling, A.H. Antagonistic growth-
    activating and growth-inhibiting principles in serum.
    J. Exp. Med. 1923, 37, 653-658.

3. Barnes, D. and Sato G. Serum-free Culture: A "Unifying
    Approach" Cell, 22, 649-655.

**INCREASED EXPRESSION OF FACTOR VIII BY BUTYRATE
IN CHINESE HAMSTER OVARY CELLS**

*V.GANNE, *P.GUERIN, °T.FAURE and *G.MIGNOT
*TM Innovation, 3 avenue des tropiques F-91943 LES ULIS CEDEX FRANCE
°TRANSGENE, 11 rue de Molsheim F-67000 STRASBOURG FRANCE

INTRODUCTION

In order to design a chemically defined medium adapted for CHO TG 1020-22-12 cells, we have tested different factors. Among them, sodium butyrate was selected for its ability to multiply the specific productivity of factor VIII by about 3.
The questions which we have attempted to answer in this work are related to the mechanism of butyrate action.
Is the butyrate effect observed on factor VIII expression due to:
1) gene amplification?, 2) DNA demethylation?, 3) transcriptional or post-transcriptional effect ?

MATERIALS AND METHODS

CELLS AND MEDIUM
The CHO, TG 122020-22-12 cells were grown in selective ISCOVE medium supplemented with
hypoxanthine, thymidine, xanthine, mycophenolic acid and 5% FCS, at 37°C in 5% CO2 in a humidified atmosphere.
On day 3, the cells were fed with fresh medium with or without 3mM sodium butyrate,
and incubated for either 24 or 48 hours.

FACTOR VIII ASSAYS
Factor VIII procoagulant activity was determinated by two methods:
1) a modification of the partial thromboplastin time method (BEHRING) one stage assay with CNTS factor VIII standard
2) a chromogenic assay measuring the factor VIII dependant generation of factor Xa
from factor X (STAGO)

SOUTHERN ANALYSIS OF DNA
Total DNA was purified by phenol/chloroform procedure . The DNA was digested by the enzymes EcoRI, HindIII, and TaqI for quantitative analysis and MspI/HpaII for methylation analysis.
The DNA was electrophoresed on 1% agarose/formaldehyde gels, transferred to NYTRAN N filter and hybridized with, a P32 labeled FVIII cDNA probe.

NORTHERN ANALYSIS OF RNA
Total cellular RNA was isolated by the guanidine thiocyanate method (CHIRGWIN et al., 1979)
10 µg of RNA were electrophoresed on 1% agarose formaldehyde gels, transferred to nitrocellulose or NYTRAN N filter and hybridized with a P32 labeled FVIII cDNA probe.

SLOT ANALYSIS OF RNA
Total cellular RNA, isolated by the guanidine thiocyanate method, was transferred to nitrocellulose and hybridized with P32 labeled FVIII cDNA probe.

RESULTS

EFFECT OF BUTYRATE ON THE FACTOR VIII EXPRESSION
For incubation periods of 24 or 48 hours in the presence of 3mM butyrate factor VIII production was increased twice.
This increase was correlated with a decrease of cell proliferation.(Table I)
Specific cell productivity was increased by a factor of three.

EFFECT OF BUTYRATE ON FACTOR VIII GENE AMPLIFICATION
Cells were treated with 3 mM sodium butyrate, and 15 µg of DNA were digested by EcoRI, HINDIII and TaqI. The fragments were analysed by Southern blot hybridization.(Fig.1)
The pattern analysis did not reveal any differences between control and butyrate treated cells .
These results imply that butyrate does not induce a gene amplification of factor VIII.
EFFECT OF BUTYRATE ON GENE METHYLATION OF FACTOR VIII
The DNA of butyrate-treated cells was digested by two isoschizomer enzymes, MspI and HpaII
MspI and HpaII recognize the same sequence CCGG ; MspI cleaves if the DNA are methylated or unmethylated, whereas, HpaII cleaves, only if the C was unmethylated.
The analysis of the resultant patterns (fig.2) shows a different pattern with these two enzymes, implying that the DNA remained in a methylated state after butyrate treatment.
These results demonstrate that butyrate does not modify the methylation state of the DNA.

EFFECT OF BUTYRATE ON FACTOR VIII mRNA AMOUNT
The 48 hour butyrate treatment produced a 9kb band which corresponded to factor VIII mRNA .(fig 3), as seen the by Northern Blot.
This 9kb band did not appear with control cells or after the 24 hour butyrate treatment.
The lower species could be due to partially degraded or truncated mRNA.

INFLUENCE OF CYCLOHEXIMIDE ON THE FACTOR VIII EXPRESSION
Cycloheximide is a specific inhibitor of protein synthesis.The addition of 20 and 50µg/ml cycloheximide 1,2 or 4 hours before medium harvest, produced significant effects on the expression of factor VIII.(Table II)
The sensibilisation with cycloheximide was increased for butyrate treated cells

INFLUENCE OF CYCLOHEXIMIDE ON mRNA SYNTHESIS
After two hours cell incubation with cycloheximide at 20µg/ml, total RNA was extracted and analysed by slot blot.(fig 4)
Autoradiograms show a decrease of the intensities of the bands of the cells treated with butyrate and cycloheximide. This phenomenon was not observed with the untreated cells.

DISCUSSION

The intensity of the signal in the autoradiogram demonstrated that butyrate displays a large induction of mRNA whereas the secretion of protein remains low.
This observation could be associated with other studies (DORNER and al.1989) which shows that butyrate induces the synthesis of GRP 78 and 94 proteins.
These proteins have been reported to play an important role in the regulation of factor VIII expression in CHO cells (DORNER and al. 1987,KAUFMAN and al. 1988)
Because they are associated with the endoplasmic reticulum, they could eliminate misfolded or incompletely glycosylated factor VIII proteins.
DORNER and al. showed that butyrate induction is particularly effective for the combination of the adMLP promotor with SV40 enhancer sequence.
The clone TG 1020-22-12 has this combination adMLP/SV40.
The sensitivity of butyrate induced cells to cycloheximide suggests that butyrate induces a cycloheximide sensitive protein to activate the adMLP/SV40 promotor, leading to an increased amount of the mRNA and to the expression of recombinant factor VIII in CHO cells.
Results of mRNA and protein expression in controlled cells treated by cycloheximide indicate the difference between the butyrate enhanced protein (BEP) and GRP 78 and 94.

	COAGULATION ACTIVITY (relative values)	CELLS DENSITY (millions of cells)
CONTROL DAY3-DAY4	100	51
BUTYRATE DAY3-DAY4	153	44
CONTROL DAY4-DAY5	76	76
BUTYRATE DAY4-DAY5	158	34

<u>TABLE I</u>

Butyrate effect on the factor VIII expression and cell density.

<u>TABLE II</u>

Cycloheximide effect on factor VIII expression in the presence or absence of 3mM sodium butyrate. 2 concentrations of cycloheximide were tested (1) 20 and (2) 50µg/ml .

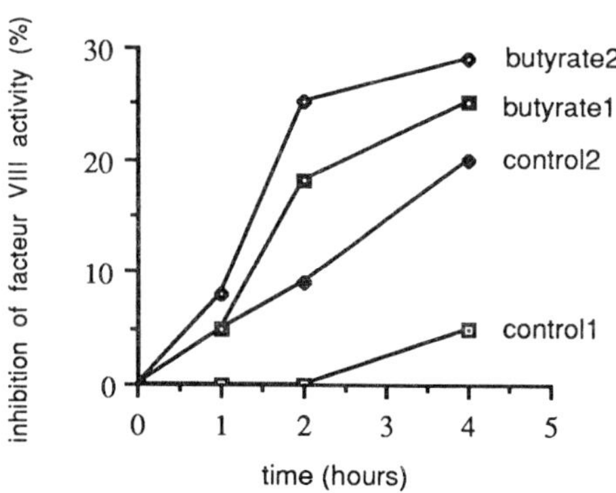

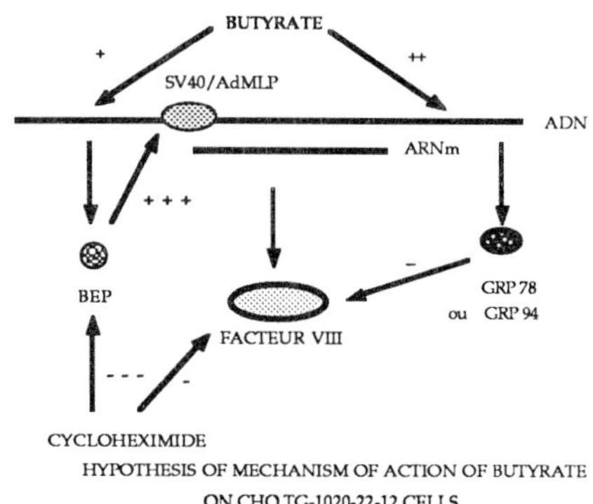

HYPOTHESIS OF MECHANISM OF ACTION OF BUTYRATE ON CHO TG-1020-22-12 CELLS

<u>**FIG1 SOUTHERN ANALYSIS OF BUTYRATE TREATED CELLS**</u>

15 µg of DNA was prepared from cells which had been grown for 24 and
48 hours with or without 3mM sodium butyrate. It was digested by
EcoRI, HindIII, and TaqI, electrophoresed on 1% agarose gel,
transferred to NYTRAN N membrane and hybridized with random
primed FVIII cDNA.
A: control, 24 hours
B: butyrate, 24 hours
C: control, 48 hours
D: butyrate, 48 hours

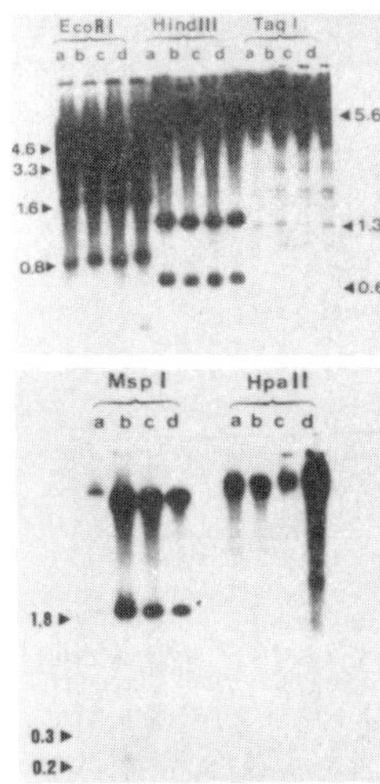

<u>**FIG2.METHYLATION ANALYSIS OF BUTYRATE TREATED CELLS**</u>

15µg of DNA was prepared from cells which had been grown for 24 and
48 hours with and without 3mM sodium butyrate. It was digested by
MspI and HpaII, electrophoresed on 1% agarose gel, transferred to
NYTRAN N membrane and hybridized with random primed FVIII
cDNA.
MspI cut if the C was methylated or not, whereas, HpaII cut only if the
C was unmethylated.
A: control, 24 hours
B: butyrate, 24 hours
C: control, 48 hours
D: butyrate, 48 hours

<u>**FIG3. NORTHERN ANALYSIS OF BUTYRATE TREATED CELLS**</u>

Total cellular RNA was prepared from cells which had been grown for
24 or 48 hours, in the presence or absence of 3mM sodium butyrate, and
then electrophoresed on 1% agarose-formaldehyde gel, transferred to
NYTRAN N and hybridized with random primed FVIII cDNA.
A: control, 24 hours
B: butyrate, 24 hours
C: control, 48 hours
D: butyrate, 48 hours

<u>**FIG4. RNA SLOT ANALYSIS OF BUTYRATE TREATED CELLS WITH
CYCLOHEXIMIDE**</u>

Total cellular RNA was prepared from cells which had been grown for
48 hours in the presence or absence of 3mM butyrate and incubated
2hours before the harvest,with 20ug/ml cycloheximide. It was
transferred to nitrocellulose and hybridized with random primed
FVIII cDNA.
A: control
B: butyrate
C: control+Cycloheximide
D: butyrate+Cycloheximide

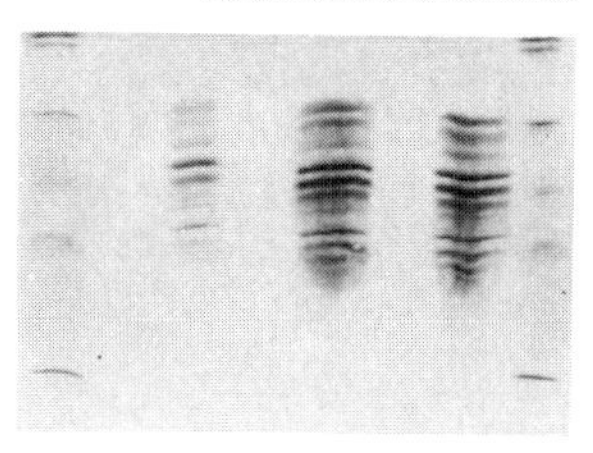

REFERENCES

1 - CHIRGWIN,J.M, PRIZYBYLA,A.E, MAC DONALD R.J, and RUTTER,W.J,(1979) biochemistry 18:5294

2 - PAVIRANI.A, MEULIEN.P, HARRER.H, SCHAMBER.F, DOTT.K, VILLEVAL D, CORDIER.Y, WIESEL.M.L, MAZURIER.C, VAN DE POL. H, PIQUET.Y, CAZENAVE.J.P.and LECOCQ.J.P.,(1987)Choosing a host cell for active recombinant factor VIII production using vaccinia virus. Biotechnology,5, 389-392

3 - KAUFMAN R.J.,WASLEY.L.C,DORNER A.J.(1988), Synthesis, processing and secretion of recombinant human factor VIII expressed in mammalian cells. J.Biol.Chem. 263 6352-6362.

4 - DORNER.A.J, WASLEY.C.W, KAUFMAN.R.J.(1989) increased synthesis of secreted proteins induces expression of glucose-regulated proteins in butyrate-treated chinese hamster ovary cells..J.Biol.Chem.264: 20602-20607

5 - DORNER,A.J.,BOLE.D.G., KAUFMAN,(1987), J.Cell.Biol.102, 2665-2674

6 - MIGNOT.G, GANNE.V,FAURE.T, PAVIRANI.A, and VAN DE POL.H. (1988). The use of a statistical approach for the optimization of culture conditions of genetically engineered cell lines. in <u>Advances in Animal Cell Biology and Technology for Bioprocess</u> ,Butterworths, SPIER et al , pp52-58.

7 - KRUH.J, (1982.). Effects of sodium butyrate, a new pharmacological agent, on cells in culture. Molecular and Cellular Biochemistry.42.65-82.

POLYAMINE ENHANCED PRODUCT EXPRESSION FROM TRANSFORMED AND RECOMBINANT
CELL LINES

Stephen J. Froud, John McLean and Andrew Mint

Celltech Ltd., 216 Bath Road, Slough, SL1 4EN, United Kingdom.

ABSTRACT

The addition of high concentrations (0.1 - 10 mM) of ornithine or
putrescine to EBV transformed human B lymphocyte or recombinant CHO rat
or mouse myeloma serum-free suspension cultures resulted in most cases
in an elevated product concentration. Under these conditions product
formation was usually enhanced with little or no increase, and in many
cases a decrease, in cell proliferation.

KEY WORDS

Putrescine, ornithine, lymphocyte, CHO, myeloma, expression,
recombinant, tPA, TIMP, antibody.

INTRODUCTION

The polyamines spermidine and spermine, the diamine putrescine, and
their precursor ornithine are present in all mammalian cells. The
polyamines bind to proteins, phospholipids, DNA, rRNA, mRNA and tRNA
(1,2). Despite extensive research efforts, the mechanisms by which
these interactions influence cellular physiology are not well
understood. Nevertheless, the cellular need for polyamines in order to
maintain cell growth and function is firmly established.

The polyamine biosynthetic pathway is highly regulated after the
synthesis of ornithine (for review see 3). In intact animals adequate
ornithine is generally available from extracellular sources. Similarly
cells cultured in the presence of serum obtain ornithine from the
action of the arginase in the serum. In serum-free culture, however,
some cells lack arginase (4) and this fact may account for the apparent
need for putrescine in many serum-free media formulations (5).
Putrescine, then, is added to such media to ensure cell proliferation.
In general, the concentration of putrescine in such media is below 0.01
mM, as high concentrations are known to inhibit cell growth.

We have studied the effects of ornithine, putrescine, spermidine and
spermine on homologous and heterologous protein production during
suspension culture of a variety of cell types, with particular
reference to relatively high concentrations of these compounds.

MATERIALS AND METHODS

Cells from a growing culture were centrifuged and resuspended in 50 ml
of medium to approximately 0.1 million cells per ml. Duplicate
suspension cultures were prepared with the test compound. Controls
contained less than 0.01 mM of that compound. The cultures were gassed
with CO /air, incubated at 37 C and agitated at 120 rpm. Viable and
total cell concentrations were determined daily by Trypan Blue
exclusion. Tissue plasminogen activator (tPA) and derivatives thereof
were assayed by S2251 amidolytic or fibrin gel dissolution assay. The
other products were assayed by ELISA.

RESULTS

The EBV transformed human B lymphocytes (see Table 1) displayed an
increase in the specific concentration (amount per cell) of antibody
produced when either 0.1 mM ornithine or putrescine was added to the
medium (Table 2). Cell line A grew to a higher cell density in the
presence of these compounds, whereas cell line B showed no such
improvement in the presence of 0.1 mM putrescine and, furthermore, it
grew poorly in the presence of 0.1 mM ornithine. The effect of 0.1 mM
putrescine on cell line B is of particular note; A large increase in
antibody concentration was obtained in the absence of an increase in
cell concentration. In all cases where an increase in antibody
concentration was seen, the value obtained was similar to that obtained
when the cells were grown in medium containing 5% foetal calf serum
(FCS).

A variety of recombinant cell types, expression systems and products
were investigated (see Table 1). All but one cell line showed an
increase in product concentration when 1 mM putrescine or ornithine
(when tested) was included in the medium (Table 2). As noted for the
lymphocytes, the effect of this high concentration of these compounds
was dependent on the cell line but in all cases where an increase in
product concentation was seen, this was associated with an increase in
the specific concentration of the product.

For the recombinant myeloma cell lines (C and G) this latter effect
became more pronounced at higher concentrations of these compounds
(Table 2), such that an increase in the product concentration was
obtained even when the cell concentration was quite markedly reduced,
until an optimum was exceeded. This indicates a marked increase in the
specific production rate in these cell lines. For example, in the
presence of 5 mM putrescine the specific production rate for cell line
G was double that of the control cultures.

As expected, when these compounds were added to a medium containing 1%
serum no increase in product concentration was observed.

Although for certain cell lines, the addition of 1-10 uM spermidine or
spermine to the culture medium did produce an increase in cell and/or
product concentration, these compounds were generally cytostatic at
relatively low concentrations, and were not investigated further.

Table 1   Cell Lines

Cell Line	Cell Type	Product	Vector Type
A	EBV transformed human B lymphocyte	Human IgG	-
B	EBV transformed human B lymphocyte	Human IgM	-
C	Rat Yo myeloma	tPA	Single copy
D	CHO	TIMP	Unamplified
E	CHO	tPA derivative	Single copy
F	CHO	tPA derivative	Single copy
G	Mouse myeloma	tPA derivative	Amplified

Table 2 The Effect of Ornithine or Putrescine on Different Cell Lines

Results are expressed as percentage change from controls of maximum cell concentration, product concentration and specific product concentration (amount per cell).

Cell Line	Compound	Conc. (mM)	Cell Conc.	Product Conc.	Specific Conc.
A	Putrescine	0.1	+36%	+133%	+71%
A	Ornithine	0.1	+29%	+139%	+85%
B	Putrescine	0.1	0	+64%	+64%
B	Ornithine	0.1	-29%	-17%	+17%
C	Putrescine	1	0%	+30%	+32%
D	"	"	-3%	+170%	+175%
E	"	"	+3%	+14%	+10%
F	"	"	+3%	-6%	-8%
G	"	"	+7%	+14%	+7%
C	Ornithine	1	-8%	+22%	+33%
C	Putrescine	1	0	+30%	+32%
"	"	2	-7%	+53%	+65%
"	"	5	-30%	+29%	+83%
"	"	10	-31%	+22%	+76%
"	Ornithine	1	-8%	+22%	+33%
"	"	2	-8%	+22%	+33%
"	"	5	-13%	+60%	+80%
"	"	10	+5%	+5%	0
G	Putrescine	1	+7%	+14%	+7%
"	"	2	0	+37%	+37%
"	"	5	0	+104%	+104%
"	"	10	Not Determined		

REFERENCES

1   Feurstein, B.G. and Marton, L.J. In: The Physiology of Polyamines Vol. 1 (ed, Bachrach, V. and Heimer, Y.M.) CRC Press, 1989, pp109-124.
2   Pegg, A.E. Cancer Res. 1988, 48, 759-774.
3   Heby, O. and Persson, L. Trends Biochem. Sci. 1990, 15, 153-158.
4   Holtta, E. and Pohjanpelto, P. Biochim. Biophys. Acta 1982, 721, 321-327.
5   Ham, R.G. Proc. Natl. Acad. Sci. USA 1965, 53, 288-293.

THE DEVELOPMENT OF A PROCESS FOR THE PRODUCTION OF HIV1 GP120 FROM
RECOMBINANT CELL LINES.

S.J. Froud, G.J. Clements, M.E. Doyle, E.L.V. Harris, C. Lloyd, P.
Murray, A. Preneta, P.E. Stephens, S. Thompson and G.T. Yarranton.

Celltech Ltd., 216 Bath Road, Slough, SL1 4EN, United Kingdom.

ABSTRACT

The HIV1 envelope glycoprotein gp120 has been expressed in CHO and
myeloma cell lines. The glutamine synthetase system was used for gene
amplification. After immunopurification, the identity of the 120 kd
protein was confirmed by SDS-PAGE, amino-acid analysis, N-terminal
sequencing, and antibody and CD4 binding. Some of the purified gp120
had been specifically cleaved to two disulphide-linked polypeptides.
This cleavage was caused by a trypsin-like serine protease, released
from the CHO cells possibly as a result of depletion of certain
amino-acids. Optimisation of the cell culture process resulted in the
production of essentially uncleaved HIV1 gp120.

KEY WORDS

HIV1, gp120, recombinant, expression, CHO, myeloma, purification,
protease, suspension culture.

INTRODUCTION

The Human Immunodeficiency Virus (HIV) has been identified as the major
etiological agent of Acquired Immunodeficiency Syndrome (AIDS). The
virus infects susceptible cells after interaction between the HIV
envelope glycoprotein and the cell surface marker CD4. The HIV
envelope protein is expressed from the _env_ gene as a single polypeptide
chain consisting of a 30 amino-acid leader sequence and the precursor
protein gp160. Post translational processing results in the removal of
the leader sequence to reveal an amino terminal threonine residue and
the cleavage of the polypeptide into the large extracellular gp120 and
the small transmembranous gp41; the gp120 is highly glycosylated, half
of its molecular weight being due to carbohydrate residues. A key tool
for research into AIDS is a supply of the individual proteins of HIV1
virus. This work describes the development of a process for the
production of recombinant HIV1 gp120.

<u>MATERIALS AND METHODS</u>

The plasmid pSP64 BH10 was kindly provided by R.C. Gallo (National Cancer Institute, USA). This plasmid contains a <u>Sst</u> 1 fragment of the proviral HIV clone BH10, which itself was derived from unintegrate linear DNA from H9 cells acutely infected with HIV1 IIIB. The 5' end of the <u>env</u> gene was reconstructed using oligonucleotides to allow incorporation into the vector. A translational stop codon was introduced at the cleavage site between gp120 and gp41 by site directed mutagenesis[1]. The DNA encoding gp120 was introduced into the vector EE6 HCMV[2]. The glutamine synthetase gene was introduced[3] and CHO K1 cells were transfected by calcium phosphate precipitation[4]. Cell lines were plated in increasing concentrations of methionine sulphoximine (MSX) to select for amplification events[3]. The selected cell line was incubated at 37°C in 850cm^2 roller bottles. The growth medium was as described previously[3] and the base medium was changed to DMEM for harvesting. The immunopurification matrix was a sheep anti–peptide antibody (D7324 from Aalto Bioreagents) coupled to CNBr–activated sepharose. SDS–PAGE was performed using 7.5% or 10% polyacrylamide. Amino–acid analysis was performed on a Biotronik LC500 analyser. Amino terminal sequence analysis of electrophoresed proteins was performed on an Applied Biosystems 470A protein sequencer after blotting and excision. Culture supernatant and purified gp120 was assayed by ELISA. This consisted of a murine anti gp120 monoclonal antibody (9284/7054 from Dupont) for capture, the sheep antibody from Aalto and a rabbit anti–sheep F(ab)'$_2$ peroxidase conjugate (313–035–006 from Jackson Immuno Research). Glucose and lactate were assayed by HPLC after deproteinisation by precipiation.

RESULTS AND DISCUSSION

Expression of HIV1 gp120

An expression vector for CHO cells was constructed by reconstruction of the 5' end of the <u>env</u> gene, the insertion of a translational stop codon at the cleavage site between gp120 and gp41 and the introduction of the glutamine synthetase gene. Stable CHO cell lines expressing gp120 were obtained upon transfection and selection in the presence of the glutamine synthetase (GS) inhibitor methionine sulphoximine (MSX). The gene copy number was increased to 100–300 per cell with a concomitant increase in the production of gp120.

The highest producing GS amplified CHO cell line, 17.1, produced only 1–3 mg L^{-1} of gp120, considerably less than is usually found for this system (20–200 mg L^{-1}). The reason for this low level of expression has not yet been elucidated but is probably the result of poor mRNA transport from the nucleus to the cytoplasm.

Characterisation of purified gp120

Gp120 was recovered from clarified culture supernatant by immunopurification and concentration. The protein appeared as a single band of 120 kd and was more than 90% pure when analysed by SDS-PAGE under non-reducing conditions. The identity of the gp120 was confirmed by amino acid analysis and amino terminal sequencing. The results obtained agree with published data[5,6] and the latter confirmed that the expressed, purified gp120 had been correctly processed during secretion.

In addition, gp120 could be detected in a twin site ELISA utilising a mouse anti-gp120 monoclonal antibody and a sheep anti-gp120 peptide antibody. Furthermore, the biological activity was confirmed in a sCD4 sandwich ELISA and CD4 cell-based assay[7,8]. In the former the binding affinity of gp120 for sCD4 was similar to that for gp120 obtained from virion preparations, whereas in the latter the specificity of binding was confirmed by competition with sCD4.

Reduction of the purified protein followed by SDS-PAGE, however, revealed that some of the gp120 had been cleaved to two disulphide linked polypeptides of relative molecular mass 70 kd and 50 kd. This cleavage has also been reported with gp120 obtained from both viral and other recombinant sources[9-12]. Amino-terminal sequence analysis indicated that the cleavage was highly specific, occurring between arginine 315 and alanine 316 at the tip of the V3 loop. Inhibition studies have demonstrated that this specific cleavage is due to a trypsin-like serine protease (data not shown).

In order to investigate the significance of this cleavage, it was necessary to identify conditions from which uncleaved gp120 could be obtained.

The effect of culture conditions on the cleavage of gp120.

The effect of culture conditions on the cleavage of gp120 was investigated by product, nutrient and metabolites analysis during a 7 day culture of cell line 17.1.

Gp120, as detected by ELISA, steadily accumulated through the culture period (Fig. 1). Western blot analysis of the culture medium, however, showed that after day 2 a small but increasing proportion of the gp120 was cleaved.

During the culture period lactate did not accumulate to a concentration that might be expected to have an adverse effect upon the cells, nor was glucose depleted from the medium (Fig. 2). The onset of cleavage, however, coincided with the depletion of certain amino-acids from the medium, notably asparagine, glutamate, aspartate and serine (Fig. 3).

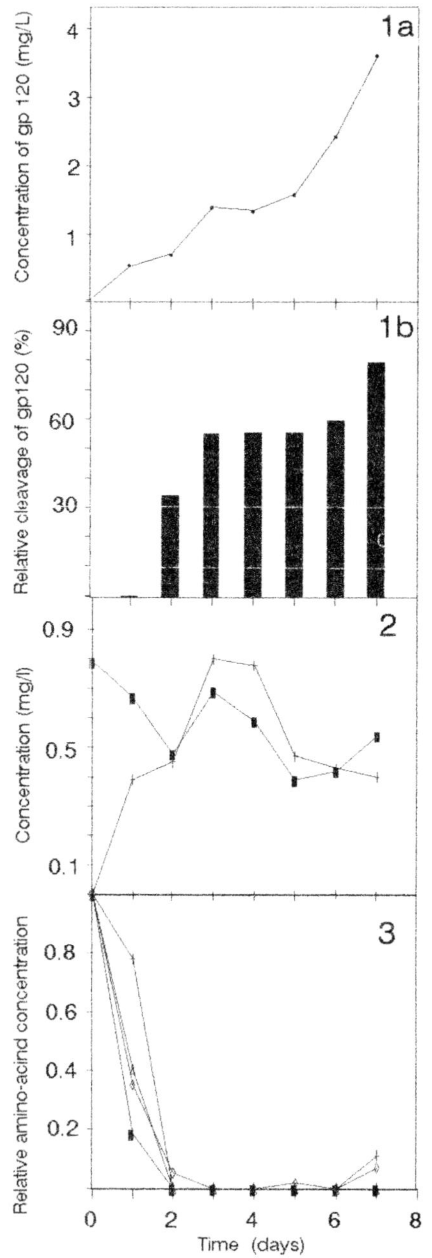

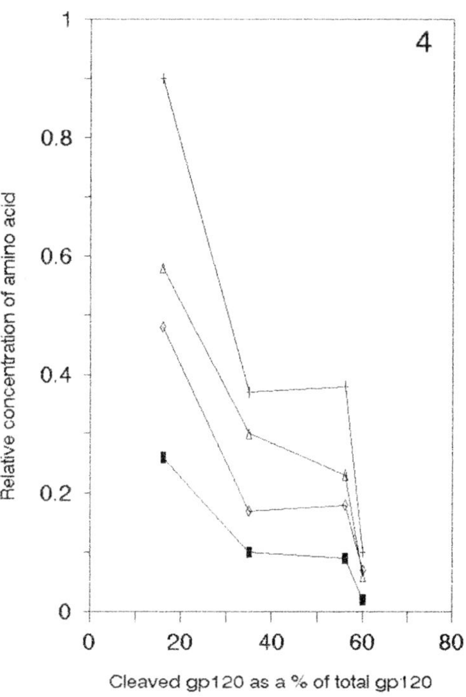

Fig. 1-3 Medium analysis of a 7-day culture of cell line 17.1. Fig.1a, gp120 concentration (by ELISA). Fig. 1b, relative cleavage of gp120 as determined by Western blot analysis.

Fig. 2, (+) lactate concentration (mg/l), (■) glucose concentration relative to the initial value. Fig. 3, amino-acid concentration relative to the initial concentration.

Fig. 4, The relation ship between the concentration of amino-acids measured 24h after adding medium to cultures of different cell densities. and the cleavage of the gp120 purified after a further 48h.

(■) Asparagine, (◇) serine (△) glutamate, (+) aspartate.

This relationship was confirmed by comparing cell cultures of different
cell density, incubating these for 3 days and subsequently purifying
the gp120. The results demonstrated that the amount of cleavage is
inversely proportional to the amount of these amino-acids remaining in
the medium after the first day of incubation (Fig. 4) and, by
inference, that the amount of cleavage is proportional to the length of
time of the incubation after these amino acids have been depleted.
This has led to the hypothesis that depletion of one or more key amino
acids from the culture medium results in the release of a trypsin-like
serine protease from the CHO cells This release may be due to
induction, secretion, cell death or lysis.

Optimisation of culture conditions

Modification of the culture conditions has resulted in the production
of essentially uncleaved purified HIV1 gp120. This was achieved in
roller bottles by shifting to the harvest medium at a low cell density,
by reducing the time between harvests and by of improving the efficacy
of the purification process. Under these conditions it is likely that
amino-acids are not being depleted from the medium and protease release
is diminished. Although reasonable quantities of essentially uncleaved
gp120 were produced, this roller bottle procedure was labour intensive
and low in yield (0.3 mg 1^{-1}).

For subsequent scale-up, however, the amino-acids could be maintained
in excess in fed-batch suspension culture. Consequently the CHO cell
line 17.1 has been adapted to suspension culture and a GS amplified
murine myeloma cell line has been constructed. Both of these cell
lines produce HIV1 gp120 in suspension culture.

ACKNOWLEDGEMENTS

Most of this work was funded by the MRC AIDS directed programme. We
thank Johnathan Karn (Laboratory of Molecular Biology) and Geoffrey
Schild (NIBSC) for helpful discussion, John Moore (Chester Beatty
Laboratories) and Lesley Walker (Northwick Park Hospital) for CD4
binding assays, Alan Benett for plasmid constructs, and Peter Dumbell,
Sandy Carne and Christopher Sutton for amino acid sequencing and
analysis.

REFERENCES

1. Kramer, W., Drutsa. V., Jansen, H.W., Kramer, B., Pflugfelder, M.
    and Firtz, H.J. _Nucleic Acids Res_. 1984, _12_, 9441-9456.

2. Stephens, P.E. and Cockett, M.I. _Nucleic Acids Res_. 1989, _17_, 7110.

3. Bebbington, C.R. and Hentschel, C.C.G. In: _DNA Cloning_; _A
    Practical Approach_ Vol. 3 (Ed, Glover, D.M.) IRL Press, Oxford,
    1987, pp.163-188.

4. Graham, F.L. and Van der Eb, A.J. _Virology_ 1973, _52_, 456-467.

5. Allan, J.S., Coligan, J.E., Barin, F., McLane, M.F. Sodroski,
    J.G., Rosen, C.A., Haseltine, W.A., Lee, T.H. and Essex, M.
    Science 1985, _228_, 1091-1093.

6. Ratner, L., Haseltine, W., Patarca, R., Livak, K.J., Starcich, B.,
    Josephs, S.F., Doran, E.R., Rafalski, J.A., Whitehorn, E.A.,
    Baumeister, K., Ivanoff, L., Petteway Jr, S.R., Pearson, M.L.,
    Lautenberger, J.A., Papas, T.S., Ghrayeb, J., Chang, N.T., Gallo,
    R.C. and Wong-Staal, F. _Nature_ 1985 _313_, 277-284.

7. Walker, L. personal communication.

8. Moore, J. _et al_. _AIDS_ (In Press).

9. Lasky, L.A., Nakamura, G., Smith, D.H., Fennie, L.m Shimasaki, C.,
    Patzer, E, Berman, P., Gregory, T. and Capon, D.J. _Cell_ 1987, _50_,
    975-985.

10. Dowbenko, D., Nakamura, G., Fennie, C., Shimasaki, C., Riddle, L.,
    Harris, R., Gregory, T. and Lasky, L. _J. Virology_ 1988 _62_
    4703-4711.

11. Boyle, P.O. personal communication.

12. Farrar, G. personal communication.

Wurm: With respect to the comparison of myeloma and CHO cells you only mentioned the depletion of amino acids for CHO cells. Do you see the same depletion for myeloma cells?

Froud: Investigations with the myeloma cells are at an early stage and we have not yet optimised the system.

Wurm: Would you comment on the yield from myeloma cells as well?

Froud: Again that system has not been optimised. These proteins are difficult to express and we are talking of amounts much lower than the 100-200 mg/l than we would normally get.

Wurm: A final comment. We know that gp120 is a highly glycosylated protein and it is interesting from a scientific point of view to compare the glycosylation in a mouse and CHO cell line. Are there some data on this?

Froud: We have not looked at the glycosylation patterns. In the CHO cell line the affinity for CD4 and a number of other factors, antibody binding etc., are very similar to the human viral isolate.

Munster: The data you showed indicated that very little glucose was used as a carbon source, they therefore produced very little lactate, and there is no glutamine in the medium. Do I then infer that the four amino acids are essential for growth?

Froud: The medium is based upon GMEM and to get optimal growth the concentration of asparagine and glutamine has been raised considerably. They are the key factors. We have less information on the other amino acids.

Munster: Is this a general phenomenon for this amplification system?

Froud: Yes, it is related to the fact that we have a highly amplified glutamine synthetase expression in these cell lines. Asparagine is also well known as a requirement for CHO cells.

"SAFE" ANIMAL DERIVED MEDIUM SUPPLEMENTS FOR CELL CULTURES.

Adolf Von Seefried and Paul Haffenden.
Bocknek Ltd., 165 Bethridge Road, Toronto, Ontario   M9W 1N4
                                    Canada

ABSTRACT:

Freedom of infectious agents, or components thereof, is essential in the production of biologics for human or veterinary
use. Some contaminants can be removed by filtration, physical
agents, or purification. However, any remaining contaminant
could affect the cell culture systems. Sera are still used,
or they are replaced by serum derivatives in special formulations. These medium supplements must originate from animals
known to be free of adventitious agents, and must be processed
under controlled conditions to prevent contamination.

Examples of "safe" medium supplements are those derived from
animals which have been selected, tested, maintained in isolation, and fed without animal derived supplements. The animals
must have originated from geographic areas free of endemic
diseases such as Bovine Spongiform Encephalopathy, Bluetongue,
Brucellosis, Foot and Mouth Disease, TB, Riftvalley Fever, and
others. In case of endemic diseases, the animals must be
protected by isolation and vaccination.

Using "Donor Bovine Serum", as an example of a "safe" supplement, a comparative study with "Foetal Bovine Serum" was
carried out in a wide range of cell cultures.

INTRODUCTIONS:

Sera, or serum components in special formulations, are still
essential and most economical in many cell culture systems in
diagnostic, research, and industrial use. Processing technology has been improved to achieve "sterility" beyond the
exclusion of bacterial contamination. However, the problem
remains that some infectious, adventitious agents might escape
filtration or destruction by physical means. These agents
could have an adverse effect on the cell culture system
itself, and may escape purification or inactivation procedures, presenting a risk in the final product. Any materials
collected in abattoirs, even under veterinary inspection, may
have been derived from an infected animal not having any
clinical signs of disease. It is, therefore, advantageous to
obtain all animal derived medium supplements from animals
known to be free of infectious agents, and processed by
acceptable methods.

MATERIALS AND METHODS:

Fetal Bovine Serum (FBS) was prepared from blood collected
aseptically in approved Abattoirs, and Adult Bovine Serum
(DBS) was prepared from sterile blood collected from isolated,
healthy donor animals. The sera were sterilized by membrane
filtration, and represent regular batches acceptable to international regulatory standards for the production of biologics
for human and veterinary use.

The Donor Herd was established as follows:
Healthy animals, free of adventious, infectious agents, were
selected from disease-free breeding establishments, and
maintained in disease-free environments by complete isolation
from other animals. All feed was obtained "in-house", free of
animal derived supplements. Observation by a qualified
veterinarian, and immunization against some endemic disease
(BVD, IBR, and PI-3) provided additional assurance. Furthermore, the animals are tested regularly for Bovine Leukosis,
TB, and other endemic diseases.

The basic cell culture medium was Dulbecco's Minimal Essential
Medium at PH 7.2, adjusted with sodium bicarbonate and Hepes
buffer. The growth factors were purchased from Waitaki,
Toronto. The cell culture strains were examples of those used
in the industry, which are also available from any public cell
culture collection. Using standard techniques, cell cultures
were initiated at sufficiently low densities to obtain confluent growth, or the end of the logarithmic growth phase,
within seven days.

RESULTS AND DISCUSSION:

Table I shows examples of bovine viruses known to (a) be
endemic worldwide and (b) to cause persistent or latent
infections, frequently without any clinical signs. BIV is
genetically, structurally, and immunologically related to
human immunodeficiency viruses, and is known to infect human
cell cultures. The disease could manifest itself through
immunological disorders, lymphocytosis, and CNS lesions,
but could remain undetected in the slaughter house situation.
Similarly BLV, another retrovirus, may present itself in
less than 5% of infections with lymphosarcomas and tumors,
but otherwise would not show clinical signs. It is known
that in most parts of the world 15 - 20% of the cattle have
been infected and remain infectious for life. Potential
cross-over to humans or mutations to human viruses are
possible.

BVD, IBR, and P1-3 are frequently present not only as persistant, long lasting infections, but are also introduced through live-virus vaccines. The five viruses listed in Table I can be eliminated only if the blood originates from selected animals, as in the donor herd described above.

TABLE I

BOVINE VIRUSES, ENDEMIC WORLDWIDE

	Disease		Elimination From Serum		
Name		Virus	Testing	Irradiation[1]	Animal Selection
BIV	Immunodeficiency	Lenti, Retro	?[2]	?	+
BLV	Leukosis	Retro	?	?	+
BVD	Diarrhea, Mucosal	Pesti	?	+	+[3]
IBR	Rhinotracheitis	Herpes	+	+	+[3]
P1-3	Parainfluenza	Myxo	+	+	+[3]

Notes: (1) 1.5 - 2.5 Megards
      (2) Nucleic acid probes, infection of human astrocytes
      (3) Select "negative" animals and immunize with <u>inactivated</u> vaccines

Some infectious agents are found only in certain areas, which is an advantage in the establishment of a disease-free herd. The examples shown in Table II are diseases which have either never occurred in certain geographic regions, or have been eliminated by vaccination or eradication. For instance, Canada is, with the exception of a certain region in British Columbia, free of these diseases except rabies. Rabies is easily preventable by immunization with inactivated vaccine or by isolation of the donor animals. Of particular concern in this group of diseases is BSE, which is caused by a highly heat and irradiation resistant prion, which is difficult to detect, and is the cause of a slow disease affecting the central nervous system. Unless animals have been kept in isolation for long periods of time, or known to have been derived from disease-free stock, they are not qualified "blood donors". Prions are known to cross the species barrier, eg. from sheep to cattle and perhaps to man. Similar diseases (Kuru and Creutzfeldt-Jacob) occur in man. Infection may occur through contact or ingestion of infected tissue, and prions could conceivably be present in blood of infected animals and contaminate the final, biological product. Regions with dense populations of sheep have to be considered as high risk.

119

Pleuropneumonia is an example of a disease caused by mycoplasmas, which are not desirable in cell culture systems.
Filtration, even at 40 nm pore-size, would not remove the organisms. Bluetongue is endemic in many parts of the world.
There are many antigenically different strains and adequate
tests are not available. A serious cell culture contaminant fo
any research, diagnostic, or production cell culture systems.

It is possible to keep healthy donor animals in isolation
assuring freedom from these infectious agents.

TABLE II

ADVENTITIOUS, INFECTIOUS (BOVINE) AGENTS ENDEMIC IN SPECIFIC GEOGRAPHIC AREAS

Disease		Elimination From Serum		
Name	Agent	Test-ing[1]	Filtra-tion	Irradi-ation[2]
Aujesky's	Herpes Virus	+	−	+
Blue Tongue	20 Orbiviruses	+[3]	−	+
Foot and Mouth	67 Picornaviruses	+	−	+
Pleuropneumonia	Mycoplasma	+	−	+
Q-Fever	Rickettsia	?	+	+
Rabies	Rhabdovirus	?	−	+
Rift-Valley F.	Enveloped RNA virus	+[4]	−	+
Rinderpest	Paramyxovirus	+	−	+
B. Spongiform Encephalopathy	Prion (Protein)	?[4]	−	−[5]

Notes: (1) USDA − test protocols not available
       (2) 1.5 − 2.5 Megarads
       (3) Testing in chick embryos (death) or sheep
            (serology)
       (4) Animal tests
       (5) Highly resistant

The following 5 tables show cell culture results obtained with
Foetal Bovine Serum (FBS) and Donor Bovine Serum (DBS).

Table III compares results of FBS versus DBS for the growth of
the Human Diploid Cells WI-38 in three subcultivations. In
order to use equivalent protein concentrations, the serum
concentrations had been adjusted. Similarly, as shown in
Table IV, the growth of Hybridoma Cells was adequately supported with (DBS) as compared to FBS at the optimum
concentrations. In this case 12% DBS could be used to replace
20% FBS.

TABLE III

GROWTH COMPARISONS OF HUMAN DIPLOID CELLS (W1-38)
IN MEDIUM SUPPLEMENTED WITH FOETAL OR DONOR BOVINE
SERUM AT EQUAL PROTEIN CONCENTRATIONS

| SERUM | | Cell X 10^6 Per Subcultivation | | | Total |
TYPE	$\%^{(1)}$	1	2	3	Population Doublings
FBS	10	4.8	4.2	5.3	9.8
FBS	7	4.8	4.8	4.5	9.7
DBS	6	3.6	4.0	5.2	9.6

Note: (1) To achieve final protein concentration = 0.37%

TABLE IV

GROWTH OF HYBRIDOMA CELLS ATCC # 2.43
IN DULBECCO'S MEM PLUS FBS AND/OR DBS

| FBS % | DBS % | POPULATION DOUBLINGS/PASSAGE | | |
		1	2	Total
20	–	3.1	3.8	6.9
–	20	2.5	3.9	6.4
–	16	3.1	3.8	6.9
–	12	3.0	4.1	7.1
–	10	2.2	4.2	6.4
10	12	2.8	4.2	7.0
5	12	2.8	3.7	6.5
2	12	2.4	4.0	6.4
0.5	12	2.8	3.7	6.5

Note: Cell inoculum = 1 X 10^6 cells per 12 ml medium (25 cm^2)

The growth of CHO cells required the addition of growth
factors, as shown in Table V. The combination of transferrin,
fetuin, and albumin was particularly beneficial when DBS was
used to replace FBS.

TABLE V

**GROWTH OF CHINESE HAMSTER OVARY (CHO) CULTURES
IN DBS\FBS AND GROWTH FACTORS**

DBS %	FBS %	T	F	A	I	1	2	3	Total
						Population Doublings\Passage			
–	10	–	–	–	–	5.6	4.2	3.9	13.7
6	–	–	–	–	–	4.9	2.8	2.9	10.6
6	–	+	+	–	–	5.7	3.2	3.5	12.4
6	–	+	+	+	–	5.5	3.6	4.3	13.4
6	–	+	+	–	+	5.2	3.8	3.3	12.3

Notes: T = Transferrin 50 ug/ml   F = Fetuin 50 ug/ml
A = Albumin 2 ug/ml   I = Insulin 10 ug/ml

TABLE VI

**GROWTH OF HUMAN FORESKIN
FIBROBLAST CELL CULTURES IN
MEM PLUS FBS, DBS, AND CS[1]**

DBS %	FBS %	CS %	1	2	3	Total
			Population Doublings/Passage[2]			
10	–	–	2.8	3.0	3.0	8.9
–	6	–	2.9	2.7	2.7	8.2
2	6	–	3.0	2.6	3.1	8.7
–	–	10	3.0	2.7	2.9	8.6
2	–	8	3.0	3.3	2.4	8.7
2	–	5	2.9	3.0	3.0	8.9

Notes: (1) FBS = Foetal Bovine Serum, DBS = Donor Bovine
Serum, CS = Calf Serum
(2) Cell inoculun = 0.4×10^6 cell/25 cm^2

Table VI shows the growth obtained with Human Foreskin
Cultures with either FBS, DBS, OR CS (Calf Serum). These
cells appeared to be less fastidious, and all serum
combinations were satisfactory. Vero Cells, as shown in Table
VII, did particulary well in 4 subcultivations, when DBS was
used, 6% and 4% successfully replaced FBS at a 10%
concentration.

122

<u>TABLE VII</u>

<u>GROWTH OF VERO CELLS IN MEM</u>
<u>SUPPLEMENTED WITH EITHER FETAL, CALF, OR</u>
<u>ADULT (DONOR) BOVINE SERUM. (JUNE 1989)</u>

| <u>Serum</u> | | Population Doublings [1]Per Passage | | | | |
<u>Type</u>	%	1	2	3	4	Total
Foetal	10	4.7	3.1	4.5	4.5	15.4
Donor	6	5.1	4.3	2.3	5.0	16.7
Donor	4	4.5	4.3	3.1	4.8	16.7
Donor	2	3.0	3.3	2.5	4.3	13.1
Fetal/ Donor	2/4	4.9	4.0	2.7	4.0	15.6

Notes: (1) Population Doublings in 25 cm^2 cultures, initiated
with 0.4 X 10^6 cells/flask

CONCLUSION:

Cell culture systems used in industry, diagnostics, and
research cannot be maintained free of adventitious agents, if
one of the medium components contains a contaminant. The risk
of contamination is high, if these medium components (serum or
growth factors) have been derived from animals, which have
been brought to the abattoirs, particularly in geographic
areas known to be burdened with endemic diseases. The "safe"
low risk alternative is a source of raw materials from healthy
animals, which are kept in isolation and constantly monitored
for health and freedom of adventitious, infections agents. As
an example of such a material, Donor Bovine Serum (DBS)
successfully replaced Foetal Bovine Serum (FBS) in the
cultivation of diploid, heteroploid, primary, and hybridoma
cell cultures. Similarly, so-called serum-free media contain
animal derived materials, particularly albumin, which are
obtainable from healthy donor animals. In the past, serious
contamination originated from animals, whose tissue had been
used to establish cell cultures. It has now become mandatory
to avoid the addition of contaminants to clean cell culture
systems.

ACKNOWLEDGEMENTS:

The technical assistance in the cell culture work by
Mr. Paul Junor, and the management of the Donor Herd by
Mr. Dave Gillespie is greatly appreciated.

<u>Paper of Seefried</u>

Munster: The idea of isolated herds of animals is a good idea;
               does this have any impact on the cost of the serum.

Seefried: It is cheaper; it is one-third of foetal in cost and
               you use it at about 8%.

Vournakis: Have you considered the problem of bovine parvovirus
               which are a problem for CHO cells.

Seefried: They have not been a problem in our area.

EFFECT OF DESFERRIOXAMINE ON TRANSFERRIN RECEPTOR EXPRESSION, GROWTH &
IgG PRODUCTION OF THE RAT HYBRIDOMA MAC57.

N.J. Tomlinson[*], L. Davis[+], J. Craig-Gray[+], N. Jenkins[*].

[*]University of Kent, Canterbury, Kent, CT2 7NJ, U.K. and
[+]Glaxo Group Research, Greenford, Middlesex, UB6 OHE.

ABSTRACT

The potential of the iron chelator, desferrioxamine (DFX), to induce
transferrin receptor (TfR) expression in hybridomas was investigated, and
the consequences for cell growth and IgG production monitored. Cells
were sampled every 12h following 10µM DFX treatment and compared to
control cultures. Double-fluorescence labelling and a fluorescence
activated cell sorter were used to determine TfR levels at different
stages of the cell cycle. After 36h and 48h a significant increase in
the surface TfR levels was observed, and the proportion of cells in the
G_2/M phase of the cell cycle decreased. A slower cell growth rate in
DFX-treated cells was reflected in the lower rate of ^{3}H-thymidine
incorporation, and reduced cell counts over the same time period. There
was also a 38% higher rate of ^{35}S-methionine incorporation into the IgG
in DFX-treated cells. Together these data indicate that although DFX
induces the expression of surface TfR in hybridomas, this does not result
in a higher growth rate. However, specific production of IgG was
increased, which may be a consequence of the slower growth rate.

INTRODUCTION

The iron-binding protein transferrin has been shown to be one of the
growth requirements of hybridoma cells cultured in serum-free medium (1).
A relationship between the surface levels of the transferrin receptor and
the S/G_2/M stages of the cell cycle has been well documented (2,3). The
expression of the TfR is regulated at the translational level by the
stability of the mRNA. The half life of the TfR mRNA is controlled by
the binding to specific 3'untranslated sequences of a cytoplasmic protein
whose activity is iron dependent (4). Chelation of the free iron with
DFX therefore produces an increase in the surface expression of TfR (5).
In order to investigate the relationship between TfR levels, cell growth
and IgG production this drug was used to induce the expression of surface
TfR in the rat hybridoma, MAC57.

MATERIALS AND METHODS

All materials were purchased from Sigma Chemicals unless otherwise
stated.

Cell culture and treatment with DFX

MAC57 rat hybridoma (ECACC 86036310) were maintained in 30ml RPMI
medium (Imperial Laboratories) supplemented with 2mM glutamine and 10%
FCS (Gibco). Cells were grown in 75cm^2 tissue culture flasks in a wa-
ter-saturated incubator at 37°C, 5% CO_2/95% air. Cells were treated by

the addition of 10µM DFX (Ciba-Geigy) and the various cell parameters assessed every 12h in triplicate from each flask. All treatments were carried out in quadruplicate.

Cell counts were determined by the Trypan Blue exclusion method.

Comparison of Surface TfR levels

Cells were harvested and washed three times in ice cold PBS and resuspended in either 500µl PBS (control) or 500µl OX26, mouse anti-rat TfR monoclonal antibody and incubated on ice for 1h. After washing the cells were incubated for 1h on ice in 500µl fluorescein isothiocyanate (FITC) conjugated goat anti-mouse IgG (1:40). Following washing the cells were fixed in fresh ice cold 50% ethanol in water and the DNA stained with 50µg ml^{-1} propidium iodide in the presence of 0.3mg ml^{-1} RNase for 30 mins. at 37°C. Single cells were analysed using a Coulter EPICS fluorescence-activated cell sorter (FACS) operated at 448nm, photomultiplier tubes 600 (green) and 393 (red) with gains of 20 and 5 respectively.

^{3}H-thymidine incorporation

Cells were harvested, counted and resuspended at 10^{6} cells per ml. 200µl aliquots were placed in wells of 96 well tissue culture plates and 0.5µCi ^{3}H-thymidine (Amersham) in 50µl medium added to each well. The cells were incubated at 37°C for 4h with the label then the well contents were transferred to LP$_{4}$ tubes and the cells washed onto glass fibre paper (Whatman) using a DynaTech cell harvester and the paper discs counted in a liquid scintillation counter (Beckman).

^{35}S-methionine incorporation and IgG precipitation

The cells were treated as for labelled thymidine incorporation except that 10µCi of ^{35}S-methionine (ICN) was added per well. After incubation the cells were removed by centrifugation and 150µl of 50mM Tris-HCl (pH 8.2), 5mM EDTA, 5mM EGTA, 0.5% Na deoxycholate added. 30µl Protein-A Sepharose (10% suspension) was then used to bind the IgG by incubation at 4°C on a rotating wheel for 2h. The Sepharose beads were then washed twice in 50mM Tris-HCl, 5mM EDTA, 0.5% Nonidet P-40, 0.1% bovine serum albumin, 0.5M NaCl and again in 50mM Tris-HCl, 5mM EDTA, 0.5% Nonidet P-40 before resuspending in 200µl distilled H$_{2}$0. 3ml of scintillant fluid was then added and the samples counted in a liquid scintillation counter.

Measurement of secreted IgG

This was achieved using a standard sandwich ELISA technique.

RESULTS AND DISCUSSION

The surface TfR levels of the MAC57 rat hybridoma were increased threefold after treatment with the ferric chelator, desferrioxamine (Fig. 1). This did not appear to stimulate the growth of these cells, in fact the growth rate was reduced and the maximum viable cell number was 50% lower in treated cells than in the controls (Fig. 2, open symbols). The incorporation of ^{3}H-thymidine, which reflects the rate of DNA synthesis, was also decreased significantly after 48h (p < 0.001; Fig. 2, closed symbols). This reduction in the growth rate may be due to inhibition of

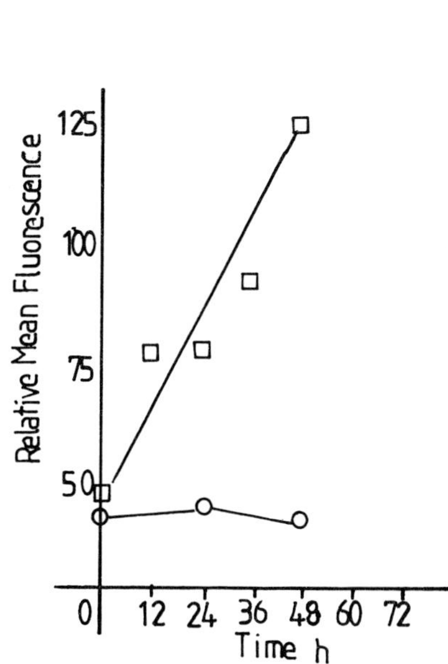

Fig. 1. Relative mean surface fluorescence after labelling with anti-TfR monoclonal antibody

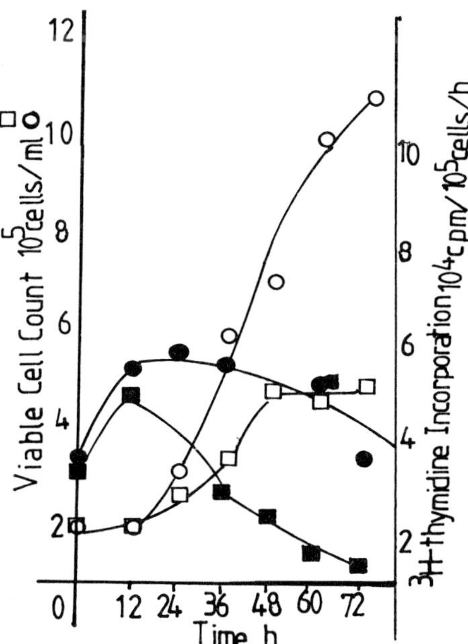

Fig. 2. Viable cell number (open symbols) and ^{3}H-thymidine incorporation (closed symbols)

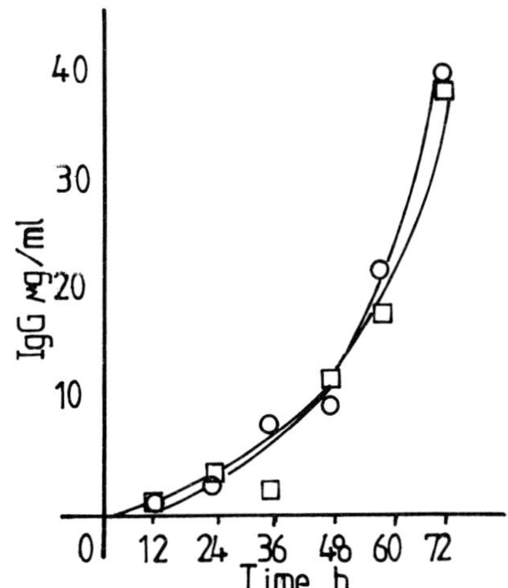

Fig. 3. Concentration of IgG in culture supernatant

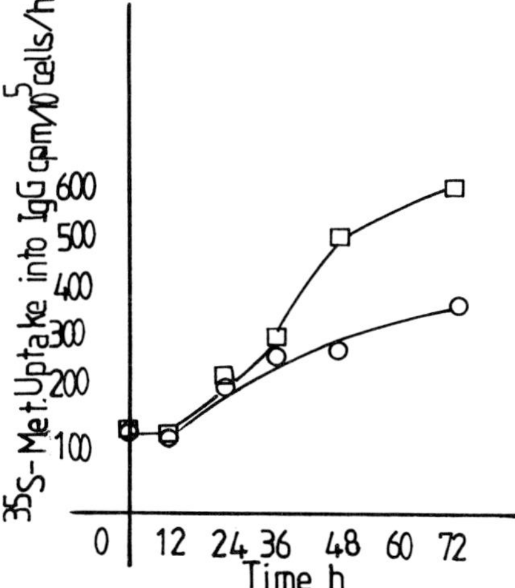

Fig. 4. ^{35}S-methionine incorporation into IgG

127

DNA synthesis by DFX since it was shown by FACS analysis that the treated cells were predominantly in the G_1 and S phases of the cell cycle (data not shown).

Antibody production was maintained in both treated and control cultures and similar antibody titres were reached in each case (Fig. 3). However, the specific IgG production rate was increased by 38% in treated cultures as measured by incorporation of ^{35}S-methionine into immunoglobulin (Fig. 4). This increase in specific IgG production rate in the treated cells may be due to a perturbation of the cell growth since other groups have also observed this phenomenon (6,7,8). It has been suggested that these effects are due to cell cycle regulation of the antibody production with Ig synthesis restricted to the G_1 and S phases of the cell cycle (9). The findings of this investigation are possibly consistent with such a hypothesis since the DFX treated cells were predominantly observed in the G_1 and S phases and had an elevated antibody production.

ACKNOWLEDGEMENTS

NT was supported by a SERC Biotechnology Directorate research studentship. The authors would like to thank Dr. Butcher and the AFRC, Animal Physiology Research Station, Cambridge for the gift of the hybridoma cells.

REFERENCES

1. Kovar, J. and Franek, F. Hybridoma cultivationin defined serum-free media: growth supporting substances. I. Transferrin. Fol. Biol. (Praha) 1985, 31, 67-175
2. Trowbridge, I.S. and Omary, M.B. Human cell surface glycoprotein related to cell proliferation is the receptor for transferrin. Proc. Nat. Acad. Sci. USA 1981, 78, 3039-3043
3. Sutherland, R., Delia, D., Schneider, C., Newman, R., Kemshead, J. and Greaves, M. Ubiquitous cell-surface glycoprotein on tumour cells is proliferation-associated receptor for transferring. Proc. Nat. Acad. Sci. USA 1981, 78, 4515-4519
4. Koeller, D.M., Casey, J.L., Hentze, M.W., Gerhardt, E.M., Chan, L.N.L., Klausner, R.D. and Harford, J.B. A cytosolic protein binds to structural elements within the iron regulatory region of the transferrin receptor in mRNA. Proc. Nat. Acad. Sci. USA 1989, 86, 3574-3578
5. Rao, K.K., Shapiro, D., Mattia, E., Bridges, K. and Klausner, R.D. Effects of alterations in the cellular iron on biosynthesis of the transferrin receptor in K562 cells. Mol. Cell Biol. 1985, 5, 595-600
6. Dalili, M. and Ollis, D.F. The influence of the cyclic nucleotides on hybridoma growth and monoclonal antibody production. Biotech. Lett. 1988, 10, 781-786
7. Glassy, M.C., Tharakan, J.P. and Chau, P.C. Serum-free media in hybridoma culture and monoclonal antibody production. Biotechnol. Bioeng. 1988, 32, 1015-1028
8. Oyaas, K., Berg, T.M., Bakke, O. and Levine, D.W. In: Advances in Animal Cell Biology and Technology for Bioprocesses (Eds. Spier, R.E., Griffiths, J.B., Stephenne, J. and Crooy, P.J.) Butterworths, Kent, England, 1989, pp. 212-220
9. Suzuki, E. and Ollis, D.F. Cell cycle model for antibody production kinetics. Biotechnol. Bioeng. 1989, 34, 1398-1402

Gerbert: Why do you think the effect on your cells is due to chelate action and not to iron shortage? It would be of interest to deprive the cells of iron using chelate and then some time afterwards adding transferrin.

Tomlinson: I did a control experiment by adding iron loaded chelators and we still saw the synthetic effect which makes us think it is not just iron deprivation. Iron is required by DNA synthetic enzymes, ie is required for growth, which is why I concluded the chelator was toxic.

Al Rubei: Am I right is suggesting that the observed increase in specific IgG production is due to an increase in the death rate and the release of stored product, rather than the accumulation of cells in G1 phase? Recent surveys of the literature would support this.

Tomlinson: No. I didn't go through the protocol in detail but in fact cells were removed from the culture and 2 x 10^5 viable cells were re-suspended in the labelling medium. The measurement of IgG was therefore from viable cells only.

Section 3
Serum free and protein free media

DEVELOPMENT OF SERUM-FREE MEDIA FOR MAMMALIAN CELL CULTURE

Kierulff, J., Persson, B., Rexen, P., Morcel,[*]C. & Emborg, C.

Department of Biotechnology, Centre for Food and Process Biotechnology, The Technical University of Denmark, DK-2800 Lyngby, Denmark.
[*]Department of Biochemical and Food Engineering, I.N.S.A. - Avenue de Rangueil, 31077 Toulouse, France.

ABSTRACT

The MTT method has proved to be a usable screening system for development of serum-free media for murine hybridomas using factorial assays. Results obtained by the MTT method have been compared to results from cell counting and found to agree. A TSP system for screening for IgG production has been tested and found usefull.

INTRODUCTION

Serum-free media have already been reported, but because of the great differences in nutritional requirements even for genetically identical cells, development of cell specific medium is often necessary. This is very labour and cost intensive due to the large number of media formulations needed to be tested. Quick and easy screening methods are therefore needed in addition to "clever" screening plans (1). The MTT method (3-(4,5-diMethylThiazolyl-2-yl)-2,5diphenylTetrazolium bromide) already described (2,3) seems to fit the requirements. MTT is a yellow, water soluble salt which is biologically active. It enters the mitochondria in the cells where it is reduced to a blue, water insoluble formazan, which can be extracted from the cells (e.g. with SDS, 20 % w/v in H_2O/DMF (1:1)). The reduction will only take place in living cells, and a cell with a high level of activity will give a higher response than a resting cell due to a higher level of activity/higher number of mitochondria. It can therefore be used as a viability/activity test. Because of the ease in which the assay can be performed, it is usefull in screening for new mediaformulations. However, screening methods for product (e.g. IgG) are also needed. This can be done with the TSP system (Transferrable Solid Phase) (4). The TSP system basically consists of a lid for a microtiterplate. It is supplied with 96 tips fitting the wells of the plate. The tips are made of polystyrene and have affinity for proteins. The TSP is simply exchanged for the lid on the microtiterplate soaking the tips in the media. During incubation the proteins in the media will adsorb to the tips. The tips can then be analysed for IgG by an ordinary sandwich ELISA technique. This allows easy screening of 96 samples in one step. The method is not quantitative, but semi-quantitative which is all needed for screening purpose.

MATERIALS AND METHODS

Cell lines: Four murine hybridoma cell lines were used (all derived from myeloma x63-Ag8.653/BALB c) producing IgG_1.
Media: DME with additional 6 mM glutamine and 15 mM HEPES but without antibiotics and serum was used as basal medium. To this medium the different compounds were added making full factorial assays testing up to 6 factors at a time.
Growth assay: 100 μl of medium was added to each well on a microtiterplate (Nunc, Denmark) and innoculated with 25 μl of cell suspension (with 0.1 - 0.8 % serum) to a final concentration of 0.4×10^5 living cells/ml. The cells were grown for up to 7 days at 36.5°C and 5 % CO_2. At the end of incubation 25 μl of MTT (4 mg/ml in PBS) was added to each well for two hours, followed by 150 μl of SDS (20 % w/v in H_2O/DMF (1:1), pH 2) overnight. $OD_{570-690}$ was measured and the total of the three wells was calculated. The increase in OD from day 0 or 1 for each media formulation was used for further calculations.
IgG assay (TSP assay): A TSP plate (Nunc, Denmark) was exchanged for the lid of a microtiterplate and incubated together with the microtiterplate. When the plate was analysed for cell growth by the MTT method the TSP was analysed for IgG by an ordinary sandwich ELISA technique.
Experiments in shakeflasks: The cells were grown in basal medium with 0.8 % serum and different factors in 300 ml shakeflasks with 50 ml of medium at 50 rpm. Samples were taken dayly and the cell density determined by counting (trypan blue exclusion) and by the MTT method.

RESULTS

The MTT method has been evaluated comparing $OD_{570-690}$ to cell counting. We have done preliminary experiments showing a linear dependence between the cell number and $OD_{570-690}$.

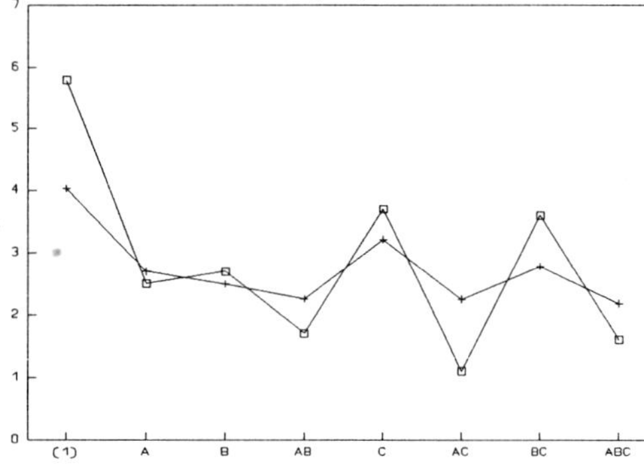

Fig. 1: Results obtained from shakeflasks on day 2.
A: Na2HPO4/NaH2PO4, B: Pleuronic F68, C: Tracemetals.

We have also performed factorial assays in shakeflasks. The experiment showed that the results obtained by the MTT method on the samples from the shakeflasks and the results obtained by cell counting led to the same conclusion, as did an experiment growing the cells in the microtiterplate. The results are showed in fig. 1. To determine if any of the tested factors gave a significant increase or decrease of the cell growth/cell activity or the production of IgG, the results were first evaluated qualitatively. Most of the main effects (single factor effects) were strong enough to be visualised in this way. To visualise the possible interactions Yates algorithm was performed.

Table 1 shows some results obtained by the TSP method culturing two different hybridoma cell lines in microtiterplates. The size of the numbers depends of the time of the final colour reaction and can therefore differ from day to day, However, the proportion of the numbers will fit the proportion of the IgG concentration.

cell line	HYB 1-2	HYB 66-4	HYB 1-2	HYB 66-4	HYB 1-2	HYB 66-4
day	1	1	3	3	3-1	3-1
basal media	1008	1266	808	1342	-200	76
FeSO4	855	1441	830	1449	-25	8
FeCl3	853	1629	894	1491	41	-138
FeSO4+FeCl3	981	1730	1127	1493	146	-237

Table 1: IgG concentration obtained by the TSP method (OD_{492} total of 3 wells x 1000)

It can be seen from the table, that HYB 66-4 produced more IgG than HYB 1-2. This have been verified in several experiments making quantitative IgG analysis. From the last column (day 3-1) it can be seen that the two cell lines don't respond identically. Addition of both $FeSO_4$ and $FeCl_3$ causes a significant increase in the IgG concentration for HYB 1-2, but causes a dramatic decrease in the IgG concentration for HYB 66-4.

CONCLUSION

The MTT and TSP method have proved to be usefull tools in preliminary screening revealing candidates worth for further investigation. The experimental design and way of handling the data revealed several (surprising) interactions which would probably not have been discovered in the case of an "one factor at a time" approach. By incorporating the cell line as one of the factors in the experimental design, we have discovered differences in the response for hybridoma cell clones made during the same fusion (from the same mouse), i.e. genetically identical cells.

ACKNOWLEDGEMENTS

This study was supported by a grant from the Danish Technical Research Council and by a grant from Centre for Food and Process Biotechnology.

REFERENCES

1   Emborg, C. et al., Two-level factorial screening of new plasmid/strain combinations for production of recombinant-DNA products, <u>Biotechnol. Bioen.</u> 1989, <u>33</u>, 1393

2   Mosmann, T., Rapid colorimetric assay for cellular growth and survival: Application to proliferation and cyto-toxicity assays. <u>J. Immunol. Methods</u> 1983, <u>65</u>, 55

3   Hansen, B.H. et al., Re-examination and further develop-
    ment of a precise and rapid dye method for measuring cell
    growth/cell kill. <u>J. Immunol. Methods</u> 1989,
    <u>119</u>, 203

4   Løvborg, U. Guide to solid phase immuno assays. <u>Published
    by A/S Nunc, Roskilde, Denmark</u> 1984

CONCEPT AND STRATEGY FOR THE DEVELOPMENT OF A GENERAL PURPOSE
SERUM-FREE MEDIUM FOR ANCHORAGE-DEPENDENT CELLS

L. Kaspi D. Fiorentini, R. Talmon, R. Levi, and G. Bennett

Biological Industries, Kibbutz Beit HaEmek, Israel

ABSTRACT

Most so called multi-purpose serum-free media (SFM) are expensive
sophisticated mixtures of many hormones and growth factors, or contain
inexpensive, undefined ingredients. This work is based on the concept
that different anchorage-dependent cell types might share basic
requirements, and thus a simple general purpose medium could be turned
into specific media for individual cell types by the addition of a few
defined ingredients. The SFM developed supports long-term growth of
chosen anchorage-dependent epithelial and fibroblast-type cells.

Keywords: Anchorage-dependent cells, Primary cells, Cell longevity,
Long-term growth, Serum-free medium, Defined medium.

INTRODUCTION

The ideal SFM, suitable for long term growth of all cells, should be
completely defined, standardized, and inexpensive. Previous experiments
performed with BS-C-1 cells (1) showed that similar serum-free growth of
a particular anchorage-dependent cell can be attained in different
media. Such a finding is contrary to the concept of specific media for
specific cells. We therefore engaged in the development of a unique SFM
which would support the growth of many, if not all, anchorage-dependent
cells.

MATERIALS AND METHODS

Cells: A549 (ATCC-CCL 185), BGM, BHK-21 (CCL 10), BS-C-1(CCL26), CHO
DHFR⁻ (CRL 9096) HEp2 (CCL23), 3T3 clone A31 (CCL 163), Vero (CCL 81),
MA10(2), Primary epithelial cells from human thymus (ET). Primary chick
embryo fibroblasts (CEF) were prepared by the method of Rubin (3)
directly in serum-containing medium or SFM. All media were prepared in
house. All chemicals were obtained from Sigma.
Trypsinization was performed with crystalline trypsin as described
elsewhere (1). Trypsinized cells were counted by the trypan blue
exclusion method (hemocytometer).

RESULTS

Preliminary expreriments were performed, with representative cells
chosen for their wide use in industry or research (BHK, CHO, A549, 3T3,
CEF). Five media differing from each other with respect to amino acid,

salt and vitamin concentrations, as well as the basal medium recommended for each cell, were supplemented with serum at low concentration (0.5-1%), and their ability to support the growth of the cells was tested (growth curves). The medium which gave the best results for all five cells was chosen as a unique basal medium. A minimal SFM (MSFM) was prepared by adding transferrin, ethanolamine, selenium, putrescine, linoleic acid and insulin to the basal medium. Serum-free growth of the representative cells was attained by a combination of specific additions (BHK, A549 and CHO: Fibronectin (FN); 3T3: Bombesin), high density seeding ($5x10^5$ cells/T25 flask) and weaning (CHO, 3T3). After at least three passages in MSFM with specific supplements, optimization of the medium was attempted with albumin, various hormones, lipids, metabolites, trace elements and growth factors. Besides hormones and growth factors, which were subsequently avoided, lipids (lecithin + cholesterol) were the only addition to the MSFM (LSFM) which improved the growth of all representative cells.

The range of cells tested was then enlarged and serum-free growth was attained in the same way as for the representative cells. Both MSFM and LSFM were used. Optimization was attempted, but no addition improved LSFM, which was superior or equivalent to MSFM.

Long-term growth of cell lines in LSFM has been undertaken (Table 1)

Cells	Weeks in SFM	Doubling time(hrs)	Maximal density (cells/cm^2,T25)	Additions to LSFM
A549	12	30	2×10^5	Fibronectin
BGM	13	30.5	$2.5x10^5$	-
BHK-21	28	13	$2.2x10^5$	Fibronectin
BS-C-1	33	33	$1.8x10^5$	-
CEF	12	39	$8x10^4$	-
CHO	7	14.5	$3.2x10^5$	Fibronectin
ET	Primary	Not tested	$1.4x10^5$	EGF, HC(*)
HEp-2	12	20	$2.8x10^5$	Fibronectin
MA10	6	Not tested	$2x10^5$	Fibronectin
3T3	26	15.5	$3.2x10^5$	-
Vero	14	18	$2.1x10^5$	-

Table 1 Growth of Anchorage - dependent Cells in SFM
(*) Epidermal Growth Factor, Hydrocortisone.

CEF were grown from primary culture until senescence in parallel in MSFM, LSFM and serum-containing medium (Fig 1). Total population doublings was about 70% in LSFM as compared to serum- containing medium, and lower in MSFM.

Preliminary qualitative experiments to assess production of biologicals showed positive results with CEF (vaccines),with ET (Interleukin 3 - like factor), and with MA10 (progesterone).

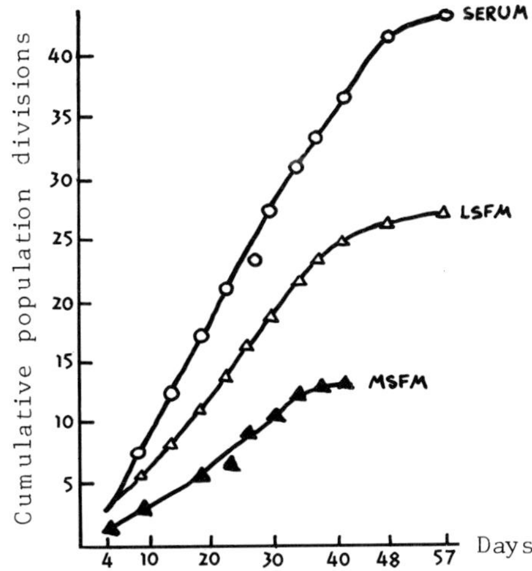

Figure 1   Longevity of CEF in Different Media
1 - 3 x 10^5 cells were seeded in T25 flasks and counted in situ to quantitate attachment (4). Every 5-7 days, cells were trypsinized, counted and reseeded, until senescence.

DISCUSSION

This work shows that a unique, unsophisticated and defined SFM can easily be adapted to support the growth of widely different anchorage-dependent cells by the addition of a few specialized components. Long term growth was attained without use of albumin, growth factors or hormones, besides insulin. The experiments with CEF show a striking effect of lipids on longevity of diploid cells. Although the doubling time of CEF was longer in SFM than in serum, these cells might reach a higher number of population doublings in SFM if growth factors and/or hormones were added to the medium, and if the effect of trypsin was countered in a more thorough way (experiments in progress).

ACKNOWLEDGEMENTS

MA10 cells were provided by M. Ascoli through Drs. Barkey and Ber: Medical School, Technion, Haifa.

REFERENCES

1   Fiorentini, D., Kaspi, L., Talmon R. and Bennett, G. Development of a series of versatile serum-free media formulations. _Proc. of the second annual meeting of the JAACT_. 1990, In Press

2   Ascoli, M. Characterization of several clonal lines of cultured Leydig tumor cells: gonadotropin receptors and steroidogenic responses, _Endocrinol_. 1981, _108_: 88

3   Rubin, H. Preparation of primary chick embryo cells, _Tissue Culture Methods and Applications_. Acad. Press, NY, 1973, p. 119

4   Litwin, J. The growth of human diploid fibroblasts in serum-free medium, _Develop. Biol. Standard, Vol 55_. S. Karger, Basel, 1984, pp. 261-266

GROWTH OF MAMMALIAN CELL LINES UNDER SERUM-FREE CONDITIONS

Bente Rasmussen and Claus Koch

Research Centre for Medical Biotechnology
Statens Seruminstitut, Artillerivej 5, 2300 Copenhagen S, Denmark

ABSTRACT

The myeloma cell line X-63Ag8.653 has been adapted to growth in serum-free media, DMEM + 2% ultroser (X-63$_{ultroser}$) and DMEM + 10% BMS (X-63$_{BMS}$). These adapted cell lines have been used in fusions to form hybridoma cell lines.
The hybridoma formation was carried out in the serum-free media and the results show, that this procedure is a useful strategy to develop hybridoma cell lines, adapted to growth under serum-free conditions.

INTRODUCTION

Growth of mammalian cell lines under serum-free conditions has several advantages as compared to cultivation of cells in the presence of foetal calf serum (FCS). It reduces the risk of microbial contamination, it simplifies the purification of protein products from the cell culture, and it reduces the production costs.

In particular, if the product, secreted by the cell line, is developed for therapeutic use in humans it is necessary to use a synthetic medium for the growth of the producing cell line, in order to avoid unknown and potentially harmful factors from the medium. We have assayed various adaptation strategies using two different, commercially available synthetic media.

Several studies have been reported with established hybridoma cell lines being adapted to serum-free media. An alternative approach is to produce hybridoma cell lines under serum-free conditions from the fusion step.

For this study we have adapted the myeloma cell line X-63Ag8.653 to the serum-free media DMEM + 2% ultroser HY and DMEM + 10% BMS. These adapted cell lines (X-63$_{ultroser}$, X-63$_{BMS}$) have then been used in the cell fusion procedure. The rationale behind this approach is that the characteristics that X-63$_{ultroser}$ and X-63$_{BMS}$ have developed during the adaptation to the serum-free media will be transferred to the hybridoma cell line and make it more probable that this cell line can be established in serum-free medium.

MATERIALS AND METHODS

Media: DMEM is Dulbeccos MEM-Modification DMEM-Powdered Media (Biochrom, Germany) to which is added to final concentration: 3.7 g/l NaHCO$_3$, 2 mM L-glutamine, 1 mM Na-pyruvate, 10 mM Hepes buffer, 5x10^{-5} M mercaptoethanol, 100 IU/ml penicillin, 100 microgram/ml streptomycin.

"

The foetal calf serum is from Biochrom (Germany).

Ultroser HY (IBF, France) is a serum substitute which consist of substances required for the growth of hybridoma cell lines. These substances include: albumin, transferrin, lipids, insulin, vitamins (C and B12) and selenium. The final concentration in the medium is proprietary but the protein concentrations in the final medium (0.6 mg/ml) is about 1/10 of the protein concentration in medium containing 10% FCS.

Basal Medium Supplement (BMS) (Biochrom, Germany) is a serum substitut produced from defined components by using bovine organ extracts. The protein concentration in the final medium (1.5 mg/ml) is about 1/5 of the protein concentration in medium containing 10% FCS.

Fusion-protocol: Different antigens were used for immunizations of (CF1X Balb/c) female mice. Fusions were carried out according to Köhler and Milstein (1) with slight modifications. For each fusion either $X-63_{FCS}$, $X-63_{ultroser}$ or $X-63_{BMS}$ were used, ratio spleen cells/myeloma cells 5:1. The cells used for the fusion (total number 4×10^8) were then divided into the three media (DMEM + 10% FCS, DMEM + 2% ultroser, DMEM + 10% BMS). For each medium the cells were distributed in 5 microtiterplates with 96 wells each. Only 60 wells on each plate were used, which gives a total of 300 wells for each medium.

RESULTS AND DISCUSSION

Cell lines which usually grow in serum supplemented medium can be adapted to medium supplemented with synthetic substances. In this study X-63Ag8.653 has been adapted to medium containing 2% ultroser or 10% BMS by progressively reducing the proportion of serum over a few passages:
1st passage: 50% serum supplemented medium + 50% synthetic medium. 2nd & 3rd passages: 25% serum supplemented medium + 75% synthetic medium. 4th & 5th passages: 10% serum supplemented medium + 90% synthetic medium. 6th passage: 100% synthetic medium.

Figs. 1,2 and 3 show that it is possible to develop hybridomas in the two serum-free media used in this study. If the myeloma cell line is adapted to growth in medium containing 10% FCS (Figs. 1) there is no differences between the results obtained in the two media containing ultroser or BMS regarding the number of wells with hybridomas or the ratio between number of wells with hybridomas and number of wells with antigen specific antibodies. However, the number of wells with hybridomas is significantly higher in FCS than in serum-free media in four out of five experiments, ultroser being slightly better than BMS.

If the myeloma cell line is adapted to medium containing ultroser (Fig.2) there is no significant differences in the number of wells with hybridomas in the three media, and with respect to the number of wells with antigen specific antibodies it is also quite similar in the three media. In general, there are more wells containing hybridomas in all media than in the previous experiments.

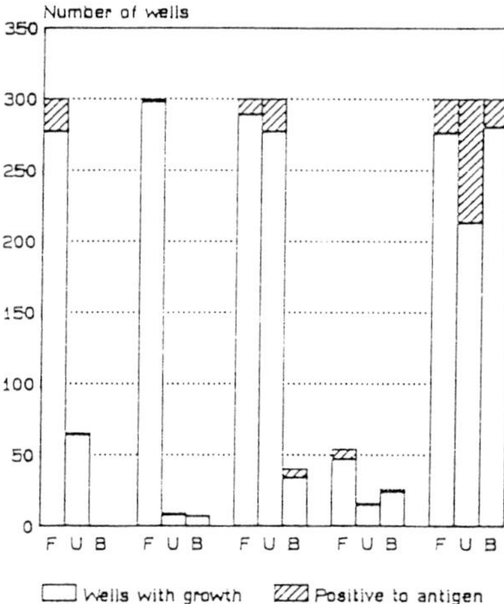

Figure 1. X-63 FCS used for five different fusions which were divided into the three media F:DMEM + 10% FCS, U:DMEM + 2% ultroser, B: DMEM + 10% BMS.

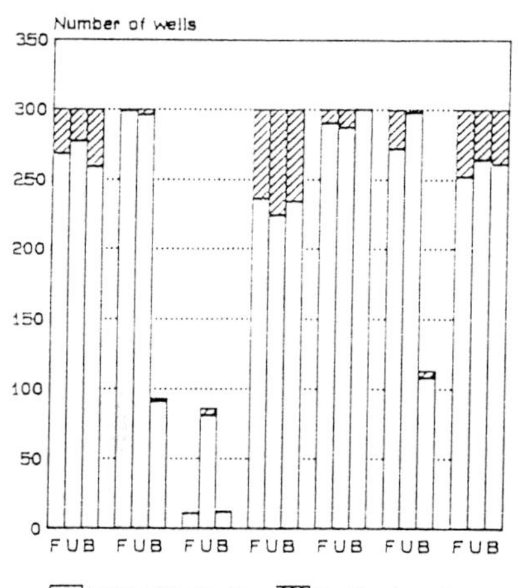

Figure 2. X-63 ultroser used for seven different fusions which were divided into the three media F:DMEM + 10% FCS, U:DMEM + 2% ultroser, B: DMEM + 10% BMS.

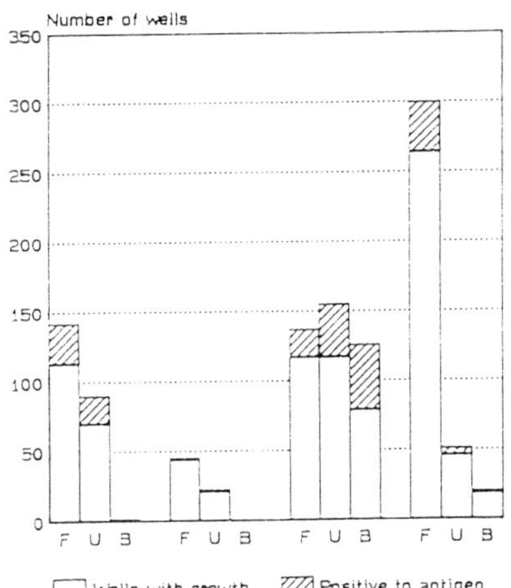

Figure 3. X-63 BMS used for four different fusions which were divided into the three media F:DMEM + 10% FCS, U:DMEM + 2% ultroser, B: DMEM + 10% BMS.

When the myeloma cell line is adapted to medium containing BMS (Fig.3) the number of wells with hybridomas is lower compared to when the other myeloma cell lines were used. In medium containing FCS or ultroser there is no difference in the number of wells containing hybridomas and the number of wells with antigen specific clones is almost identical. In medium containing BMS the cells did not grow well; only in one out of four fusions there was a significant number of hybridomas.

We have thus found, that adaptation of myeloma cells to serum-free media will in some cases give better growth characteristics of hybridoma cells (ultroser), whereas in other cases (BMS) cell growth characteristics turn out to be less advantageous.

REFERENCES

1 Köhler, G., Milstein, C.: Continuous cultures of fused cells secreting antibody of predefined specificity. Nature 1975, 256, 495

DEVELOPMENT OF A LOW-SERUM GROWTH MEDIUM FOR PRODUCTION OF A HUMAN GLYCOPROTEIN BY RECOMBINANT BHK CELLS

G. Schmid[#], H. Zilg[*], and R. Johannsen

Cell Culture Development Group and [*]Research Laboratories of Behringwerke AG, P.O. Box 1140, D-3550 Marburg 1, FRG. [#]Present address: Central Research Laboratories, ZFE/MB, F. Hoffmann-La Roche AG, CH-4002 Basle, Switzerland

ABSTRACT

For anchorage-dependent recombinant BHK cells stimulatory effects of transport proteins, trace elements, hormones, and lipid sources on cell growth and product formation were established. We determined metabolic quotients for glucose, amino acids, lactate, ammonia, fatty acids, and product as well as molar yield coefficients. Cell growth in medium with 0.1% or 0.025% FBS plus supplements was found to be stable for at least 6 weeks (i.e., 6 passages) with a specific growth rate μ_{max} of 0.80 ± 0.05 d^{-1}.

INTRODUCTION

Medium costs account for a substantial amount of the manufacturing costs for therapeutic or diagnostic proteins by mammalian cell culture (1). The design of optimal production media for repeated-batch or continuous culture of hybridomas and recombinant cell lines is therefore an important component in any scale-up process. Besides the need to use low-serum/serum-free media it is important to know specific consumption and production rates for substrates and by-products such as glucose, lactate, pyruvate, glutamine, ammonia, other amino acids, fatty acids, etc. Although knowledge of these requirements will lead to improved media there currently is limited data available on metabolic quotients (2-8).

MATERIALS AND METHODS

Cell lines

Construction of recombinant baby hamster kidney (rBHK) cell lines expressing human antithrombin III (rhATIII) was performed as described before (9,10).

Medium composition and culture conditions

Adherent rBHK ATIII cells were grown in T25 flasks in a 37°C incubator with 5% CO_2 in air. Cultures were seeded at $2.5 \cdot 10E4$ viable cells/mL ($1 \cdot 10E4$ cells/cm^2). Throughout the study Iscove's Modified Dulbecco's medium (IMDM) was used as the basal medium. It was supplemented with 10% FBS (control) or in case of low-serum growth media with 0.1% or 0.01% FBS plus the following additional factors: human transferrin (30% iron-saturated), insulin, monoethanolamine, trypsin inhibitor, fibronectin, and linoleic, oleic, and palmitic acids bound to fatty acid free bovine serum albumin. Details on the medium composition can be found in (8).

Prior to the experiments the tissue culture plastic was treated with 2 mL human fibronectin (50 mg/L) for 1 h at room temperature. Any excess fibronectin was removed by aspiration before the addition of culture medium. The trypsinizing solution contained trypsin at 0.25% (w/v) and EDTA at 0.03% (w/v) in phosphate-buffered saline (PBS). Viable cell concentrations and viability were determined by the trypan blue exclusion method using a hemacytometer.

Metabolite and product analyses

Determinations of amino acid concentrations were performed using a High Performance Amino Acid Analyzer 6300 (Beckman Instruments). Glucose and lactate were assayed with enzymatic analyzers. Free fatty acids (FFA's) were quantitated by gas liquid chromatography of fatty acid methyl esters as reported by Schmid et al. (8). For the analysis of product concentrations culture media were submitted to a specific EIA assay using 98% pure ATIII from human plasma as standard (11).

Estimation of metabolic quotients

Metabolic quotients were estimated from a plot of the metabolite consumption or production vs ($e^{\mu t} - 1$) by using an approach developed by Smiley et al. (12) as previously described (8).

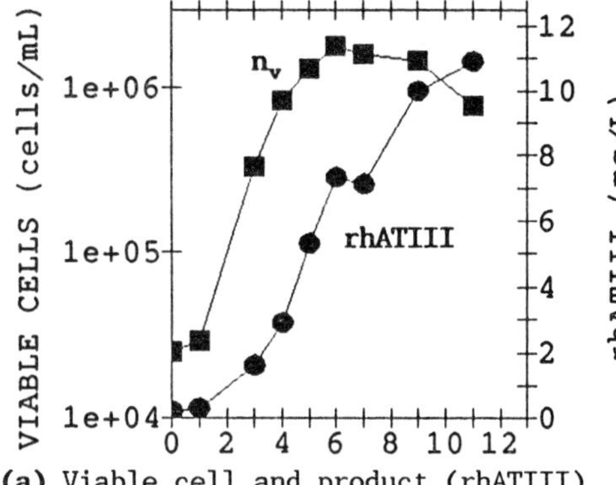

(a) Viable cell and product (rhATIII) concentrations vs culture time

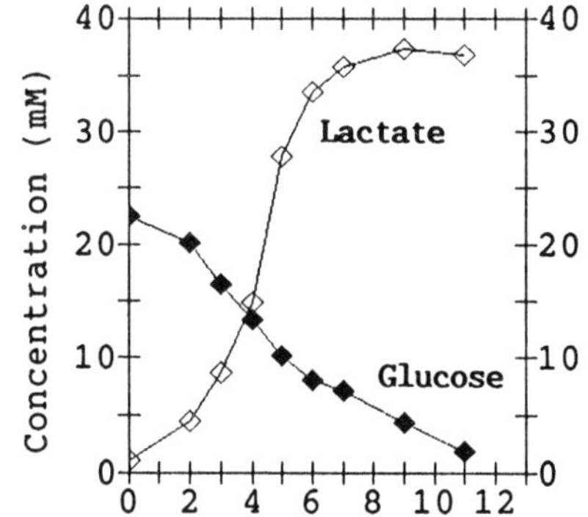

(b) Glucose and lactate concentrations vs culture time

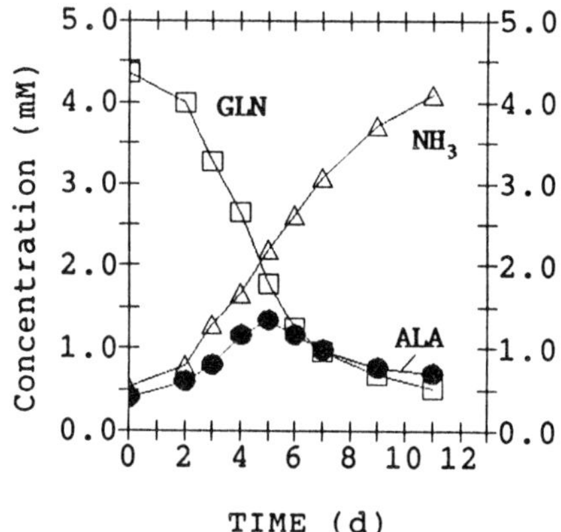

TIME (d)

(c) Glutamine, alanine, and ammonia concentrations vs culture time

Figure 1

Batch growth of adherent rBHK cells producing human antithrombin III

Culture conditions: Iscove's modified Dulbecco's medium with 10% FBS, T25 flasks in a 5% CO_2 incubator at 37°C

METABOLIC QUOTIENTS (mmol/billion cells·d)		
Cell Line IMDM w/	rBHK ATIII 10% FBS	0.1% FBS
μ_{max} (d^{-1})	1.09	0.73
Gluc.	11.29	12.30
Lact.	+14.45	+13.80
GLN	1.57	1.53
NH$_3$	+1.40	+1.28
ASP	0.72	0.23
THR	0.13	0.15
SER	0.37	0.41
ASN	0.01	ND[a]
GLU	0.94	0.35
PRO	0.06	ND[a]
GLY	0.06	0.09
ALA	+1.07	+0.94
VAL	0.21	0.26
CYS	0.04	0.07
MET	0.08	0.08
ILE	0.20	0.26
LEU	0.27	0.31
TYR	0.08	0.13
PHE	0.08	0.10
TRP	0.03	ND[a]
LYS	0.21	0.23
HIS	0.07	0.06
ARG	0.19	0.11

[a] not detectable

Table 1

Specific consumption/production rates for rhATIII producing BHK cells

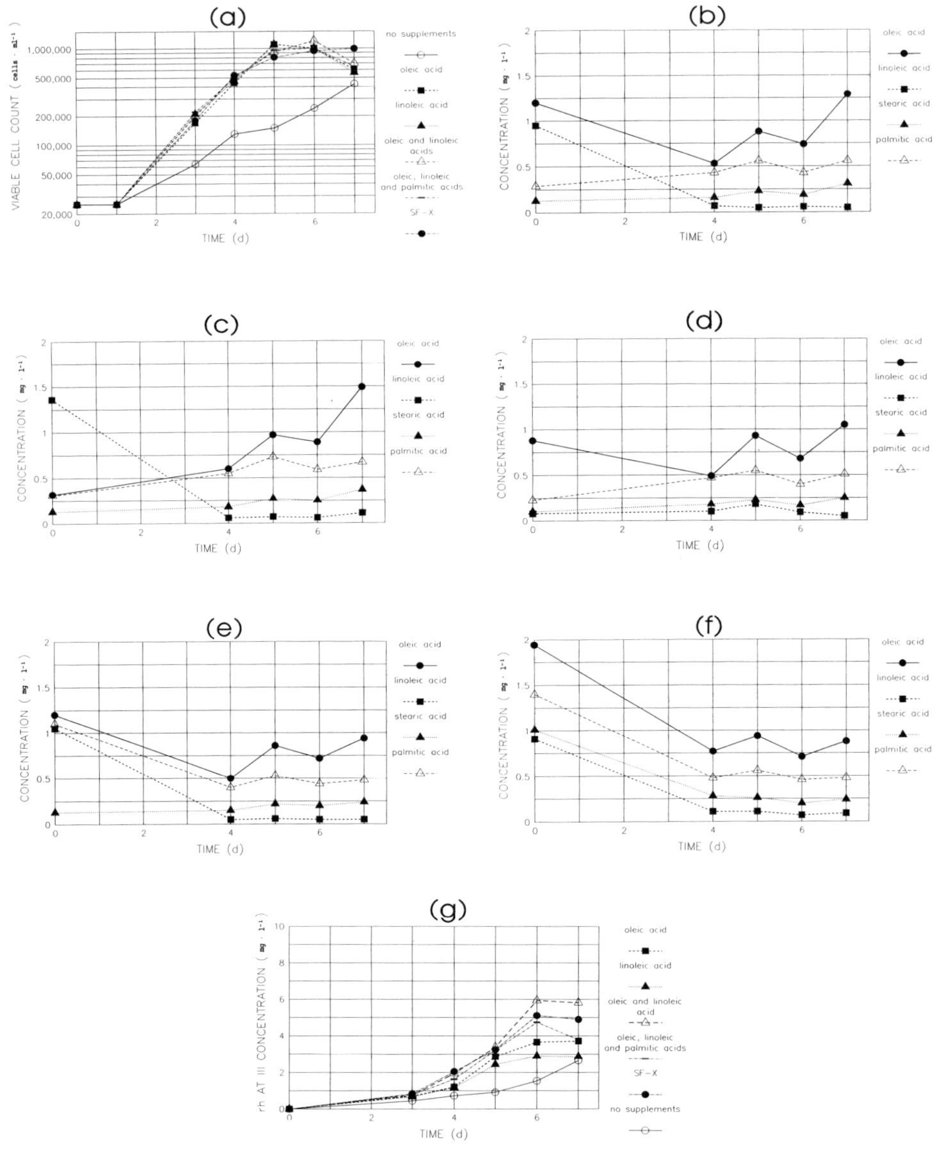

Figure 2

(a) Batch growth curves for recombinant baby hamster kidney (rBHK) cells cultivated in low-serum medium supplemented with free fatty acids in different combinations **(b)-(f)** Utilization of fatty acids for 5 different initial combinations of free fatty acids **(g)** Product (rhATIII) concentration vs time under these conditions

RESULTS AND DISCUSSION

Using an adherent BHK cell line that produces a recombinant human glycoprotein
we did establish the stimulatory effects of (various combinations and concentrations of) transport proteins, trace elements, peptide and steroid hormones, and
lipid sources on cell growth/product formation (data not shown). In our approach
we performed transient experiments whereby cells grown in 0.5% or 0.25% FBS were
seeded at 2.5·10E4 cells/mL in 0.1%, 0.025%, 0.01%, and 0% FBS containing basal
medium plus the respective supplements. From studies in tissue culture flasks we
determined metabolite/byproduct consumption and production rates for glucose,
lactate, ammonia, GLN, amino acids, fatty acids, and product as well as apparent
molar yield coefficients (Figures 1 and 2, Table 1). We observed differences in
metabolic quotients as function of specific growth rate, FBS concentration, and
type of recombinant cell line. Stability of cell growth/product formation was
further assessed in medium with 0.1%, 0.025%, and 0.01% serum plus supplements
over a period of at least 6 weeks (i.e., 6 passages) and found to be impaired
below 0.025% FBS (Figure 3).

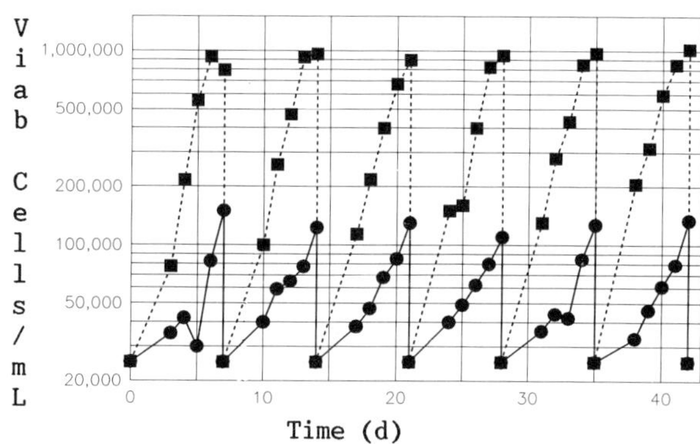

Figure 3

**Stability of rBHK cell growth
in T25 flasks under low-serum
conditions** Cells were passaged
weekly in medium containing
0.1% FBS [circles] or 0.1% FBS
plus supplements (see above)
[squares]; μ_{max} = 0.80±0.05 d^{-1}

ACKNOWLEDGEMENTS

We would like to thank K. Linne–Archinal and M. Weigel for excellent technical
assistance with the tissue culture experiments and A. Tobelander and D. Wehr-
stedt for performing amino acid, fatty acid, and phospholipid analyses.

REFERENCES

1 Griffiths, J. B. TIBTECH 1986, 4, 268
2 Griffiths, J. B., and Pirt, S. J. Proc. Roy. Soc. B. 1967, 168, 421
3 Schmid, G., and Johannsen, R. Biotech. Lett. 1990, in press
4 Miller, W. M. Ph.D. Thesis 1987, University of California, Berkeley, CA
5 Miller, W. M., Blanch, H. W., Wilke, C. R. Biotechnol. Bioeng. 1988, 32, 947
6 Schmid, G., Wilke, C. R., and Blanch, H. W. American Chemical Society National Meeting, Aug 30–Sept 1, 1987, New Orleans, paper no 74
7 Wagner, R., Ryll, T., Krafft, H., and Lehmann, J. Cytotechnol. 1988, 1, 145
8 Schmid, G., Zilg, H., Eberhard, U., and Johannsen, R. J. Biotechnol. 1990,
   in press
9 Zettlmeissl, G., Wirth, M., Hauser, H., and Küpper, H. Behring Inst. Res.
   Comm. 1988, 82, 26
10 Wirth, M., Bode, J., Zettlmeissl, G., and Hauser, H. Gene 1988, 73, 419
11 Zettlmeissl, G., Ragg, H., and Karges, H. Bio/Technology 1987, 5, 720
12 Smiley, A. L., Hu, W.–S., Wang, D. I. C. Biotechnol. Bioeng. 1989, 33, 1182

OPTIMALISATION OF A SERUM FREE MEDIUM FOR LARGE SCALE
CONTINUOUS GROWTH AND IMMUNOGLOBULIN PRODUCTION BY A MOUSE
HYBRIDOMA

Kristin Heirwegh, Toon De Kesel, and Peter De Waele
N.V. INNOGENETICS, Industriepark 7, B-9710 Gent, België

Our aim is the development of a serum free medium that would
contain the lowest possible concentration of added proteins
and would allow the cells to continuously grow and produce
antibody.

Cells adapted to DMEM + 10% serum were seeded three-fold,
without adaptation, in a serum free mixture (SF mix)
containing common additives such as insulin, transferrin, Na-
selenite, glutamine, and BSA. DCCM (Biological Industries,
Israel) with or without a mixture of lipids (LM1) was added.
Total cell counts, viability and immunoglobulin (Ig)
production were determined daily until day 9, when viability
approached zero. Ig production was found to be proportional
to total cell concentration, and could be increased from 30 to
60 μg/ml by adding DCCM; amounts up to 250 μg/ml were reached
by adding DCCM and LM1.

Cells were subcultured for about 30 generations in SF mix +
DCCM +/- LM1. In SF mix alone, adaptation did not occur.
Growth and Ig production were evaluated after this adaptation.
Although growth had slown down slightly, Ig production
remained proportional to total cell concentration. Up to 160
μg/ml Ig was detected in an antigen independent ELISA. This
decline in production was not due to instability as the mouse
hybridoma was shown to be stable for over 250 generations in
DMEM + 10% serum. The same production levels were reached in
both media: on Day 6 with DCCM + LM1, but only on Day 9 with
DCCM alone, and were again reflected by the growth curves.

The same trend of parallel growth and Ig production (up to 160
μg/ml at Day 8 was found when replacing DCCM by completely BSA
free low protein medium (LPM, developed by Dr. L. Kaspy of
Biological Industries) and simultaneously eliminating BSA from
the SF mix for easy downstream processing. Another LM
composition (LM2) seemed to stimulate growth and Ig production
even more, up to 220 μg/ml at Day 8.

Adaptation of cells to different basic media + 10% serum with
the aim of ulteriorly combining them without serum along with
the selected serum free additives revealed that growth could
be improved by replacing our SF mix in DMEM/Ham F-12, High GEM
(Flow Labs) and PFHM-2 (Gibco). Ig production almost equalled
cell growth except for High GEM whereby production tended to
be lower than cell growth, and for PFHM-2 which showed a
tendency towards higher production/cell. In a serum free
combination with DCCM or LPM and a lipid mixture, DMEM/Ham F-
12 and PFHM-2 seem to be most promising (work in progress).

Longterm Serum-Free Culture of Murine Hybridomas

*S.A. Clark, A. J. Racher and J.B. Griffiths : The Animal
Cell Technology Group, Division of Biologics, The Centre for
Applied Microbiology and Research, Public Health Laboratory
Service, Porton Down, Salisbury, Wilts. UK.*

Abstract

We have established a sub-clone of the murine hybridoma
C1E3, termed C1E3.10. This sub-clone was derived by
adaptation to the serum-free/defined medium Excell 300 (1),
followed by recloning for high antibody secretion.
Production of monoclonal antibody in stationary flask
cultures gave similar results in both serum containing and
EXCELL 300 medium.
Using this cell line we have monitored the production of
monoclonal antibody in EXCELL 300 over an extended period of
culture, greater than 75 days, in a small scale cell
entrapment bioreactor, (Dynacell).
The levels of glucose, lactic acid and glutamine in the
reservoir of the bioreactor were monitored and analysed.
Variations in concentration of lactic acid, in particular,
had a profound effect on the rate of antibody production.

Introduction

The adaptation of most hybridomas to grow and secrete
monoclonal antibody (McAB) in serum-free/defined media is
possible providing care is taken in the adaptation
procedure. The best results are generally seen when a
stepwise adaptation method is used (1).
The level of McAB secreted in the adapted cell line is often
substantially lower than the original. By cloning the
adapted cell line we have successfully selected high
secreting clones from recently adapted cell lines.
We have been studying a hybridoma (C1E3) which secretes an
IgG_3 McAB which binds to *Toxoplasma gondii* (2) and is
currently incorporated in a diagnostic screening kit.

Methods

Media : Two media were used in this study. The basal medium
for the hybridomas was RPMI 1640 containing 10mM HEPES
(Imperial Labs, UK.). EXCELL 300 (JR Scientific,
California) was supplied with or without Phenol red as a
powder which was reconstituted in water. A liquid
supplement was then added and the medium sterile filtered.
The protein concentration in EXCELL 300 is 7-10ug/ml (1).

<u>Figure (1) : Spinner Culture of C1E3.10.</u>

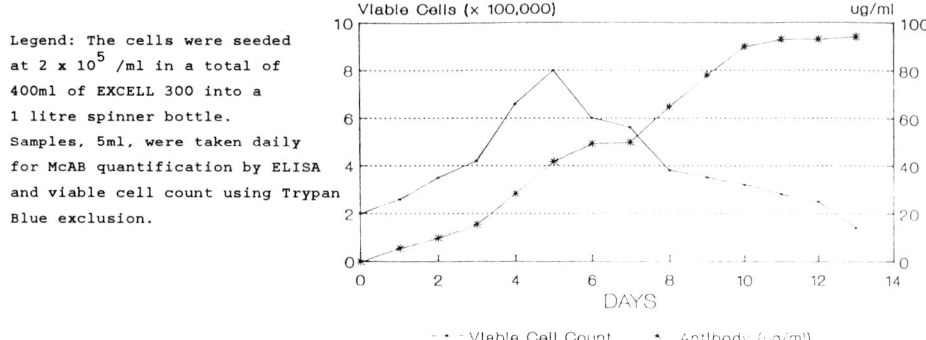

Legend: The cells were seeded at 2 x 10^5 /ml in a total of 400ml of EXCELL 300 into a 1 litre spinner bottle. Samples, 5ml, were taken daily for McAB quantification by ELISA and viable cell count using Trypan Blue exclusion.

Adaptation and selection of clone C1E3.10 : The hybridoma cell line C1E3 was adapted to grow in the serum-free/defined medium EXCELL 300 (JR Scientific) some time ago (1). Briefly, a stepwise approach from 10% FCS was taken. The cell line was grown for three to four weeks in basal medium containing 5% Control Process Serum Replacement (CPSR1) (Sigma, UK), which has an equivalent protein content to 1% FCS. The medium was then changed to EXCELL 300 and the growth of the cells monitored over a further four weeks. Having established a culture which was growing in EXCELL 300, cloning in serum containing medium with mouse macrophage feeder cells was undertaken to select a high McAB secreting clone, termed C1E3.10.
The characteristic McAB secretion pattern of the new clone was assessed in a spinner culture (Techne, UK), see Fig 1.

Quantification of Monoclonal Antibody Levels : The concentration of McAB in the culture supernatants was assessed by a quantitative ELISA assay, which has previously been described (1). ELISA plates were coated with a truncated version of Staphyloccocal Protein-A, produced as a recombinant product in E. coli (Porton Products), at 100 ng/ml. The conjugate was sheep F(ab)$_2$ anti-mouse Ig coupled to horseradish peroxidase (HRP) and the chromogen was tetramethylbenzidine.
Each sample was tested over 10 doubling dilutions and the concentration assessed against standard C1E3 McAB purified by a cationic exchange column MonoS (Pharmacia, Sweden) on FPLC.

Metabolite Assays : The daily samples from the bioreactor were assayed for glucose and lactate concentration by a glucose/lactate analyser (Yellow Springs Instruments, USA). Glutamine concentration was assessed using an assay based on glutamine synthetase (3).

<u>Figure (2) : Key Parameter Levels in C1E3.10 DYNACELL Culture.</u>

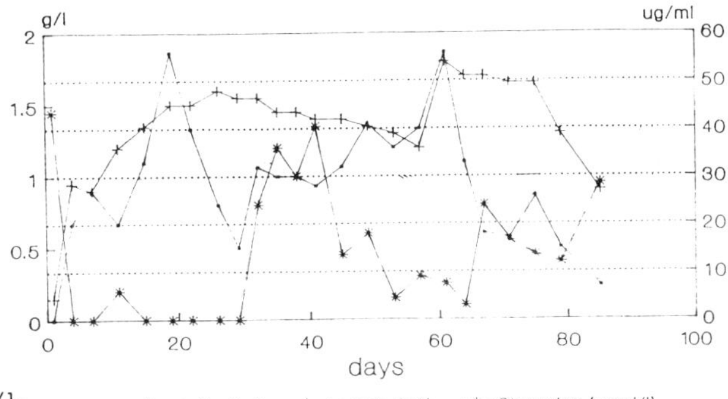

Culture of C1E3.10 in the DYNACELL Cell Entrapment Bioreactor : The Dynacell (Millipore, UK) is a small cell entrapment bioreactor. The cell cassette has a total volume of 12.5 ml and is fed by a reservoir of 1 litre of medium which is continually perfusing the reactor.
Initially, the cassette was perfused with 500ml of basal medium containing 5% FCS overnight, the next day the reactor was seeded with 10^8 C1E3.10 cells in basal medium containing 5% FCS.
Samples, 5ml, were taken daily from the media reservoir and assessed for glucose, lactate, glutamine and McAB concentration, see Fig 2.

Results

Analysis of McAB Secretion by C1E3.10 in Spinner Culture : The spinner culture was run for 13 days, by which time the percentage of viable cells had dropped to 11%. The secretion of McAB and growth curve seen in this culture demonstrated that C1E3.10 is a hybridoma which secretes McAB all through the culture and does not produce increased amounts during the stationary/decline phase of growth. The decline in growth of the culture started to occur as the glutamine became exhausted, this was accompanied by a burst of lactate production (data not shown). The steady McAB production rate during both growth and stationary phases of C1E3.10 made it an ideal hybridoma to use in a continuous batch production system like the Dynacell, see Fig 1.

<u>Figure (3) : Summary of Antibody Production in the Longterm
C1E3.10 DYNACELL Culture.</u>

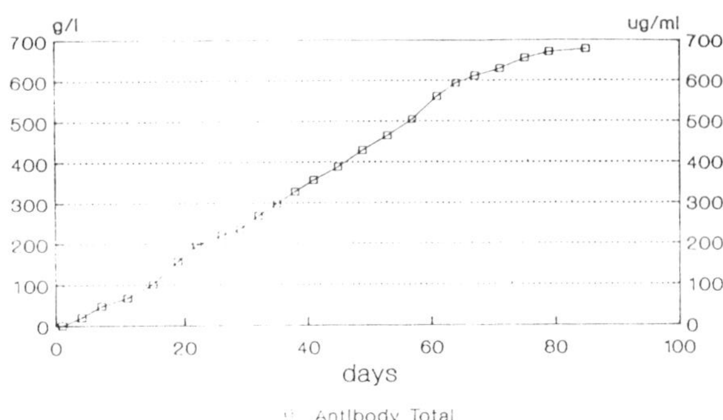

Antibody Secretion of C1E3.10 in the DYNACELL: During the
initial establishment period of the culture, 8 days, the
perfusion medium was RPMI1640 containing 5% FCS.
2 litres of supernatant were generated in that period at a
mean McAB production rate of 5.9 mg/day.
During the subsequent period of culture, 72 days, EXCELL 300
medium alone was used. The rate of McAB production in EXCELL
300 varied considerably, a maximum rate of 14.5 mg/day was
achieved in the third EXCELL 300 media change, see Fig 3.

Metabolic Status of C1E3.10 in the DYNACELL : The variations
in McAB production rate can be related to the metabolic
status of the cells in the bioreactor. Using the key
metabolic indicators, lactate and glutamine the culture was
monitored throughout, see Fig 2.
Lactate levels in the reservoir increased gradually during
the first 20 days of culture with no apparent effect on the
increasing rate of McAB production. When the lactate
concentration reached 1.5g/l, a rapid decline in the rate of
McAB production was seen.
A high lactate concentration was occurring concomitantly
with low glutamine concentrations, suggesting that the cells
had switched carbon source from glutamine to glucose. To
reduce the lactate concentration it was decided to provide
the cells with more glutamine to delay the switch between
carbon sources. Consequently, 4 mmoles of glutamine was
added to each litre of medium used from day 32.

This had the desired effect as the rate of McAB production began to rise and the concentration of lactate began to decline until by day 57 there was only 1.2 g/l of lactate in the end culture supernatant. The next litre of EXCELL 300 produced a peak of McAB but the lactate again rose sharply, despite the presence of the additional glutamine. From that point on the culture rapidly declined in glucose consumption rate and McAB production until it stopped turning over glucose on day 84.

Discussion

The Dynacell bioreactor has been shown, in this study, to be an ideal system for batch production of McAB on a small scale. Due to the low level of turbulence in the system the hybridoma cells do not require agents such as Pluronic, to protect them from shear forces.
From an initial inoculum of 10^8 cells over 0.6 grams of McAB was obtained in 20-25 litres of EXCELL 300 over a period of 2-3 months ie. 50-100 mg/week.
The relationship between the consumption of glutamine and the production of lactate appeared critical to the continued survival of the culture. By supplementing the medium with excess glutamine the level of lactate production was controlled for a time. However, this was only a temporary measure because the glutamine utilisation rate increased so that eventually the higher levels were utilised in the same time span as the original glutamine levels. When all of the glutamine was being consumed the control of lactate production was again lost and a sharp rise detected.
Therefore, the maintenance of a high enough glutamine concentration to ensure that the rate of lactate production is kept in check appears to be an essential factor in the establishment of a longterm hybridoma culture in the Dynacell bioreactor.
Further work with this bioreactor system is planned in which other hybridomas are used and the level of glutamine is varied to design the best conditions for longterm growth and stable McAB secretion.

Acknowledgements

The authors wish to thank Anita Bone for technical assistance, Porton Developments for financial contributions and Jayne Gosney in the preparation of this manuscript.

References

(1) S.A. Clark, D. Looby and J.B. Griffiths. (1989) In
    "Advances in Animal Cell Biology and Biotechnology for
    Bioprocesses", pp. 291-297, Ed. Spier, R.E.,
    Butterworths, UK.
    Title : The adaptation of hybridoma cell lines to grow
            and secrete monoclonal antibody in serum-free/
            defined medium.

(2) J.P. Wright and A.H. Balfor (1983) Parasitology 87:LXVI
    Title : Monoclonal antibodies to *Toxoplasma gondii*.

(3) Mecke, D. (1984) In "Methods of Enzymatic Analysis"
    Volume VIII, Metabolites 3: Lipids, Amino Acids and
    Related Compounds, pp. 364-369, Eds. Bergmeyer, H. U.,
    Bergmeyer, J and Grayssl, M. Verlag Chemie, Weinheim.

Serum-free media suitable for upstream and downstream processing

Volker Jäger

Gesellschaft für Biotechnologische Forschung mbH, Mascheroder Weg 1, D-3300 Braunschweig, Fed. Rep. Germany

Abstract

During the past decade the use of serum-free media has become a standard method for the cultivation of most mammalian cell lines which are of importance for the production of biotechnologically relevant products such as biopharmaceuticals. More recently, there have been also successful efforts in the development of protein-free media for various cell lines. Ideally these media should facilitate and simplify downstream processing, reduce costs and minimize risk of virus and bacterial contamination. In addition, productivity of several cell lines could be increased. However, not all media which support the growth of cells in culture flasks are suitable when used in large-scale fermenters, which expose the cells to mechanical stress and to homogeneous conditions without microenvironments. Downstream processing is indeed simplified in protein-poor or protein-free media, but the lack of protective carrier proteins leads to increased product degradation by proteases released from the cells, which occurs even in viable cultures. Thus, necessary compromises have to be made between the requirements for upstream and downstream processes in order to facilitate an optimal product quality.

Supplements for serum-free media

The major advantage using serum as a medium supplement is its universality as a source of nutrients, growth factors, carrier proteins and attachment factors. Serum-free media have to be tailored according to the individual requirements of the cell lines. A wide variety of supplements have been described to support growth and production of mammalian cell lines (Barnes, 1987). Some of the most frequently used factors are listed in Table I:

Table I: *Supplements for serum-free media*

		Carrier:
1.	Carrier proteins and peptides	
	Albumins (BSA, HSA, Ovalbumin)	
	Lipoproteins (HDL, LDL)	
	Transferrin (human, bovine)	
	Glycyl-histidyl-lysine (GHL, Liver growth factor)	
2.	Lipids, steroids, fatty acids and precursors	
	Phospholipids: Phosphatidyl ethanolamine, – choline	HDL
	Cholesterol	LDL
	Oleic acid, linoleic acid, linolenic acid	Albumin
	Ethanolamine, Phosphoethanolamine	

3.   Growth factors and hormones

PDGF	(platelet-derived growth factor)
EGF	(epidermal growth factor)
bFGF	(fibroblast growth factor)
Interleukin-2	(T-cell growth factor)
Interleukin-6	(B-cell growth factor, hybridoma growth factor)
IGF-I	(insulin-like growth factor)
Insulin	

Hydrocortison, Dexamethason, Testosteron, Progesteron, Triiodothyronin, Somatostatin, Prostaglandins, etc.

---

4.   Attachment factors

In media:	Matrix precoating:
Fibronectin	Collagen
Fetuin	Poly-L-lysine
Laminin	
Fibrinogen	
Serum spreading factor	

---

5.   Protease inhibitors

Soy bean trypsin inhibitor (SBTI)
Pancreatic secretory trypsin inhibitor (PSTI)
α_1-Antitrypsin
Aprotinin

---

6.   Improvements of basic media

Vitamins: Alphatocopherol, Biotin
Inorganic Salts: Mg^{2+}, Ca^{2+}, Zn^{2+}, SeO_3^{2-}, various trace elements
Components influencing redox potential:
        Ascorbic acid, Glutathion, 2-Mercaptoethanol,
        α-Thioglycerol, etc.

Carrier proteins are one of the most important factors in serum-free media. Components which are toxic to cells in an unbound form (e.g. fatty acids), which are highly insoluble in aquous solutions (e.g. cholesterol) or which cannot penetrate the cellular membrane in normal concentration (e.g. iron), can be incorporated by the cells by means of specific carrier proteins.

Albumins, mostly of bovine or human origin, are mainly used as a carrier for lipids, steroids and fatty acids (Yamane, 1978; Sato *et al.* 1984), but have also protective functions because of their capacity to bind heavy metal ions, detergents and endotoxins. Bovine or human lipoproteins are carriers of a variety of lipids, high density lipoprotein contains mainly phospholipids, low density lipoprotein contains mainly cholesterol. They are only essential for cells with high requirements of lipids and cholesterol or cell lines which cannot synthesize these compounds *de novo* (Kawamoto *et al.* 1983) and need a specific carrier for receptor mediated endocytosis. Transferrin is responsible for the supply of cells with iron. In contrast to lipoproteins, which are mostly degraded after incorporation, transferrin can be recycled by the cells (Dautry-Varsat *et al.,* 1983). Holotransferrin binds to the receptor and the complex is incorporated by endocytosis. The endocytic vesicle is transported to a lysosom where iron is released under acidic conditions. Apotransferrin has a much lower affinity to the receptor and will be released into the medium after the vesicle has reached again the outer membrane of the cell. Glycyl-histidyl-lysine, better known as liver growth factor, is a copper binding peptide which supports growth of several cell lines (Pickart *et al.*, 1973).

Fatty acids, steroids and lipids are essential for a number of cell lines (Yamane, 1978; Sato *et al.* 1984; Murakami *et al.* 1982b) and have to be added normally in combination with a carrier protein. Lipid precursors such as ethanolamine or phosphoethanolamine are also found to be essential for growth of several cell lines (Murakami *et al.* 1982a).

Growth factors and hormones are used in a wide variety for the cultivation of mammalian cells and only the most important factors are listed in Table I. Normally, the spectrum of growth stimulatory activity is limited to a specific type of cells but not to a certain species, which is in contrast to carrier proteins, where the species plays an important role for receptor binding and biological activity. On the contrary, growth factors are relatively conservative molecules and only slight variations between different species could be observed. Platelet-derived growth factor, epidermal growth factor and fibroblast growth factors are growth promoting for most fibroblast-like cell lines but porcine bFGF has also been found to stimulate growth of a human myeloma cell line (Jäger *et al.* 1988). Interleukin-2 is essential for T-cells and some T-cell derived lymphomas, interleukin-6 stimulates growth of B-cells and some hybridomas. In contrast to these proteins, insulin-like growth factor and insulin have a broad spectrum of activity as they increase the metabolic activity and DNA replication of most mammalian cell lines. The hormones listed in Table I are found to be important for several cell lines but are of debatable value for most cell lines used for large-scale processes (e.g. hybridomas, BHK-21, CHO).

Attachment factors are necessary for all anchorage dependent cells or cells which grow spreaded on a matrix when grown in serum-supplemented media and which should grow with a similar morphology under serum-free conditions (i.e. not suspended). Some of these factors are dissolved in the medium whilst others are precoated on the matrix (e.g. culture flask, microcarrier, etc.).

Protease inhibitors are essential for serum-free inactivation of trypsin after detachment of cells from the matrix. Some of them have exhibited growth promoting activities.

Finally, a number of low molecular weight compounds like vitamins and trace elements could be essential when serum is omitted. Therefore, improved basic media have been developed which already include these components (Table II) and which are routinely used for serum-free cell culture. The most widely used media composition DMEM/Ham's F12 was shown to be inferior to IMDM/Ham's F12 which is now used at GBF in a slight modification as basic medium for serum-free culture (Table III).

Table II: *Common basic media for serum-free cultivations*

DMEM	:	Ham's F12		1 : 1
RPMI 1640	:	DMEM	: Ham's F12	2 : 1 : 1
DMEM	:	RPMI 1640		1 : 1
IMDM	:	Ham's F12		1 : 1

A useful serum-free medium should provide comparable growth to serum-supplemented medium, not only in culture flasks but also under the conditions of a large-scale production process (Fig. 1) which is often more rigorous to cells in view of the fact of mechanical stress by agitation and gas bubbles. This stress can be reduced by protective proteins (e.g. BSA) or carbohydrate polymers (e.g. PEG, dextran) which increase the viscosity of the medium. Most of anchorage-independent cell lines are now routinely cultivated in serum-free media for industrial-scale processes, irrespective whether they normally grow in suspension such as hybridomas or have to be adapted to suspended growth such as recombinant CHO or BHK-21 cell lines.

However, efforts have to be made for the development of serum-free media for large-scale cultivation of either anchorage-dependent cell lines or other cells which should grow attached to a matrix as part of the production process. The attachment of standard production cell lines such as CHO or BHK-21 on non-porous microcarriers is drastically reduced in serum-free media. Attachment of the cells can be achieved by using a serum-supplemented medium during the initial growth phase and a subsequent medium exchange to serum-free culture conditions (Blasey *et al.*, 1988). The disadvantages of such a method are the remaining agents of serum origin, and very often attachment to the carriers is markedly reduced after serum is totally removed. An alternative is the addition of defined attachment factors to the media composition (e.g. fibronectin, fetuin, laminin, thrombospondin, fibrinogen, serum spreading factor) and precoating of the matrix material (e.g. with collagen, poly-L-lysine). Unfortunately, most cell lines require several factors for good attachment which increase the media costs tremendously.

Significantly higher production in serum-free medium is normally resulted by high producing subclones. In these cases it is useful to establish master cell banks after adaption to serum-free medium and subsequent testing. Slight increases of production can be observed also if serum components have diminished product formation and secretion or if they have affected product yield by inactivating the product.

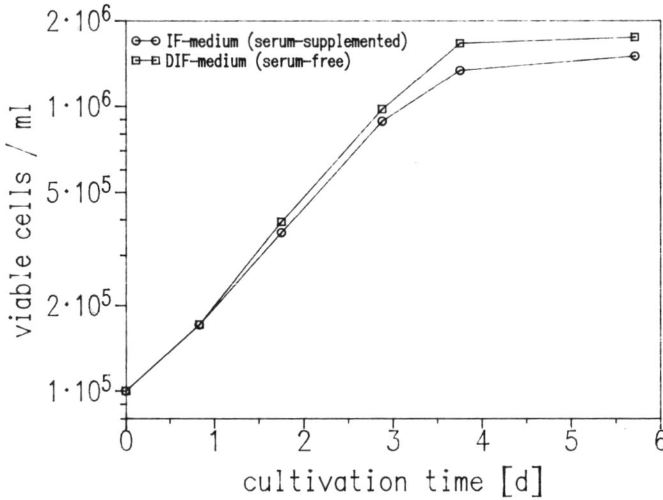

Fig.1:   Growth of Ag8.653 myeloma cells in serum-supplemented and serum-free DIF-medium.

Media requirements for production and genomic stability

Another important parameter, which is mostly overlooked, is the stability of the cell line under serum-free culture conditions. Hybridoma cells showed a reduced stability in product formation compared with their production in serum-supplemented media. To give an example, the rat-mouse heterohybridoma 187.1 (ATCC HB58), cultivated in our laboratory for more than 1½ years (more than 230 passages) was absolutely stable in antibody production when grown in medium supplemented with 10% FCS. The same cell line, which could be adapted easily to our serum-free 'DIF-medium' (Jäger *et al.* 1988) at comparable growth rates, ceased production after 3 - 6 months (40 - 80 passages) of cultivation in this medium. The growth rate of the cells was slightly increased at this time indicating that a non-producing subclone started to overgrow the producing cells. The same phenomenon was observed with a number of other hybridomas. Obviously, serum contains factors which protect these cells against genomic instability. The identification of these stabilizing components could result in further improvements in the development of serum-free media.

Strategies for reduction of media costs

One of the most important reasons for the efforts in development of serum-free media is unquestionably the reduction of media costs. The use of commercially available media is commonly not profitable because most of these media are more expensive than standard media supplemented with 10% FCS. In addition, the self-development of the medium results mostly in better growth and productivity due to the individual tailoring according to the requirements of the cell line, which is not possible with a medium of unknown composition. Costs of a process medium for large-scale production of monoclonal antibodies is listed in Table III.

Table III: *Costs of a process medium for large-scale production of monoclonal antibodies (without filtration, water, manpower, etc.)*

Component		Costs per 1000 litres
Basic medium:		
50% Iscove's MDM wo. Hepes buffer		529.00 $
50% Ham's medium F12		
NaHCO$_3$	(3.61 g$\cdot$l^{-1})	17.00 $
Sodium pyruvate	(2 mmol$\cdot$l^{-1})	50.00 $
L-glutamine	(3 mmol$\cdot$l^{-1})	65.00 $
Ethanolamine	(20 μmol$\cdot$l^{-1})	0.14 $
Suppl. amino acids according to the individual consumption rate of the cell line		36.86 $
Protein supplements:		
Human serum albumin (HSA)	(833 mg$\cdot$l^{-1})	1740.00 $
Human transferrin (iron saturated)	(4.2 mg$\cdot$l^{-1})	395.00 $
Bovine insulin	(10 mg$\cdot$l^{-1})	735.00 $
Total:		3568.00 $

Compromises have to be made using expensive growth factors (e.g. bFGF, EGF, PDGF, IGF-I, IL-6, etc.) Although used in very low concentrations, supplementation of these factors increase media costs drastically and if not essential for cell growth and maintenance they should be omitted whenever posssible, even when the growth rate is slightly reduced. However, in the near future recombinant growth factors at reasonable prices will offer new chances in development and optimization of serum-free media in large-scale mammalian cell culture.

Once successfully cultivated in a bioreactor, cells can often be adapted to growth in media with reduced protein concentrations (Fig.2). A further reduction can be achieved at higher cell concentrations in perfusion culture due to accumulation of autocrine growth factors which can stimulate cell division in media without exogenous growth factors. Unfortunately some of these growth factors are not yet identified. Comparison of four recombinant BHK-21 cell lines producing interferon-ß, interleukin-2, antithrombin III or platelet derived growth factor AA dimers and routinely cultivated in our laboratory showed that the PDGF-AA producing cell line grew significantly faster than the other cell lines indicating that the product also acts as an autocrine growth factor. Retention of carrier proteins within the bioreactor could be an attractive method because some of them can be recycled by the cells. In hollow fibre bioreactors albumin and transferrin can be retained within the extracapillary space together with cells and product and have to be replenished only when product is harvested from this compartment (Jäger et al., 1989).

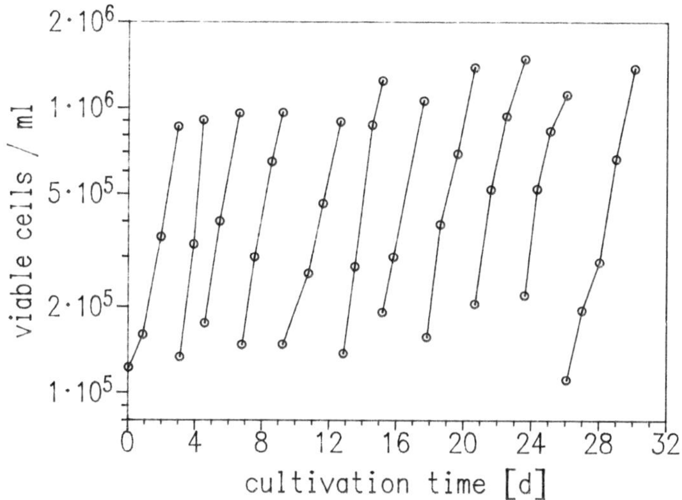

Fig.2:   Repeated batch fermentation of hybridoma cell line 187.1. BSA content of the medium was reduced from 1 g/l to 0.5 g/l on day 9. The growth rate decreased from 0.058 h⁻¹ to 0.027 h⁻¹ combined with a reduced viability (from 92% to 65%). After one batch cells had adapted to the modified culture conditions and the growth rate increased again to 0.058 h⁻¹.

Most cell lines which are used for large-scale cultivation are of rodent or primate origin. Despite of this fact most of the protein supplements are of bovine origin because they are available in large quantities at low costs. Rodent proteins are too expensive due to the limited size of the donors, but human proteins appear to have higher affinities to receptors of rodent cells than their bovine analogues. Therefore media costs could be significantly reduced using carrier proteins from the right species (which might be more expensive on a per gram basis) at reduced concentrations. For the cultivation of several murine hybridomas which did not grow without transferrin even in the presence of high concentrations of ferric citrate (500 μM), human transferrin could be reduced down to 200 μg/l. About 100 mg/l of bovine transferrin had to be added to reach comparable growth.

In other cases carrier proteins can be replaced by low molecular weight substitutes. Transferrin can be substituted by iron chelates or high concentrations of highly soluble iron salts (Kovar and Franek, 1987; Kovar, 1988; Merten et al., 1989) but in contrast to human cell lines most murine cell lines are dependent on the protein. Albumin which acts mainly as a carrier of fatty acids can be replaced by cyclodextrin- fatty acid complexes (Yamane et al., 1982). However, growth is most often significantly reduced indicating that albumin plays also a lot of other important roles such as detoxification of the medium by absorption of detergents and heavy metal ions.

The use of protein-free media in large-scale bioreactors is still an exception. A BHK-21 cell line producing interleukin-2 was cultivated successfully in our laboratory using a protein-free medium (Lucki-Lange and Wagner, 1990) but shear forces are extraordinary low in this stirred tank bioreactor. Other recombinant BHK-21 cell lines although transfected identically did not grow in this medium. Several other protein-free media have been developed for cultivation in culture flasks but they did not work in stirred tanks without additional protein supplements (Cleveland et al., 1983; Merten et al., 1989), demonstrating that the role of autocrine growth factors, individual media tailoring and design of bioreactors is becoming of major importance using protein-free media.

Media requirements for downstream processing and strategies to optimize product quality

Another reason for the efforts to establish routinely serum-free cultivation processes for industrial scale production of biopharmaceuticals is the ease of product purification. Serum-free media also eliminate or at least reduce significantly the risk of contamination of virus or other infectious agents derived from serum and therefore simplify the validation of the production process according to GMP guidelines and acceptance by regulatory organs.

The requirements for media in downstream processes are normally contrary to the requirements for upstream processes in view of the total protein concentration. Media should not contain contaminating proteins with a structure, size or IEP similar to the product. To give an example, bovine IgG is a problematic contaminant in a purification process for mouse, rat or human monoclonal antibodies, but also transferrin can cause difficulties, especially when the IEP of the monoclonal antibody is in a similar range. These reasons indicate again, that an ideal serum-free medium is a medium totally free of protein supplements. Nonetheless cell derived proteins cannot be eliminated. Depending on the culture conditions, the viability of the culture and the specific behaviour of the cell line itself the cell derived protein concentration is in a range from 50 to 500 mg/l. Cellular proteins normally contain a variety of proteases which may cause problems and have to be considered to optimize product quality. Supplemented proteins (e.g. albumins) could be necessary as protectants against product degradation by proteases serving as a substrate in competition with the product. Protease concentration was thought to be a problem related with decreasing cell viability but recent data indicate that most of these proteases are released actively into the medium by viable cells (Lind et al. 1990). This secretion is associated with cell growth and cannot be influenced by the cultivation process, so it might be useful to add protease inhibitors for inactivation of these cell derived proteases. Another important parameter for protease activity is the pH of the supernatant. A low protease activity at neutral pH does not indicate a low protease content in the supernatant (Schlaeger *et al.* 1987; Rudge *et al.* 1987; Karl *et al.* 1990). During purification of the product it might be necessary to shift the pH to alkaline or acidic conditions (e.g. affinity chromatography) resulting in an increased protease activity (Rudge *et al.* 1990).

Sera naturally contain large amounts of protease inhibitors, mainly α_1-antitrypsin, keeping the protease activity in serum-supplemented media low.

A number of protease inhibitors such as pancreatic secretory trypsin inhibitor (PSTI), soy bean trypsin inhibitor (SBTI) or aprotinin could be used as a supplement in serum-free media, but only aprotinin appeared to have a sufficient stability and a spectrum wide enough for efficient inhibition of most serine proteases. Nevertheless aprotinin inhibited only parts of the total protease activity in the supernatant as shown in Table IV.

Table IV: *Inhibition of protease activity by aprotinin (Data from Lind et al., 1990)*

Cell line	Percentage of maximum inhibition of total protease activity by aprotinin
BHK-21pSVIL2	50 %
Hybridoma 412	20 %

References

Barnes, D.W. (1984) Attachment factors in cell culture. In: J. Mather (ed.) Mammalian cell culture: The use of serum-free hormone supplemented media, Plenum Press, NY, pp. 195 - 237

Barnes, D.W. (1987) Serum-free animal cell culture. BioTechniques **5**, 534 - 542

Blasey, H.D., W. Grossebüter, J. Lehmann, H. Giehring, D. Schwengers (1988) Beta-Interferon production in serum-free medium on a new type of microcarrier. Proc. of the Engineering Foundation Conference on Cell Culture Engineering, Palm Coast, Florida, p. W10

Chatzisavido, N., K. Lie, E. Lindner-Olsson (1989) Insulin-like growth factor I (IGF-I) stimulates the production of monoclonal antibodies in serum-free medium. In: R.E. Spier, J.B. Griffiths, J. Stephenne, P.J. Crooy (eds.) Advances in animal cell biology and technology for bioprocesses. Butterworths, pp. 283-286

Cleveland, W.L., I. Wood, B.F. Erlanger (1983) Routine large-scale production of monoclonal antibodies in a protein-free culture medium. J. Immunol. Methods **56**, 221 - 234

Dautry-Varsat, A., A. Ciechanover, H.F. Lodish (1983) pH and the recycling of transferrin during receptor-mediated endocytosis. Proc. Natl. Acad. Sci. USA **80**, 2258 - 2262

Eichner, W., V. Jäger, D. Herbst, H. Hauser, J. Hoppe (1989) Large-scale preparation of recombinant platelet-derived growth factor AA secreted from recombinant baby hamster kidney cells. Eur. J. Biochem. **185**, 135 - 140

Flier, J.S., P. Usher, A.C. Moses (1985) Monoclonal antibody to the type I insulin-like growth factor (IGF-I) receptor blocks IGF-I receptor-mediated DNA-synthesis: Clarification of the mitogenic mechanisms of IGF-I and insulin in human skin fibroblasts. Proc. Natl. Acad. Sci. USA **83**, 664 - 668

Jäger, V., J. Lehmann, P. Friedl (1988) Serum-free growth medium for the cultivation of a wide spectrum of mammalian cells in stirred bioreactors. Cytotechnology **1**, 319 - 329

Jäger, V., W. Eichner, J. Lehmann (1989) Production of human PDGF-A in a stirred tank perfusion reactor and in a hollow fiber reactor system. In: R.E. Spier, J.B. Griffiths, J. Stephenne, P.J. Crooy (eds.) Advances in animal cell biology and technology for bioprocesses. Butterworths, pp. 323 - 326

Karl, D.W., M. Donovan, M.C. Flickinger (1990) A novel acid proteinase released by hybridoma cells. Cytotechnology **3**, 157 - 169

Kawamoto, T., J.D. Sato, A. Le, D.B. McClure, G.H. Sato (1983) Development of a serum-free medium for growth of NS-1 mouse myeloma cells and its application to the isolation of NS-1 hybridomas. Anal. Biochem. **130**, 445 - 453

Kovár, J., F. Franek (1987) Iron compounds at high concentrations enable hybridoma growth in a protein-free medium. Biotechnol. Lett. **9**, 259 - 264

Kovár, J. (1988) Growth-stimulating effect of ferric citrate on hybridoma cells: Characterization and relation to transferrin function. Hybridoma **7**, 255 - 263

Lind, W., V. Jäger, M. Lucki-Lange, R. Wagner (1990) Characterization of protease activity in serum-free culture supernatants of hybridomas and recombinant mammalian cells. *This volume.*

Lucki-Lange, M., R. Wagner (1990) Conditions for the production of recombinant IL-2 in stirred suspension culture using a protein-free medium. *This volume*

Merten, O.W., H. Keller, L. Cabanie, J. Litwin, B. Flamand (1989) Development of a serum-free medium for hybridoma fermentor cultures. In: R.E. Spier, J.B. Griffiths, J. Stephenne, P.J. Crooy (eds.) Advances in animal cell biology and technology for bioprocesses. Butterworths, pp. 263 - 268

Murakami, H., H. Masui, G.H. Sato, N. Sueko, T.P. Chow, T. Kano-Sueko (1982) Growth of hybridoma cells in serum-free medium: Ethanolamine is an essential component. Proc. Natl. Acad. Sci. USA **79**, 1158 - 1162

Murakami, H., H. Masui, G.H. Sato (1982) Suspension culture of hybridoma cells in serum-free medium: Soybean phospholipids as the essential components. In: G.H. Sato, A.B. Pardee, D.A. Sirbasku (eds.) Growth of cells in hormonally defined media. Cold Spring Harbor Conferences on Cell Proliferation Vol. 9, Cold Spring Harbor, NY, pp. 711 - 715

Penhallow, R.C., A. Brown-Mason, R.C. Woodworth (1986) Comparative studies of the binding and growth supportive ability of mammalian transferrins in human cells. J. Cell. Physiol. **128**, 251 - 260

Pickart, L., L. Thayer, M. Thaler (1973) A synthetic tripeptide which increases survival of normal liver cells, and stimulates growth in hepatoma cells. Biochem. Biophys. Res. Commun. **54**, 562 - 566

Rudge, J., M.A. Desai, S.A. Shojaosadaty, A. Lydiatt (1987) Continuous culture of murine hybridomas with integrated recovery of monoclonal antibodies. In: R.E. Spier, J.B. Griffiths (eds.) Modern approaches to animal cell technology. Butterworths, pp. 556 - 574

Ryll, T., M. Lucki-Lange, V. Jäger, R. Wagner (1990) Production of recombinant interleukin-2 with BHK cells in a hollow fibre and a stirred tank reactor with protein-free medium. J. Biotechnol. *in press*

Sato, J.D., T. Kawamoto, D.B. McClure, G.H. Sato (1984) Cholesterol requirement of NS-1 mouse myeloma cell for growth in serum-free medium. Mol. Biol. Med. **2**, 121 - 134

Shintani, Y., K. Iwamoto, K. Kitano (1988) Polyethylene glycols for promoting the growth of mammalian cells. Appl. Microbiol. Biotechnol. **27**, 533 - 537

Schlaeger, E.J., B. Eggimann, A. Gast (1987) Proteolytic activity in the culture supernatants of mouse hybridoma cells. Develop. biol. Standard. **66**, 403 - 408

Titeux, M., U. Testa, F. Louache, P. Thomopoulos, H. Rochant, J. Breton-Gorius (1984) The role of iron in the growth of human leukemic cell lines. J. Cell. Physiol. **121**, 251 - 256

Yamane, I. (1978) Role of bovine albumin in a serum-free culture medium and its application. Natl. Cancer Inst. Monogr. **48**, 131 - 133

Yamane, I., M. Kan, Y. Minamoto, Y. Amatsuji (1982) Alpha-cyclodextrin: A partial substitute for bovine serum albumin in serum-free culture of mammalian cells. In: G.H. Sato, A.B. Pardee, D.A. Sirbasku (eds.) Growth of cells in hormonally defined media. Cold Spring Harbor Conferences on Cell Proliferation Vol. 9, Cold Spring Harbor, NY, pp. 87 - 92

<u>Paper of Jager:</u>

Pouradier: Do you really consider the use of albumin or human
              albumin for cell culture. The first is allergenic and
              the second has to be heated for 20 hours and stabilized
              by Caprillate and tryptophane and both of these
              processes are detrimental to cell culture.

Jager: We used human serum albumin which is manufactured as a
              pharmaceutical and we observed better growth results
              with this particular cell line but we have other cell
              lines where we normally use bovine serum albumin and
              get better results this way.

Pouradier: The human albumin you mentioned is stabilised and
              heated?

Jager: The human albumin we use is made by the German Red
              Cross and it's produced as a therapeutic and stabilized
              with tryptophane.

Reuveny: What about the proteins which are either secreted by
              the cells or which enter the protein-free medium
              following cell lysis.   How much protein is derived
              from this source.

Jager: The total concentrations of protein released from the
              cells is 50-500 mg/L into a totally protein -free
              medium,. A minimum of 30-40 cell derived proteins can
              be detected.   Most of these are actively released and
              are not there by cell lysis.

Hofmann: Do you see any changes in the quality of your products
              dependent on whether they are produced in serum
              containing or serum-free media - such as glycosylation
              pattern or IEF pattern. We have seen such differences.

Jager: Normally the glycosylation is not influenced by the
              serum-free medium.   It depends on the particular
              recombinant protein.   For example with IL-2 you have a
              normal distribution of normal glycosylated and
              unglycosylated molecules which is independent of
              whether you use serum-free or serum-supplemented
              medium.

Hofmann: In a monoclonal antibody differences can be seen.
              Mullering has also seen such differences.   There is a
              paper by Invitron where they see a change in the N-
              glycosylation.   We see a different IEF pattern
              depending on the presence of serum in the medium.

Jager: We did not look at the glycosylation pattern for each
              protein we produced for diagnostic use; but the ones we
              have checked did not show differences.

Mertens: You said that mouse hybridomas need transferrin, we
                have established a completely protein-free medium which
                we have used for a lot of mouse-mouse hybridomas
                without transferrin. You have to give enough iron to
                the cells. In some cases we used 800µm iron (Fe^{+++}
                complexed with ascorbic acid).

Jager: I have read your publication and have checked the use
                of iron salts as a substitute for transferrin and we
                have grown some murine hybridoma cells but although we
                get growth in static systems we do not get growth in a
                stirred bioreactor. Did you not also publish that when
                you go to a bioreactor you have to add transferrin.

Mertens: This was only for one cell line before the medium was
                adapted for this cell line. But when the iron was
                complexed with glycylleucine it is possible to work in
                stirred tank bioreactors without using transferrin.

Jager: It depends on the parental myeloma cells in our hands
                we could only get down to 200ng/L

PRODUCTION OF HUMAN FIBRONECTIN FROM SERUM- FREE CONTINUOUS CULTURED HUMAN HEPATOBLASTOMA CELL LINE, HUH-6

K. Nagamine(1), M. Shiraishi(1), Z. Kong(3), K. Shinohara(2) and H. Murakami(3)

1 Nichirei Research Institute, JAPAN ; 2 National Food Research Institute
; 3 Kyushu University, JAPAN

ABSTRACT

Fibronectin is known as one of cell attachment factors effective for the growth of anchorage cells. We have studied on the production system of the human fibronectin from serum-free cultured human cell lines. In this paper, the continuous culture system of human hepatoblastoma cell line, HUH-6 clone5 which cultured in e-RDF medium supplemented with insulin using the modified roller bottle and the purification are described.

INTRODUCTION

The serum-free culture has become an important tool for the production of bioactive molecules from various types of animal cells. In the most cases, some additional growth factors and/or cell attachment factors are indispensable for growth of the cells when cultured in serum-free media.

Fibronectin is an effective factor for the growth of anchorage cells. It has been obtained mostly from either human or bovine sera, however, it is difficult to purify the fibronectin from those sera because of their complexity. Though some cell lines are known to synthesize and secrete fibronectins, the quantity of those produced is not sufficient under the normal culture condition.

MATERIALS AND METHODS

Cell culture and fibronectin determination

The cell line used in this study was a human hepatoblastoma cell line, HUH-6 clone5 (HUH-6 cells)[1-2]. HUH-6 cells were cultured in e-RDF medium[3] supplemented with insulin (0.4IU/ml) and maintained in a humidified atmosphere of 5%CO2-95% air for 2 years.The e-RDF medium does not contain any protein.

Fibronectin produced from the cells into the conditioning media were measured by two-site enzyme-linked immunosorbent assay (ELISA) using anti-fibronectin polyclonal antibodies.

Fibronectin production

Fibronectin was produced by perfusion culture system of HUH-6 cells using the modified roller bottle (Falcon,#3007, 850 cm^2) equipped with a feed-head. The conditioning media (spent media) were continuously collected from the roller bottle.

Fibronectin purification

The conditioning media were centrifuged at 3000 rpm for 10 min. The supernatants were applied to a gelatin-Sepharose 4B (Pharmacia) column. The column was washed with 1 M NaCl in PBS and 0.8 M urea, 0.5 M NaCl in PBS. The fractions containing fibronectin were eluted with 6 M urea, 0.5 M NaCl in PBS and dialyzed against 2 mM CAPS buffer (pH 11.0).

The yield of fibronectin from conditioning media was calculated according to values measured by ELISA. The purity of fibronectin was analyzed by SDS-PAGE.

RESULTS

Serum-free culture and fibronectin production

The growth rate of HUH-6 cells in e-RDF media supplemented with insulin (0.4IU/ml) was the same as that in e-RDF media supplemented with fetal calf serum (10%v/v). The optimal concentration of insulin was 0.4 IU/ml for cell growth.

Figure 1 shows the glucose consumption rate of HUH-6 cells in e-RDF media supplemented with insulin and fibronectin production. From the glucose consumption rate, it is suggested that HUH-6 cells reached confluent density at the 21 days. The production of fibronectin increased dramatically after the cells reached confluence. The amount of fibronectin at the confluent stage was over 50 ug/ml/day in the media.

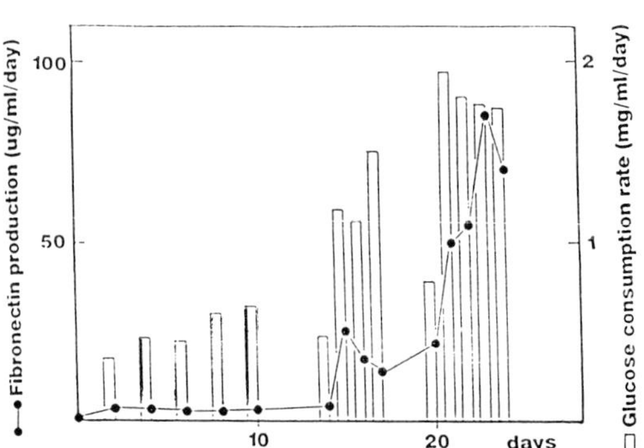

Fig.1 Fibronectin production (●) and glucose consumption rate (▫) of HUH-6 cells in e-RDF media supplemented with insulin. HUH-6 cells were inoculated 1x105cells/2ml media into 35 mm dish.

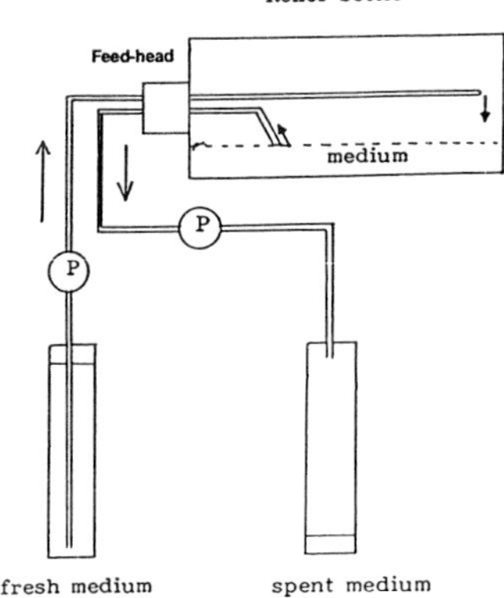

Fig. 2 Schematic drawing of continuous fibronectin production

168

Figure 2 shows schematic drawing of continuous fibronectin production system using modified roller bottle which has 2 pumps to regulate flow rate of serum-free media. Fibronectin was produced over 20 mg/day/one bottle by this system of roller bottle. At present, HUH-6 cells are being maintained for 2 months.

Fibronectin purification

Human fibronectin was purified from the conditioning media of HUH-6 cells, by the procedures with a gelatin affinity chromatography. Table 1 shows the yield of human fibronectin from the conditioning media of HUH-6 cells. From 2 L of conditioning media, 27.6mg of the human fibronectin was successfully obtained by the procedures described above. The yield of fibronectin was 31%. The purity of human fibronectin from HUH-6 cells was found to exceed 90 % by analysis of SDS-PAGE .

Table 1 Yield of fibronectin from conditioning media of HUH-6 cells

	Volume (ml)	Fibronectin concentration (ug/ml)	Fibronectin (mg)	Yield (%)
Conditioning media	2000	44	88.0	—
Elution of gelatin -Sepharose	53	520	27.6	31

DISCUSSION

HUH-6 cells were successively maintained for 2 years in serum-free media. During the period, production of fibronectin from HUH-6 cells was stable. We obtained a large amount of fibronectin by perfusion culture system using roller bottle. The fibronectin secreted in the conditioned medium was purified by gelatin affinity gel chromatography. The amount of human fibronectin purified from 1 L of conditioned media of HUH-6 cells was more than 10mg. We considered that fibronectin produced from HUH-6 cells might be cellular fibronectin. Its biological activity was the same as commercial human plasma fibronectin by cell spreading assay using BHK-21 cell.

These results would ensure consistency and predictable large scale production of fibronectin using a high cell density serum-free cell culture of HUH-6 cells.

REFERENCES

1 Tanaka, M., Kawamura, K., Frang., Higashino, K., Kishimoto, S., Nakabayashi, H. and Sato, J. Biochem. Biophys. Res. Commun. 1983, 110, pp 837-841

2 Shinohara, K., Kong, Z-L., Nagamine, K., Shiraishi, M. and Murakami, H in preparation

3 Murakami, H., Shimomura, T., Nakamura, T., Ohashi, H.,Shinohara, K. and Omura, H. J. Agricult. Chem. Soc. JAPAN 1984, 58, pp 575-583

DEVELOPMENT OF A PROTEIN-FREE MEDIUM FOR BIOREACTOR CULTURES OF HYBRIDOMA CELL LINES.

Merten, O-W, Keller, H, Cabanié, L

Institut Pasteur, Laboratoire de Technologie Cellulaire. 25, rue du Docteur Roux, F-75015 Paris/France.

ABSTRACT:

Protein-free media for cultures of mouse hybridoma cell lines in stirred tank reactors have been developed. Starting from a serum-free medium (Merten et al. (1988) 9th ESACT-meeting, Knokke/B), which contained transferrin as the only protein (MEM + additives), we have developed a protein-free medium for hybridomas, derived from SP2/0 and 653 myelomas. The replacement of transferrin had been possible by high concentrations of Fe^{3+}. This medium supported cell growth and antibody production of hybridomas in Roux bottle and spinner cultures, but not bioreactor cultures. However, the use of iron chelators, either 11mM glycylglycine (GG) or 10mM iminodiacetic acid (IDA) with different concentrations of Fe^{3+} lead to cell growth in bioreactors. For three hybridoma cell lines (1: SP2/0; 2: 653) we have found that the use of 50µM of $Fe_2(SO_4)_3$ complexed by GG or IDA have been sufficient for supporting growth and production, both, in static batch and continuous stirred tank reactor cultures. A fourth cell line (SP2/0) did not grow in this medium. The use of either GG, 50µM $Fe_2(SO_4)_3$, 2.5 µg/ml transferrin and insulin, or IDA, 400µM $Fe_2(SO_4)_3$, 20µM vitamine C lead to successful continuous stirred tank reactor cultures. The cells have been cultivated for 500-1000 hrs. By using either dexamethasone or cholesterol and varying their concentrations and the concentration of Fe^{3+}, this medium may be adapted to other hybridoma cell lines.

INTRODUCTION:

The use of serum- or even protein-free media for the production of monoclonal antibodies (mAbs) facilitates considerably the purification process and leads to a more standardized production process. Most of the published serum-free (SF)-media contain insulin, albumin, and transferrin. It could be shown, that the presence of insulin and albumin is not necessary for hybridoma cultures in bioreactors. Insulin is not stable at 37°C, it disappeares with a half life time of ca. 48 hrs. (1), in addition, its presence is not necessary for most of the mouse hybridoma cell lines (1,2,3). Albumin can pose problems in down-stream processing, and can be replaced by polymeric protectants, like Pluronic F-68 (4) or PEG-20000 (5). Dextran (6), α- (7) or β-cyclodextrin (8) can replace the lipid transporting function of albumin. Lipidic substances at low concentrations, like vitamin E or dexamethasone can be added without carriers (1,3). Transferrin, an iron carrier (9) essential for cell growth, can be replaced with between 50 and 500µM iron salts (1,10-13) for cultures in Roux bottles or spinner flasks. Chelating agents, like IDA, GG (13) or citrate/vitamin C (1,12), have been used for preventing the development of precipitates.
In spite of these developments, no protein-free medium has been used for low-density bioreactor cultures of hybridomas up to now. Therefore, we

have tried to replace transferrin by Fe3+, complexed by GG or IDA, for static hybridoma batch cultures with the aim to develop a protein-free medium which can equally be used in static batch (Roux bottles) and in agitated continuous bioreactor cultures. Using four different hybridoma cell lines, the difficulties in developing a protein-free medium for a general application will be shown and solutions will be discussed.

MATERIAL AND METHODS:

Cell lines: I.13.17 and U0208 are mouse hybridoma lines, derived from X63.653, 10/8/20 and ID2C3 are mouse hybridoma lines, derived from SP2/0. They have been received from Dr. Mazié (I.13.17), Dr. Michelson (10/8/20), Dr. Louvard (ID2C3), all Institut Pasteur, and Dr. Katinger (U0208), Universität für Bodenkultur, Institut für angewandte Mikrobiologie, in Vienna/A. All cells have been tested for the absence of mycoplasmas (Institut Pasteur, Service des Mucoplasmes). The cells have been cultivated as described elsewhere (14).

Medium: MEM (lab.-mixed, using reagents from Merck, Sigma and Gibco) was used with some modifications: arginine 105 mg/l, cystine 48 mg/l, glutamine 584 mg/l, tyrosine 72 mg/l. Before the development of the protein-free bioreactor medium, the cells had been routinely cultivated in the following medium-formulation: modified MEM: 2 g/l serum replacement concentrate 3000 (Medical & Veterinary Suppliers Ltd., Botolph Claydon, U.K.), 100µM $Fe_2(SO_4)_3$ (Serva), 1 ng/ml dexamethasone, 20µM α-tocopherol, 10exp-7M Na_2SeO_3, 10exp-5M ethanolamine, 10exp-5M 2-mercaptoethanol, 1mM pyruvate (Serva), 0.01% Pluronic F-68 (Serva)(all reagents were coming from Sigma, except those where another source is indicated).

Development of a protein-free medium for I.13.17, 10/8/20, and U0208 (only shown for I.13.17): Cells, cultivated under serum-free conditions (see above) were centrifuged (5 min, 1000 rpm, 25°C) and suspended in test or control medium in duplicate at a concentration of 3x10exp5 c/ml and cultivated in T-25 flasks for 150 hrs. Each day viable and total cell density were determined as published previously (14).

For routine cultures, modified MEM containing 50µM $Fe_2(SO_4)_3$ complexed by 11mM GG (Sigma) or 10mM IDA (Sigma) was used afterwards.

For bioreactor cultures, after development of the protein-free formulation: same medium, + 2g/l glucose, 0.025% Pluronic F-68 or 0.1% PEG-20000 (Serva).

Development of a protein-free medium for ID2C3: Cells, cultivated under serum-free conditions (above mentioned protein-free medium for routine cultures, + 2.5 µg/ml human transferrin (Sigma), 2.5 µg/ml bovine insulin (Sigma)) were centrifuged (5 min, 1000 rpm, 25°C) and suspended in test or control medium in duplicate at a concentration of 3x10exp5 c/ml and cultivated in T-25 flasks for 150 hrs. Each day viable and total cell density were determined as published previously (14).

For routine cultures of ID2C3, modified MEM containing 400µM $Fe_2(SO_4)_3$ complexed by 10mM IDA with 20µM vitamin C was used afterwards.

For bioreactor cultures of ID2C3, after development of the protein-free formulation: same medium, + 2g/l glucose, 0.025% Pluronic or 0.1% PEG.

Bioreactor culture conditions: An 1.5 l Biolafitte stirred tank reactor, equipped with a spinfilter (pore diameter: 10 µm), and a Techne Bioreactor BR-06 (for I.13.17), equipped with a sedimentation tube, were used employing the following conditions: temperature: 37°C, pO2: 10-15% air-saturation, pH 7.25, agitation: 60 rpm, Biolafitte: marine impeller, Techne:

flotating impeller. The fermentors were started from spinner cultures and switched to the continuous culture mode before having reached the stationary growth phase (dilution rate: 0.01 - 0.025 per h).
The determinations and calculations (growth rate, specific productivity, viability) were done according to Merten (14).
Fe-59 incorporation studies: In order to follow the incorporation of iron into the cells, Fe-59 studies have been performed, using 10/8/20 and ID2C3. For each cell line, cells cultivated in their protein-free routine medium have been separated (5 min, 1000 rpm, 25°C), washed once with MEM, and suspended at 8x10exp5 c/ml in MEM-SF (routine medium without iron and IDA), to which 100µM Fe-59 (Amersham IFS 1, lot 281, ferric chloride in 0.1M HCl, 1mCi/ml), complexed by 10mM IDA was added. This was done in duplicate. The cultures (T-25 flasks, 37°C) were stopped after 17 hrs. The s:ipernate was separated (5 min, 4°C, 1500 rpm), the radioactivity of 50µl was measured in a LKB-gamma-counter. The cell pellet was washed twice with 2ml PBS and frozen in 1ml at -20°C. After three cycles of freezing, thawing, and vortexing, the cell debris was centrifuged (12000 rpm, 10 min, 4°C) and the radioactivity of 50µl cytoplasma was counted in a LKB-gamma-counter. The percentage of incorporated radioactivity (= incoporated Fe^{3+}) to total added radioactivity (= total Fe^{3+}) was calculated.

RESULTS:

The hybridoma cell line I.13.17 had already been adapted to a protein-free medium for growth in Roux bottle and spinner flasks. However, this medium could not be used for stirred tank cultures, possibly because of the toxic effect of high iron concentrations ($200µM\ Fe^{3+}$)(3). Therefore, transferrin had to be used initially in stirred tank cultures (3). However, by complexing the high iron concentration with 11mM GG or 10mM IDA (13), transferrin could be replaced in the medium. The following conditions were tested: 25, 50, 100, and 200 µM Fe^{3+} as sulfate, complexed by 11mM GG, as control served a medium with non-complexed $200µM\ Fe^{3+}$. The results for I.13.17 are shown in Fig. 1 (a-d) with reference to our control medium (MEM-SF, $200µM\ Fe^{3+}$, without GG)(Fig. 1e). It is evident, that higher iron concentrations promoted cell growth (highest viable cell density: 1.5-1.6x10exp6 c/ml, viability: 70-80%), when compared to lower Fe-concentrations or the control culture, which showed reduced growth or growth inhibition and a reduced viability. For bioreactor cultures, an iron concentration of 100µM was chosen, because the iron complexing capacity of GG is limited to this concentration (3). This medium composition has been used successfully for bioreactor cultures of I.13.17. However, in order to get rid of iron precipitates, which were still present to some extent, GG has been replaced by IDA. One typical bioreactor culture is shown in Fig. 2. This culture was started with 4x10exp5 c/ml (viability: 75%) and lasted for about 500 hrs. Two different media have been tested: 1) MEM-SF (3g/l glucose, 0.025% Pluronic F-68), and 2) MEM-SF (3g/l glucose, 0.1% PEG-20000). They were similar for supporting cellular growth, however it seemed that medium 2 augmented the IgG-productivity to some extent, which is in accord with Shintani et al. (5). The reduced growth between 106 and 127 hrs. was due to a reduced pH.
Fig. 3 and 4 present the fermentations of 10/8/20 and U0208 in MEM-SF (IDA, 0.1% PEG-20000) and MEM-SF (IDA, 0.025% Pluronic F-68), respectively. Both cultures were inoculated with 2.5 and 5.5x10exp5 c/ml, respectively, and had a duration of more than 500 hrs. The large variations of the

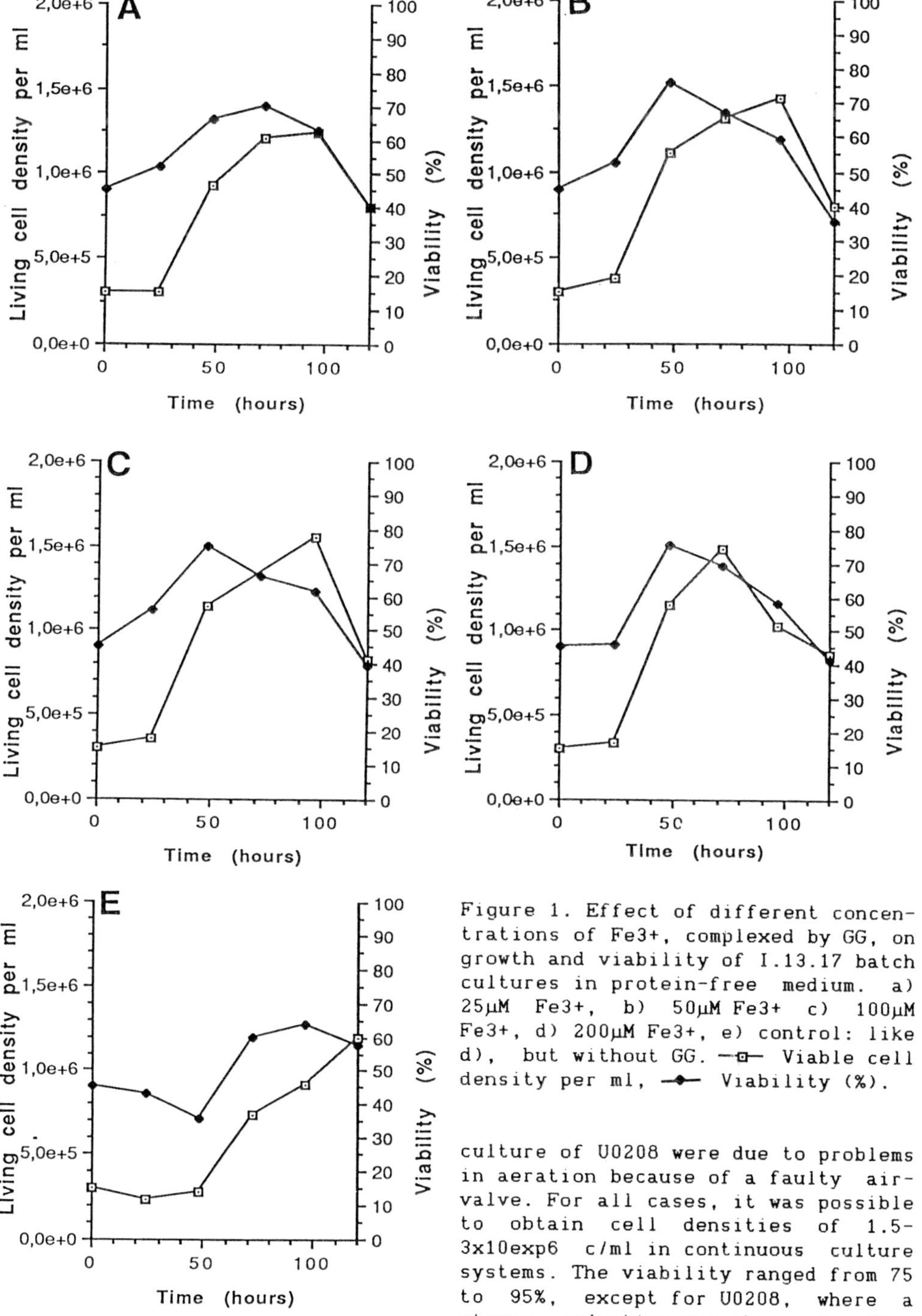

Figure 1. Effect of different concentrations of Fe3+, complexed by GG, on growth and viability of I.13.17 batch cultures in protein-free medium. a) 25μM Fe3+, b) 50μM Fe3+ c) 100μM Fe3+, d) 200μM Fe3+, e) control: like d), but without GG. —□— Viable cell density per ml, —◆— Viability (%).

culture of U0208 were due to problems in aeration because of a faulty air-valve. For all cases, it was possible to obtain cell densities of 1.5-3x10exp6 c/ml in continuous culture systems. The viability ranged from 75 to 95%, except for U0208, where a strong reduction was observed after 160 hrs. due to aeration problems.

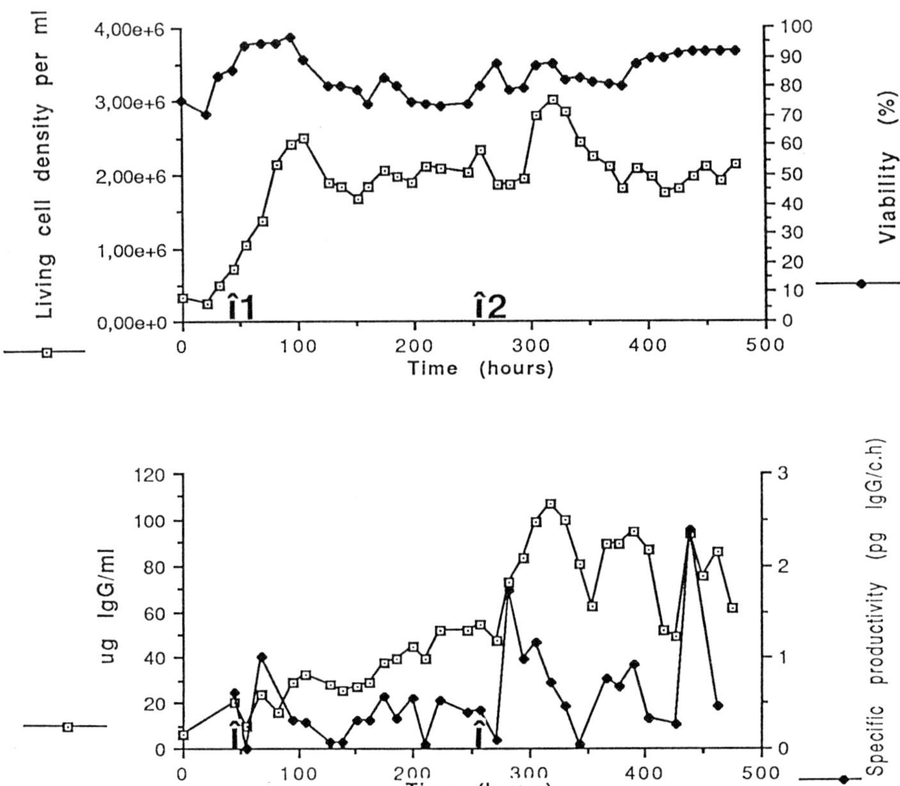

Figure 2. Continuous culture of I.13.17 in a 1.5 l stirred tank reactor using protein-free medium: 1) MEM-SF (IDA, 100µM Fe3+) + 0.025% Pluronic F-68 (0-250 hrs.), 2) MEM-SF (IDA, 100µM Fe3+) + 0.1% PEG-20000 (after 250 hrs.). The upper diagram shows the development of viable cell density (c/ml) and viability (%), the bottom diagram shows the accumulation of IgG in the supernatant (µg/ml) and the specific productivity (pg IgG/ml).

For I.13.17 and 10/8/20, an IgG-accumulation of up to 130 mg/l could be observed. The production of U0208 was low and not stable, probably due to a certain unstability of this cell line.
A fourth cell line (ID2C3) did not grow in this medium, containing 100µM Fe3+ and 11mM GG, without the presence of transferrin and insulin (both at 2.5µg/ml), which was probably due to difficulties in iron incorporation by this cell line. Therefore, we tested higher concentrations of iron (100-800µM)(12), complexed by IDA (10mM), with or without 20µM vitamin C, with respect to standard conditions (100µM Fe3+, 2 µg/ml transferrin)(Fig. 5). The cells were able to grow well at higher iron-concentrations, with or without vitamin C, although at 400 (Fig. 5 c,d) and 800µM (Fig. 5 a,b), the presence of vitamin C lead to a somewhat higher living cell density and a slightly increased growth, when compared to vitamin C-free, standard, or low iron (100µM Fe3+, +/- vitamin C)(Fig. 5 e,f) conditions. The SF-medium, containing 0.025% Pluronic F-68 and 800µM Fe3+, complexed by 10mM IDA and 20µM vitamin C has been used for bioreactor cultures of ID2C3

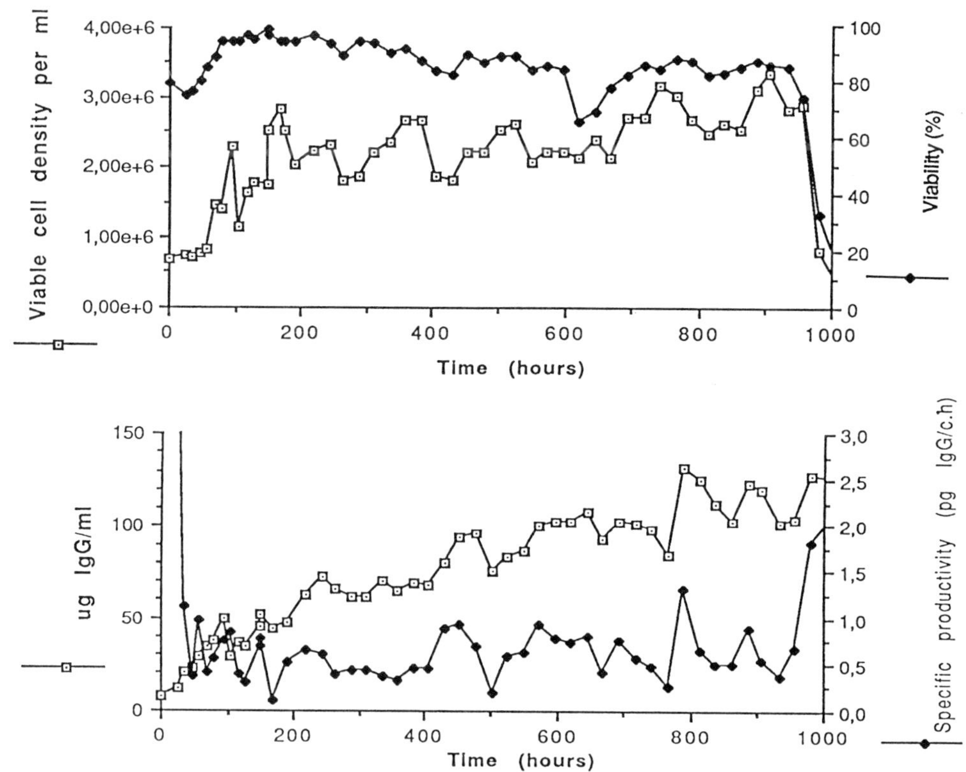

Figure 3. Continuous culture of 10/8/20 in a 1.5 l stirred tank reactor using protein-free medium (MEM-SF (IDA, 100µM Fe3+) + 0.1% PEG-20000).

(Fig. 6). The variations in cell density, viability, and specific productivity were due to aeration problems. The continuous culture lasted for about 500 hrs., cell density, viability, and product accumulation were equal to the other cultures, previously presented.
For the different iron requirement of these four cell lines, we compared the incorporation of Fe-59 for 10/8/20 and ID2C3, growing and producing well at 100µM and 400-800µM Fe3+, respectively. The incubation of both cell lines in MEM-SF (IDA) during 17 hrs. in the presence of 100 µM Fe-59 revealed that both cells incorporated about 0.95% of the total radioactivity into the cytoplasma (14850/1562590 cpm and 4350/457150 cpm for 10/8/20 and ID2C3, respectively). This proved that both cell lines have the same capacity of incorporating Fe3+; however, they have certainly a different capacity of utilizing the incorporated iron. This issue is being investigated further.

DISCUSSION:

Serum-free media have already been used for several years (for review:

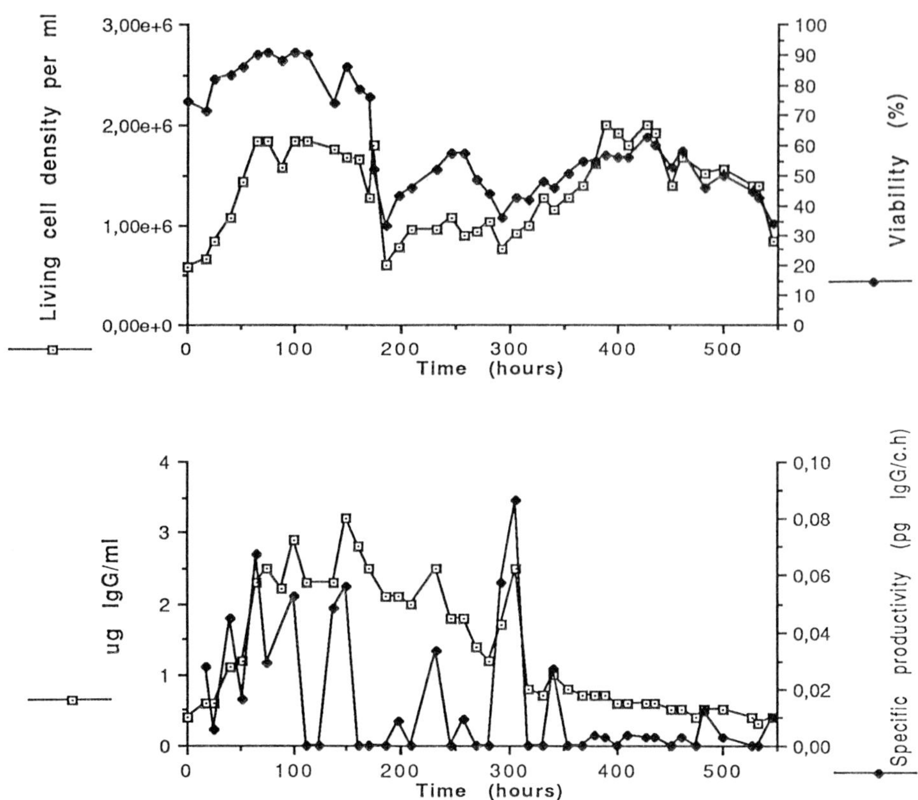

Figure 4. Continuous culture of U0208 in a 1.5 l stirred tank reactor using protein-free medium (MEM-SF (IDA, 100µM Fe3+) + 0.025% Pluronic).

15), however, protein-free hybridoma media are a more recent development. In 1987, Yabe et al. (13) tested systematically high concentrations of iron, complexed by various chelators, for replacing transferrin in static batch cultures of mouse hybridoma cell lines. In the same year, Kovár and Franĕk (12) used 500µM Fe3+, as citrate, and vitamin C successfully for several types of mouse hybridoma and myeloma cell lines. Recently, a protein-free medium has been used for spinner cultures (1). We (3,16) were able to grow hybridomas in protein-free high iron concentration medium (no transferrin, no Fe-chelator) in Roux-bottle and spinner cultures, however we failed to grow these cells in stirred tank reactors in a continuous mode in absence of transferrin (3), probably because of a toxicity due to iron or the incapacity of the cells using the iron. However, the use of iron-chelators, like IDA or GG, allowed us to cultivate mouse hybridoma cell lines and other cell lines, like YAC-1, M1 or the suspension clone of BHK-C13 (not shown), in bioreactors (1-12 l, stirred tank, airlift) using the protein-free medium presented. Most of these cell lines can grow with complexed 100µm Fe3+, however in some cases, like for ID2C3 (this paper) or other hybridoma cells (1,17) higher Fe-concentrations (up to 800µM) were necessary for cellular proliferation.
It is not clear, how the cells can handle these very high non-physiologi-

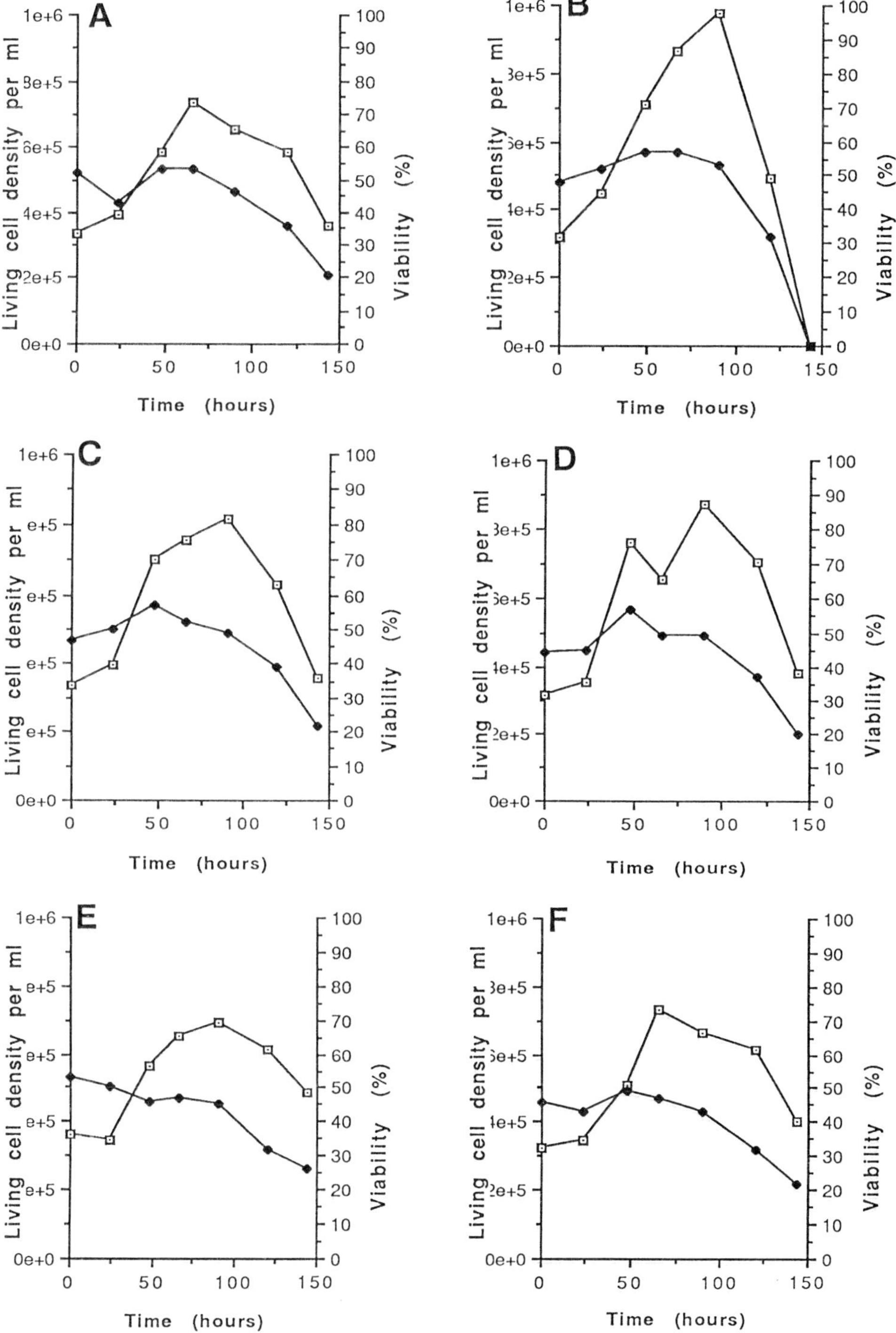
A
Living cell density per ml
Viability (%)
Time (hours)
B
C
D
E
F
1e+6
3e+5
1e+5
0e+0
100
90
80
70
60
50
40
30
20
10
0
0
50
100
150

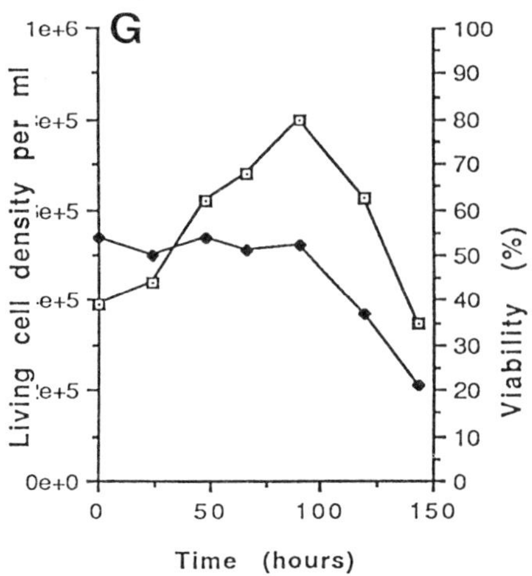

Figure 5. Development of a protein-free medium for cell line ID2C3. The effect of different concentrations of Fe3+, complexed by IDA with or without 20µM vitamin C, on growth and viability of ID2C3 batch cultures in protein-free medium. a) 800µM Fe3+, no vitamin C, b) 800µM Fe3+, with vitamin C, c) 400µM Fe3+, no vitamin C, d) 400µM Fe3+, with vitamin C, e) 100µM Fe3+, no vitamin C, f) 100µM Fe3+, with vitamin C, g) control: like e), but with 2 µg/ml transferrin. —□— Viable cell density per ml, —◆— Viability (%).

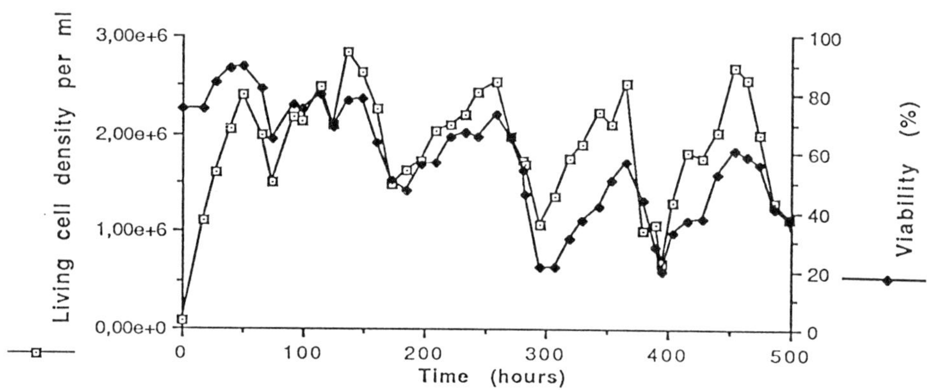

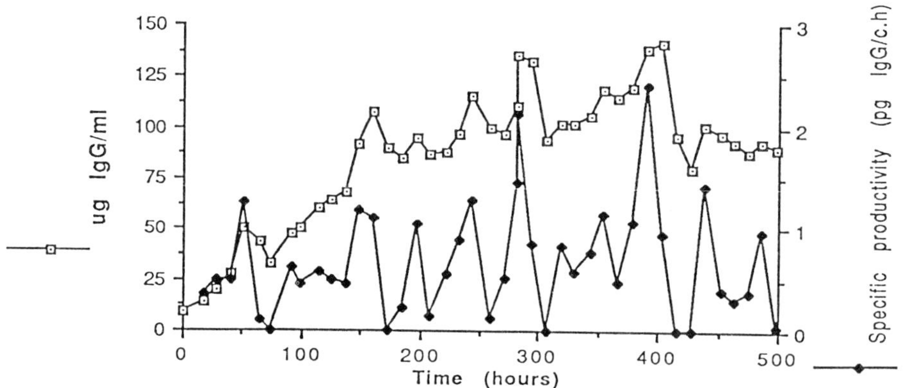

Figure 6. Continuous culture of ID2C3 in a 1.5 l stirred tank re-actor using protein-free medium (MEM-SF (IDA, 800µM Fe3+) + 0.025% Pluronic F-68).

cal Fe-concentrations, and why different cells need different Fe-concentrations. Three possible explanations can be suggested, that 1) the cells can incorporate and use Fe in a non-complexed or complexed form, when high Fe-concentrations are available; 2) there is still a certain residual transferrin-concentration, which cycles from medium to cell, unloads Fe^{3+}, and cycles back to the medium (18)(not probable, because the transferrin would have been diluted out due to the use of continuous culture systems from 500-1000 hrs.), and 3) the cells might be able to produce transferrin, which is known for certain proliferating T-lymphocytes (19) or siderophores (20).

Finally, for the first time it could be shown, that mouse hybridoma cells can grow in low cell density bioreactor cultures using protein-free media. By using, either dexamethasone (3,16) or cholesterol (21,22,23) and varying their concentrations and the concentration of Fe^{3+}, this medium can be adapted to other hybridoma cell lines.

REFERENCES:

1 Schneider Y-J (1989) J Immunol Method 116, 65-77.
2 Jäger V, Lehmann J, Friedl P (1988) Cytotechnology 1, 319-329.
3 Merten O-W, Keller H, Cabanié L, Litwin J, Flamand B (1989) In "Advances in Animal Cell Biology and Technology for Bioprocesses", eds. Spier RE, Griffiths JB, Stephenne J, Crooy PJ, pp. 263-268, Butterworths, Borough Green, Sevenoaks/UK.
4 Mizrahi A (1977) Biotechnol Bioeng 19, 1557-1561.
5 Shintani Y, Iwamoto K, Kitano K (1988) Appl Microbiol Biotechnol 27, 533-537.
6 Chessebeuf-Padieu M, Mignot G, Tsaconas C, Fischbach M, Padieu P Mack G (1985) Presented at the Symposium "Quo Vadis?", Group Sanofi, pp. 385-397, MEDSI Pub., Paris/F.
7 Yamane I, Kan M, Minamoto Y, Amatsuji Y (1981) Proc Japan Acad 57B, 385-389.
8 Ohmori H (1988) J Immunol Method 112, 227-233.
9 Octave J-H, Schneider Y-J, Trouet A, Crichton RR (1983) Trends Biochem Sci 8, 217-220.
10 Titeux M, Testa U, Louache F, Thomopoulos P, Rochant H, Breton-Gorius J (1984) J Cell Physiol 121, 251-256.
11 Brock JH, Stevensen J (1987) Immunol Lett 15, 23-25.
12 Kovář J, Franek F (1987) Biotechnol Lett 9, 259-264.
13 Yabe N, Kato M, Matsuya Y, Yamane I, Iizuka M, Takayoshi H, Suzuki K (1987) In Vitro Cell Develop Biol 23, 815-820.
14 Merten O-W (1988) Cytotechnology 1, 113-121.
15 Merten O-W, Litwin J (1990) Cytotechnology, in press.
16 Litwin J (1989) In "Advances in Animal Cell Biology and Technology for Bioprocesses", eds. Spier RE, Griffiths JB, Stephenne J, Crooy PJ, pp. 273-275, Butterworths, Borough Green, Sevenoaks/UK.
17 Kovář J (1989) In Vitro Cell Develop Biol 25, 395-396.
18 Huebers HA, Finch CA (1987) Physiol Rev 67, 520-582.
19 Lum JB, Infante AJ, Makker DM, Yang F, Bowman BH (1986) J Clin Invest 77, 841-949.
20 Fernandez-Pol JA (1983) Microbiology 1983, 313-317.
21 Sato JD, Kawamoto T, McClure DB, Sato G (1984) 2, 121-134.
22 Sato JD, Kawamoto T, Okamoto T (1987) J Exp Med 165, 1761-1766.
23 Myoken Y, Okamoto T, Osaki T, Yabumoto M, Sato GH, Takada K, Sato SD (1989) In Vitro Cell Develop Biol 25, 477-480.

CONDITIONS FOR THE PRODUCTION OF RECOMBINANT IL-2 IN STIRRED SUSPENSION CULTURE USING A PROTEIN FREE MEDIUM

Mona Lucki-Lange, and <u>Roland Wagner</u>

Arbeitsgruppe Zellkulturtechnik, Gesellschaft für Biotechnologische Forschung mbH, Mascheroder Weg 1, D-3300 Braunschweig, FRG

ABSTRACT

A suspension culture in a homogeneous stirred bubble free aerated system with continuous medium exchange was established for the cell line BHK 21 pSVIL2. High cell densities of up to $3 \cdot 10^7$ ml^{-1} were reached. The production of IL-2, which did not exceed 1 mg d^{-1} in previous microcarrier processes based on 1-l-bioreactors, was increased to 4 mg d^{-1}. Using a cell specific supplementation of amino acids IL-2 production increased to 6 mg d^{-1} at high cell densities for 4 weeks of cultivation. Compared with other previous serum-free medium formulations cultivation with the protein-free medium had the lowest costs and also lowered the burden on downstream processing. Data are shown concerning the further optimization of the production process going from a microcarrier to a suspension culture.

INTRODUCTION

Interleukin 2 (IL-2) is an important protein of the body protective system. It is the growth faktor for activated T-lymphocytes and plays a central part in the mobilization and control of the cellular immune response. These effects were responsible for the potential therapeutical application of IL-2 in cases were T-cell deficiencies occur as in Aids [4,5,7,14], leukemia [18] and several forms of cancer [12,13]. A production process based on a high producing cell line BHK 21 pSVIL2 grown on microcarriers in a stirred tank double membrane bioreactor under serum-free medium conditions has already been established [15-17]. The specific productivity of the cell line was 0.3 pg d^{-1} in culture flask. Here the cultivation and production of this cell line in stirred suspension culture under protein free medium condition are compared with the previous production process with a serum-free microcarrier culture.

MATERIALS AND METHODS

Cell line

The cell line provided by our genetic engineering department has been manipulated by genetic methods to produce human interleukin 2 constitively under the control of the SV 40 promotor [2].

Medium formulations

The basal medium was composed of a 1:1 mixture of DMEM and Ham's F12 (Gibco BRL, Eggenstein). It was supplemented with 2.3 g l^{-1} NaHCO$_3$, 1.3 g l^{-1} D(+)-glucose-monohydrate, 0.4 g l^{-1} glutamine, 0.11 g l^{-1} Na-pyruvat (Serva, Heidelberg), 2.0 g l^{-1} dextran T 70 (Pharmacia, Uppsala). Otherwise dextran was removed and amino acids were added according to the cell specific consumption rates as followed: 1.5 g l^{-1} glutamine, 0.027 g l^{-1} tryptophane, 0.04 g l^{-1} asparaginic acids, 0.08 g l^{-1} serine (all chemicals not specified in the text were purchased from Merck, Darmstadt).

Analysis of fermenter samples

Glucose and lactate were determined with YSI 27A glucose and lactate analysers (Yellow Springs Instruments, Ohio).
Free amino acids were quantified by means of a reversed phase HPLC system with pre-column derivatisation with o-phthaldialdehyde (OPA) (Serva, Heidelberg) [8].
For determination of the total cell number, nuclei were fixed and stained with 0.1% crystal violet in 0.1 mol l^{-1} citrate and subsequently counted by means of an hemocytometer.
The proportion of dead cells was estimated by trypan blue exclusion.
Protein was determined according to Bradford (Bio-Rad, Munich) [1].
IL-2 activity was tested by (^{3}H)-thymidine incorporation assay using the IL-2 dependent murine CTLL as described [6] and employing an internal laboratory standard IL-2 preparation for comparison. The specific activity of the purified IL-2 amounts to 10^7 U mg^{-1} [3].
SDS-gelelectrophoresis was carried out with the Phast Development System (Pharmacia, Uppsala) using prepared 10-15% polyacrylamide slap gels [10]. Samples were heat-denaturated with 100 mmol l^{-1} sodium dodecyl sulfate (SDS, Serva, Heidelberg) and 0.7 mol l^{-1} ß-mercaptoethanol. Finally gels were stained with silver stain method [11, modified]. It was not necessary to purify and to concentrate the fermenter samples.

Reactor system and culture conditions

Preculture was performed in roller bottles (Falcon, Becton Dickinson, N.J.) with DMEM/F12 medium supplemented with 5% NCS (Kraeber and Co, Hamburg). One day before inoculation, medium in the roller bottles was replaced by medium without proteins. All cultivations were carried out at 37°C and pH 6.9-7.3. For cultivation of the cells a 1.4-l-double membrane stirrer bioreactor was used [9]. The stirrer speed was adjusted to 50 rpm and the oxygen concentration amounted to 2.7 mg l^{-1} corresponding to a potentional of 40% air saturation.

RESULTS AND DISCUSSION

Cells were trypsinized from the roller bottles, washed twice with protein-free medium and then transferred for protein-free inoculation into the reactor resulting in an initial cell density of 3.75$\cdot 10^5$ ml^{-1} (Fig. 1a) and 3.8$\cdot 10^5$ ml^{-1} (Fig. 2a) respectively. The protein content in both cultivations was 120 μg ml^{-1} due to cell specific proteins caused by release from secretion and cell lysis. The cell density rapidly increased to 2.1$\cdot 10^7$ ml^{-1} and 1.5$\cdot 10^7$ ml^{-1} respectively. 90% of these cells were viable. Medium perfusion was adjusted according to glucose and amino acid concentrations which were not limited during the whole cultivation. Both processes showed nearly identical reproducible results with respect to specific metabolic rates. Production increased by a factor of 1.5 when using amino acid supplemented medium (Fig. 2b). Lactate concentration did not exceed 1 g l^{-1} indicating that there was no detectable inhibition resulting from this compound and no influence on the pH. The cell specific IL-2 productivity decreased continuously from 1.3 mg 10^{-9} d^{-1} at the beginning to a final constant value of 0.14 mg 10^{-9} d^{-1}. 26 (26.7) mg IL-2 were produced with 40 (58) l of medium consumption corresponding to a product specific medium consumption of 1.54 (2.17) l mg^{-1}.

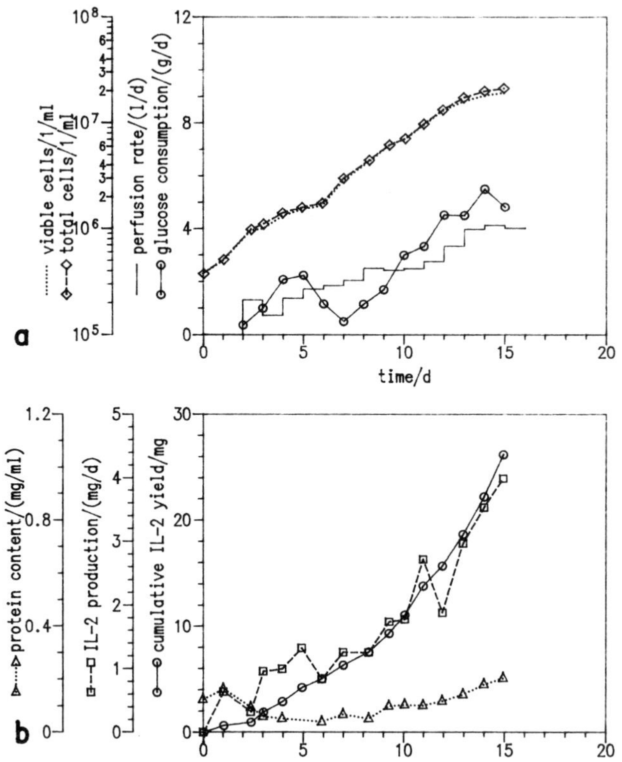

Fig.1
Cultivation with dextran supplemented medium as indicated in the text. At day 12 amino acids as specified in the text were added as a result of reduced production.

basal medium plus	costs per liter	cultivation method
10 % FCS	25-30 $	standard cultivation in cell culture
5 % NCS	3.10 $	pre culture in roller bottles
10 mg l^{-1} insulin 2 g l^{-1} dextran T70	3.90 $	microcarrier culture
protein-free special amino acids	0.55 $	suspension culture

Table I:
Comparison of medium cost in both production systems and in the precultures.

The addition of insulin and dextran increased medium costs by a factor of 6
when compared with the basal formulation. It was of the same order as the NCS
supplemented medium which, however, is affected by the problems of serum
containing media.

As shown in table I, the microcarrier culture had 7 fold higher medium costs
per liter than the suspension culture resulting from the necessary use of
expensive compounds such as insulin and dextran which were responsible for
adaequate cell growth and adherence in this process.

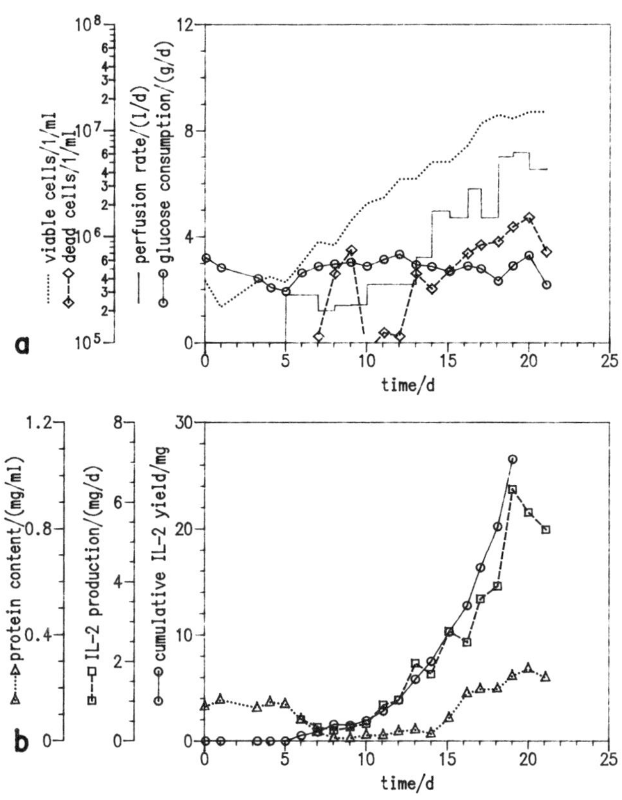

Fig.2
Cultivation with amino
acids supplemented medium
as indicated in the text.

Product specific medium consumption was in the same magnitute of 1.5 l mg⁻¹
for both systems (Table. II). But due to the higher medium costs for the microcarrier culture there were also higher product specific expenditures which were
7 times the costs for the suspension culture as already shown for the medium
costs (Table I). But both production systems were more efficient than conventional roller bottles. One roller bottle contained 200 ml medium so that it could
be calculated that 10 and 15 roller bottles are needed to obtain the same
amount of product as in a 1.4-l microcarrier and suspension reactor respectively.
The experiments demonstrated that a well advanced and optimized production
process is able to increase the product yield to a factor of about 15 with
respect to the medium concentration and the costs.

cultivation	spent medium / product [l mg^{-1}]	medium cost / product [\$ mg^{-1}]	average production [mg l^{-1} d^{-1}]
suspension	1.5	0.75	1.24
microcarrier	1.4	5.24	0.80
roller bottle	3.7	11.56	0.6

Table III:
Comparison of the specific efficiency of the various production processes with regard to medium cost.
The suspension culture had the lowest product specific expenditure of only 0.75 \$ mg^{-1} IL-2 compared with 5.24 \$ mg^{-1} for the microcarrier culture. Medium cost for the roller bottle relied on the use of 5% NCS as indicated in table I.

REFERENCES

[1]   Bradford, M.M. 1976. A Rapid and Sensitive Method for the Quantitation of Microgram Quantities of Protein Utilizing the Principle of Protein-Dye Binding. Anal. Biochem. 72, 248-25.

[2]   Conradt, H.S., Nimtz, M., Dittmar K.E.J., Lindenmaier, W., Hoppe J. and Hauser, H. 1989. Expression of Glycosylated Human Interleukin-2 in Recombinant Mammalian Cell Lines. J. Biol. Chem. 264, 17368-17373.

[3]   Conradt, H.S., Geyer, R., Mohr, H., Mühlradt, P.F., Plessing, A. and Stirm, S. 1985. Biochemical Characterization (Partial Amino Acid Sequence and Carbohydrate Structure) of Interleukin-2 from Human Peripheral Blood Lymphocytes. In: Cellular and Molecular Biology of Lymphokines, Academic Press 121-126.

[4]   Dopfer, R., Niethammer, D., Peter, H.H., Kniep, E.-M., Monner, D.A. and Mühlradt, P.F. 1984. In vivo Effects of Interleukin 2 on Lymphocyte Subpopulations in a Patient with a Combined Immunodeficiency. Immunobiol. 167, 452-461.

[5]   Flomenberg, N., Welte, K., Mertelsmann, R., Kernan, N., Ciobanu, N., Venuta, S., Feldman, S.P., Kruger, G., Kirkpatrick, D., Dupont, B. and O'Reilly, R. 1983. Immunologic Effects of Interleukin 2 in Primary Immunodeficiency Deseases. J.Immunol. 130, 2644-2650.

[6]   Gillis, S., Ferm, M.M., Ou, W. and Smith, K.A. 1978. T Cell Growth Factor: Parameters of Production and a Quantitative Microassay for Activity. J. Immunol. 129, 2027-2032.

[7]   Gramatzki, M., Burmester, G.R., Heyden, N., Rödel, W., Mühlradt, P.F. and

Kalden, J.R. 1984. Interleukin-2 Treatment of a Patient with Hemophilia B and AIDS. <u>Blood</u> <u>49</u>; 222.

[8] Larsen, B.R. and West, F.G. 1981. A Method for Quantitative Amino Acid Analysis Using Precolumn o-Phthalaldehyde Derivation and High Performance Liquid Chromatography. <u>J. Chromatogr. Sci.</u> <u>19</u>, 259-265.

[9] Lehmann, J., Vorlop J. and Büntemeyer, H. 1988. Bubble-free Reactors and Their Development for Continuous Culture with Cell Recycle. <u>In: Animal Cell Biotechnology (R.E. Spier and J.B. Griffiths eds.) Academic Press Vol. 3</u> pp. 221-237.

[10] Olsson, I., Axiö-Fredriksson, U.B., Degerman, M. and Olsson, B. (1988a) Fast Horizontal Electrophoresis I. Isoelectric Focusing and Polyacrylamide Gel Electrophoresis Using PhastSystem™. <u>Electrophoresis</u> <u>9</u>, 16-22

[11] Olsson, I., Wheeler, R., Johansson, C., Ekström, B., Stafström, N., Bikhabhai, R. and Jacobson, G. (1988b) Fast Horizontal Electrophoresis II. Development of fast Automated Staining Procedures Using Phast System™. <u>Electrophoresis</u> <u>9</u>, 22-27

[12] Rosenberg, S.A., Lotze, M.T., Muul, L.M., Leitman, S., Chang, A.E., Etting-hausen, S.E., Matory, Y.L., Skibber, J.M., Shiloni, E., Vetto, J.T., Seipp, C.A.,; Simpson, C. and Reichert, C.M. 1985. Observations on the Systemic Admini-stration of Autologous Lymphokine-Activated Killer Cells and Recombinant Interleukin-2 to Patients with Metastatic Cancer. <u>N. Engl. J. Med.</u> <u>313</u>, 1485-1492.

[13] Shu, S., Chou, T. and Rosenberg, S.A. 1986. In vitro Sensitization and Expansion with Viable Tumor Cells and Interleukin 2 in the Generation of Specific Therapeutic Effector Cells. <u>J. Immunol.</u> <u>136</u>, 3891-3898.

[14] Vaith, P., Mass, D., Feigl, D., Hauke, G., Lang, B., Oepke, G., Stierle, H.E., Bross, K.J., Andreesen, R., Gross, G., Monner, D.A., Grote, W. and Mühlradt, P.F. 1985. In-vitro und in-vivo Studien mit Interleukin-2 und verschiedenen Immunstimulanzien bei einem Patienten mit AIDS. <u>Immun. Infekt.</u> <u>13</u>, 51-63.

[15] Wagner, R., Krafft, H. and Lehmann, J. 1989. The Production of Human Interleukin 2 by Recombinant Mammalian Cells. <u>In: Advances in Animal Cell and Biology and Technology for Bioprocesses (R.E. Spier, J.B. Griffiths, J. Stephenne and P.J. Crooy, eds.), Butterworths Pub.</u>, pp. 374-377.

[16] Wagner, R. and Lehmann, J. 1988. The Growth and Productivity of Recombinant Animal Cells in a Bubble-Free Aeration System. <u>Trends Biotechnol.</u> <u>6</u>, 101-104.

[17] Wagner, R., Ryll, T., Krafft, H. and Lehmann, J. 1988. Variation of Amino Acid Concentrations in the Medium of HU ß-IFN and HU IL-2 Producing Cell Lines. <u>Cytotechnology</u> <u>1</u>, 145-150.

[18] Welte, K., Venura, S., Wang, C.Y., Feldman, S.P., Ciobanu, N., Kruger, G., Feickert, H.J., Merluzzi, V.J., Flomenberg, N., Moore, M.A.S. and Mertelsmann, R. 1983. Human Interleukin 2: Physiology, Biochemistry and Pathophysiology in Lymphoblastic Leukemias and Immunodeficiency Syndromes. <u>In: Haematology and Blood Transfusion Vol. 28, Modern Trends in Leukemia V (Neth, Gallo, Greaves, Moore, Winkler, eds.), Springer Verlag Berlin</u>, pp. 369-379.

<u>**Paper of Wagner**</u>:

Hofmann: When we grow hybridomas in protein-free medium we
             see an increase in sensitivity to mechanical
             stress - they may lyse when you stir them. Do you
             see the same effects with BHK, or do you do
             anything to the medium to prevent this?

Wagner: No, we have not seen stress effects but I think
             it depends upon the adaptation of our cell line
             because it has been in cultivation for over 2 1/2
             years.

A PROTEIN-FREE SERUM REPLACEMENT (SSR) FOR CELL CULTURE

Hans Ingolf Nielsen[1] and Kjell Bertheussen[2]

[1]Medi-Cult a/s, Kanalholmen 12, DK-2650 Hvidovre, Denmark, and
[2]Dept. of Clinical Medicine, University of Tromsø, Norway.

ABSTRACT

A synthetic, protein-free serum replacement (SSR) has been
developed which in its basic form contains the principles
necessary to keep cells alive and in good condition, yet at the
same time does not induce growth, attachment or differentation.
This allows a total control over the experimental conditions
and the cells in culture.
Keywords: Serum replacement, Protein-free media, Serum-free
media, Defined media, Cell culture.

INTRODUCTION

In modern cell biological research it is of utmost importance
to be able to control the cells and to know exactly what they
are exposed to. An ideal medium for research purposes should
therefore contain the basic principles which can keep cells
alive for an appropriately long periode of time, and at the
same time not give growth, attachment or differentiation unless
the right growth, attachment or differentiation factors are
present. This paper describes a synthetic serum replacement
(SSR) which fulfills these requirements.

MATERIALS AND METHODS

In the development of a serum replacement as described , some
of the properties and functions of serum and its components
must be avoided, some must be controlled, and some must be
replaced by simpler and controlable systems.

Among the disadvantages of serum which can be avoided in serum-
free culture are:
- Batch to batch variations
- The inflammatory and transforming effect due to blood
  platelet products
- The presence of pathogens and unknown substances
- The presence of unknown antibodies

Some components of serum are important for the behaviour of
the cells, but not necessarily for the mere maintenance. This
is true for a number of hormones, growth factors and attachment factors. Such signal molecules should therefore not be
present in the basic serum replacement, but should be used
selectively in order to control cell behaviour.

Some of the functions of serum are essential for the maintenance of living cells, and must therefore be provided by the serum
replacement, as well:

- Iron and trace elements must be kept in solution at physiological pH, and made available to the cells
- The correct surface tension and viscosity of the medium must be present
- The cells often need an environmental buffer which prevents toxic effects due to (heavy) metal ions, free radicals, proteases, and toxic impurities.

In order to fulfill these requirements, the Medi-Cult® Synthetic Serum Replacements contain a low molecular weight metal ion buffer and chelating system and a non-toxic surfactant.

Certain nutrients (e.g. lipids) cannot be synthesized by all cells and must therefore often be present. Since lipids are water insoluble, a lipid carrier (e.g. albumin) may be required, as well. Because of the fact that not all cells need these molecules, it is considered an advantage not to add them to the basic SSR Synthetic Serum Replacement, but rather add them to the medium, if needed.

Cells in culture are exposed to a much higher oxygen tension than they are *in vivo*. They are therefore subject to oxydation damages, unless protected by antioxidants. Such antioxidants are found in serum. In serum-free culture, pyruvate has proven to be an important antioxidant. Due to its degradability, it is not included in the SSR serum replacement, but is added to the medium.

The above described basic Medi-Cult® SSR Synthetic Serum Replacement (SSR1) is usually supplemented with insulin which is required by practically all cells. This makes it SSR2. Media with SSR2 and pyruvate are named with the suffix -SR2 (e.g. RPMI-SR2, DMEM-SR2). SSR3 is especially made for hybridoma cells, and consists of SSR2 and a low molecular weight compound. All components of SSR are dialyzable.

RESULTS AND DISCUSSION

With the appropriate additions of pyruvate, signal molecules and possibly lipids/albumin, SSR2 has been shown to support a wide range of cell types, e.g.:

Vero (RPMI-SR2 + EGF + HSA + coating)
HeLa (RPMI-SR2 + EGF + dexamethasone + HSA + coating)
HeLa S3 (RPMI-SR2 + coating)
HL 60 (RPMI-SR2 + coating)
3T3 (IMDM-SR2 + dexamethasone + HSA + fetuin (+ FGF) + coating)
SV40 3T3 (IMDM-SR2 + FGF (or fetuin) + HSA + coating)
L929 (RPMI-SR2 + coating)
CHO-K (IMDM-SR2 (+ HSA) + coating)
Fibroblasts (normal) (IMDM-SR2 + EGF + dexamethasone + HSA + fetuin + coating)
Endothelial cells (Guinea pig) (RPMI-SR2 + EGF + coating)
(the coating mentioned above is gelatine + serum)
Hybridoma cells (human and murine) (RPMI-SR3, sometimes with

dexamethasone and/or HSA)
Monocytes (RPMI-SR2 + HSA)
Macrophages (RPMI-SR2)
Langerhans islets (RPMI-SR2)
Oocytes and embryos (human and murine) (EBSS-SR2)

Figures 1 - 3 show examples of growth curves for cells in SSR media and serum-containing media.

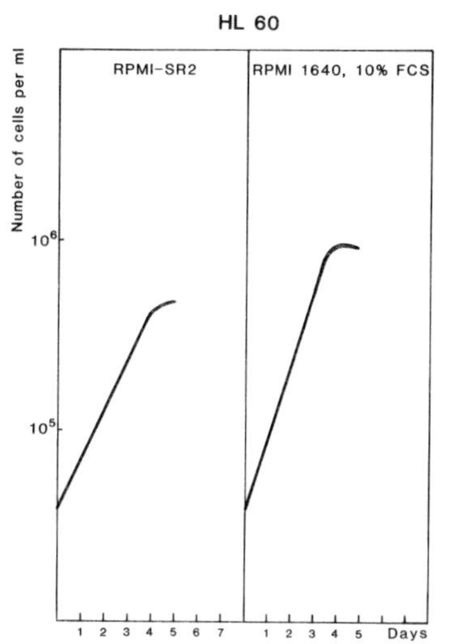

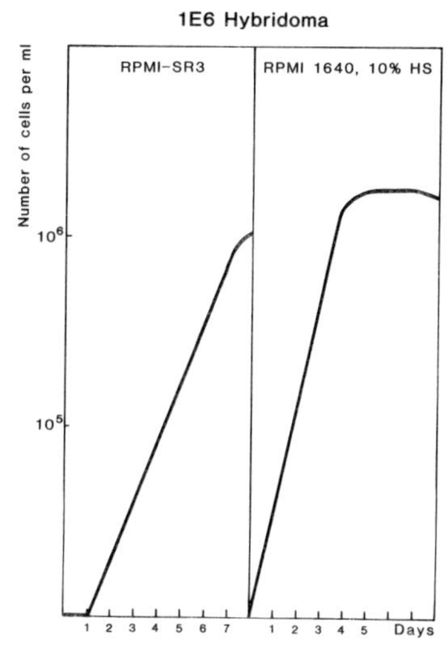

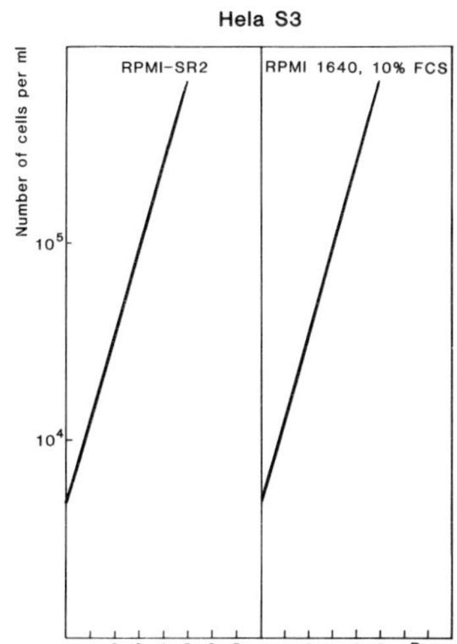

Figure 1. HL 60 cells.

Figure 2. 1E6 Hybridoma cells.

Figure 3. Hela S3 cells.

It is concluded that the Medi-Cult® SSR synthetic serum replacements provide the researcher with a valuable tool in his attempt to control the cell culture conditions. An added advantage in biotechnological research and production is the absence of all but the most important proteins. This obviously facilitates purification and thereby reduces the expenses.

Adaptation and Characterization of Hybridomas Growing in Low Protein and Protein-Free Medium

Frieder Hofmann & Kathie Fritchman

BioTechnetics, 4116 Sorrento Valley Blvd., San Diego, Ca 92121, USA

Abstract:

An adaptation and selection schedule for murine hybridomas is described that results in growth of cells in protein-free basal nutrient that is completely chemically defined. Hybridomas that have passed through the selection process exhibit the same generation times and viabilties combined with higher specific productivity compared to unaltered cells grown in FBS supplemented medium. The protein-free clone is stably transformed to grow in this medium and does not appear to autocrinely secret growth factors required by the original cell line. Judged from SDS-PAGE the secreted antibody is >90% pure. The IEF pattern of the antibody secreted by the protein-free clone does not change with changing the growth condition. However, it is significantly different from the IEF pattern of the antibody secreted by the original cell line.

Introduction:

Hybridomas grow readily in serum supplemented media. However, for the production of injectable grade monoclonal antibodies (MAb) addition of serum presents serious problems as even fetal sera contain a significant amount of immunoglobulin that is difficult to purify away from the MAb of interest. Serum further shows lot to lot variability of cell growth promotion and can be a source of adventitious agents in the final product. Due to these and other problems attempts have been made to formulate serum-free media [1].

A conservative approach for the development of serum-free nutrient is to identify and isolate those individual serum components that are required for cell growth and antibody production and then add them back to the basal media formulation. This, however, will result in media that are more expensive than the serum supplemented nutrient and that are highly customized.

On the other hand, hybridomas can be readily adapted to decreased serum levels. Following this line of thought we developed an adaptation and selection schedule that finally leads to continuous growth of hybridomas in basal nutrient that is completely protein-free.

Materials & Methods:

Murine hybridomas KS1/4 and 9.2.27 and target cell lines UCLA-P3 (human lung adenocarcinoma) and A375 (human melanoma) were kindly provided by Dr. Ralph Reisfeld, Scripps Clinic and Research Foundation, La Jolla, CA, USA. Murine hybridoma OKT-3 was obtained from the ATCC, Rockville, MD, USA.

RPMI 1640 (Irvine Scientific, Irvine, CA, USA) supplemented with selenite, putrescine, pyruvate, ascorbic acid, ethanolamine and ferric nitrate was used as basal nutrient. Fetal Bovine Serum (FBS) (Gibco, Gaithersburg, MD, USA), bovine serum albumin (BSA) (Sigma Chemical Co., St. Louis, MO, USA) and human transferrin (ibid.) were added to the basal medium as indicated in the text.

Cell culture was performed in T-flasks and multi-well plates (Costar, Cambridge, MA, USA) at starting titers of 10^5 cells/ml.

Limited dilution cloning was executed using 96-1/2-well plates with starting titers of 10, 5, and 0.5 cells per 50 µl and well. Cultures were incubated at 37 °C in a 5 to 7% CO_2 atmosphere with the exception of low protein and protein-free media which required >10% CO_2 in air.

For transwell plate experiments cell lines were washed three times in the nutrient of interest and then placed in either the top or bottom well of the transwell plate. 48 hours later the cell titer of each well was determined.

MAb concentration of culture supernatants was quantified by ELISA using goat-anti-mouse-Ig affinity purified serum (Organon Teknika-Cappel, West Chester, PA) as capture antibody and horseradish peroxidase labeled goat-anti-mouse-Ig affinity purified serum (ibid.) as detecting antibody. Blocking agent was 0.5% BSA. The enzyme reaction was carried out in 100 mM phosphate-citrate buffer pH 5.0, 10 mM H_2O_2, 1 mg/ml o-phenylenediamine. The optical density of wells was determined by an ELISA plate reader (Flow Laboratories, MacLean, VA, USA) at 490 nm.

MAb 9.2.27 in the presence of MAb KS1/4 was determined by specifically capturing the 9.2.27 antibody in 0.5% BSA on dried $5 \cdot 10^4$ A375 cells/well. Bound antibody was detected following the ELISA procedure. MAb KS1/4 in the presence of MAb 9.2.27 was determined accordingly using dried UCLA-P3 cells to specifically capture the KS1/4 antibody.

SDS-PAGE of culture supernatants and IEF analysis of KS1/4 MAb were carried out on a PhastSystem (Pharmacia LKB Biotechnology, Piscataway, NJ, USA) using 10-15% gradient PhastGels and PhastGels IEF 5-8, respectively. Gels were stained with PhastGel Blue R. Samples for IEF were purified on a 47 mm Protein A affinity membrane (Memtek, Billerica, MA). The membrane was equilibrated with regeneration buffer (2.5 M NaCl, 50 mM glycine, pH 8.9) prior to loading the sample in regeneration buffer. The membrane bound antibody was extensively washed with regeneration buffer before it was eluted with 50 mM Acetate, pH 4.0. The eluant was immediately neutralized with 200 mM trisodium phosphate and concentrated on Centricon microconcentrators (Amicon, Danvers, MA, USA).

Table 1: *Result of limited dilution cloning of hybridoma OKT-3 in low   protein (100 ng/ml) basal nutrient. Figures indicate number of clones in each class.*

MAb Concentration [μg/ml]

Cell Confluence [%]	<5	5	10	15	20	25	30	35	40
10	27								
20	29	3							
30	11	7		1					
40		6	2						
50		4	5	1					
60	1	3	2	1					
70			1	2	1		1	1	
80			1	3			1	1	
90			1	1			1	2	
100							1		

Results & Discussion:

Adaptation of cell lines to reduced levels of growth factors began by exposing the cells which were previously cultivated in 1 to 10% FBS to serum-free basal medium supplemented with 0.5% BSA and 10 μg/ml of human transferrin. All of the eight murine hybridoma lines that have so far undergone this treatment showed good growth in this medium after an initial reduction in viability. Depending on the cell line, viability could be reduced to 60% for the first two to three passages. However, after two weeks all cell lines showed viability values comparable to culture in FBS containing medium.

After the cell line had recovered it was subjected to limited dilution cloning in the serum-free medium. Two to three weeks into the cloning procedure the relative cell confluence of each well was estimated and the MAb concentration of the cell supernatant determined (Table 1). Five to six of the highest producing and fastest growing clones were proliferated to the 6-well plate stage and their production and generation time monitored for two weeks.

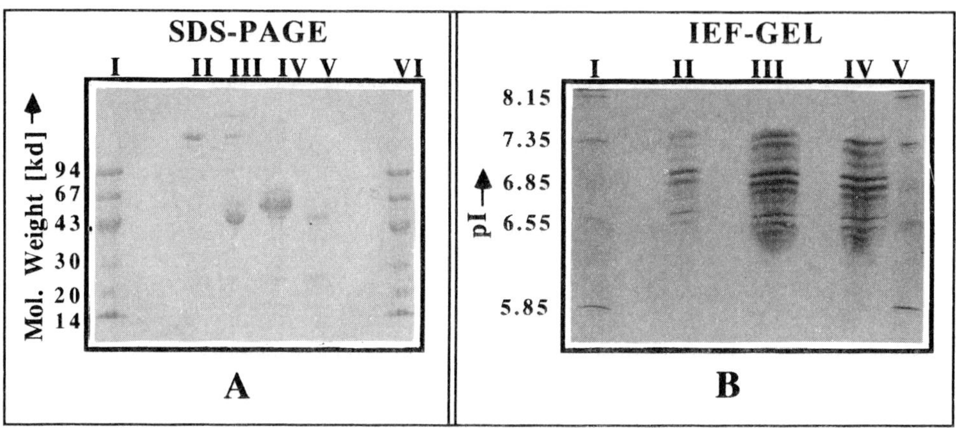

Figure 1: *Electrophoretic analysis of antibody preparations.*
A) SDS-PAGE of 20-fold concentrated KS1/4-71 (Lane II: non-reduced; Lane V: reduced) and KS1/4-OL (Lane III: non-reduced;Lane IV: reduced) culture supernatant. KS1/4-71 was cultivated in protein-free medium. KS1/4-OL was grown in 1% FBS supplemented nutrient.(Lane I and VI: mol. weight standards)
B) IEF pattern of Protein A purified KS1/4 antibody. Lane II: Antibody secreted by KS1/4-OL in 1% FBS supplemented medium. Lane III: Antibody secreted by KS1/4-71 in protein-free medium. Lane IV: Antibody secreted by KS1/4-71 in 1% FBS supplemented medium. Lane I and V: pI standards.

The clones that exhibited stable production in the new medium were then subjected to nutrient that had further reduced levels of albumin and/or transferrin. The nutrient where a clone could just survive was used for the next limited dilution cloning step. Depending on the individual cell line requirements, three two six cloning steps were required to reduce the protein content of the basal medium to 100 ng/ml of transferrin. Stably growing clones in this low protein medium served as the basis for final adaption and selection for growth in the protein-free basal nutrient formulation.

In all cases the cloning procedure had a beneficial side effect in that cell productivity increased by a factor of two to six when compared to the original cell line. Generation time and viability of the new clones were not significantly different from that of the parent line. However, cells growing in the low (100 ng/ml) protein and protein-free media showed increased sensitivity to mechanical stress and toxic impurities in chemicals used in the formulation of basal medium. The sensitivity to mechanical agitation could represent a disadvantage depending on the production system in place. However, it could potentially be overcome by the addition of macromolecules that enhance media viscosity (not tested).

An immediate obvious advantage of growing hybridoma in low protein and protein-free medium is the initial antibody purity in the culture supernatant. Judged from SDS-PAGE results purity of the cell free supernatant of a hybridoma grown in protein-free basal medium can be greater than 90% (Fig. 1a). Initial purity of MAb in low protein medium is not detectably different from that of protein-free medium (result not shown). This is expected as the protein contamination introduced through extraneous transferrin in low protein medium amounts to less than 1% of the secreted MAb concentration of an average producing hybridoma. However, the advantage of protein-free medium is that no foreign protein is introduced into the process.

Table 2: *Mixed culture of KS1/4-OL (OL) and KS1/4-71 (#71) in transwell plates. Figures indicate cell titer after 48 hours. Starting titer was $1 \cdot 10^{5}$/ml. Dashed line indicates membrane separator.*

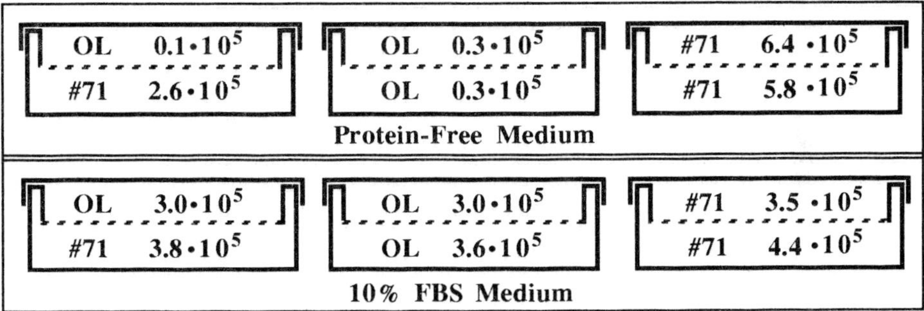

Line KS1/4-71 isolated from limited dilution cloning in protein-free medium was most thoroughly characterized. This clone was in continuous culture in basal medium for over six months without exhibiting a significant decrease in growth rate or viability (generation time: (21.3 ±0.4) h; viability: (89 ±1.2)%; original line: generation time: (20.3 ±0.7) h; viability: (91 ± 2.5)%). However, this cell line showed about a two-fold higher specific productivity when compared to the original cell line (productivity: (92 ±6) pg/(cell·day) vs. (48 ±6) pg/(cell·day)).

The original KS1/4 cell line (KS1/4-OL) had been weaned to grow in 1% FBS supplemented basal medium. When KS1/4-OL was exposed to protein-free medium it stopped growing and died off within three to four days.

In contrast, KS1/4-71 did not lose its capability to thrive in protein-free medium even after a one month passage in 1% FBS medium. This strongly indicates that KS1/4-71 is stably transformed rather than transiently physiologically adapted to grow in protein-free medium.

To decide whether this clone has gained the capability of autocrinely secreting growth factors required by the original cell line three experiments were performed.

In the first experiment clone 71 was cultivated for three days in protein-free medium to a titer of $8.6 \cdot 10^{5}$ cells/ml. The cell-free supernatant was harvested and 1:1 diluted with fresh protein-free nutrient. The parent cell line and clone 71 were exposed to this nutrient mixture and to fresh protein-free and 1% FBS containing medium. Clone 71 exhibited similar growth in all three media. In contrast, parent KS1/4 only proliferated in 1% FBS and died off in both protein-free media without showing any difference between the conditioned and fresh formulation.

In a second experiment clone 71 and the parent cell line were co-cultivated but separated by a 0.4 µm membrane in 10-transwell plates . As indicated by the results shown in Table 2 clone 71 did not support growth of the parent cell line in protein-free medium.

In a third experiment clone 71 was directly co-cultivated with non-protein-free adapted hybridoma 9.2.27. This hybridoma secretes an antibody that binds to a different antigen. The cells were grown together and separately in protein-free and 1% FBS nutrient for a total of six passages. Dilution of cultures with fresh nutrient at time of passage was identical for all combinations based on the cell count in the KS1/4-71 /.9.2.27 mixed culture in protein-free medium. Although 9.2.27 antibody was detected in the supernatant of 1% FBS supplemented medium of both the 9.2.27 culture and KS1/4-71 / 9.2.27 mixed culture it was not discovered in any of the protein-free culture supernatants (Table 3).

Table 3: *Specific binding results of culture supernatants of KS1/4-71 and 9.2.27 hybridomas grown in 1% FBS supplemented and protein-free medium (PFM). KS1/4 and 9.2.27 were cultivated separately and combined. KS1/4 antibody binds specifically to cell line UCLA-P3 (P3) and 9.2.27 binds specifically to cell line A375.*

Culture Condition		Specific Binding to:		Culture Condition		Specific Binding to:	
1% FBS		**P3**	**A375**	**PFM**		**P3**	**A375**
Culture	KS1/4	yes	no	Culture	KS1/4	yes	no
	9.2.27	no	yes		9.2.27	no	no
	Combined	y e s	y e s		**Combined**	y e s	**<u>no</u>**

These three experiments suggest that the protein-free media clone KS1/4-71 is unlikely to support its growth with autocrinely secreted growth factors. The results rather support the view that KS1/4-71 is a growth factor independent mutant.

It is noteworthy that the low protein and protein-free growing clones do not require unsaturated fatty acids or cholesterol as these compounds were not included in the basic nutrient formulation.

There is a concern that the IEF pattern of antibodies changes with the culture condition of the hybridoma. Moellering et al.[2] showed that the differences in the IEF pattern of an antibody secreted by a hybridoma proliferated in serum-free culture and ascites were due to enzymic modification of the antibody in ascitic liquid. In contrast, we found that the IEF pattern of KS1/4-71 antibody did not change with the growth condition (Fig. 1b). However, the antibody IEF pattern of the selected protein-free medium clone was significantly different from the antibody IEF pattern of the original cell line. This means that the different conditions of *in vitro* culture have no influence on the secreted product of a stable clone that has been selected for growth in protein-free medium. However, care should be taken in the case of weaning cells to serum-free or protein-free conditions. In all our cloning experiments we saw a great heterogeneity in terms of growth and productivity of the previous clone when exposed to new growth medium (Fig. 1). It appears possible that there may also be differences in post-translational modifications of the antibody hidden in this scheme. Currently, it is not known how important the IEF pattern of a therapeutic antibody might be in terms of efficacy and *in vivo* stability. Product consistency, however, is important and can apparently be achieved by cloning the hybridoma in the final production nutrient.

In summary, it is possible to adapt and select murine hybridomas to grow in completely protein-free media. Besides the benefit of high initial antibody purity the selection process also delivers clones that secret antibody at a significantly higher level. In addition, the cost of the medium described is that of regular basal nutrient - the lowest possible. On the down side, these clones are more shear sensitive and it usually takes four to six months until the final clone is isolated.

References:

1) Murakami, H. "Serum-Free Media for Cultivation of Hybridomas" (1989) in "Monoclonal Antibodies: Production and Application", Advances in Biotechnological Processes, Vol. 11, Mizrahi, A., ed., Alan R. Liss, Inc., New York, NY, USA, pp 107-141

2) Moellering, B.J., Tedesco, J.L., Townsend, R.R., Hardy, M.R., Scott, R.W. & Prior, C.P. "Electrophoretic Differences in a MAb Expressed in Three Media" (1990), BioPharm 3,2:30-38

CHARACTERIZATION OF PROTEASE ACTIVITY IN SERUM-FREE CULTURE SUPERNATANTS OF HYBRIDOMAS AND RECOMBINANT MAMMALIAN CELLS.

Waldemar Lind, Volker Jäger, Mona Lucki-Lange, and Roland Wagner

Arbeitsgruppe Zellkulturtechnik, Gesellschaft für Biotechnologische Forschung, Mascheroder Weg 1, D-3300 Braunschweig, FRG

ABSTRACT

[^{3}H]-labelled Casein was used for a quantitative determination of protease activity in cell culture supernatants during long-term cultivation of BHK and hybridoma cells. They produced recombinant human interleukin 2 an IgG$_{2a}$-antibody respectively in serum- or protein free medium. Protease activities were characterized by inhibitor studies and specific p-NA derivates. Only 20% of the total protease activity in hybridoma cells and up to 50% in BHK cells is based om serine type proteases.

Key words: Protease activity, serum- or protein free medium, serine proteases, protease-inhibitor, LDH-activity, long-term cultivation.

INTRODUCTION

Proteolytic enzymes, or proteases, are enzymes which catalyze the cleavage of peptide bonds in other proteins. They have many physiological functions, ranging from generalized protein digestion to more specific regulatory functions such as the activation of zymogens, blood coagulation and the lysis of fibrin clots, the release of hormones and pharmacologically active peptides from precursor proteins, and the transport of secretory proteins across membranes [10]. During cultivation of animal cells proteases are released into the medium. Cultures of transformed cells often show a higher protease activity than those of normal cells [2,4]. Medium supplemented with serum inhibits proteases as the total protein content in serum consists of up to 10% inhibitors. In cultures with serum-free medium proteases can have a negative influence upon cell prolife-ration as well as causing protein substrate loss [9]. Additionally, a low protein content may cause a higher protease activity [12].

MATERIAL AND METHODS

Media

The serum-free medium DIF for the cultivation of hybridomas consists of a 1:1 mixture of Iscove's modified Eagle and Ham's F-12 medium (Gibco-BRL) supplemented with 10 mg/l iron saturated human transferrin, (Behringwerke, Marburg), 10 mg/l bovine insulin (I 5500 Sigma) and oleic acid complexed by BSA (Serva 11924). The preparation of these supplements has been described by V. Jäger [5].

The protein-free medium for the cultivation of transformed BHK cells is based on a 1:1 mixture of DMEM and Hams's F-12 medium (Gibco-BRL) and some organic and inorganic supplements as described by Lucki-Lange and Wagner (1989) [8].

Cell lines

The rat-mouse-hybridoma 412 (Institut für Neurobiologie, Heidelberg) is a hybridoma of the myeloma X63-Ag 8.653 and the spleen of the Spraque-Dawley-rat. It produces an IgG_{2a}-antibody.

The BHK 21 pSVIL2-cell line provided by the genetic engineering department of the GBF was manipulated by genetic methods to produce human interleukin 2 constitutively under the control of the SV 40 promoter (Conradt *et al.* 1986 [1]).

Reactor systems

For the cultivation of the cells in suspension 1.4-l-double membrane reactors were used (Lehmann *et al.* 1988 [7]). Dense cell cultivation of the hybridoma cells was performed in the hollow fibre bioreactor system according to Jäger (1988) [5].

Analysis of samples

Viable and dead cell numbers were estimated by trypan blue exclusion.

Lactate dehydrogenase (LDH) activity was determined as described previously [11]

Immunoglobulin concentrations were determined by using a standard sandwich-ELISA [5].

Protease-inhibitors

SBTI (Soybean Trypsin Inhibitor, Sigma, Deisenhofen) specifically inhibits trypsin. The specific activity of the inhibitor was 6000 U/mg. In the assay the inhibitor was used at a concentration of 1 mg/ml ($\equiv$ 6000 U/ml)

Aprotinin (Bayer, Leverkusen) is a basic protease inhibitor. It inhibits a broad spectrum of serine proteases and shows an unusual stability to proteolytic degradation [6]. The specific activity of aprotinin was 5850 KIU/mg. One KIU (Kallikrein-Inaktivator-Unit) corresponds to an aprotinin amount, which is able to decrease the activity of two biological Kallikrein-Units about 50%. In the assay the inhibitor was used at a concentration of 26 mg/ml ($\equiv$1500 KIU/ml).

ϵ-aminocaproic acid specifically inhibits plasmin and plasminogen activators. The inhibitor concentration in the assay was 10 mg/ml.

Substrates for the determination of protease activity

The protease assay is based on the measurement of trichloroacetic acid (TCA) soluble peptides which are released from isotopically labelled protein substrates, according to Hatcher *et al.* (1976) [3]. The [³H]-labelled Casein is prepared by irradiation of Casein nach Hammarstan (Serva Feinbiochemica, Heidelberg) with Tritium according to the Wilzbach-Method (Amersham International plc., England), followed by a removal of labile Tritium. This method includes a partly damage of the substrate and it was therefore purified through separation on Sephadex G-25 (PD 10) and additionally on Sephadex G-75 Medium columns (Pharmacia, Uppsala). The Tritium labelled Casein has a specific activity of

$1.055 \cdot 10^5$ Bq/μg. In the assay a Casein concentration of 6.66 μg/ml with a total activity of $3 \cdot 10^5$ cpm was used.

Supernatants of cell cultivation in the hollow fibre system were also tested for protease activity with the chromogenic substrate S-2288 (H-D-Ile-Pro-Arg-p-NA$\cdot$2HCl), (Kabi Vitrum, Sweden). This substrate is particularly specific for a broad spectrum of serine proteases such as thrombin, urokinase, plasmin etc.
In the assay S-2288 was used in a 2 mmol/l concentration. The release of p-NA was determined in a kinetik photometer (Ultrospec K, LKB, Freiburg) at a wavelength of 405 nm (t = 1 min; T = 37°C).

RESULTS AND DISCUSSION

Proteolytic activities in the presence of inhibitors

The influence of inhibitors on protease activities was proved on supernatants from suspension cultures of the BHK 21 pSVIL2 cell line (sample Nr. 1, 2) and in supernatants of the hetero-hybridoma cell line cultivated in the hollow fibre bioreactor (sample Nr. 3, 4). High inhibitor concentrations were chosen, so that all target proteases would be inhibited.
As shown in the table the serine protease inhibitors were able to inhibit only a part of the total protease activity. The transformed BHK cell line released more serine proteases than the hetero-hybridoma cells. Since ϵ-aminocaproic acid showed no inhibitory effect, the serine protease activities are due to other proteases than plasmin or PA.

Sample-Nr.	1	2	3	4
$\mathrm{cpm}_{[\mathrm{sample}]} \cdot 10^{-2}$	383	428	364	530
$\mathrm{cpm}_{[\mathrm{sample}]} \cdot 10^{-2}$ + SBTI	170 -56%	200 -53%	300 -17%	435 -18%
$\mathrm{cpm}_{[\mathrm{sample}]} \cdot 10^{-2}$ + Aprotinin	200 -47%	210 -51%	290 -20%	405 -23%
$\mathrm{cpm}_{[\mathrm{sample}]} \cdot 10^{-2}$ + ϵ-aminocap.	no inhibition			

Table: Data are expressed in percent of protease inhibition

Proteolytic activities during long-term cultivation

At the beginning of the cultivation of BHK cells (see fig. 1b) the protease activity was high due to the previous trypsinization step for releasing the cells from the surface of the culture flasks. The cells were transferred under protein-free conditions, which necessitated the termination of trypsin-activity by supplementation with SBTI. Inhibition could not be completely suppressed but when perfusion was started after 48 hours the remaining trypsin could be washed out and protease activity which was released from the cells remained at a constant low level. As a result of process control with respect to perfusion a constant enzyme activity level could be maintained between 120 and 320 hours of cultivation (fig. 1b). The effect of perfusion on medium proteins could be demonstrated after 100 h when the continuous mode was stopped for a short time and protease activity dramatically increased.

LDH-activity remained constant during cultivation and correlated with the small portion of dead cells. An increase at the end of fermentation when oxygen limitation occured could be found and more cells died. Whereas the LDH-activity is linearly correlated with the number of dead cells the protease-activity depended on the ratio of viable to dead cells and their cell cycle phase. The higher product concentrations and protease activities at the end of cultivation are based on membrane clogging of the perfusion system.

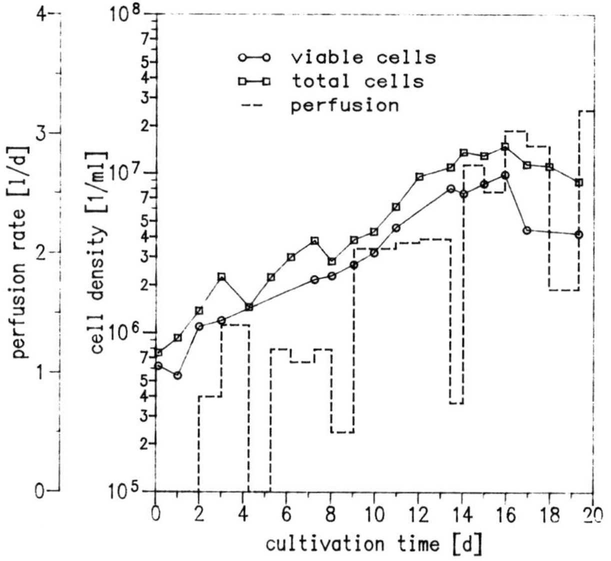

Fig. 1a: Viable and total cells during long-term cultivation of BHK 21 pSVIL2 cells

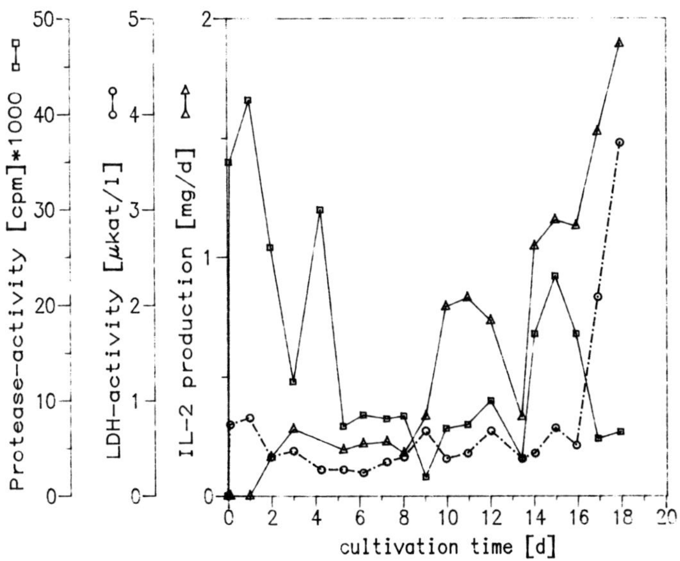

Fig. 1b Progress of protease-activities, LDH and IL-2 production during cultivation of BHK 21 pSVIL2 cells.

Production process for monoclonal antibodies was characterized by the separation of the cell propagation phase in a 1.4-l-stirred tank and the cell maintenance phase in a hollow fibre reactor. At the beginning of the cell propagation protease-activity was approx. 9000 cpm and with the beginning of perfusion was decreased to approx. 4000 cpm (fig. 2b). With increasing cell density protease activities also increased, whereas the dilution effect of the perfusion caused a maintanence at an intermediate level. After 11 days of cultivation $1.5 \cdot 10^{10}$ cells were harvested resulting in a reduced mass of $3.66 \cdot 10^6$ cells per ml. At the end of the propagation process protease-activity and LDH-activity increased. In contrast to LDH-activity, which showed a direct correlation to the number of dead cells, there is no such correlation between proteolytic activity and the amount of dead cells. At the end of the process protein concentration and enzyme activity increased as a result of membrane clogging as mentioned before. After 18 days of cultivation cells were transferred into the extracapillary space of the hollow fibre cartridge. The high cell density and the ultrafiltration membrane caused higher protein concentrations (see fig. 3). A proteolytic activity of 6.3 μkat/l could be determined within the shell side of the reactor for serine proteases using the specific substrate S-2288. Characterization of protease activities with specific inhibitors demonstrated that only a portion of approx. 20% was caused by serine proteases in hybridoma cells. Due to our results with specific enzyme inhibitors as shown in the table it can be assumed that total protease activity was several times higher and may therefore cause serious problems in high density cell cultivation.

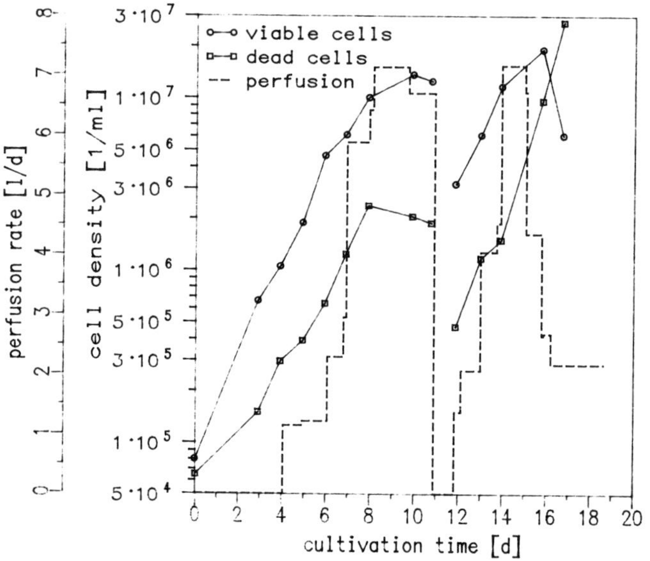

Fig. 2a Viable and dead cells during the cultivation of the hybridoma cells.

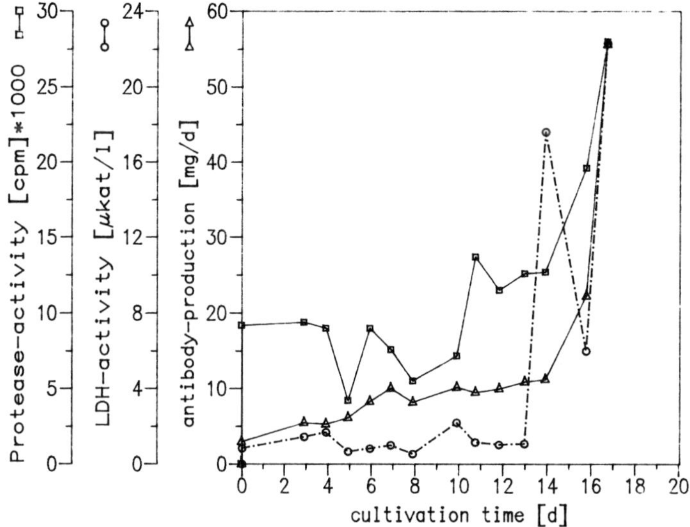

Fig. 2b Progress of protease-activities, LDH and MAb-production during cultivation of hybridoma cells.

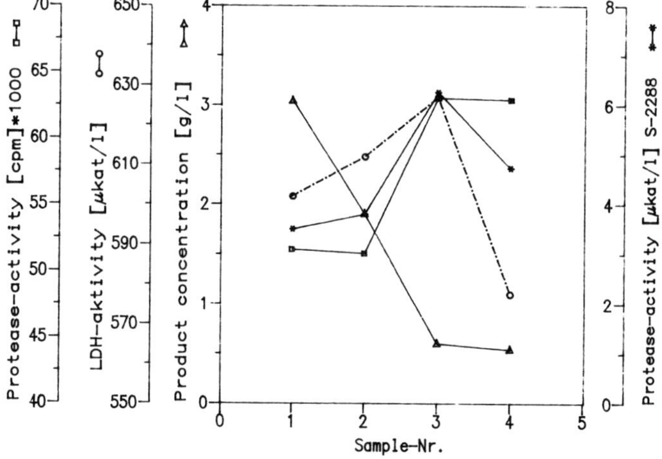

Fig. 3 Cultivation of hybridoma cells in the hollow fibre bioreactor.

REFERENCES

[1]   Conradt, H. S.; Ausmeier, M.; Dittmar, K. E.; Hauser, H. J.; Lindenmaier, W. Secretion of Glycosylated Human Interleukin-2 by Rekombinant Mammalian Cell Lines. <u>Carbohydrate Research</u> 1986, <u>149</u>, pp 443-450

[2]   Goldberg, A. R. Increased Protease Levels in Transformed Cells: A Casein Overlay Assay for the Detection of Plasminogen Activator Production. <u>Cell</u> <u>1974</u>, 2, pp 95-102

[3]   Hatcher, V. B.; Wertheim, M. S.; Rhee, C. Y.; Tsien, G.; Burk, P. G. Relationship between Cell Surface Protease Activity and Doubling Time in Various Normal and Transformed Cells. Biochim. et Biophys. Acta 1976, 451, pp 499-510

[4]   Hatcher, V. B.; Obermann, M. S.; Wertheim, M. S.; Rhee, C. Y.; Tsien, G.; Burk, P. G. The Relationship between Surface Protease Activity and the Rate of Cell Proliferation in Normal and Transformed Cells. Biochem. and Biophys. Res. Comm. 1977, 76, pp 602-608

[5]   Jäger, V. Entwicklung eines Hohlfaser-Perfusionsreaktor-Systems zur Produktionsoptimierung monoklonaler Antikörper, Dissertation, Universität Hannover, 1988

[6]   Kassel, B.; Wang, T.-W. The Action of Thermolysin on the Basic Trypsin Inhibitor of Bovine Organs; in: Proc. Int. Res. Conf. of Proteinase Inhibitors, München, WdG Verlag, Berlin, 1971, pp 89-94

[7]   Lehmann, J.; Vorlop J.; Büntemeyer H. Bubble-free Reactors and their Development for Continuous Culture with Cell Recycle. In: Animal Cell Biotechnology (R.E. Spier and J.B. Griffith eds.) Vol. 3, 1988, pp 221-237

[8]   Lucki-Lange, M.; Wagner, R. Conditions for the Production of Recombinant IL-2 in Stirred Suspension Culture Using a Protein-Free Medium. In: Production of Biologicals from Animal Cells in Culture Research, Development and Achievements (Spier, R. E.; Griffiths, J. B.; eds.) 1990, Butterworths, submitted

[9]   Murakami, H. Serum-Free Media Used for Cultivition of Hybridomas. In Monoclonal Antibodies: Production and Application 1989, pp 107-141; Alan. Liss Inc.

[10]   Neurath, H. Evolution of Proteolytic Enzymes. Science 1984, 224, 350-357

[11]   Ryll, T.; Lucki-lange, M.; Jäger, V.; Wagner, R. Production of Recombinant Interleukin 2 with BHK Cells in a Hollow Fibre and a Stirred Tank Reactor with Protein-Free Medium. J. Biotechnology in Press 1990

[12]   Schlaeger, E. J.; Eggimann, B.; Gast, A. Proteolytic Activity in the Culture Supernatants of Mouse Hybridoma Cells. Develop. Biol. Standard 1987, 66, pp 403-408

<u>**Paper of Lund:**</u>

<u>**Jenkins:**</u>	Have you looked at the chromogenic substrates you can get from Kabi which have a narrow range of specificity to try and identify which target residue the protease(s) are working on.
<u>Lind:</u>	I have tried it but the substrates were not sensitive enough. I will test it.
Jenkins:	It will help you define which proteases you are looking at if you used more specific substrate.

Section 4
Cell physiology

ANIMAL CELLS IN CULTURE MAKE SECONDARY METABOLITES TOO.

R.E. Spier,
Wolfson Cytotechnology Laboratory,
University of Surrey, Guildford, Surrey, GU1 2PS. U.K.

1. Objectives of this paper;.

The three points I wish to make in this paper are that,

1. animal cells in culture are not significantly different in kind from other microorganisms in culture,

2. animal cells in culture make secondary metabolites in an equivalent manner to other microorganisms and

3. animal cell physiologists wishing to understand the mechanisms which control the production of secondary metabolites in animal cells may well be able to learn some lessons and get some ideas from studies which have been done on other microorganisms making antibiotics or enzymes not needed for the growth and replication of the producing cell.

2. Animal Cells and Other Microbes.

That animal cells in culture are equivalent to other microbes found in nature is a concept that is thrust upon an Animal Cell Biotechnogist working in a traditional department of Microbiology. It is not a new idea. In 1962 a review appeared on this subject (1). In summary the essential arguments supporting this contention are that;

1. animal cells are small, (needing a microscope for their visualisation), organisms which grow and divide in the artificial conditions of a culture using biochemicals and physicochemical structures which have homologues in all cellular life forms,

2. the techniques for manipulation, measurement, sterility and quality control, scale-up and product generation are similar to those used for bacteria, yeast, penicillia etc.,

3. each of the different classes of microorganism has a macroform: bacteria have the stromatolites, fungi have the mushrooms, algae have the seaweeds, protozoa have the slime moulds, (viruses have the least in common with other microorganisms, (though Virology is nearly always included in microbiology texts !), their parasitic nucleic acid becomes active only as a cellular entity in which case they become an element in giving a particular character to a cellular and conventional microorganism),

4. most microorganisms can exist in clonal forms; in low-aqueous environments this form of existence would be the norm particularly for fungi and soil organisms and it is important to realise that within a clone there will be , of necessity, some form of differentiation as the different cells of the clone experience differing microenvironments due to concentration gradients of nutrients, oxygen and the materials secreted by the local cells.

That most microorganisms can live in clonal forms is crucial to the understanding of the nature of, and reason for, the production of secondary metabolites. (Incidentally, it is as well to recognise that we, humans, are clones of 10^13-10^14, almost, (taking into account somatic mutation), genetically identical, microbial cells).

2. What are Secondary Metabolites ?

There is not a consensus as to what constitutes a secondary metabolite. Some 17 definitions are presented in reference 2. However, Table 1 presents this author's view of the essential characteristics of secondary metabolites.

Table 1.

2.1. Particular molecular species produced by cells

2.2. The cells which produce them do not need or use them for their own regulation or growth, (were the cell to be mutated to cease to produce such a metabolite then the normal consequence would be that the cell would grow and divide at a faster rate than previously)

2.3. Their functionality is usually dependent on generating an advantage for a collection, (usually, a clone), of cells operating as an organism

2.4. They can be small or large molecules made by single enzymes or multiple enzymes in sequence whose aminoacid composition can be coded for on either chromosomes or episomes in a linked or non-linked array of genetic information

2.5. They are generally secreted, (to the advantage of the other cells of the clone or the clone in its totality), or stored to similar effect

2.6. They are unique to the producing cells and can often be used to characterise the producing clone

2.7. They are made at a particular time in the life history of a clone in a spatially localised subsection of the clone

2.8 Their functions can include those of;

      *providing protection by killing other microorganisms,
      *metal complexing agents, (which can be functional in the killing sense by depriving other organisms of essential nutrients), or making essential nutrients available intracellularly,
      *a commodity which enables the mutually beneficial interaction of plants and bacteria, nematodes and insects, insects and bacteria, (3)
      *sex hormones
      *effectors of differentiation and on occasion of the death and dissolution of particular sectors of the clone
      *promoters of the sexual process by generating smells, tastes and colours

2.9. Examples of such secondary metabolites are given in Table 2

Table 2

EXAMPLES OF NON-ANIMAL CELL SECONDARY METABOLITES, (culled from 3)

Material	Producing Organism	Function
Streptomycin	Actinomycetes bacteria	Antibiotic
Penicillin	Penicillium Fungi	Antibiotic
Prodigiosin	Serratia Bacteria	Antiamoeba
Tabtotoxin-b-lactam	Pseudomonas Syringae	Chlorosis in H. Plants
Peptide lactones	Alternaria Fungus	Black Spot in Apples
Aflatoxin	Aspergillus Fungus	Insecticide
Tunicamycin	Corynebacterium	Rye grass toxicity of L. Animals
Siderophores	Nocardia	Fe,Cu,Zn uptake in competitive situations
Diatretylnitrile	Leucopacillus ectomycorrhiza	Resistance to plant pathogen Phytophtora
Tryptophan Derivatives	Xenorhabdus	Insecticide for Nematodes
Polymyxin	Bacillus	Antibiotic for Insects
Trisporic Acids	Mucales	Sex hormones
Gramicidin	Bacillus	Spore differentiation
Odour, Taste Colour Materials	H.Plants	Sexual reproduction

2.10. Table 3 for animal cell products (4) .

Table 3

Examples of Secondary Metabolites produced by Animal Cells.

Steroids	Hyaluronic Acid
Collagen	Chondroitin Sulphate
Laminin	Fibronectin
Heparin	Chitin
Gonadotrophin	Haemoglobin
von Willebrand Factor	Macrophage and Granulocyte Stimulating Factors
Interferons	Interleukins
Phosvitin	Tyrosine transaminase
Crystallin	Immunoglobulins
Casein	Histamine
Serotonin	Dopamine
Acetyl Choline	Choline esterase
Adrenalin	noradrenalin
Cyclic ketones	Oxygen radicals
Melanin	Dopaoxidase
Myosine	Creatine kinase
Elastin	Insulin
Triiodothyronine	Growth hormone
Prolactin	Hyaline

2.11. The products derived from the insertion of genes into a host cell or by the infection of a host cell by viruses may not be considered to be secondary metabolites but may rather be termed either Tertiary Metabolites or Parasitic Metabolites

3. The Physiology of the production of Secondary Metabolites in non-animal cell .

While there is a defined biochemistry which is implicated in the production of each and every metabolite generated by a cell, there is also a physiology which defines the quantitative, (rate and amount), and qualitative aspects of that production, its spatial localisation, the time at which the production occurs and the way external or environmental factors are implicated in that production. For the secondary metabolites produced by non-animal cells in culture extensive studies have been done to determine, in particular, the way in which external factors can, for instance, increase the production of antibiotics. In parallel with these studies , investigators have sought to unravel the control mechanisms affecting such production with identical objectives in mind. Such work has tended to consider the producing cell as the element for the focus of attention. However the definition of a secondary metabolite as developed in section 2 above would shift the focus of that attention to the situation wherein the producing entity is A CELL AS A MEMBER OF A CLONE OF CELLS operating in a manner which would confer benefit to the colony as a whole rather than the producing cell as an isolated, independent entity. It is however heuristic to survey the hypotheses which have been adduced to account for the way secondary metabolites have been produced in non-animal cell microbes for from such conjecturings may come the more successful hypotheses of the future.

Early work showed that the ability of an organism to produce a secondary metabolite could be markedly influenced by the nature of the culture. Surface cultures would perform differently from cultures of cells held in monodisperse form in suspension which again would be different from clumps of cells homogeneously distributed about the three dimensional space of the bioreactor, (2,5). It is particularly striking in this vein to note that a colony of a fungus growing on a surface will show marked differentiation such that an outer zone or peripheral zone can be discerned where growth takes place at the hyphal tips. The next innermost zone is one where secondary metabolites are produced but sporulation does not take place. More centrally yet, the third zone is where fruiting and sporulation takes place while at the centre of the colony there is an aged zone of necrosis. (5). This organisation of the colony can demonstrate that an antibiotic produced by such a fungus may have the function of killing its own cells in the centre of the colony in order to provide nutrients for the adjacent cells which are producing the fruiting and sporulating bodies which would enable the cells of the colony to escape from the nutrient depleted situation to colonise new ground following the dispersal of the spores, (see also 10).

The concept that the fungus produces antibiotics to kill off local bacteria which would otherwise deplete nutrient reserves may not be tenable for; (i), the secondary metabolite is not formed at the periphery of the colony where the bacteria are likely to be encountered in the first instance, (ii), the local concentrations of secondary metabolite are insufficient to kill microorganisms outside the domain of the colony itself, (c), the antibiotics produced are often specific to a type of bacterium which would give others a free reign to grow and replicate and (d), the organisms which produce the antibiotics make enzymes which hydrolyse the antibiotics as they are produced. (Successful commercial variants of antibiotic producing organisms are those which have lost the ability to hydrolyse their own antibiotic and/or which are immune to its action by decreasing the passage of the antibiotic across the cell membrane into the cell). It is likely that the cells at the centre of the colony where nutrients have been depleted longest are no longer able to make the hydrolytic enzymes and therefore succumb to the toxic effects of the antibiotic and make the materials of which those cells are made available to the other, adjacent, cells of the colony for spore formation.

Nutrient limitation is alleged to be the cause of the production of secondary metabolites by a substantial subset of non animal cell microbial physiologists. They cite evidence that when either carbon, nitrogen or phosphorous sources are in short supply the cells switch to secondary metabolite production. Oxygen depletion may operate in a similar way, (5). The argument is developed to hypothesise that the limitation of such nutrients relieves a "catabolite repression" of the production of the secondary metabolite thus enabling the efflorescence of such metabolites. However, there are examples when secondary metabolites are produced in conditions where nutrients are in plentiful supply, (2).

A further development of the idea of the critical influence of the nutrient state is that which posits that it is the level of a key energy rich intermediate which controls the physiology of secondary metabolite production. To this end the levels of energy charge, $((ATP+0.5ADP)/(ATP+ADP+AMP)$ which is 1 when there is only ATP and lower values, typically 0.8 to 0.95 when ADP and AMP are present), or the level of ATP or of the Triphosphonucleotides can be taken as an index of the cellular state. While there are indications that correlations of such parameters with the time of the production of the secondary metabolite can be obtained (5), there is not a universal situation which can be accepted by all who work in this area.

More recent work has shown that there are molecules whose concentration changes with the level of secondary metabolite production. Such a material is ppGpp (magic spot). This can be shown to rise when the cells of Streptomyces griseoflavus produce bicozamycin and aerial mycelium, (6). This author asserts that this molecule is involved in the signalling system which leads to differentiation and secondary metabolite formation. A second molecule which is involved in the signal transmission could be that of cAMP, (7). In addition there has been defined an A-Factor, (8) which is a butyrolactone which when added to Streptomyces in the presence of non-limiting nutrients is capable of making those cells produce the secondary metabolite and differentiate into the sporulating form of the organism.

Considerable attention has been given to the exploration of the concept that secondary metabolites are produced when cells are growing at a rate which is intermediary between that of full exponential growth and the zero growth rate of the stationary phase. (Before a decline in cell viability or numbers has set in), (Reference 5 quotes an example for Streptomyces based production of oleandomycin where it is clear that the maximum rate of antibiotic biosynthesis is when the cells are in the transition between the exponential and stationary growth phases). This phenomenon is translated into the "Fed-Batch" system of culture for the production of secondary metabolite antibiotics. The system seeks to maintain the cells in this transition growth rate situation by periodicaliy removing a relatively small fraction of the culture (5-10%), and replacing the same with fresh nutrients.

4. The Physiology of the Production of Secondary Metabolites from Animal Cells in Culture.

Work over the last five years, particularly that focused on the production of monoclonal antibodies from hybridoma cell lines has repeatedly demonstrated that the cells generate product at a higher cell specific rate when the cells are stressed in any of a number of wholly unrelated ways. The production of these less than optimal (for cell growth) conditions can be achieved by such physical stresses as an increase in osmolarity from 300 to 400 mOsmols, an increase in the hydrodynamic stress, a decrease in the pH to about 6.8, or a decrease in the temperature to 32 degC. Further stresses can be inflicted by nutritional or chemical means. Such insults can be levied by lowering the dissolved oxygen concentration, decreasing the level of a key nutrient, (glucose, glutamine), adding a metabolic inhibitor, increasing the cell concentration or by decreasing the serum level. This phenomenology promotes the questions; do all these stresses act in the same way to increase the cell specific productivity of antibody and what is that mechanism if it is common to the different situations ?

A cursory investigation of the situation can show that it is unlikely that the levels of exogenous metabolites are implicated in the control mechanism. As evidence one can cite the cells of the skin where the epidermal layer is dividing continually while the nextmost layer differentiates into a keratinocyte which ceases to divide; both layers of cells are well within range of supplies of nutrients adequate for their metabolism yet one layer differentiates while the other divides yet again. Secondly, cells in the liver (hepatocytes) do not show differences dependent upon their distance from the capillaries which supply them with nutrients. This makes it unlikely that cells in the body depend on exogenous nutrient levels to effect their differentiation. Rather it is well known that molecules involved in the attachment of cells to surfaces have a profound effect on the differentiation of the cell.

In experiments where the level of adenine nuceotides and energy charge have been measured in relation to the cell specific productivity of an antibody it was found that energy charge did not correlate with high cell specific productivity whereas the overall level of adenine nuceotides did so correlate. (Unpublished work of the author and K. Modha). Bushell et al, on the other hand has found that antibody is produced within a window of values of energy charge and growth rate when these are plotted against one another over the time course of the culture,(9).

The possibility remains that secondary metabolism in animal cells is controlled by the level of particular signal molecules within the cell which operate by controlling the switch mechanism which determines whether a cell makes biomass for growth and reproduction or whether the cell ceases to reproduce and concentrates its efforts on the production of a secondary metabolite. The level of such signal molecules could be dependent on the concentrations of key intermediary metabolites which may either induce or relieve catabolite repression of particular genes which code for the signal molecules or the derepression of the genes could be a response to the state of the cell as determined by the perceived level of stress that cell is experiencing which could be either nutritional, chemical or physical. A summary of the possible interactions is presented as a model which could promote the development of such hypotheses. (Figure 1).

The situation is clearly complex. But the model does lend itself to experimental investigation based on concepts which include an additional dimension; that of the signal molecules and their effects. There is little doubt that cells can be switched on to produce certain secondary metabolites, (antibodies, haemoglobin, pepsin etc.), and that once they have been so designated it is that metabolite and not any other which is produced beyond the requirements of the producing cell. This means that signal molecules can and do switch particular genes on and off and that it is but a minor extension of this concept to envisage such gene switching mechanisms to be implicated in the control of secondary metabolite production of animal cells in culture. These considerations would turn the thinking away from the easily measurable glucose, lactate, glutamine, ammonia axis towards the potentially more rewarding signal cascades which permeate the cell's operating systems. Although such cascades were most extensively worked out in animal cell systems it now becomes clear that they exist in bacteria too and what is more they can be involved in the control of differentiation, (11). Such a juxtapositioning of the physiology of all the microbial organisms leads to concepts and hypotheses which reflect back and forth between the special interest areas of the investigators. Antibiotic producers and antibody producers have more in common than either of them realise. Both such investigators can use this common ground to progress their subject areas and develop models and operating systems which will give us better and more effective control over the biosynthetic machinery of the cellular life forms that we have had bequeathed to us.

5. References.

1. Ross, J.D., Treadwell, P.E., Syverton, J.T.   (1962)
Cultural Characterisation of Animal Cells,
Ann Rev. Microbiol vol 16   pp141-188

2. Vanek, Z., Blumauerova, M. (1986)
Physiology and Pathophysiology of Secondary Metabolite Production
In; Overproduction of Microbial Metabolites
Ed. Vanek, Z., Hostalek, Z.
Butterworths, London pp 3-26

3. A.L. Demain, 1989
Functions of Secondary Metabolites
In; Genetics and Molecular Biology of Industrial Microoranisms
American Society for Microbiology, pp 1-11

4. Weinberg, E.D, 1984
Comparative aspects of secondary metabolism in cell cultures of green plants , animals and microorganisms
In; Secondary Metabolism and Differentiation in Fungi
Ed. Bennet, J.W., Ciegler,A.
Marcel Dekker, New York. pp 73-94

5. Bushell, M.E., (1988)
Growth, Product Formation and Fermentation Technology
In; Actinomycetes in Biotechnology,
Academic Press, London, pp 186-217

6. Ochi, K., (1988)
Nucleotide pools and stringent response in regulation of Streptomyces differentiation
In; Biology of Actinomycetes '88
Ed. Okami,Y., Beppu, T., Ogawara,H.
Japan Scientific Society Press, Tokyo, pp 330-337

7. Bushell, M.E., (1989)
The process physiology of secondary metabolite production
In; Society of General Microbiology Symposium 44
Ed. Banmberg, S., Hunter,I., Rhodes,M.
Cambridge University Press, pp 95-119

8. Beppu,T. (1986)
Pleiotropic Regulatory Mechanisms of Secondary Matabolism in Streptomyces
In; Overproduction of Microbial Metabolites
Ed. Vanek, Z., Hostalek, Z.
Butterworths, London pp 165-182

9. Bushell, M.E., Scott,M., Bell,S., Wardell,N., Spier, R.E.,
These proceedings.

10. Postgate, J., (1989)
A microbial way of death
New Scientist, May, 43-47

11. Stock, J.B., Stock, A.M., Mottonen, J.M. (1990)
Signal Transduction in Bacteria
Nature vol 344 395-400

FIGURE 1:

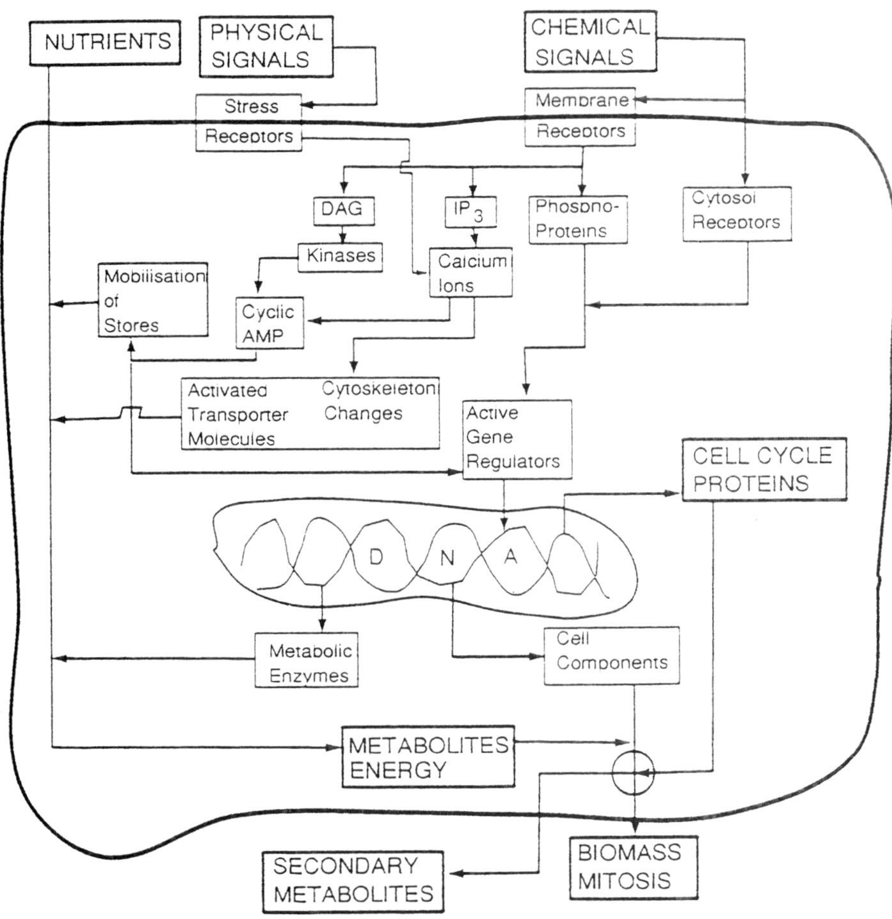

NUTRIENTS
PHYSICAL SIGNALS
CHEMICAL SIGNALS
Stress Receptors
Membrane Receptors
DAG
IP3
Phospho-Proteins
Cytosol Receptors
Kinases
Calcium Ions
Mobilisation of Stores
Cyclic AMP
Activated Transporter Molecules
Cytoskeleton Changes
Active Gene Regulators
CELL CYCLE PROTEINS
D N A
Metabolic Enzymes
Cell Components
METABOLITES ENERGY
SECONDARY METABOLITES
BIOMASS MITOSIS

Petri: I want to comment on motility and adhesion of
            embryonic and cancer cells (from Terry's talk).
            It was reported in 1978 that a histiocytic lymphoma
            cell line expresses a urokinase receptor on its
            surface and expression of this receptor can be
            stimulated several 1000-fold by the tumour
            promoting agent phorbol acetate. We have produced
            5×10^{11} phorbol ester treated U937 cells from which
            the receptor has been purified to homogeneity,
            characterised for N-terminal sequences. This has
            enabled us to clone the receptor. It has been
            suggested that such a receptor helps metastatically
            active cells to capture circulating urokinase,
            activating circulating tPA, and thus helping
            metastatic cells to penetrate the extracellular
            matrix for metastasis formation.

Spier: We might create a problem for ourselves in that in
            switching that gene off for the receptor we might
            turn on metastasis.

Miller: I can't think that of the list of secondary
            metabolites you gave, collagen, fibronectin and
            such molecules can be considered as secondary
            metabolites. Also, we have found the signals, the
            cytokines, so you don't have to look for small
            adenylic derivatives.

Spier: I think collagen and fibronectin are secondary
            metabolites because a B cell for instance doesn't
            need them to grow. Although some other cells do
            need them, it is not necessarily the cells that
            produce the collagen or fibronectin that take
            advantage of its presence eg liver produces
            fibronectin but doesn't need it. Secondary
            metabolites are produced because the cells are
            acting as part of an organism, and not just for
            their own requirements. On signals there was a
            paper in Nature recently on signal molecules of
            bacteria which controlled growth and
            differentiation etc. These are very analogous to
            receptors on animal cells eg instead of
            phosphorylation on tyrosine they use histidine.
            So we have phosphate cascades in bacteria as well
            as animal cells.

Al Rubei: Your concept of a switch between biomass or
            secondary metabolites I find difficult to support.
            There are only a few genes which control nuclear
            proteins that are cell cycle dependent. Even those
            genes are not switchable. Secondly, secondary
            metabolites, although not needed by the producing

cells, are needed by other cells for synthesis and regulation. These cells have evolved in a multicellular body so how do you reconcile this with your concept? Thirdly, when cells do not produce what we expect them to, it is probably because we exaggerate viability. These cells are continuously nearly dead, or dead, but we count them as viable. Thus specific productivity values are underestimated.

Spier: On your first point I am posing a question, not giving you the answer of what genes are turned on or off. I am suggesting that we recognise there is a switch which has to determine whether the chemicals available to the cell go into biomass, or into secondary metabolites. On the second point secondary metabolites in nature have an effect on other cells, even in the same clone. On specific productivity and cell death evaluation I am unsure. Certainly trypan blue stained cells can be revived eg cells taken out of the freezer, so I am uncertain whether cell death is meaningful or not in this context.

REMOVAL OF INHIBITORY FACTORS FROM HYBRIDOMA CELL CULTURES BY GEL FILTRATION

Øystein W. Rønning and Mona Schartum,

Dept. of Biotechnology, Center for Industrial Research, Blindern,
N - 0314 OSLO 3, Norway.

ABSTRACT

A new approach for removing inhibitory or toxic factors from cell cultures has been investigated. Given that these factors are of relatively low molecular weight, it should be possible to separate them from the high molecular weight growth factors by passing the spent medium through a gel filtration column. Results obtained so far, show that after passing the spent medium once through a Sephadex G-25 column, the life span of the culture was increased by several days, while the amount of antibody produced by the culture was doubled compared to untreated bach cultures. This method of removing inhibitory factors from the culture is an alternative to dialysis based systems using microporeus membranes.

INTRODUCTION

The growth curves of hybridoma cells in batch cultures are characterized by a rapid decline in cell viability after maximum cell density is reached (figure 1). Other cell types often show a period of stationary phase before cell death occurs. The rapid decline in cell viability is probably caused by accumulation of inhibitory or toxic factors in the growth medium [1].

One way of increasing the total outcome of the culture would be to increase its lifespan. This can be achieved by <u>e.g.</u> removing the inhibitory factors from the culture medium at a stage where the cell number is maximum. Since the major inhibitory factors are of small molecular weight, it should be possible to separate them from the high molecular weight growth factors and antibodies by passing the spent medium through a gel filtration column using the principle of group separation.

We have investigated this approach for murine hybridoma cells grown as static cultures in tissue culture flasks.

MATERIALS AND METHODS

<u>Cells:</u> Murine hybridoma cells (6c5), producing monoclonal antibody (IgG) against the K88 antigen on *E. coli* variants, were produced as described previously [2].

The cells were grown in tissue culture flasks (Costar) in a humidified incubator (37^0C, 5% CO_2). In the present experiments 1-2 x 10^5 cells/ml were seeded per flask into 50 ml of DMEM (Dulbecco's modified Eagles medium, Gibco).

<u>Gel filtration:</u> A glass column (inner diameter: 5,0 cm) was packed with Sephadex G-25 medium (gel hight: 30 cm). The column was equilibrated with DMEM. Spent growth medium (170 ml) was applied to the column and eluted with DMEM. The OD at 280 nm was monitored and the fractions containing the macromolecules were collected and filtered through a 0.2 µm membrane filter and returned the same cells it was taken from.

RESULTS AND DISCUSSION

Figure 1 shows a grow curve of 6c5 cells as measured by the MTT-test[3]. It shows the typical course of hybridoma cells: A rapid decline in viability after maximum cell density is reached.

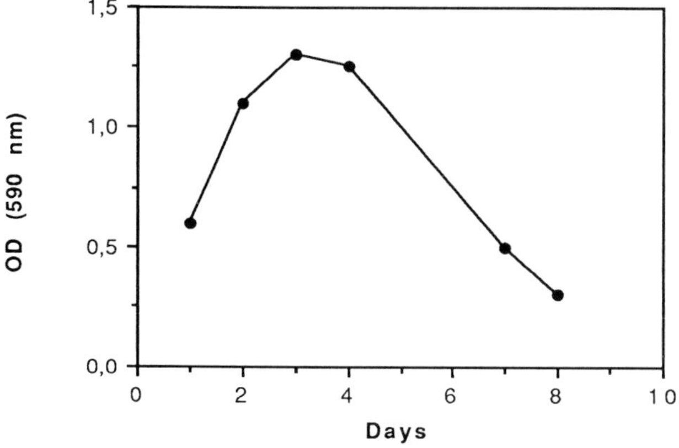

Figure 1.
MTT-test applied to cultures of 6c5 cells at various days after seeding 2x10^5 cells per ml of growth medium (DMEM , 15% FCS).

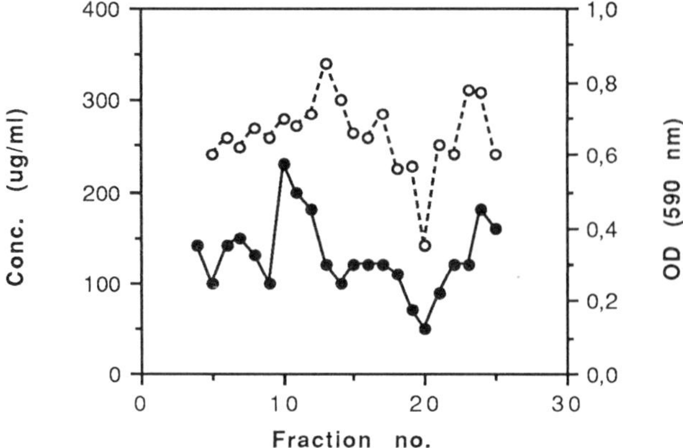

Figure 2.

The concentration of monoclonal antibody (●) and the OD from the MTT-test (O) in cultures of 6c5 cells grown on fractions of spent medium passed through a Sephacryl S-300 column. Each fraction was supplemented with 15% FCS. The assays were performed after three days of culture.

The growth medium was taken from such a culture at day 5, i.e. after the decline has started, and passed through a column of Sephacryl S-300, that was equlibrated with DMEM. The eluted fractions (in DMEM) was supplemented with 15% FCS and assayed for the ability to support growth of fresh cells. Figure 2 shows the activity of these cultures 3 days after addition of 10^5 cells/ml to each fraction. Fraction 20 clearly contains some substance that inhibits cell growth, while maximum cell growth (or activity) was observed in fraction 13.

The concentration of antibody was measured in each fraction with an ELISA-method (Fig.2). Fraction 20 also contained the least amount of antibody, while the highest concentration was found in fraction 10-12. This coinsided with the fraction where the antibody contained in the spent medium was eluted (data not shown). The peak at fraction 10-12 thus represents the sum of the antibody already present in the growth medium and the amount produced during the assay period (3 days). The fractions containing most antibody (10-12) was close to the fraction supporting cell growth the most (13), while the fraction containing the inhibitory factors (20) was distant from these.

This observation led to the idea that perhaps a gel filtration colum could be used in a production situation, if the separation characteristics of Sepacryl S-300 were exchanged with a gel used for group separations. Sephadex G-25 is such a gel (exstensively used for desalting, buffer exchanges etc.)

6c5 cells were allowed to grow to maximum cell densites in T-150 tissue culture flasks. This is usually achieved after 3 days if the staring concentration is $2 \cdot 10^5$ cells/ml. At this time four cell cultures containing $2\text{-}3 \cdot 10^6$ cells/ml (200 ml each) were centrifuged to concentrate the cells in 30 ml of medium. The remaining medium (170 ml) was:

Culture 1:   run through a Sephadex G-25 columm as desribed in
             materials and methods.
Culture 2:   returned to the same cells (Spent medium)
Culture 3:   replaced with fresh DMEM
Culture 4:   replaced with fresh DMEM + 15% FCS

Figure 3 shows the growth curves, of these four cultures starting from the day of the above treatments (day 0). The culture with the untreated spent medium (culture 2) showed an immediate decline in cell viability, while the culture with the spent medium that had been passed through the Sephadex G-25 column (culture 1) showed an almost steady state value for 4 days before the decline started. The cultures given fresh medium showed values between these extremes.

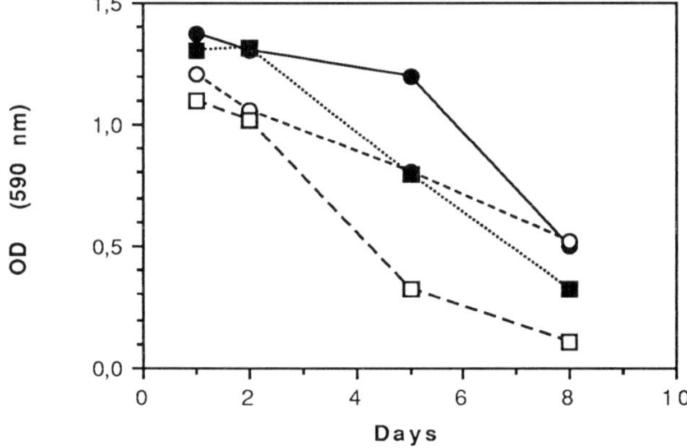

Figure 3.
MTT-test applied to cultures of 6c5 cells that had reached maximum cell density (approx. $3\text{x}10^6$ cells/ml). Cultures were given spent medium that had been passed through a Sephadex G-25 column ($\bullet$) or was untreated.($\square$) and other cultures were given fresh medium with ($\blacksquare$) or without (O) 15% FCS.

Type of medium	Day 0	Day 8
Treated by gel filtration	48 +/- 9	146 +/- 64
Untreated	62 +/- 12	73 +/- 9
DMEM	0	67 +/- 25
DMEM + 15% FCS	0	81 +/- 17

Table 1
Concentration of monoclonal antibody (μg/ml) in cultures of 6c5 cells grown in different types of media.

The concentration of antibody in the medium was analyzed when the cultures were made (on day 0) and at the end of the experiment (on day 8). Table 1 shows these values for the four cultures. In the culture with the untreated spent medium (culture 2) there was an unsignificant increase in antibody concentration, while in the culture with the spent medium treated by gel filtration (culture 1) the concentration at day 8 was about twice that of the other cultures.

The primary effect of removing the inhibitory factors by gel filtrattion is probably that the viability of the culture is prolonged. This is illustrated in figure 4 where the growth curve, of the culture 1 and 2 in figure 3 are superimposed onto the curve shown in figure 1.Although not taken from the same experiment, the curve for culture 2 (spent untreated medium) followed the declining part of the growth curve completely, while for culture 1 (medium treated by gel filtration) maximum cell viability was attained for several days.

In conclusion, the following advantages are achieved by culturing, hybridoma cells with the described meth.

1. Inhibitory of toxic factors are effictively removed
2. Expensive growth factors are returned to the culture
3. The product (monoclonal antibodies) is returned to the culture yielding a more concentrated starting material for downstream processing.

The technique offers an alternative to microporeous membranes for achieving the same goals, however, scale up technology is well known making the principle usable in connection with larger, stirred tank reactors.

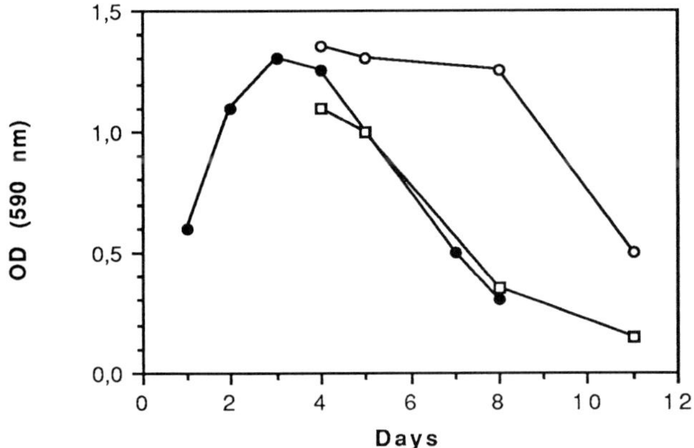

Figure 4.
The results from figures 1 and 3 are superimposed to illustrate the prolonged lifespan of the culture grown on spent medium passed through a Sephdex G-25 column. For details see legends to these figures.

AKNOWLEDGEMENT

This study was performed with grants from the Norwegian council for industrial and scientific research (NTNF).

REFERENCES

1   Lindberg, G. and Rønning, Ø. Production of an inhibitory factor by hybridoma cells grown *in vitro*. Engineering Foundation meeting 1988.

2   Lund, A., Hellemann, A. L. and Vartdal, F. Rapid isolation of K88 *Escherichia coli* by using immunomagnetic particles. J. clin. microbiol. 1988 26, 2572

3   Mosmann, T. Rapid colorimetric assay for cellular growth and survival: Application to proliferation and cytotoxicity assay. J. immunol. methods 1983, 65, 55

<u>**Paper of Ronning**</u>

Litwin: You show that you can prolong the life of hybridoma
            cells by passing the spent medium through a column
            and putting it back. Have you tried to enrich the
            spent medium to get even better growth?

Ronning: No, we have enriched the medium but not with using
            the column. Adding amino acids, glucose and other
            constituents of the basal medium had no effect.

Munster: Can you say what the inhibitory compounds were?

Ronning: No, we have not analysed them.

Munster: I hear that mammalian cells are far more complex
            than bacteria but the whole session this morning
            has focused on glucose, glutamine, lactate and
            ammonia. If they are so complex should we not be
            looking further afield for different metabolites
            and inhibitors. There should be many analogies in
            the bacterial world.

Spier: For three years we made concentrates of materials
            that could be exuded from cells in the simplest
            possible medium that could keep 10^8 cells for 4
            hours. Several chromatographic peaks were
            identified after fractionation, some of which had
            inhibitory effects on cell growth. So, to answer
            the question there is far more to it than just
            lactate and ammonia, which are probably the least
            of our problems.

Munster: What about the various metabolites? In one talk
            asparagine was shown to be important for antibody
            production yet everybody still focuses on glucose
            and glutamine.

Spier: Again you are looking at small molecules, we are
            looking at things of 30KD. We are still looking
            for the factors that control the switching system,
            the relationship and interactions between signal
            molecules and the levels, concentrations and
            activities of metabolites that we see on the
            Boehringer chart.

Handa-Corrigan:
            We should be trying to determine metabolic
            parameters in order to optimise our production
            strategy. We find in the literature so many amino
            acids, and known and unknown toxic products, that
            we have to look just at the key ones. The ones
            used the most are glucose and glutamine so as long
            as other ingredients are supplied by the medium we

can get away with just monitoring these, and dealing with accumulating toxic metabolites.

Ronning: We have done our experiments with other cell lines and it seems the inhibitory factor comes from the myeloma cell. Other cells did not show this inhibitory fraction so it comes from the parent myeloma.

Vournakis: The increased medium perfusion rates I reported resulting in increased bioreactor output probably related to the removal of inhibitory substances. We have attached dialysis systems to the perfusion cultures and, using different molecular sizes, are trying to determine whether they are small or large molecular weight compounds. Mammalian cells have mitochondria and their interaction with cytoplasmic metabolic pathways is very complex and interesting. This is an area which will prove to be fruitful and raise the mammalian cells to its appropriate level of complexity in comparison to prokaryotes.

THE EFFECT OF METABOLIC BY-PRODUCTS ON ANIMAL CELLS IN CULTURE

Michael Butler, Thomas Hassell, Christopher Doyle, Susan Gleave and Philip Jennings

Department of Biological Sciences, Manchester Polytechnic, U.K.

ABSTRACT

1. Eight independent cell lines which were examined showed considerable variation in sensitivity to added ammonia. The growth of some cell lines was not inhibited by the concentrations of ammonia that normally accumulate in culture. 2. The growth inhibitory effect of ammonium chloride increases at higher culture pH values. This data suggests that NH_3 rather than NH_4^+ may be the toxic form of the molecule in the culture medium. 3. Although the addition of lactate upto 20 mM can cause some growth inhibition, lower concentrations can have a sparing effect on ammonia toxicity. Data indicates that this may be related to the intracellular sequestration of ammonia and formation of alanine.

INTRODUCTION

Animal cells grown in culture will release ammonia and lactate into the medium as by-products of energy metabolism (1,2). We have addressed several questions related to the effect of these compounds on cell growth.

MATERIALS and METHODS

Anchorage-dependent cell lines were cultured in 25 cm^2 T-flasks in a medium of GMEM supplemented with 10% bovine serum. Cells were harvested by exposure to 2ml trypsin (0.25%) in phosphate buffered saline. The anti-paraquat secreting hybridoma (PCXB1/2) was routinely cultured in 25 cm^2 T-flasks in RPMI 1640 supplemented with 10% new born calf serum. Experimental cultures were performed in T-flasks or in 24-well plates with each well containing 0.5-2.0 ml cultures.

RESULTS and DISCUSSION

1. <u>Is accumulated ammonia growth inhibitory to all cell cultures or are certain cell lines more sensitive?</u>
The growth inhibitory concentrations of NH_4Cl were determined for eight cell lines by additions to the culture medium. The cell lines were classified into three groups depending on their response to 2 mM added ammonium chloride. This is the concentration that typically accumulates in batch cultures. The first group of cells were relatively unaffected by this concentration of ammonium whereas the second group showed final cell yields reduced by 50-60% compared to controls. The third group (HeLa and BHK) showed particular sensitivity to ammonium with cell yields reduced by >75%. The concentrations of NH_4Cl which inhibit cell growth by 50% (IC-50) are tabulated and further illustrate the sensitivity of some cell lines, with the yield of HeLa cells reduced by 50% at 0.8 mM NH_4Cl. The IC-50 values of some of the insensitive lines (HDF, Vero and 293) were not

determined as they were beyond the concentration range tested.

TABLE 1
The effect of added ammonium chloride on cell yields

Cell line	% decrease in cell yield at 2mM NH_4Cl	IC-50 (mM)
HDF	0	>2.5
Vero	0	>2.5
293	8	>2.5
PQXB1/2	14	5.1
MDCK	50	1.8
McCoy	60	1.7
HeLa	75	0.8
BHK	80	1.3

The anchorage-dependent cells ($3.5 - 5.5 \times 10^5$) were inoculated into 10 ml of GMEM and grown for 3 days. The hybridoma (PQXB1/2) cultures (2ml) were inoculated with 1.4×10^5 cells/ml and grown for 3 days. The pH of the media (7.4) was unaffected by the NH_4Cl additions.

2. Can the inhibitory effect of ammonia be related to the NH_3 or NH_4^+ form of the molecule?

The ratio of NH_3/NH_4^+ in solution increases with pH and at $37^{\circ}C$ has a pK value of 9.27. Therefore in order to determine the relative effect of the ionised and unionised forms of ammonia, the toxicity of NH_4Cl was determined at various pH values.

Cultures of PQXB1/2 cells were grown for 4 d at initial pH values of 6.8 to 7.8 and at NH_4Cl concentrations of 0-15mM. Changes of pH during cell growth were minimised by a medium buffer which consisted of 24mM bicarbonate/ 5% CO_2 plus 25mM HEPES. The IC-50 of NH_4Cl at each pH value was determined from the final cell densities (Table 2). The results show that pH has a significant effect on ammonia toxicity which increased at high pH values. The ratio of NH_3/NH_4^+ calculated at each pH showed a significant negative correlation with the IC-50 value. This data suggests that NH_3 is the toxic species in the media.

TABLE 2
The effect of pH on the growth inhibition of NH_4Cl

Initial pH	NH_3/NH_4^+	IC-50 (mM)
7.8	.0912	4.0
7.6	.0575	4.8
7.4	.0363	6.7
7.2	.0229	7.5
6.8	.0091	7.6

3. Does lactate affect the growth inhibition by ammonia?

The interactive effects of lactate and ammonia were determined on the growth of PQXB1/2 cells. A matrix of cultures was established on a multi-well plate in which the lactate concentration was varied from 0-24 mM and the NH_4Cl concentration from 0-6 mM. (Table 3). Results show that added lactate concentrations upto 8mM had a sparing effect on ammonia toxicity and this has a considerable effect on cell yields of cultures containing 4-6 mM NH_4Cl.

TABLE 3

The interactive effect of added NH_4Cl and lactate on the final cell yield of PQXB1/2 cells

Lactate (mM)	NH$_4$Cl (mM) 0	2	4	6
0	100	100	100	100
4	100	118	120	165
8	98	100	138	150
12	92	58	75	115
16	85	50	60	75
20	75	48	50	65
24	70	30	30	30

Media (2 ml) containing varying concentrations of NH_4Cl and sodium lactate were inoculated with PQXB1/2 cells ($2x10^5$ cells/ml). Cell yields were determined after 4 d growth.   The final yield of the control culture (no additions) was $1.1x10^6$ cells/ml.   Results are expressed as relative values compared to controls at each added NH_4Cl concentration   (n=2).

Analysis of the specific rates of substrate consumption and by-product formation in these cultures (Table 4) showed that the addition of NH_4Cl increases the specific consumption of glucose and the production of alanine.   This is consistent with the hypothesis (3) that ammonia may be de-toxified by complexation with α-keto acids such as pyruvate and may explain the extracellular release of alanine.   The pyruvate may originate by intracellular glycolysis which could result in an excessive demand on energy metabolism.   The effect of the exogenous addition of lactate may be to provide an alternative substrate for the sequestration of ammonia and so reduce the demand on cellular metabolism.

TABLE 4

Specific rates of glucose consumption and alanine production

Additions to media	Glucose	Alanine
	(pmole/ cell–day)	
Control (no addition)	6.5	1.69
+NH$_4$Cl (6mM)	14.6	4.61
+lactate (3mM)	5.8	2.81
+NH$_4$Cl (6mM) + lactate (3mM)	8.9	3.15

REFERENCES

1 Butler,M.; Imamura,T.; Thomas,J. and Thilly,W.G. High yields from microcarrier cultures by medium perfusion. J. Cell Sci. 1983, 61, 351

2 Reuveny,S., Velez,D., Miller,L. and Macmillan,J.D. Factors affecting cell growth and monoclonal antibody production in stirred reactors. J. Immunol. Meth., 1986, 86, 53

3 Hassell,T. and Butler,M. Adaptation to non–ammoniagenic medium and selective substrate feeding lead to enhanced yields in animal cell cultures. J. Cell Sci. 1990, in press.

CYTOSKELETAL MICROFILAMENT NETWORK AND ENERGY
METABOLISM AFFECT ABILITY OF ANIMAL CELLS TO
RESIST SHEAR INJURY

E. Terry Papoutsakis*, J.F. Petersen[†] and L.V. McIntire[†]
*Department of Chemical Engineering, Northwestern University
2145 Sheridan Road, Evanston, IL 60208-3120, USA
†Rice University, Department of Chemical Engineering
Houston, PO BOX 1892, TX 77251-1892, USA

Abstract: Our earlier experimental findings have shown that suspended animal cells are more sensitive to shear and other fluid-mechanical forces under conditions of reduced growth and energy metabolism. Here we employ a battery of effectors (drugs) to specifically probe the involvement of the cell's cytoskeletal structure and energy metabolism in the ability of cells to resist shear injury. Cell injury was quantitated by the fractional normalized cell viability and the release of lactate dehydrogenase after exposing the cells for a short time period (10 min) to well-defined, laminar shear in a rotational Couette viscometer. Treatment of our model hybridoma cells with either cytochalasin E or B, which disrupt the microfilament (actin) network, resulted in a marked increase in shear sensitivity. On the contrary, treatment with colchicine, which disrupts the microtubule network, did not affect the cell's shear fragility. When glycolysis was inhibited by treatment with deoxy-D-glucose, or when respiration was separately inhibited with KCN treatment, small effects were observed on the cell's shear sensitivity. A combined inhibition of glycolysis and respiration resulted in larger increases in shear injury.

INTRODUCTION

We have discussed earlier (1-4) that understanding the cell injury (damage) of freely suspended animal cells due to agitation and/or aeration in various bioreactors is a problem of both fundamental and practical value in animal-cell biotechnology. This understanding has two major components: a fluid-mechanical component and a biological component. Regarding the fluid-mechanical component, we have shown recently that the damage of freely-suspended cells in agitated bioreactors in the presence of a gas phase is due exclusively to the instabilities of the formed vortex and the associated bubble entrainment and breakup (2). The biological component of the problem would address issues such as, (i) what determines the shear sensitivity of the cells, and (ii) what cell-biological processes are affected and how by fluid forces. We have observed earlier (1) that the shear sensitivity of CRL-8018 hybridoma cells (a model cell line for studying fluid-mechanical cell injury) is affected by a variety of factors including the agitation history of the cells, the concentration of specific metabolites, and the age of the cells in batch cultures. Specifically, the cells were more sensitive to well defined viscometric shear during the lag and stationary phases than during the exponential phase of the batch cultures. These and additional studies (3) suggest that the cell's shear sensitivity may be linked to the cell's energy metabolism and may thus depend on cellular components that are immediately affected by the energy metabolism. One such component is the cellular cytoskeleton. The cytoskeleton is probably an important mediator of the mechanical properties and consequently the shear sensitivity of cells. Of fundamental importance in investigating the shear sensitivity of cultured cells is establishing if and which of the cell's cytoskeletal components or structures affect the mechanical properties. Two major components of the cytoskeleton are the microtubules and the microfilaments. Microtubules are formed by the polymerization of the protein tubulin and are important in a number of cellular functions including mitosis. Microfilaments are formed by the polymerization of actin and various actin binding proteins. Both microtubules and microfilaments are dynamic assemblies; polymerization and depolymerization of these structures occur constantly in the cell. Polymerization in both structures requires energy from ATP (microfilaments) or GTP (microtubules).

Normal assembly and disassembly of the microtubules and microfilaments can be altered by a number of factors including temperature change, Ca^{2+} concentration, and several different drugs. Colchicine, an alkaloid, inhibits further addition of tubulin monomers to microtubules, resulting in depolymerization of the microtubules. The cytochalasins are a family of metabolites excreted by some species of molds. These drugs inhibit the addition of actin molecules to microfilaments, leading to depolymerization of the microfilaments. In the experiments reported here, the role of the cytoskeleton in cellular shear sensitivity was investigated by disrupting the cytoskeleton of cells with either colchicine or cytochalasin E or B prior to shearing in the viscometer.

We have also carried out experiments to investigate the role of energy metabolism in shear sensitivity by chemically inhibiting the two major energy-producing pathways in the cell, glycolysis and respiration. Glycolysis was inhibited by addition of deoxy-D-glucose (DDG), a glucose analog which competes with glucose for transport into the cell but is not metabolized. Since DDG competes with glucose, the relative amounts of DDG and glucose determine the degree of inhibition. KCN was used as an inhibitor of respiration in the cells. It acts by binding tightly to cytochrome a_3, which prevents oxygen electron transport.

MATERIALS AND METHODS

Cultures and use of effectors (drugs). ATCC CRL-8018 mouse-mouse hybridoma cells, which produce an IgM antibody against hepatitis B surface antigen, were grown in T-flasks in a serum-free medium (5) as previously described (1-4). The cultures were routinely subcultured every three days by 1:8 dilution with fresh medium. Cells from the same culture were split into two samples of 10 ml volume each. For experiments using colchicine, one sample was given an addition of 0.1 ml of PBS (control) while the other sample received 0.1 ml of PBS containing colchicine (test) at a working concentration of 10^{-4} and 10^{-3} M. For experiments with cytochalasin E, one sample was given an addition of 0.1 ml of dimethyl sulfoxide (DMSO, control) while the other sample received 0.1 ml of DMSO containing cytochalasin E (test) at a working concentration of 0.005 mg/ml (10^{-5} M) or cytochalasin B (test) at a working concentration of 10^{-4} M. Each sample was pre-incubated with the drug or control for 30 min prior to shearing. The samples were then sheared in a viscometer (1,3) at a stress of 50 dyne-cm^{-2} for 10 min. For each sample, the viable cell density before and after shearing was determined by trypan-blue dye exclusion by counting in a hemacytometer, and percent cell lysis was determined by lactate dehydrogenase (LDH) release (1,3). For each drug or control, three cultures were sheared each day over a three day period.

For the experiments to investigate the effect of the cellular-energy metabolism on shear sensitivity, cells from the same culture were split into two samples of 10 ml volume. One sample was given an addition of 0.1 ml of PBS (control) while the other sample received 0.1 ml of PBS containing the inhibitor (test). Each sample was pre-incubated for 60 min prior to shearing. The samples were sheared at a stress of 50 dyne-cm^{-2} for 10 min. For each sample, the viable cell density and cell lysis were determined as above before and after shearing. DDG and KCN were used at working concentrations of 0.01 M. Each experimental condition was repeated three times per day over a three day period.

Data analysis. In these experiments, test and control samples were derived from the same culture, eliminating random variation resulting from differences between individual cultures. Since each test was paired with its control experimentally, it is also appropriate to pair them in the data analysis (as opposed to comparing the average of all test samples with the average of all control samples). The convention used here to compare test and control samples is:

$$RESULT_{LYS} = FL_{CONTROL} - FL_{TEST}$$

$$RESULT_{VIAB} = NV_{TEST} - NV_{CONTROL}$$

where FL is fractional lysis and NV is normalized viability. Use of this convention gives a result between -1.0 and 1.0 for each run. A result less than zero implies a harmful effect on the cells by the drug while a positive results implies a beneficial effect. A result of zero indicates no effect by the drug. A sample of results (effect of cytochalasin E) is presented in Table 1, which will be discussed below. The results for each day are displayed by column and for replicate tests by row. (Note, however, that flask $\underline{a}$ on day 1 and flask $\underline{a}$ on day 2 are replicate cultures, but not the same culture.) Following these three rows are rows giving μ, the mean result of the three replicate cultures, and the p-value associated with μ. The p-value here is the probability that the hypothesis "μ is equal to zero" is false; a small value of p relative to 1 indicates that μ is probably not zero and that the result is statistically different from zero.

RESULTS

The effects caused by the addition of colchicine were generally small (no detailed results are shown, but the average effect in one experiment is shown in Fig. 1). It almost certainly has no important effect at a 0.1 mM concentration. At 1.0 mM, larger effects were occasionally seen with one of the assays, but the other assay indicated a much smaller effect. Also, a small harmful effect was observed on day 1, while small beneficial effects were observed on days 2 and 3. Colchicine may affect membrane transport, causing such differences, or they may be due to scatter in the data. The most likely interpretation of these results is that colchicine does not significantly change the shear sensitivity of the cells. This implies that the microtubules do not play an important role in protecting the cells from mechanical damage. No positive control experiments were done, so that the effect of increasing microtubule stability is unknown.

The results for cultures treated with cytochalasin E are shown in Table 1. These cultures were substantially less able to withstand shear in the viscometer. In these experiments, both assays techniques produced similar results, and the results were significant both physiologically and statistically. Under the conditions of these experiments, there was typically 20% more cell death/lysis (ranging from 7% to 26%) when the cells were pre-incubated with cytochalasin E. The p-values in the table are the probability that the hypothesis "μ is greater than zero" fails. The results imply that the microfilaments or other structures of polymerized actin are important in protecting the cells against mechanical damage. It appears that cytochalasin E may have a lesser effect on the third day of culture. However, the overall effect of culture age may have been below the detection limit of our assay method. These findings were confirmed by experiments using cytochalasin B, which was found to have a more profound effect on the cell's shear sensitivity (no detailed results are shown). Figure 1 summarizes the effects of the three drugs, by plotting the average decrease of the normalized cell viability due to the drug for one set of experiments each.

The results from experiments with DDG are summarized in Fig. 2. Again, there was good agreement between the two assay techniques (detailed results not shown). DDG did not have a significant effect on the shear sensitivity of the cells. The average effect of respiration inhibition by KCN on shear sensitivity from one set of experiments is shown also in Fig. 2. In general, incubation with KCN prior to shearing made the cells more sensitive to shear ($\mu<0$). The lone exception was the lysis data on Day 1, where μ was approximately zero. There was typically 10% more cell death/lysis compared to controls (ranging from -0.6 to 17.2%) after pre-incubation with KCN. The p-values were somewhat large, so that additional data will be needed before a stronger conclusion can be made. The clear trend is that pre-incubation of the cells with KCN makes them more shear sensitive.

When treated with both DDG and KCN, the cells became more sensitive to shear (Fig. 2). There was on the average 17% more cell death/lysis (ranging from 7.9 to 22.8%) than in controls. There is some scatter in the data from Day 1, but the results from Days 2 and 3 were quite reproducible.

DISCUSSION

The cytoskeletal components of the cell are prime candidates for mediators of the cell's mechanical properties. It is possible to interfere with normal cytoskeleton function by treating the cells with certain drugs. Colchicine and cytochalasins (E and B) interfere with normal assembly of the microtubules and microfilaments, respectively. Using these drugs to selectively inhibit specific components of the cytoskeleton, the microfilament network was implicated as an important contributor to the cells' ability to withstand shear. The microtubule network does not appear to play an important role. This observation implies that the microfilaments are important mediators of the structural and mechanical properties of the cells. This observation is consistent with the results of studies of platelets in plasma clots. The microfilaments in platelets were shown to be important mediators of structural and contractile properties in plasma clots, while microtubules had no affect (6,7). Also, it is known that shear stress induces actin stress fibers in endothelial cells (8,9). It follows that the shear forces must act in some way on the microfilaments. Since the microfilaments are important to cell shape and macromolecular metabolism (10,11), shearing may affect these and other cellular functions.

When respiration in the hybridoma cells was inhibited by addition of KCN, an increase in shear sensitivity was observed. In contrast, inhibition of glycolysis using DDG did not appear to affect shear sensitivity. However, later experiments employing another glycolysis inhibitor (iodoacetate) have shown that glycolysis inhibition results in substantial increase of shear sensitivity (results not shown). It appears that for the present cells and used concentration, DDG is not an effective inhibitor of glycolysis. The combined inhibition due to DDG and KCN, however, resulted in substantial increase of the shear sensitivity.

ACKNOWLEDGEMENTS. This research was supported by the National Science Foundation (USA) under Grant ECE-8896100, and matching grants from the Monsanto Corp. and the Eastman Kodak Company, and by the National Institutes of Health (USA) under Grants HL-17437 and HL-18672.

REFERENCES

1 Petersen, J.F., McIntire, L.V. and Papoutsakis, E.T. Shear sensitivity of cultured hybridoma cells (CRL 8018) depends on mode of growth, culture age and metabolite concentration. *J. Biotechnol.* 1988, **7**, 229-246.

2 Kunas, K.T. and Papoutsakis, E.T. Damage mechanisms of suspended animal cells in agitated bioreactors with and without bubble entrainment. *Biotechnol. Bioeng.* 1990, in press.

3 Petersen, J.F., McIntire, L.V. and Papoutsakis, E.T. Shear sensitivity of hybridoma cells in batch, fed-batch, and continuous cultures. *Biotechnol. Progr.* 1990, in press.

4 Papoutsakis, E.T. and Kunas, K.T. Hydrodynamic effects on cultured hybridoma cells CRL 8018 in an agitated bioreactor. In: Adv. in Cell Biology and Technology for Bioprocesses (Eds. Spier, R.E. et al.) Butterworths, 1988, p. 203-208.

5 Petersen, J.F. Shear stress effects on cultured hybridoma cells in a rotational Couette viscometer. Ph.D. thesis, Rice Univ., Houston, TX (USA), 1989.

6 Jen, C.J. and McIntire, L.V. The structural properties and contractile force in a clot. *Cell Motility* 1982, **2**, 445-455.

7 Kirkpatrick, J.P., McIntire, L.V., Moake, J.L. and Cimo, P.L. Differential effects of cytochalasin B on platelet release, aggregation and contractility: evidence against a contractile mechanism for the release of platelet granular contents. *Thrombos. Heamostas.* 1979, **42**, 1483-1489.

8 Franke, R.P., Graefe, M., Schnittler, H., Seiffge, D. and Drenckhahn, D. Induction of human vascular endothelium stress fibres by fluid shear stress. *Nature,* 1984, **307**, 648-649.

9 Wechezak, A.R., Viggers, R.F. and Sauvage, L.R. Fibronectin and F-actin redistribution in cultured endothelial cells exposed to shear stress. *Lab. Invest.* 1985, **53**, 639-647.

10 Fulton, A.B., Wan, K.M. and Penman, S. The spatial distribution of polyribosomes in 3T3 cells and associated assembly of proteins into the skeletal framework. *Cell* 1980, **20**, 849-857.

11 Cervera, M., Dreyfuss, G. and Penman, S. Messenger RNA is translated when associated with the cytoskeletal framework in normal and VSV-infected HeLa cells. *Cell,* 1981, **23**, 113-121.

Table 1. Results from experiments testing the effects of cytochalasin E on shear sensitivity. The cells incubated in cytochalasin E for 30 min at a concentration of 0.005 mg/ml prior to shearing in the viscometer, and the shear sensitivity was compared to untreated controls. μ is the average of the three replicates for each day. Replicates of the same experimental condition are denoted by a, b, and c. The p-value is the probability that μ is greater than zero.

Cytochalasin E Lysis data:

Flask	*Day 1*	*Day 2*	*Day 3*
a	-0.215	-0.352	-0.067
b	-0.153	-0.222	-0.007
c	-0.210	-0.220	-0.081
μ	-0.193	-0.265	-0.052
p	<0.01	<0.025	<0.1

Cytochalasin E Viability data:

Flask	*Day 1*	*Day 2*	*Day 3*
a	-0.255	-0.305	-0.261
b	-0.188	-0.285	-0.191
c	-0.373	-0.199	-0.121
μ	-0.262	-0.263	-0.191
p	<0.025	<0.005	<0.025

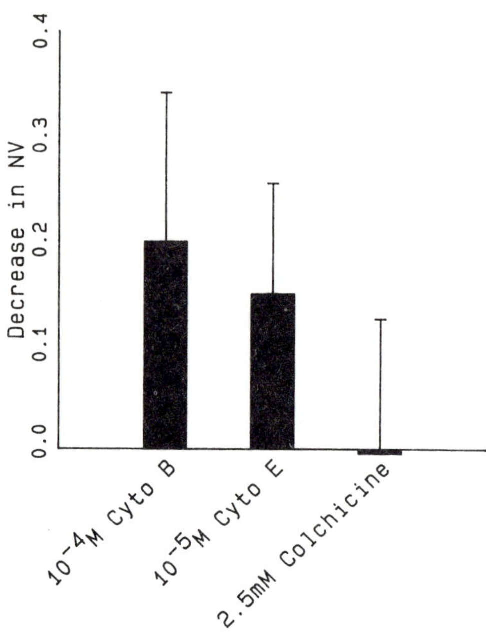

FIG. 1. Effect of cytochalasins B and E, and colchicine on cell shear sensitivity as measured by the normalized viability.

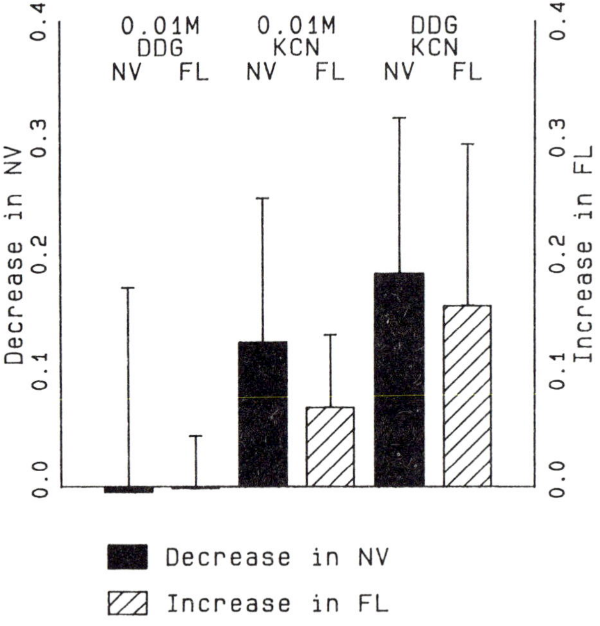

FIG. 2. Effect of DDG and KCN on cell shear sensitivity as measured by the normalized viability and fractional lysis.

<u>**Paper of Papoutsakis:**</u>

Al Rubei: Could some of the differences in response to
             cytochalisin and cholchicine be time and
             concentration dependent?

Papoutsakis:
             We have seen their effects with a range of
             haemopoetic cells using a standard protocol so what
             you suggest may be right, I don't know.

Clarke: Did you consider that heat or stress shock proteins
             might be involved in your system?

Papoutsakis:
             We couldn't see anything obvious. We looked at the
             major proteins on 2D gels. We only exposed cells
             for 30 minutes and this might not have been long
             enough for these proteins to be induced.

INTRACELLULAR CONCENTRATION OF ATP AND OTHER NUCLEOTIDES DURING CONTINUOUS CULTIVATION OF HYBRIDOMA CELLS

Thomas Ryll, Volker Jäger, Roland Wagner
Arbeitsgruppe Zellkulturtechnik, Gesellschaft für Biotechnologische Forschung, D-3300 Braunschweig, FRG.

Abstract

A murine hybridoma cell line, which produces a monoclonal murine IgG_{2a} antibody, was cultivated in a stirred reactor equipped with a bubble-free aeration and a continuous perfusion system. During growth of up to $3.1 \cdot 10^7$ viable cells per ml, intracellular amounts of ATP, ADP, AMP, NAD, GTP, UTP and CTP were measured by ion-pair HPLC technique after perchloric acid extraction of sedimented cells. We found very stable values for adenylate energy charge, whereas the ratio of trinucleotides of the purine pool to these of the pyrimidine pool changed rapidly during different growth phases.

Keywords: Adenylate energy charge; nucleotide triphosphates; purine-pyrimidine ratio; growth cycle; ion-pair HPLC

Introduction

The growth of mammalian cells is dependent on many physical and chemical parameters. These cells show pleiotypic responses to different culture conditions so that in many cases no direct relation can be made between nutrients and growth characteristics. Normally, the growth of a culture is ceased by limitation of an essential nutrient or by inhibition with a secreated endproduct. In the case of mammalian cell cultures it is often difficult to detect the limiting component. Since the information about nutrients and waste products in culture supernatants is insufficient to explain the behaviour of a cell culture, it is necessary to analyse additional parameters of the intracellular metabolism. Correlations between intracellular conditions and growth characteristics should give better explanations about the cause of growth behaviour in cell cultures.

Nucleotides were shown to be one of the most important substances for cell metabolism. They are involved in a number of cellular processes and have widespread regulatory potential (1). They participate as substrates, products, effectors or energy donators in many cellular reactions. Fluctuations of pool size could affect alterations in transport processes, macromolecular synthesis and cell growth. Some evidence has been found, that the pool size of ATP, the adenylate energy charge (AEC) or the ratio of purines to pyrimidines, influences or are dependent upon the cell cycle (2), the stimulation of quiescent cells with serum (3) or colchicine (4) and the growth control (5), respectively.

Our interest is dominantly focused on processes for the production of monoclonal antibodies and recombinant proteins with hybridoma and recombinant animal cells, respectively. Cells were cultured in bioreactors with perfusion systems, to achieve high cell densities. In order to predict the behavior of cell growth a method for detection of intracellular nucleotides has been established based on perchloric acid extraction followed by ion-pair high-performance liquid chromatography. First results from a continuous culture of a murine hybridoma are presented.

Material and Methods

Cell line and cell propagation

A murine hybridoma cell line, which produces a monoclonal murine IgG_{2a} antibody was used. Cells were propagated in a stirred reactor (1.3 l working volume) with bubble-free aeration and a continuous perfusion system (6). Oxygen content was maintained at 25 % of air saturation (1.7 mg l^{-1}). PH was controlled off line and maintained between 6.9 and 7.3. We used serum free medium consisting of a mixture of Iscoves and Ham's F12 supplemented with 3.61 g/l $NaHCO_3$, 0.18 g/l sodium pyruvate, 10 mg/l insulin, 10 mg/l transferrin and 1 g/l HSA.

Analysis of samples

Viable and dead cells were estimated using the trypan blue exclusion method. Glucose and lactate contents were determined with YSI 27A glucose and lactate analysers (Yellow Springs Instruments, OH). Amino acids were quantified by means of a reversed-phase HPLC system with pre-column derivatisation with o-phthaldialdehyde (OPA, Serva, Heidelberg).

Cell extraction procedure

Intracellular nucleotides were estimated by centrifugation of $2\text{-}3 \cdot 10^6$ cells for 1-2 min at 0°C and 187·g, immediately after sampling from the reactor. The supernatant was discarded and cells were homogenized in 500 μl of cold 0.5 mol/l perchloric acid (PCA). After cooling on ice for 1 minute we removed the precipitated macromolecules by sedimentation for 3 min at 0°C and 1680·g. The supernatant was put on ice and the protein pellet was reextracted a second time with 500 μl cold 0.5 mol/l PCA. After recentrifugation the supernatants were pooled and adjusted to pH 6.5 by adding cold 0.5 mol/l K_2HPO_4 in 1.5 mol/l KOH. The potassium phosphate precipitate was subsequently removed by sedimentation at 0°C and 1680·g for 2 minutes. The clear supernatant was filtered through a 0.45 μm filter (Milipore, type SJHVLO4NS) and stored in liquid nitrogen until analysis. The total procedure extended about 20 minutes from the fermentor sample to liquid nitrogen storage. Recoveries were tested using standard substances and spiked samples, and were in the range off 80-90 % for ATP, ADP, AMP, GTP, NAD, UTP and CTP, respectively.

Analysis of cell extracts

Analysis of cell extracts was performed by a HPLC system at a detection wavelength of 254 nm and 0.1 AUFS, consisted of 2 pumps model 64 (Knauer, Berlin), a mixing chamber (Knauer, Berlin) and a UV detector model D 430 (Kontron Instruments, Hamburg). Process control and evaluation was carried out by the MT 450 data system (Kontron Instruments, Hamburg) running on a IBM compatible computer (Kontron Instruments, Hamburg). Column temperation was realized by a column oven model K-1 (Techlab, Evessen) at 28°C. Sample were injected by an injector model 7125 (Rheodyne, Cotati, Calif.). Routinely 100 μl of cell extracts, corresponding to $2\text{-}3 \cdot 10^5$ cells, were injected into the column. We used a Supelcosil LC-18T column (15 cm · 4.6 mm i.d., 3 μm particle size) combined with a guard column cartridge (5 μm particle size, both from Supelco, Bad Homburg). Both columns contained octadecyldimethylsilyl phases and gave good performance and high theoretical plates with our elution condi tions. A typical chromatogram is shown in Fig. 1. Elution buffers were prepared with highly purified water (Millipore water system, Milipore, Eschborn). Buffer A consisted of 100 mmol/l K_2HPO_4/KH_2PO_4 (Merck, Darmstadt) + 8 mmol/l tetrabutylammonium hydrogen sulfate (Fluka, Buchs) as ion-pair reagent, pH 5.3 (KOH or H_3PO_4). Buffer B consisted of Buffer A + 30 % methanol (Baker, Deventer, Netherlands), pH 5.9 (KOH or H_3PO_4). The elution profile was composed of an initial isocratic phase of 100 % A (2.5 min) and linear methanol gradients of 0-40 % B (14 min), 40-100 % B (1 min), followed by an isocratic elution with 100 % B (6 min). Column reequilibration was performed by changing back to 100 % A (1 min) followed by an isocratic phase of 100 % A (8 min). The flow rate was 1.5 ml/min. Peaks were identified by comparison of retention times with standard nucleotides, spiked samples and on-line scanning of UV spectrums. They were quantified by integration of the areas. Standard curves were achieved with standard nucleotides (Boehringer, Mannheim) in the range of 100 - 10000 pmol. In this range the area to amount factor was linear for all substances and was taken for quantification.

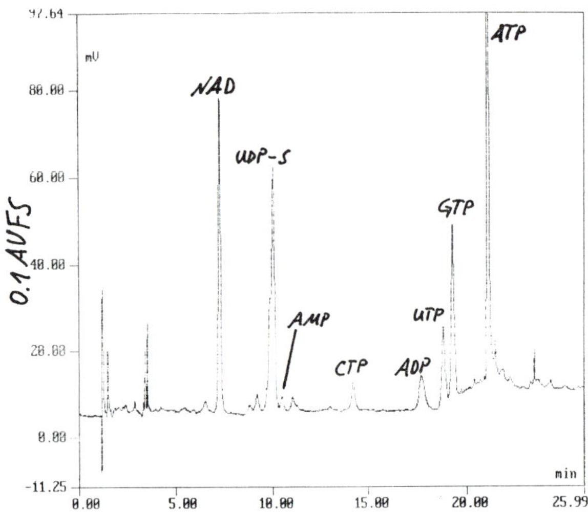

<u>Fig 1:</u>   Chromatogram of a cell extract corresponding to $3 \cdot 10^5$ cells taken from the stationary growth phase. UDP-S are UDP-Sugars. For elution conditions see material and methods.

Results and Discussion

The reactor was inoculated with $6 \cdot 10^8$ cells from roller bottles (92 % viability). After a short lag-phase of about one day the cells started the exponential growth for about four days. After they reached $1.1 \cdot 10^7$ viable cells/ml, growth slowed down and at day 8 of cultivation the cell concentration reached a stationary phase of approx. $3.1 \cdot 10^7$ viable cells/ml. The perfusion rate was increased up to 3.8 reactor volumes per day. At the end of fermentation perfusion rate dropped down caused by membrane clogging. The viability of cells was about 90 % during lag-phase and 90-95 % during log-phase. Subsequently, it decreased to 85 % during the phase of reduced growth to reach finally 65 % at the end of stationary phase (see Fig. 2).

At day 4, before end of log-phase, aspartate, glutamate, tryptophane and methionine reached low levels of approx. 10 μmol/l which might cause limited growth. Glucose still remained at 4 mmol/l at the end of log-phase and decreased below 1 mmol/l at day 8. Lactate concentration increased up to more than 20 mmol/l at the end of log phase and, therefore, it became potentially inhibitory. Fig. 3 and 4 show the progress of intracellular amounts of ATP, NAD, GTP, UTP and CTP. The cell specific amounts of all five nucleotides increased during lag-phase and reached maximum values at the early log-phase. Thereafter they remained constant or dropped down slowly during log-phase. After this phase the purine pools decreased until the end of process. Pyrimidine pools decreased during phase of reduced growth and remained constant during stationary phase. The pool of NAD was less affected than these of the trinucleotides.

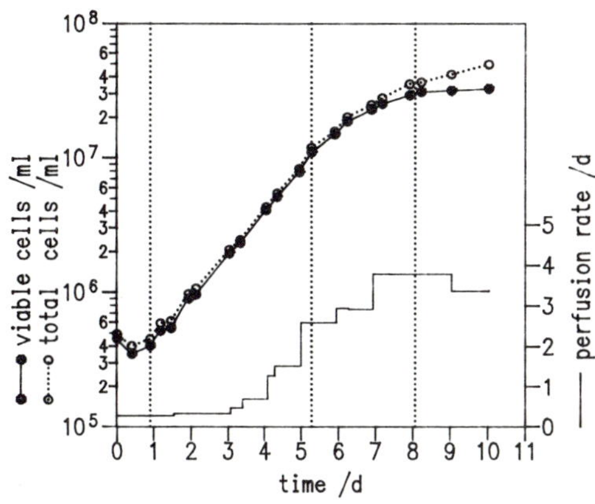

Fig. 2: Growth curve of a murine hybridoma cell line. The perfusion rate is expressed as reactor volumes per day. The growth curve is separated into 4 phases, chracterized with dotted lines. Phase 1: lag-phase; 2: log-phase; 3: phase of reduced growth; 4: stationary phase.

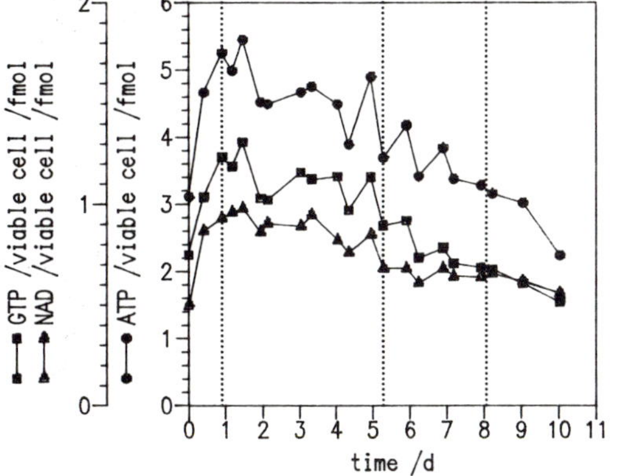

Fig. 3: Intracellular amounts of ATP, NAD and GTP during growth of a murine hybridoma cell line. Fmol = 10^{-15} mol.

The adenylate energy charge (AEC) (ATP + 0.5 ADP / ATP + ADP + AMP; [7]) was maintained at high values between 0.95 and 0.97 during the whole cultivation time (see Fig. 5). Such a high AEC was also shown to be characteristic for lymphocytes (8) and seems to be specific for mammalian cells. This is in contrast to cultured plant cells (9) or *E. coli* (10), for which values of 0.8 or less were detected.

The ratios of ATP to GTP and UTP to CTP remained normally constant under physiological conditions since their biosynthesis is dependent on reciprocal regulation which could be confirmed in our experiment (see Fig. 6). The ratios remained constant at 4.5 for ATP/GTP and 2.5 for UTP/CTP. In accordance to results from Meyer and Wagner (9, 11) for suspension cultures of plant cells, the constant ratio between purines and pyrimidines in cells has gained acceptance, because pyrimidine biosynthesis is aktivated by ATP. The UDP-sugar moiety was included in their calculation which was the dominant pool in plant cells. UDP-sugars were also found in hybridoma cells (see Fig. 1) but they were not quantified here. Hence the ratio of nucleotide triphosphates of purine and pyrimidine pools (ATP + GTP / UTP + CTP) were calculated. High variations of this ratio were found during growth cycle characteristic to the particular growth phases (see Fig. 7). The ratio dropped down from 3.9 to about 2.5 during lag-phase, remained constant during log-phase and increased when cells stopped exponential growth. When the cells reached their stationary growth phase, the ratio decreased again caused by stable intracellular pyrimidine concentrations and a decrease of the purines. This was resulted by the fact that the pyrimidine pool was more variable than the purine pools especially before and after the exponential growth of the cells.

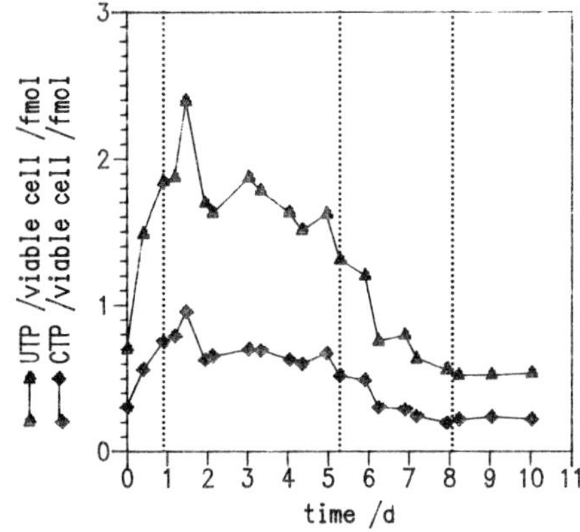

Fig. 4: Intracellular amounts of UTP and CTP during growth of a murine hybridoma cell line. Fmol = 10^{-15} mol.

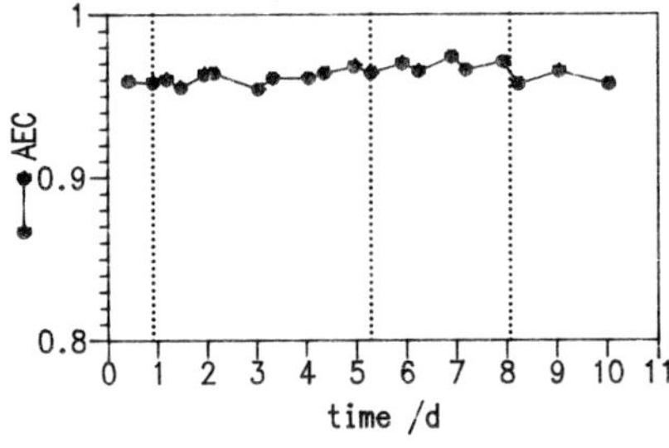

Fig. 5: Adenylate energy charge (AEC; ATP + 0.5 ADP / ATP + ADP + AMP; [7]) during growth of a murine hybridoma cell line.

Chou et al. (4) found that the ATP/UTP ratio decreased in colchicine-induced cells before initiation of DNA synthesis. Results of our experiment suggested that such a decrease of the purine to pyrimidine trinucleotide ratio was necessary to start exponential growth, if starved cells were used as inoculum. When using cells from the logarithmic phase of the preculture, no such lag-phase could be observed. Therefore it might be possible, that pyrimidine pools are more sensitive to detect the culture conditions than purine pools. If limitation or inhibition phenomena are the cause of reduced growth of hybridoma cells, the pyrimidine metabolism has to be considered to be growth controlling. Otherwise, it should be assumed that a minimum intracellular ATP amount is necessary to promote pyrimidine biosythesis, until a well-balanced ratio induced cell proliferation. Finally, it has to be concluded that investigations of the alterations of intracellular metabolite concentrations are important conditions to analyse, to control and possibly to predict the complex regulatory system of cell growth and behavior.

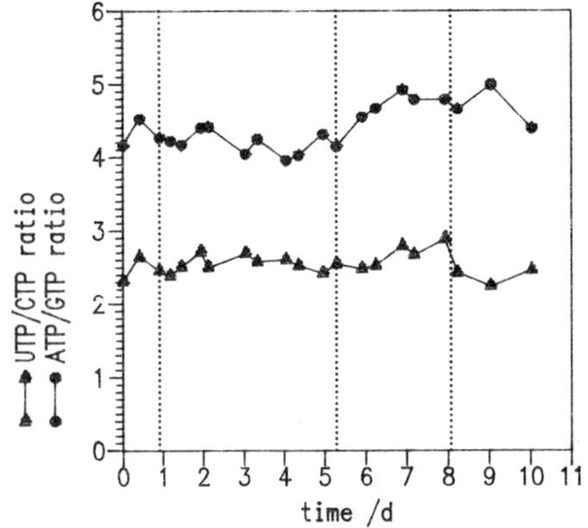

Fig. 6: Ratios of ATP/GTP and UTP/CTP during growth of a murine hybridoma cell line.

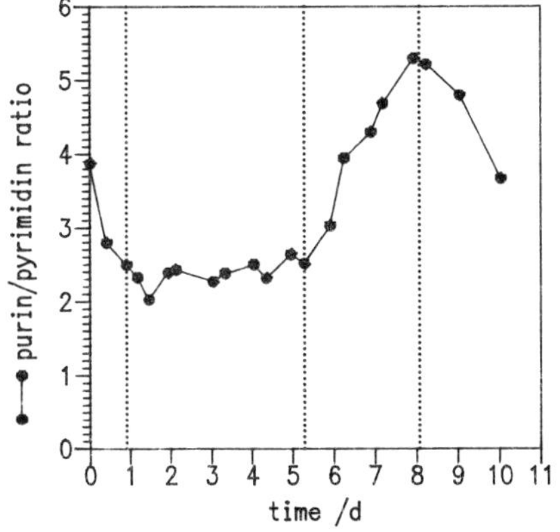

Fig. 7: Ratio of triphospates from the purine pool and the pyrimidine pool (ATP + GTP / UTP + CTP) during growth of a murine hybridoma cell line.

References

1. Atkinson, D.A. Cellular energy metabolism and its regulation (1977). Academic Press New York

2. Papaport, E.; Garcia-Blanco, M.A.; Zamecnik, P.C. (1979) Regulation of DNA replication in S phase nuclei by ATP and ADP pools. Proc. Natl. Acad. Sci. USA 76, 1643-1647

3.   Grummt, F.; Paul, D.; Grummt, I (1977) Regulation of ATP pools, rRNA and DNA synthesis in 3T3 cells in response to serum or hypoxanthine. Eur. J. Biochem. 76, 7 - 12

4.   Chou, I-N.; Zeiger, J.; Rapaport, E. (1984) Imbalance of total cellular nucleo-tide pools and mechanism of the colchicine-induced cell activation. Proc. Natl. Acad. Sci. USA 81, 2401 - 2405

5.   Murphree, S.; Moore, E.C.; Peterson D. (1974) Temporal variation of adenine ribonucleotides during the cell cycle of chinese hamster fibroblasts in culture. Experimental Cell Research 83, 189-190

6.   Lehmann, J.; Vorlop, J.; Büntemeyer, H. (1988) Bubble-free reactors and their development for continuous culture with cell recycle. In: R.E. Spier and J.B. Griffiths (eds.) Animal Cell Biotechnology Vol. 3, pp. 221-237

7.   Atkinson, D.E.; Walton, G.M. (1967). Adenosine triphosphate conversation in metabolic regulation. J. Biol. Chem. 242, 3239

8.   De Korte, D.; Haverkort, W.A.; Van Gennip, A.H.; Roos, D. (1985) Nucleotide profiles of normal human blood cells determined by high-performance liquid chromatography. Analytical Biochemistry 147, 197 - 209

9.   Meyer, R.; Wagner, K.G. (1985a) Nucleotide pools in suspension-cultured cells of *datura innoxia*. I. Changes during growth of the batch culture. Planta 166, 439-445

10.   Chapman, A.G.; Fall, L.; Atkinson, D.E. (1971) Adenylate energy charge in *Escherichia coli* during growth and starvation. Journal Bacteriology 108, 1072 - 1086

11.   Meyer, R.; Wagner, K.G. (1985b) Analysis of the nucleotide pool during growth od suspension cultured cells of *nicotiana tabacum* by high performance liquid chromatography. Physiol. Plant. 65, 439-445

Bushell: You said that adenylate energy charge was a constant parameter through the various phases of a batch cycle. As you had a continuously perfused system don't you think you were inducing a quasi-steady state where you would expect most of the physiological parameters to be constant?

Ryll: It is not really a steady state.

Bushell: Not really, but nearly!

Lehmann: To the cells I think it is a batch culture.

Merten: What is the effect of different oxygen concentrations, pH variability on ATP concentrations?

Ryll: It is a good question which I have only just started to look into.

Spier: We have found in a batch culture that when the cells have been placed under a chemical stress which has prevented their replication and ability to produce proteins, the energy charge has remained constant. However the level of ATP was elevated in the cells that were under stress. A phenomenon we don't understand at the moment, but there are things going on with ATP that are not with the energy charge.

Merten: I would expect ATP to be part of the switch mentioned in Spier's secondary metabolite talk, as with hybridomas between growth and production (low growth/high production, high growth/low production).

Werenne: A comment on stress and elevation of ATP. 2'5'asynthetase which is induced by stress needs a lot of ATP, so it makes sense.

DETERMINATION OF THE "CRITICAL SHEAR STRESS LEVEL" FOR ADHERENT BHK CELLS

Gerlinde Kretzmer, Andreas Ludwig, and Karl Schügerl

Institut für Technische Chemie, Universität Hannover
Callinstrasse 3, 3000 Hannover 1, F.R.G.

ABSTRACT

The influence of shear stress on adherent BHK cells was investigated. In order to determine the "critical shear stress level", the influence of shear stress between 0.5 and 4.5 N/m^2 on the morphology, the viability, the LDH-release and the size distribution was studied. First effects on these parameters were observed within the range of 1.4 and 1.7 N/m^2, which seemed to be the critical level for an exposure duration of 24 hours.

Key words: Adherent cells, shear stress, critical level,
           morphology

INTRODUCTION

Animal cells do not have a cell wall like other microorganisms have, therefore, they are very sensitive to mechanical stress as it appears in bioreactors.
To investigate the influence of shear forces, a flow chamber was developed, which made it possible to expose the cells to a certain shear stress.

METHODS

Cells

 Adherent Baby Hamster Kidney (BHK) cells were chosen as a model cell line. The cells were cultivated in DMEM (Gibco) supplemented with 10% FCS (Gibco) and 10% tryptose phosphate broth (Difco). Cells used for the experiments were grown on glass slides.

Flow chamber

The flow chamber was desribed before (1). A few improvements
made it possible to study low shear forces and to vary the
temperature.The exposure duration was set to 24 hours.

RESULTS

Morphology

The influence on the morphology was followed by optical
microscope and photographs. Exposing BHK-cells to shear
forces, the appearance and form of the cells changed. They
first lost their longish form and became shorter, triangular,
and finally spherical. Even in this state, they were able to
remain attached to the surface for some time before they
detached. The changing of the appearance could be observed
above 1.5 N/m^2.

Viability

The viability test was carried out by staining the cells with
trypane blue dye.
The viability of the cells decreased with increasing exposure
level. Up to a stress level of 1.3 N/m^2, there was no
influence.

LDH-analysis

If the cell membrane is damaged, the content of the cells
leakes out into the medium. For example the LDH-concentration
could be analysed and used as an indicator for the extent of
the cell damage.
The LDH-value increased within the range of 1.2 to 1.5 N/m^2.

Cell size distribution

Within the range of 0.5 to 4.5 N/m^2 of shear stress exposure,
the cell size distribution was measured by means of a laser
flow cytometer. The average cell size of unstressed cells is
about 10 to 12 um. By exposing the cells to shear stress, the
cells were damaged and the peak of the cell debris increased.
A significant increase of the cell debris was observed at
shear forces of about 1.5 N/m^2.

Cell parameter	Critical shear stress level
Morphology	1.5 N/m^2
Cell size distribution	1.5 - 1.75 N/m^2
Cell number	1.3 - 1.6 N/m^2
Medium Compounds	
LDH - value	1.2 - 1.5 N/m^2
GOT - value	1.8 - 2.1 N/m^2
Glucose	1.0 - 1.5 N/m^2

Table 1: Summary of the measured Parameters

DISCUSSION

Table 1 shows a summary of the measured parameters. These results suggest, that the "critical shear stress level" is in the range of 1.4 to 1.7 N/m^2. Exposing the cells to a shear force up to 1.4 N/m^2 there should not be an influence within 24h of exposure.
These results correspond with studies carried out by Tramper and Vlak (2). They found a critical level of 1.5 N/m^2 for Spodoptera frugiperda. Whereas Stathopoulos and Hellums (3) found a significant influence on the viability of epithelial kidney cells within the range of 0.65 to 1.3 N/m^2. They also observed the morphology changing, whereas Levesque and Nerem (4) found an elongation of endothelial cells.
These results indicate that the influence of shear force is depending on the cell line and the culture conditions.
Recent results showed that lowering the cultivating temperature might have a protective influence.
Further investigations will study these influences as well as the role of serum and supporting substratum.

REFERENCES

1   Kretzmer, G. and Schügerl, K. Development of Methods for the Investigation of the Influence of Physical Stress on Adherent Cells Dechema Biotechnology Conferences 1989, 3

2   Tramper, J. and Vlak, J. In: Upstream Processes: Equipment and Techniques Alan R. Liss, Inc., 1988, p. 199-228

3   Stathopoulos, N.A. and Hellums, J.D. Shear Stress Effects on Human Embryonic Kidney Cells in Vitro, Biotech. Bioeng. 1985, 27, 1021

4   Levesque, M.J. and Nerem, R.M. The Elongation and Orientation of Cultured Endothelial Cells in Response to Shear Stress J. Biomech. Eng. 1985, 107, 341

EFFECTS OF DISSOLVED OXYGEN SUPPLY AND GLUCOSE CONCENTRATION ON HUMAN LYMPHOBLASTOID CELL GROWTH AND METABOLISM IN CONTINUOUS CULTURE.

DERAMOUDT,F-X.* ; MIGNOT,G.* ; MERTEN,O.W.[+] and DROUET, X.[(*)]

* F. N.T S. 6 rue Alexandre Cabanel 75015 PARIS
+ Institut Pasteur 28 Rue du Docteur Roux 75015 PARIS
(*) Present address: Transia 8 Rue St-Jean-de-Dieu 69007 LYON

ABSTRACT

Human lymphoblastoid cells, which secrete monoclonal anti-Rh (D) antibody (Mab), were cultivated in a chemostat using a stirred bioreactor with serum-free medium. We analyzed the response of lymphoblastoid cell growth rate, metabolism, and Mab production to stepwise changes in oxygen supply and to the decrease of glucose feeding rate. The steady-state concentration of viable cells increased until dissolved oxygen (D.O.) reached 60% saturation, or with decreasing D.O. until the critical value of 15 to 5% saturation. The optimum D.O. for Mab production was 30%. Glucose consumption and glycolysis were enhanced at lower oxygen concentrations. Reduction of glucose concentration in the bioreactor, by means of an independent glucose feeding, enhanced growth but did not significantly affect Mab production. Furthermore, the fraction of glucose converted to lactate was reduced. Alterations in amino acid metabolism were observed. Experiments were carried out in order to study the effect of the concentration of basal medium constituants on cell growth and Mab production, and demonstrate an effective dissociation between growth and Mab production. Amino acids and vitamins have a synergistic effect on cell growth and Mab production. A general strategy for continuous cell culture will be discussed.

<u>Key words</u>: Human monoclonal antibodies, continuous cell culture, chemostat, serum-free medium, cell physiology, glycolysis, energetic metabolism, glucose feed, amino acids, vitamins.

INTRODUCTION

The large-scale production of therapeutical monoclonal antibodies needs well-standardized culture conditions. Many studies have involved optimized bioreactor design and culture system processes[1,2] but there is little information concerning the relationship between cell environment and cell physiology. This knowledge is a prerequiste for optimal culture conditions and maximal bioreactor productivity. The use of a continuous suspension culture (chemostat[3]) provides constant environmental conditions, which allow the modeling of cell growth and metabolism[4]. Such kinetic analysis has been well documented for hybridomas[5678]but little published information exists about human lymphoblastoid cells. Both cultured cells exhibit high rates of aerobic glycolysis[91011]. The glycolytic pathway produces 2mol ATP/mol glucose metabolized while the tricarboxylic acid (TCA) cycle produces 36 mol ATP/mol glucose oxidized. This lack of efficiency in the energetic metabolism seems to play a great role in mammalian cell culture properties[12]. Many studies demonstrate that the energetic metabolism is affected by the concentration of glucose[1314] and D.O.[1516] Previously , we have studied different dilution rates and have demonstrated that the theorical calculated dilution rate, according to the doubling time, is higher than the experimental observed[1718]. This difference is probably due to the autoregulatory-autocrine properties of the human lymphoblastoid cells[1920]. In the present work we analyse the metabolic effects of sequentially changing dissolved oxygen (D.O.) and glucose feed in a continuous chemostat culture.

M ATERIALS AND METHODS

Cell line and media

Human lymphoblastoid EBV-transformed cells, described by Goossens,D.[21] and provided by the
INTS, produce a Ig G1 antibody to the Rh(D) blood group antigen. Cells were adapted to grow in
the Iscove Modified Dulbeco Medium (IMDM) supplemented with chemically defined serum
substitute (without insulin or humoral hormones), described by Drouet,X.[22]. Glucose-free
medium was prepared with special IMDM Seromed).Concentrated feeding medium was prepared
by a 30% increase in feeding powder concentration Concentrated amino acid and vitamin medium
was prepared with concentrated solutions (Gibco). Glutamine medium concentration remained
constant (4mM) during all experiments. All media was supplemented with 100U/ml penicilline
and 100 µg/ml streptomycine (Gibco)

Bioreactor System:

A 2 liter glass reactor (Setric), with 1300 ml working volume, was used . Agitation was provided
by a cellascencer axial impeller operating at 30 rpm. Gas exchange was carried out by oxygen
surface aeration and air sparging (bubbling) inside the bioreactor vessel. The D.O. was monitored
by an O_2 probe (Ingold) and a Setric controller. Temperature was maintained at 37°C with hot air,
and pH was monitored at 7.4 by varying the CO_2 concentration in the bioreactor headspace. A
three-chanel peristaltic pump (P3:Pharmacia) was used for medium addition, and product removal
was regulated at a 0.3 day^{-1} dilution rate. A separate (LKB) peristaltic pump with a rate of 1ml/h
was used to feed glucose in glucose-limited experiments.

Analytic methods

Samples were removed every day. Cell concentration and viability were determined by trypan blue
exclusion method with an Hemocytometer. Glucose, lactate and ammonia were measured
enzymatically using a commercial kit (Boehringer Manhein). The amino acid concentration
measurement was performed by a procedure adapted from Sparkman[23] with a Biotromik LC 5001
analyser. This method did not allow separation of glutamine and threonine. Total
immunoglobuline concentration was determined by enzyme linked immunosorbent assay
(ELISA).

R ESULTS AND D ISCUSSION

Effect of dissolved oxygen

As shown in Figure 1, viable cell concentration decreased when D.O. reached 30% air saturation,
then markedly increased with lower D.O. Mab concentrations increased by 27% at 30% D.O. but
dramatically decreased at 5% D.O. The optimum D.O. level for Mab production, according to
specific production rate presented in Table I, is 30% air saturation. Glucose consumption and
lactate production (Table I) increased in conjunction with decreased oxygen supply, but the effect
on the fraction of glucose converted to lactate was not significant. Although alanine production
was enhanced, serine consumption decreased. Glycine was consumed at 60% and 45% D.O. and
then was produced at lower D.O. These modifications probably result from an increase in amino
acod production from glycolitic intermediates : alanine from pyruvate, serine from 3-
phosphoglycerate, and glycine from serine, all reflecting the stimulation of glycolysis and the
accompanying decrease in serine consumption. The drop in glutamine consumption at 5% D.O.
results, as observed by Miller for hybridomas, from insufficent oxygen aviability for complete
glutamine oxydation. As reported by Frame and Hu[24] ,we observe an increased demand for D.O.
at about 30%. A similar modification in glycolysis metabolism was observed for hybridoma cells,
in batch[25] and continuous culture[26] . For human lymphoblastoid cell culture, Mizrahi et al[27] have
also observed that cell growth and Mab production, in batch culture, is D.O.-dependent. The
higher glucose consumption rate observed at lower D.O. may be related to increased glycolytic
enzymes[28]

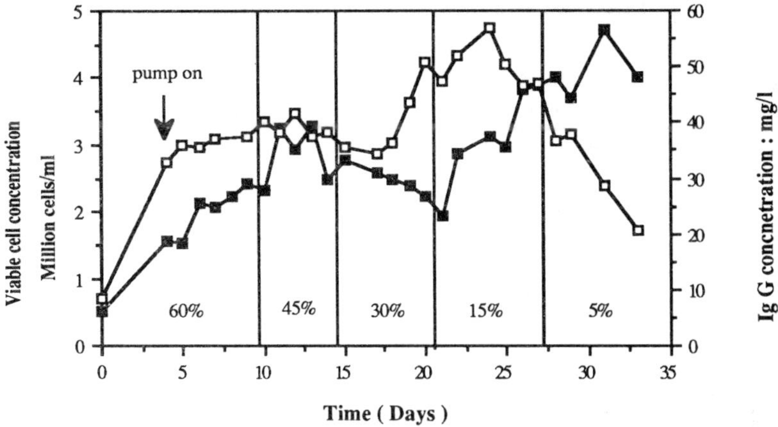

<u>Figure 1</u> Evolution of viable cells (black squares) and Mabs (white squares) concentration with stepwise decrease in D.O. supply. Initially set at 60% saturation, D.O. was sequentially changed every six days to 45%, 30%, 15% and 5% air saturation.

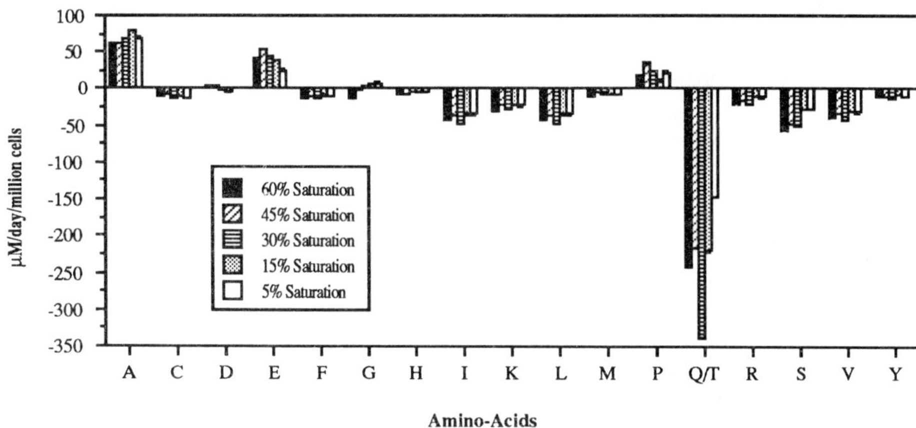

<u>Figure 2</u> Specific consumption rate of selected amino acids in response to stepwise decrease in DO supply. Data are the mean of three values at the end of each oxygen phase A: Ala, C: Cys, D:Asp, E:Glu, F: Phe, G: Gly, H: His, I: Ile, K:Lys, L: Leu, M:Met, P:Pro, Q:Gln, R: Arg, S:Ser, T:Thr, V: Val, Y: Tyr.

<u>Effect of glucose concentration</u>

The experiment was carried out in a two-phase continuous culture. During the first phase the culture was fed with standard medium and, by day 10, the glucose concentration in the bioreactor was decreased from 12 mM (Pase 1) to 1.6 mM (phase 2) by feeding the reactor with special medium without glucose. Low glucose concentration was maintained by means of independent glucose feeding. The D.O. was monitored at 30% air saturation throughout this experiment and all other conditions, including dilution rate, remained constant.

<u>Table I</u> Metabolic effects of decreased D.O. supply. Data are the mean of three values at the end of each oxygen phase.

% air sat.	Mabs production mg/10⁶ V.cell/d	Glucose consumption mM/D	Glucose consumption mM/10⁶ V.cell/d	Lactate production mM/d	Lactate production mM/10⁶ V.cell/d	Glucose/Lactate
60%	5.7	2.8	1.2	5.1	2.2	90%
45%	4.7	3.3	1.1	5.1	1.7	77%
30%	7.3	3.5	1.5	5.4	2.3	77%
15%	4.9	4.9	1.4	7.9	2.2	80%
5%	2.2	5.9	1.5	9.8	2.4	83%

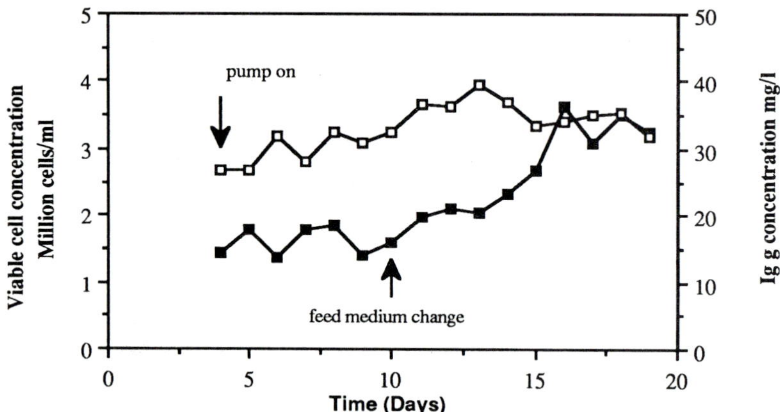

<u>Figure 3</u> Response of viable cells (black squares) and Mabs (white squares) concentration to reduced glucose feed.

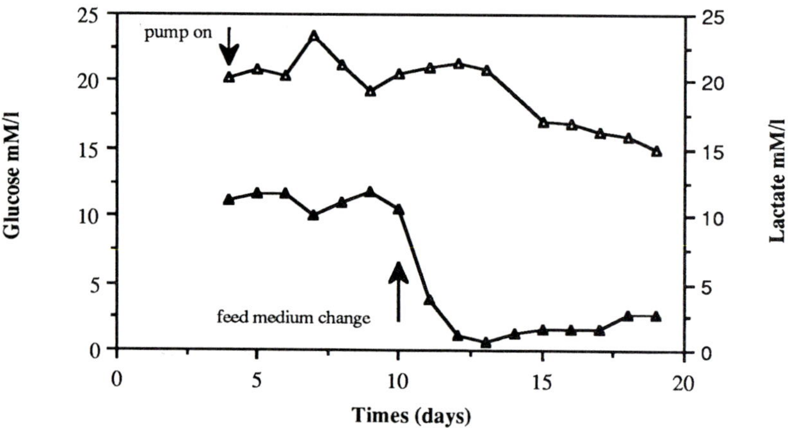

<u>Figure 4</u> Glucose (black triangles) and lactate (white triangles) concentration level in the bioreactor during glucose limited experiment.

The culture response to decreasing glucose concentration was characterised by increased cell concentration, with no effect on Mab concentration as shown in Figure 3.There was a reduction in lactate concentration from 21mM to 15mM, and the fraction of glucose converted to lactate dropped from 87% to 60%. In addition glutamine consumption and glutamic acid and proline production were increased as shown figure 3. The association of glutamine and glucose metabolism has been observed for other cell lines[29]. Increase in proline production may reflect the incomplete catabolism of glutamic acid resulting in better pyruvate oxydation through the tricarboxylic acid (TCA) cycle.These results show that under low glucose concentration a larger fraction of glucose is oxidized to carbon dioxide. This optimization of energy source utilisation is associated with increased cell growth. A similar shift in glucose metabolism resulting from controlled levels of glucose has been observed in batch culture for MDCK cells[30] and hybridoma cells[31] and, in continuous culture, similar growth enhancement association was reported for hybridomas[32].

Table II Metabolic effects of decrease in the bioreactor glucose concentration level.
Data are the mean of five values at the end of each phase.

| Phase | Mabs production | | Glucose consumption | | Lactate production | | Glucose/Lactate |
	mg/l	mg/10⁶ V.cell/d	mM/d	mM/10⁶ V.cell/d	mM/d	mM/10⁶ V.cell/d	
P1	31	7	4.3	2.7	7.6	4.7	87%
P2	34	3.6	4.7	1.4	5.7	1.7	60%

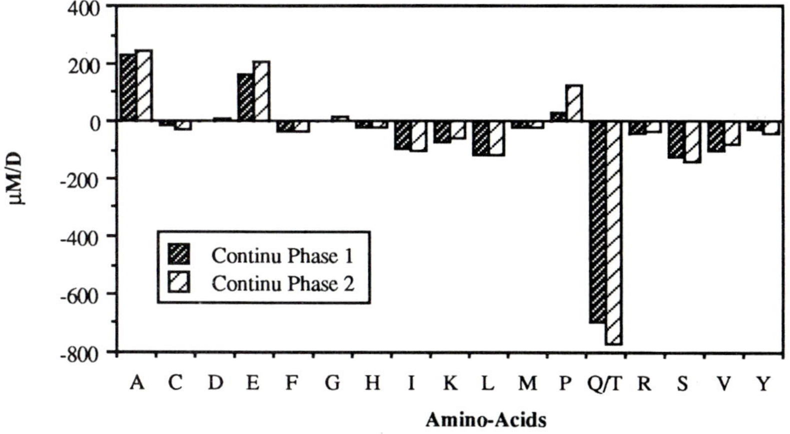

Figure 5 Consumption rate for selected amino acids in response to change in glucose supply.Data is the mean of three values at the end of each oxygen phase. A: Ala, C: Cys, D:Asp, E:Glu, F: Phe, G: Gly, H: His, I: Ile, K:Lys, L: Leu, M:Met, P:Pro, Q:Gln, R: Arg, S:Ser, T:Thr, V: Val, Y: Tyr.

In order to explain the lack of correlation between Mab synthesis and cell concentration, we investigated the role of substrate depletion. We performed the same two-phase experiment and fed the reactor with 30% concentrated glucose-free medium.

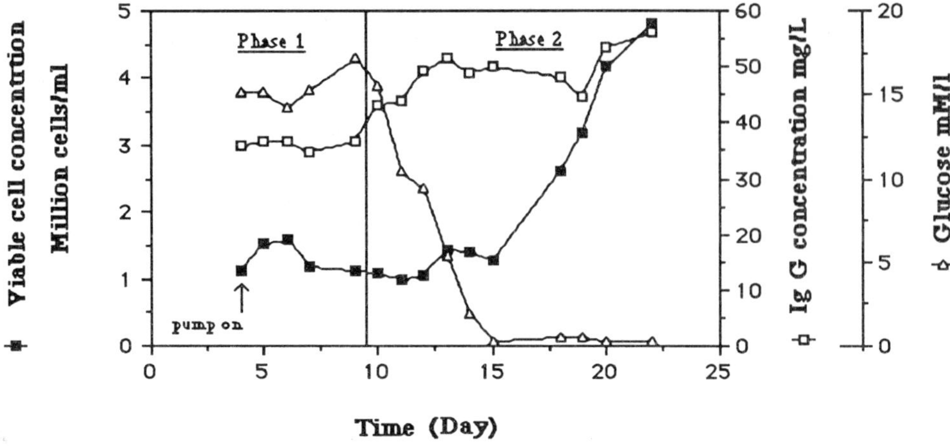

Figure 6 Response of viable cells (black squares) and Mabs (white squares) concentration to decrease in glucose concentration (white triangles) and increase in medium components concentration.

As shown in Figure 6, low glucose concentration enhances viable cell concentration but, in this case, Mab concentration was increased by 40% before cell concentration enhancement . These results indicate that Mab production is related to medium enrichment and that there is a dissociation between cell growth and Mab production. This is in accordance with results reported by Miller et al[33] ,which indicate that antibody production by hybridomas is not growth-associated in continuous culture.

Effects of amino acid and vitamin concentrations
In the last experiments, the two phenomena of glucose decrease and medium composition increase were linked.
To assess the role of amino acid and vitamin concentration in Mab production enhancement, we changed the cellular environment by doubling the concentration of standard.

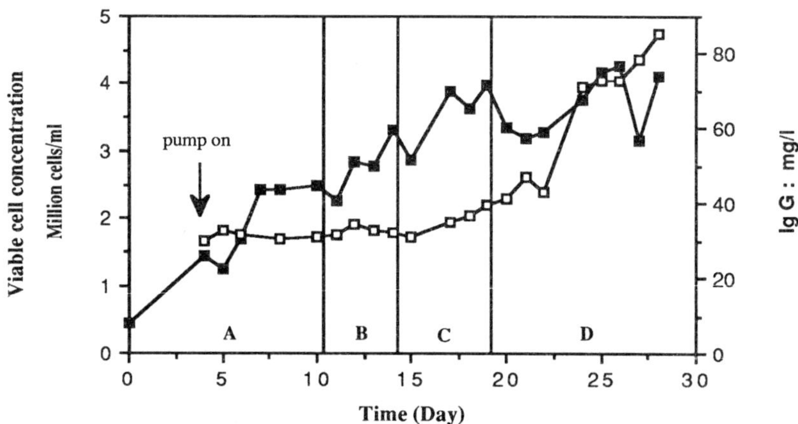

Figure 7 Response of viable cell (black squares) and Mab (white squares) concentration to stepwise increase in substrate concentration. Phase A, standard conditions; phase B, serine, leucine, isoleucine, valine, lysine and arginine concentration increase ; phase C, all essential and nonessential amino acid concentration increase;.phase D, all essential and nonessential amino acids and vitamin concentration, increase

IMDM composition in the bioreactor and feeding medium with:
- serine, leucine, isoleucine, valine, lysine and arginine during phase B,
- all essential and nonessential amino acids (without glutamine) during phase C,
- all essential, nonessential amino acids (without glutamine) and vitamins during phase D.

Phase A was performed with standard medium. All the other conditions, including dilution rate, remained constant. As shown in Figure 7, viable cell concentration increased along with amino acid concentration, and Mab concentration increased when amino acid and vitamin concentration increased. Changes in basal medium concentration also increased the osmolarity.We also determined that Mab production increase, in response to an increase in basal medium concentrate (in batch culture), is not related to medium hyperosmotic change alone (data not shown).Growth and Mab enhancement by amino acid, and vitamin supply may reflect elimination of nutriment depletion but also may be produced by synergistic effects of amino acid and vitamin metabolisms. The relation between cell environment and growth, and amino acid metabolism, are dificult to investigate. In accordance with the results reported by Tramacere et al[34] , who found that osmotic increase enhances amino acid transport by fibroblastic cells, the growth enhancement observed may also result from a synergistic effect of amino acid supply and hyperosmotic medium change.

CONCLUSION

In batch experiments, culture conditions are constantly changing and, for cell metabolism studies, may lead to erroneous conclusions. Continuous culture, such as chemostat, provides the constant environment required for precise determination of the role of changing culture conditions.

The results presented in this work demonstrate that for lymphoblastoid cells :
- Growth and Mab production are D.O. dependent, and optimum dissolved oxygen concentration for antibodies production is 30% air saturation.
- Cells are able to adapt to low oxygen or glucose concentration.
- Glucose metabolism is affected by glucose concentration.
- By controlling glucose concentration at 1mM, lactic acid accumulation can be reduced, and the fraction of glucose converted to lactate increased .
- Changing glucose metabolism, by either enhanced glycolysis or by glucose oxydation through the TCA cycle, increases cell growth but not Mab production.
- Increasing amino acid concentrations whith increase cell growth.
- Mab production is not associated with cell growth, but is strongly associated with synergistic effects of amino acid and vitamin metabolism.

An understanding of the relation between cell metabolism and cell environment permits the optimization of conditions promotingcell growth and Mab production. This information is essential for the optimisation of scale-up and the determination of efficient production strategies.

ACKNOWLEDGEMENT

We are grateful to Anne-Marie Gilles (Pasteur Institut) for performing amino acid assays.The fruitful advice and discussion of Patrick.Henno is thankfully acknowledged.

REFERENCES

[1] - REUVENY,S.; VELEZ,D.; MILLER,L.and MACMILLAN,J.D.: J.Immunol.Meth.1986, 86, 61

[2] - MERTEN,O.W. 2nd European Symposium on Proteins Purification-Technology 1986, 29Th 30Th September Nancy

[3] - MONOD,J. : Ann. Inst. Pasteur (Paris) 1950, 79, 390

[4] - TOVEY,M.G. and BOUTY-BOYE,D.: Exp.Cell.Res 1979, 118, 383

5- VELEZ,D.; REUVENY,S.; MILLER,L. and MACMILLAN,J.D.: J.Immunol.Meth. 1987, 102, 275.

6- MILLER,W.M.; WILKE,C.R. and BLANCH,H.W. : Biotechnol. Bioeng.1989, 33, 487

7- MAcMICHAEL,G.J.: Hybridoma 1989, 8 , 117

8- FAZEKAS de St GROTH,S.: J.Immunol.Meth.1983, 57, 121

9- KILBURN,D.G.; LILLY,M.D. and WEBB,F.C.: J.Cell.Sci.1969, 4, 645

10- NEWSHOLME,E.A. ; CRABTREE,B. and ARDAWI,M.S.M. : Bioscience Report 1985, 5, 393.

11- McKEEHAN,W.L. : Cell.Biol.Int Report.1982, 6, 635

12- GLACKEN,M.W. : Bio/Technol.1988, 6, 1041

13- LOW,K. and HARBOUR,C. : Develop.Biol.Standard.1985, 60, 73-

14- KROMER,E. and KATINGER,H.W.D. : Develop.Biol.standard.1982, 50, 349

15- MILLER,W.M.; WILKE,C.R. and BLANCH,H.W.: J.Cell.Physiol.1987, 132, 524

16- REUVENY,S.; VELEZ,D.; MAC MILLAN,J.D. and MILLER,L.: J.Immunol.Meth.1986, 86, 53.

17 - DERAMOUDT,F.X. Doctoral Thesis (Universite de Technologie de Compiegne) .1990

18- DROUET,X.; DERAMOUDT,F.X.; MILLAC,C.; LUILIER,M.; MIGNOT,G.; KELSCH,D.and SALMON,C. Bio-Sciences 1988, 7, 2

19- SHAW,J.E.; BAGLIA,L.A. and LEUNG,K. : J.Virol. 1988, 62 , 3415

20- GORDON, J.; LEY,S.C.; MELAMED,M.D.; ENGLISH,L.S.and HUGHES-JONES,N.C. : Nature 1984, 310, 145

21- GOOSSENS, D.; CHAMPOMIER F.; ROUGER P and SALMON C.: J.Immunol.Meth.1987, 101, 193

22- DROUET,X.; GOOSSENS,D.and ROUGER,P. Fondation Centre National De Transfusion Sanguine : 1987: European patent : EP 249 557

23- SPARCKANN,D.H.; STEIN,W.H. et MOORE,S. Anal.Chem. 1958, 30, 1190

24- FRAME,K.K. and HU,W.S. : Biotechnol.Lett.1985, 7 , 147

25- BORASTON,R.; THOMPSON,P.W.; GARLAND,S. and BIRCH,J.R.: Develop.Biol.Standard.1984, 55, 103

26- MILLER,W.M.; WILKE,C.R. and BLANCH,M.W. : Bioprocess Engineering 1988, 3, 103

27- MIZRAHI,A.; VOSSELLER,G.V.; YAGI,Y. and MOORE,G.E. : Proc.Soc.Exp.Biol.Med. 1972, 139, 118

28- SELF,D.A.; KILBURN,D.G. and LILLY,M.D. : Biotechnol.Bioeng.1968, 10, 815

29- SUMBILLA,C.M.; ZIELK,C.,L.; REED,W.D.; OZAND,P. and ZIELKH,R.:Biochem.Biophys.Acta.1981, 675,301

30- GLACKEN,M.W.; FLEISCHAKER,R.J.Jr. and SINSKEY,A.J.: Biotechnol.Bioeng. 1986, 28, 1376

31- HU,W.S.; DODGE,T.C.; FRAME,K.K. and HIME,V.B.: Develop.Biol.Standard.1987, 66, 279

32- RAY,N.G.; KARKARE,S.B. and RUNSTADLERP,W. Jr.: Biotechnol.Bioeng. 1989, 33, 724

33- MILLER,W.M.; BLANCH,H.W. and WILKE,C.R. :.Biotechnol.Bioeng. 1988 , 32, 947.

34- TRAMACERE,M.; PETRONINI,P.G. and BORGHETTI,A.F.: J.Cell.Physiol.1984, 121, 81

Paper of Deramoudt

Bushell: Your results suggest to me that a 2 stage chemostat
              with steady state conditions in 2 separate
              bioreactors would form an ideal production
              configuration for MAB production. Do you have any
              comments on this?

Deramoudt: Maybe it would work.

Merten: It depends upon the production kinetics on whether
              you can use 2 stage systems. EBV transformed cell
              lines if the system is not optimised give strict
              growth associated IgG production. So you would
              have to use a system which maintains growth ie a
              1 stage process. If you can optimise your process
              eg by adding vitamins or amino acids crucial to
              production, then a 2 stage process is possible.

THE ROLE OF DISSOLVED OXYGEN IN GROWTH OF ANIMAL CELLS

Caroline DEMANGEL, Dominique DUVAL & Isabelle GEAHEL

BERTIN & Cie, Biology and System Dept., 59 rue Pierre
Curie, ZI des Gâtines, 78 373 PLAISIR Cedex BP n°3, FRANCE.

ABSTRACT

The influence of dissolved oxygen on the growth and the
productivity of hybridoma cells was investigated in batch
cultures. To perform Kla measurements and to follow the
kinetics of dissolved oxygen during the batch, an oxygen
probe was introduced in the spinner. Kla values were found
to vary in the range 1.6-4.0 10-4 s-1. Cell cultures
maintained under different Kla were then compared. Oxygen
depletion occured about 30 hours after inoculation whatever
the Kla, but the maximum cell densities were highly
correlated with the Kla. Oxygen deprivation appears to
induce the cessation of growth by inhibiting cell division.

INTRODUCTION

Cultures of animal cells are now widely used to produce
monoclonal antibodies and recombinant proteins. In parallel
with this evolution, there is an urgent need to optimize
the culture processes, in order to improve both cell growth
and productivity.In continuous culture processes (e.g.
perfusion systems), where the cell density can reach 108
cells/ml, dissolved oxygen is known to represent the major
limiting factor of cell growth and maintenance. It is one
of the reasons why discontinuous processes (e.g. batch
systems), are still widely used, despite the fact that much
lower cell densities can be obtained (about 1-3 106
cells/ml). In this work, we have studied the influence of
oxygen on the performances of batch cultures.

MATERIALS AND METHODS

Batch cultures of hybridoma cells were performed in 500 ml
spinner flasks containing 270 ml of medium. An oxygen probe
was introduced in the axis of the magnetic stirrer to
follow the dissolved oygen tension (DOT). Cultures were
kept under continuous stirring, at various rates (40-80
rpm) and at 37°C, in a 5% CO2, 95% air atmosphere. Kla
(volumetric oxygen transfer constants, s-1) were determined
by measuring the time to reach 63% of air saturation
(1/Kla) of deoxygenated water.Cells were seeded at 2.105

cells/ml in RPMI 1640 supplemented with 10% FCS, 2 g/l D-
glucose, 2 mM L-glutamine and amino acids. At daily
intervals, aliquots of cell suspension were harvested:
     - cell count and viability were determined using the
trypan blue dye exclusion procedure.
     - glucose, glutamine, ammonia, and lactate were
assayed by enzymatic methods.
     - the IgG production was followed by an ELISA test.
     - flow cytometry was used to determine the
distribution of cells among the cell cycle.

RESULTS AND DISCUSSION

Kla measurements were performed at two different rotation
speeds (40 and 80 rpm) using a 270 ml working volume. The
corresponding Kl values (oxygen transfer constants) were
derived from these Kla using the relationship:
     Kl = (Kla x volume) / (Surface area x 100) in m.s-1
Kla values for other liquid volumes were then calculated.
The Kla values varied between (1.6-3.2) 10-4 s-1 at 80 rpm,
and between (2.0-4.0) 10-4 s-1 at 40 rpm, for working
volumes in the range 100-200 ml. These values are
consistent with those currently reported for surface
aeration.
We then examined the influence of oxygen transfer on cell
growth and productivity, by comparing the performances of
cell cultures maintained under different Kla conditions. We
found that, whatever the culture volume and the stirring
rate, cultures were depleted in oxygen as early as 30 hours
after inoculation. Moreover, the maximum cell densities, as
well as the global IgG productions, were highly correlated
with the corresponding Kla (see Figure 1).

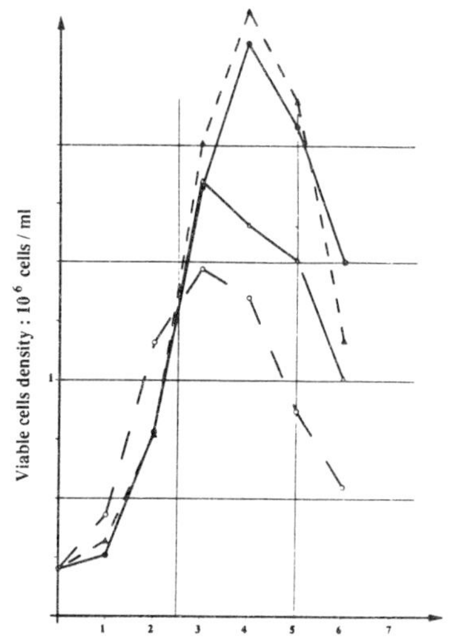

FIGURE 1 - Kinetics of
viable cell density in
batch cultures grown at
different Kla

○ kla = 1,19 10⁻⁴ s⁻¹
△ kla = 1,46 10⁻⁴ s⁻¹
● kla = 1,85 10⁻⁴ s⁻¹
▲ kla = 3,40 10⁻⁴ s⁻¹

These results demonstrate that oxygen limitation occurs at
relatively low cell densities and markedly inhibits cell
growth.
Flow cytometry analysis indicated that oxygen limitation
coincides with a decline of the percentage of cells in
S/G2/M phases (see Figure 2), while it does not appear to
influence directly cell viability. These data suggest that
oxygen depletion induces the decline phase of our batch
cultures by limiting the cell division, rather than by
enhancing cell mortality. The mechanisms of this limitation
are not yet determined and require further investigation.

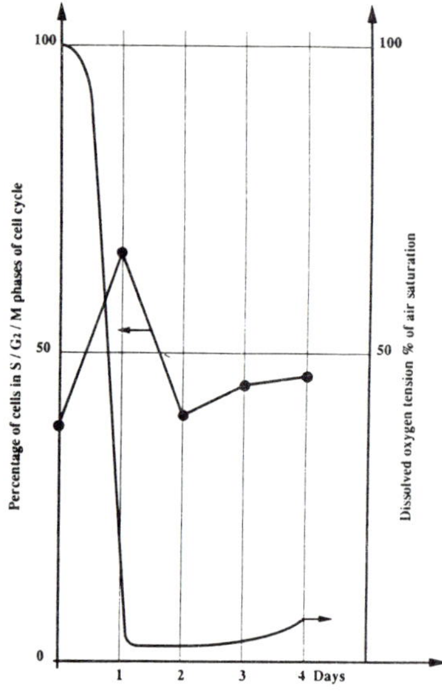

FIGURE 2 - Evolution of the
percentage of cells in
S/G2/M phases of the cell
cycle and of the dissolved
oxygen tension in a batch
culture

REFERENCES

1 W.M.MILLER, C.R.WILKE, H.W.BLANCH (1987):"Effects of
dissolved oxygen concentration on hybridoma growth and
metabolism in continuous culture. J.Cell Physiol. 132, 524-
530

2 M.LAVERY, A.W.NIENOW (1987) :"Oxygen transfer in animal
cell culture medium". Biotechnol. Bioeng. 30, 368-373

3 R.BORASTON, P.W.THOMPSON, S.GARLAND, J.R.BIRCH (1984)
:"Growth and oxygen requirements of antibody producing
mouse hybridoma cells in suspension culture". Develop.
Biol. Standard. 55, 103-111

4 R.E.SPIER, B.GRIFFITHS (1984): "An examination of the
data and concepts germane to the oxygenation of cultured
animal cells". Develop. Biol. Standard. 55, 81-92

THE EFFECT OF OSMOLARITY ON HYBRIDOMA CELL GROWTH AND ANTIBODY PRODUCTION IN SERUM-FREE MEDIA

C.L. Marshall, R. Boraston & M.E. Brown

Fermentation Technology Department, Celltech Ltd., 216 Bath Road, Slough, SL1 4EN, U.K.

ABSTRACT

In two different serum-free media, hyperosmotic and hypo-osmotic stress were detrimental to cell growth although increased concentrations of nutrients protected against hyperosmotic inhibition of growth. In one of the media tested hyperosmotic conditions resulted in increased specific yields of antibody while in the other medium antibody yields were reduced at elevated osmolarity.

INTRODUCTION

The increased application of monoclonal antibodies both in medicine and as process reagents will demand the manufacture of particular antibodies in multi-kilogram quantities. Economic and reliable manufacture of these reagents requires productive and robust culture processes.

Traditionally, design of media for mammalian cell cultures has centred on optimization of cell growth (1). However culture conditions for optimal cell growth and optimal antibody production may differ. One method reported to increase antibody production from hybridoma cells has been to expose cells to 'solute stress' by changing the medium osmolarity (2, 3)

This paper describes the influence of osmolarity on growth and productivity of a murine hybridoma cell line in two candidate serum-free media and highlights the fact that osmotic effects can be modulated by other aspects of medium design.

MATERIALS AND METHODS

Medium A was a serum-free formulation based on a modification of MEM. Medium B was developed as an alternative with substantial modifications to the nutrient content. Both were obtained as pre-prepared powders and made up in deionized water.

Osmolarity was varied by changing the water volume to powder ratio. The weight of powdered components was kept constant and the volume of water varied by up to +/- 20% of standard volume. Osmolarity ranged from 250 milliosmoles (mOs/Kg water) (120% liquid volume) to 458 mOs/Kg (80% liquid volume). Medium osmolarity was measured by depression of freezing point using a Roebling automatic microosmometer. To discriminate between the effects of osmolarity and nutrient concentration, medium was made up to standard volume and osmolarity was varied by changing the sodium chloride content of the base powder.

The cell line, a murine hybridoma (derived from the Sp2 O-Ag14 parent myeloma), secreted an IgG monoclonal antibody. Experiments were conducted using replicate shakeflask cultures. Productivity was assessed using a mouse IgG antibody-capture ELISA performed on a Zymark II robot.

RESULTS

Effects on cell growth - osmolarity adjusted by medium concentration

Where osmolarity was varied by adjusting the water to powder ratio, specific growth rate and maximum cell concentration were greatest over the range of 340-360 mOs (Figure 1). For both Media A and B, this coincided with the standard make-up volume. However satisfactory growth was achieved over a wider range, from 320 to as high as 440 mOs/Kg. In contrast, in more dilute media where the osmolarity was less than 320 mOs, maximum cell concentration and viability were dramatically reduced.

Cells cultured in medium B achieved higher concentrations than in medium A. This was due to differences in the nutrient components. Analyses of culture supernatents revealed that, in both media, glutamine was exhausted upon the cessation of growth.

Effects on cell growth - osmolarity adjusted by sodium chloride concentration

In the previous experiments, reductions in osmolarity led to a reduction in cell concentration which was greater than would be expected by simple dilution of the nutrient content. To discriminate between osmotic effects and dilution of nutrients, the osmolarity of medium B was varied by changing the concentration of sodium chloride. Concentrations of other components remained unchanged.

Results are shown in Figure 2. As before, an osmolarity of 350-360 mOs/Kg was optimal for cell growth. At lower osmolarities there was a pronounced reduction in maximum cell concentration, indicating that osmolarity, rather than nutrient dilution, was responsible for the negative effect on cell growth.

When sodium chloride was used to increase osmolarity there was a dramatic negative effect on cell growth. Thus the negative effect of high osmolarity on growth can be partially overcome by the increased concentration of another medium component or components. Some microorganisms and animal cells are known to accumulate certain non-essential amino acids such as proline and glycine under conditions of hyperosmotic stress (4) and it may be this 'osmoprotection' that allows cells to grow in medium of increased osmolarity (5).

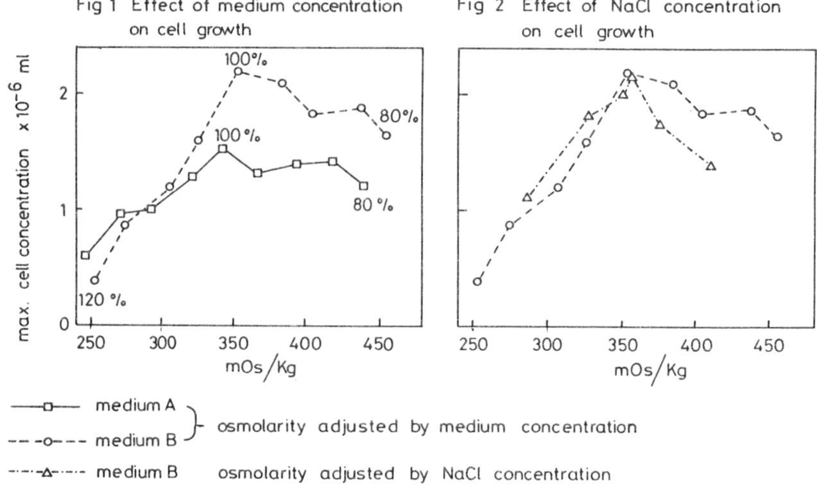

Effects of osmolarity on productivity

The effects of osmolarity on specific yield of antibody and volumetric product concentration were found to be medium-specific (Figures 3-5).

In medium A, where osmolarity was varied by changing the medium concentration, the specific yield of antibody increased with increasing osmolarity and was maximal at 440 mOs/Kg. This, combined with effects on cell growth, resulted in the highest final product concentration in medium A occuring at 440 mOs/Kg.

In medium B, where osmolarity was varied by changing the medium concentration, this trend was reversed; specific yield decreased with increasing osmolarity. The optimal conditions for volumetric product titre coincided with the optimum for cell growth resulting in the highest overall titre between media types.

In a separate experiment productivity in medium B was assessed when the osmolarity was varied by adjusting the sodium chloride concentration. Trends were found to reverse - final volumetric product concentration and specific yield increased with increasing osmolarity and were maximal at 410 mOs/Kg despite a reduction in growth rate, viability and maximum cell concentration.

DISCUSSION

Interrelationships between osmolarity and other aspects of medium design, and their effects on cell growth and antibody production, have been demonstrated.

Hypo-osmotic stress was detrimental to cell growth in both media. Hyperosmotic stress can exert a negative effect on cell growth, but increased media concentrations (or potentially specific amino acids) can overcome this effect. The results of Oyaas et al. (5) would suggest that this be due to the presence of the amino acids proline and glycine.

Osmotic stress, both low and high, can favour antibody production and the optimum osmolarity for antibody production may or may not coincide with the optimum for cell growth. These effects vary between different media, and possibly between cell lines. In medium and process design a compromise must be achieved to maximise product output.

REFERENCES

1   Waymouth, C. (1974). Journal of the National Cancer Institute 53, 1443-1448.

2   Rupp, R.G. & Geyer, S. (1985). U.K. Patent GB(11)2153830(13)B.

3   Maiorella, B., Inlow, D. & Howarth, W. (1988). International Patent PCT/US88/04068.

4   Strom, A.R., LeRudulier, D, Jakowec,M.W., Brunel, R.C. & Valentine, R.C. (1983). Basic Life Science 26, 39-59.

5   Oyaas, K., Berg, T.M., Baake, O. & Levine, D.W. (1989). Advances in Animal Cell Biology and Technology for Bioprocesses, eds. R.E. Spier, J.B. Griffiths, J. Stephenne & P.J. Crooy. U.K., Butterworths.

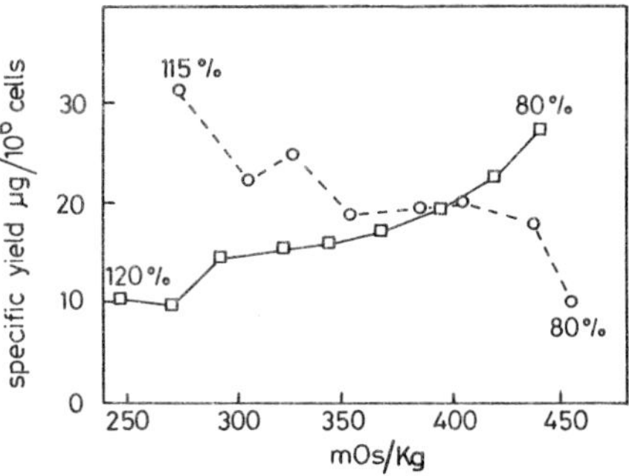

Fig. 3 Effect of medium concentration on specific yield

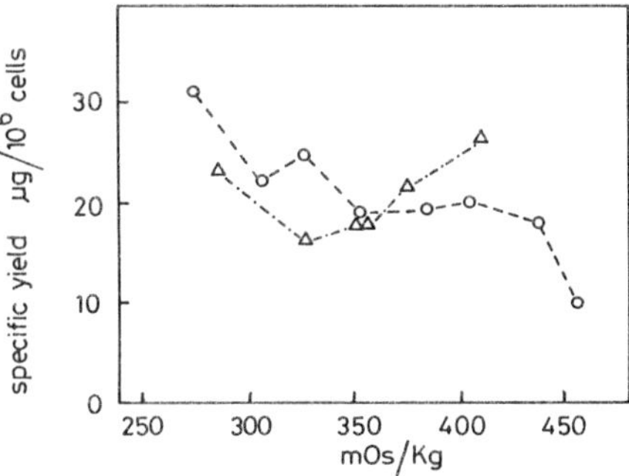

Fig. 4 Effect of NaCl concentration on specific yield

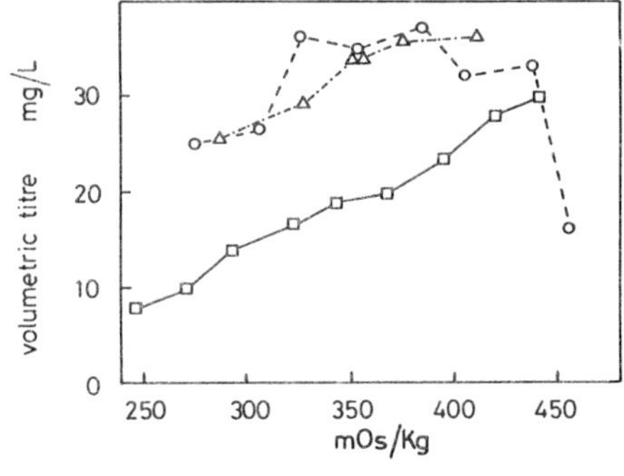

Fig. 5 Effect of medium and NaCl concentration on volumetric titre

PHYSIOLOGIGAL INVESTIGATIONS IN HIGH DENSITY PERFUSION CULTURE OF FREE SUSPENDED ANIMAL CELLS

Fenge, C.[1,2], Fraune, E.[2], Schügerl, K.[1]

1 Institut für Technische Chemie, University of Hannover, D-3000 Hannover
2 B.Braun Diessel Biotech GmbH, D-3508 Melsungen

ABSTRACT

A newly developed internal perfusion module was applied to perform a kinetic analysis of growth, metabolic activity and product formation in high density culture. Maximum viable cell densities of more than $1*10^7$ cells/ml were reached and maintained over an extended period of stationary growth. Metabolism and product formation changed significantly compared to exponential growth. Product formation could be correlated to cell growth and feed medium with regard to serum or serum supplements. Implications on production strategy were discussed.

INTRODUCTION

An increasing demand for large quantities of monoclonal antibodies stimulated investigations on cell physiology and fermentation process strategy. To improve the basic knowledge of the factors which influence productivity we started a quantitative study of cell growth and monoclonal antibody production in batch processes as well as in continuous high density perfusion cultures.

MATERIALS AND METHODS

Bioreactor and cell culture

Free suspended cells were cultivated in stirred tank bioreactors (Biostat MC,Biostat EC, B.Braun Diessel Biotech) designed for shear sensitive cells. For the physiological investigations in high cell density cultures the bioreactors were equipped with a newly developed internal perfusion module which consists of microporous hydrophilic tubular membranes (Fig.1). Consumption and production rates were calculated daily via a process data management system (microMFCS, B.Braun Diessel Biotech).
The Sp2/0-Ag14-derived mouse-mouse hybridoma cell line HB 124 (ATCC) producing an IgG 2a κ-type monoclonal antibody against insulin was used as model system. Serum containing medium and two different serum free media were investigated (Serum supplements: CPSR4 (Sigma), Nutridoma-NS (Boehringer))

Analysis

Cell number: Haemocytometer combined with Trypan blue dye exclusion. Glucose and lactate: automatic analyzer (YSI, Yellow Springs, OH). Amino acids: Ion-exchange chromatography (Biotronic, LC 2000). Antibody: enzyme linked immunosorbent assay (ELISA) for murine IgG.

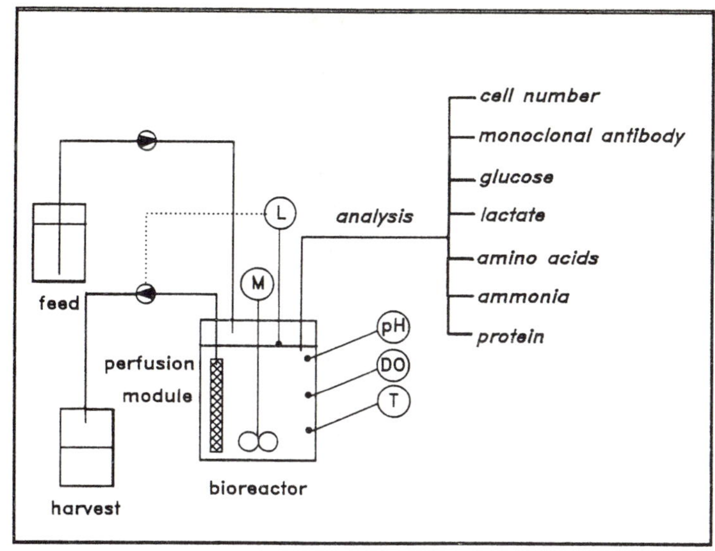

Fig.1: Set-up of perfusion bioreactor

RESULTS AND DISCUSSION

Batch cultivations

Growth, antibody production and metabolism were investigated at different dissolved oxygen concentrations (DO: 20%, 40%, 60%) in FCS containing DME-medium.
The maximum viable cell number and antibody concentration increased with increasing DO. Kinetic analysis of the data showed that the maximum growth rate μ and the maximum antibody production rate q(ab) increased with increasing DO. An increased DO, which resulted in a decreased lactate production, did not influence glucose consumption. Consequently the decreased yield coefficient Y(l/g) for the conversion of glucose into lactate indicated a more efficient glucose utilization. This phenomenon may explain high growth and antibody production rates.

Perfusion cultivation

The kinetics of different parameters of a typical high density perfusion cultivation is presented in Fig.2 and Fig.3. The concentration profile of glucose, lactate, glutamine and other amino acids reached steady state values during stationary phase due to continuous medium exchange. It was found that the exponential growth phase of the culture could be extended until the viable cell density reached $1*10^7$ cells/ml. An extensive period of stationary growth and metabolism followed. Characteristically the specific rates decreased 10 to 100 fold compared to exponential growth.
Cellular metabolism can be characterized by growth associated glucose consumption, lactate formation and amino acid consumption and production. It was found that the specific glucose consumption rate and lactate production rate reached their maximum immediately before the growth rate obtained maximum values.
During stationary phase the yield coefficient Y(l/g) decreased to Y(l/g) < 0.5, which reflects a change in metabolic pathways of energy generation from glucose as substrate compared to exponential growing cultures.

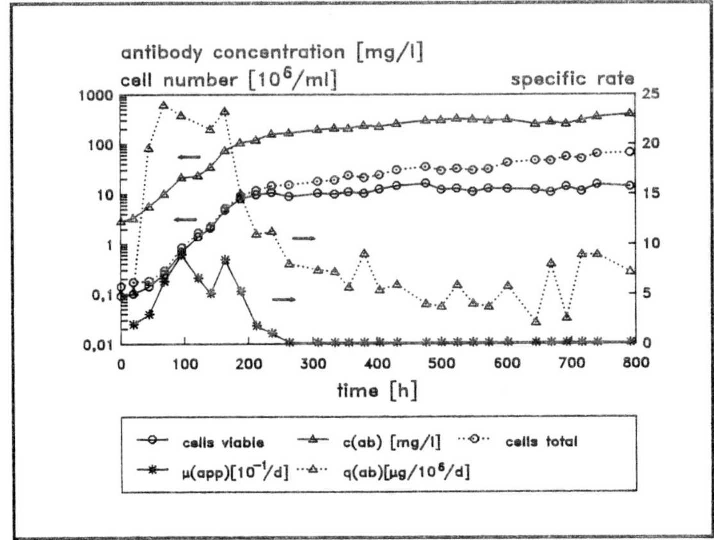

Fig.2: Growth and antibody production during high density perfusion cultivation of HB 124 cells in DMEM/HAM's F12 + 1% Nutri-doma-NS (Boeh-ringer) as serum supplement.

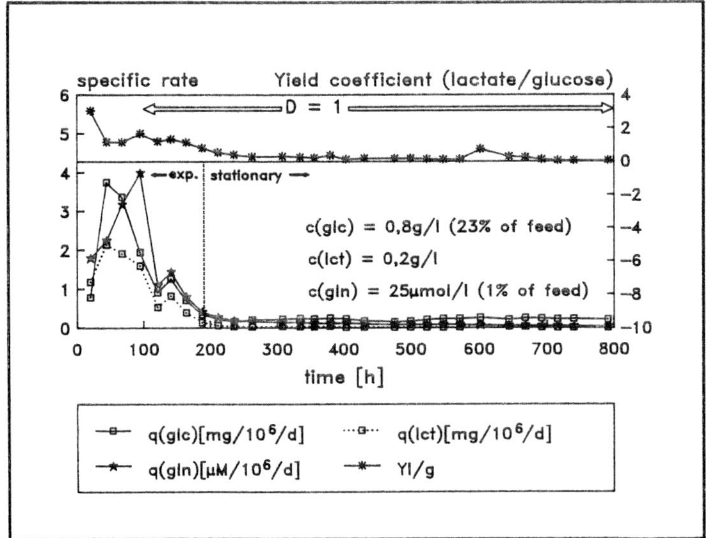

Fig.3: Changes in metabolism during high density perfusion culture (conditions see Fig.2)

Kinetic analysis of antibody production

As a prerequisite for process development and optimization antibody production kinetics in media both with serum and serum free were investigated in perfusion experiments (Fig.3). All patterns were consistent with a growth associated model and an additional non-growth associated contribution due to the release of unsecreted antibodies by lysing cells. A comparably small slope of the function $q(ab) = f(\mu)$ suggests a high cell density perfusion cultivation as the optimum production process in

CPSR4 supplemented medium. In serum containing medium cultivation processes which maintain the cells at high growth rates are appropriate (e.g. cytostat). The antibody production in Nutridoma-NS supplemented media (growth associated up to a critical specific growth rate) indicates, that a combination of perfusion and continuous cell harvest may result in high product yields.

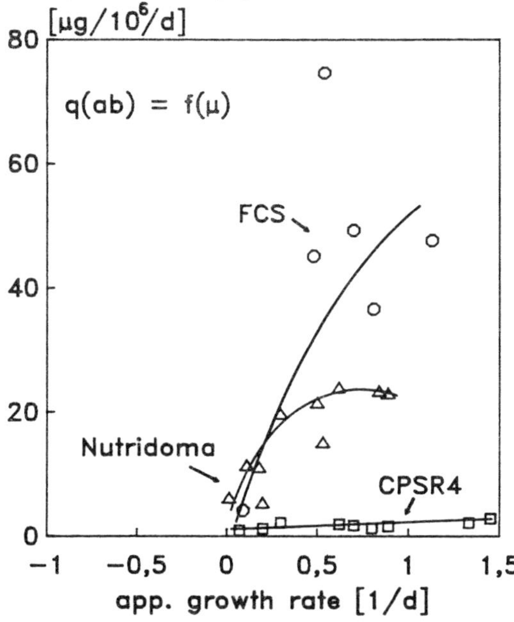

Fig.4: Antibody production patterns of HB 124 cells in perfusion culture using serum and different serum supplements.

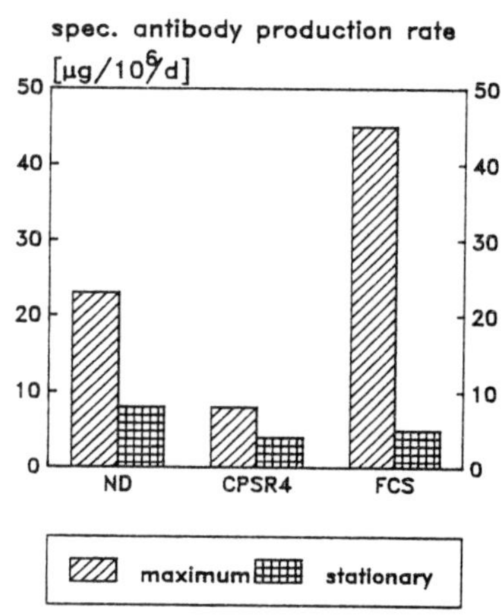

REFERENCES

/1/ Miller, W.M., Blanche, H.W., Wilke, C.R. Biotech. Bioeng. 1988, 32, 947-965
/2/ Harbour, C., Barford, J.P., Low, K.-S. Process development for hybridoma cells, In: Advances in Biochemical Engineering/Biotechnology 37 (Ed. Fiechter, A.) Springer-Verlag, Berlin 1988, pp 1-38

Acknowledgement
We would like to thank C. Müller and M. Ehrig (B.Braun Diessel Biotech GmbH) for their excellent experimental assistance.

Abbreviations:
μ: specific growth rate
q(ab): specific antibody production rate
q(glc): specific glucose consumption rate
q(lct): specific lactate production rate
q(gln): specific glutamine consumption rate
Y(l/g): Yield coefficient for the conversion of glucose into lactate
c(ab): antibody concentration

Correspondence should be addressed to: C. Fenge, B.Braun Diessel Biotech GmbH, PO-Box 120, D-3508 Melsungen

FACTORS AFFECTING HYBRIDOMA CELL ATTACHMENT TO DERIVATIZED POLYACRYLAMIDE
BEADS.

Y. Kaplan and A. Freeman, Department of Biotechnology, Faculty of Life
Sciences, Tel-Aviv University, Tel-Aviv 69978 and S. Reuveny, Israel
Institute for Biological Research, Ness-Ziona, 70450, ISRAEL.

ABSTRACT

A systematic study of factors affecting hybridoma cell attachment on
derivatized polyacrylamide (PAA) beads was conducted. Four major
parameters were tested: 1) Nature of cationic groups (primary vs.
tertiary amino groups); 2) Degree of derivatization (exchange capacity);
3) Length of the spacer arm bearing the amino groups and 4) Mean average
bead diameter. Positively charged beads (either with primary or tertiary
amines) exhibited hybridoma cell attachment within 4 hours of static
incubation. A minimal degree of exchange capacity was required for
efficient cell attachment (>80%). The threshold value of charging became
lower as the length (and hydrophobicity) of the spacer arm bearing
primary amines increased. Bead diameter (e.g. 30-80, or 80-160 μm) had
no effect on cell attachment. The most efficient carrier for hybridoma
cell attachment were PAA beads derivatized with 0.3 meq hexylamine groups
per g of dry polymer. Serum proteins had no affect on the rate of cell
attachment. Dead cells exhibited only negligible attachment. Increasing
cell to bead ratio from 1 to 5×10^5 cells per mg beads led to small
decrease in percentage of cell attachment (from 80% to 60%) indicating
that the limiting factor for achieving 100% cell attachment is not
availability of surface area, but the presence of cell population
incapable of attaching itself. Eight different hybridoma or myeloma cell
lines were tested exhibiting similar cell attachment kinetics (60-90%
cell attachment) indicating that this carrier is applicable for a wide
range of lymphoid cell lines. Scanning electron micrographs showed that
hybridoma cell attachment to the derivatived PAA beads is done by means
of small cell membrane extensions. Hybridoma propagated on derivatized
beads, with metabolic activity and antibody production rate similar to
that of a control of free cells.

KEYWORDS: Hybridoma; cell attachment; polyacrylamide beads;

INTRODUCTION

Perfusion systems were proven to be highly efficient for the production
of monoclonal antibody in culture (1,2). A major problem encountered
with perfusion cultures is continuous separation of the cells from the
growth medium (1). Efficient separation of hybridoma cells from culture
supernatant may be achieved by cell attachment onto a static matrix (non-
homogeneous system) or to small suspended particles (semi-homogeneous
systems). A ceramic matrix for the attachment of hybridoma cells in
fixed bed reactor was described by Marcipar et al. (3) and Lydersen et
al. (4). In both cases the nature of the hybridoma cell attachment was
not specified. Aunin and Wang (5) used poly-L-histidine to induce cell
flocculation. In several other systems, physical entrapment of hybridoma
cells in porous matrix (e.g. porous glass (6), polyurethane sponge (7) or
porous collagen (8)) using fixed or fluidized bed reactors, was

described. We describe here a study of factors affecting the attachment
of hybridoma cells onto series of systematically derivatized, inert
polyacrylamide microcarriers.

MATERIALS AND METHODS

<u>Cells</u>: Mouse hybridoma cell lines (F-12, producing monoclonal antibody
against bovine interferon, and G10G11, producing antibody against
carcinoembryonic antigen) were employed.
<u>Media</u>: The hybridoma cell lines were propagated in RPMI 1640 medium
supplemented with 10% fetal bovine serum (Biological Industries, Israel)
or in serum free medium - DCCM (Biological Industries, Israel).
<u>Polyacrylamide (PAA) beads</u>: PAA beads (Biogel P-150), having bead
diameter in the range of 30-80 or 80-160 µm, were obtained from BioRad
(Richmond, Ca., USA). Derivatization of the PAA beads was carried out by
direct aminolysis, as previously described (9,10). Determination of the
amino groups content, equilibration, sterilization and storage of the
derivatized beads were carried out as detailed elsewhere (9,10).
<u>Analytical methods</u>: Cells were counted by the trypan blue exclusion
method. Glucose level in culture was determined by glucose oxidase assay
(Sigma method No. 510). Lactate level was determined by the lactate
dehydrogenase assay (Sigma method No. 826). Antibody titer was measured
by the radial immunodiffusion assay (11).
<u>Determination of cell attachment and growth on derivatized beads</u>:
Appropriate amount of bead suspension was allowed to settle, the buffer
decanted and fresh growth medium added. This bead suspension was
incubated at room temperature for one hour, followed by cell inoculum
addition.
<u>Cell attachment kinetics</u>: Three ml of bead suspension (containing 4 mg
(dry weight) of beads and 6×10^5 cells per ml) were transferred to 5 ml
polypropylene tube (Nunc). The tube was stoppered and incubated under
rotation (2 rpm) at 37°C. Samples were periodically removed for
counting. Each experiment contained control of cells incubated with
underivatized beads,serving as the 100% reference for the calculation of
% of cell attachment.
<u>Cell growth</u>: Three ml bead suspension (containing 4 mg (dry weight) of
beads and 3×10^5 cells per ml) were transferred to bacterial polystyrene
Petri dish (5 cm diameter). Cultures were incubated in a CO_2 incubator
for 5 days. Culture supernatant was then assayed for glucose, lactate
and antibody.

All glassware employed in this study was presiliconized by treatment with
Sigmacoat (Sigma).

All results presented are average of at least two experiments, each in
duplicate.

RESULTS AND DISCUSSION

PAA was successfully employed by us previously for the establishment of
working system to study the effect of chemical modification on cell
attachment (9,10). This matrix is non-toxic, chemically stable, inert
(there is no non-specific adsorption of biological molecules),

transparent and autoclavable. Functional side chains carrying charged
groups on various spacers may be readily introduced into the PAA backbone
by means of controlled aminolysis via stable amide bonds. For this study
PAA beads were derivatized to generate controlled amounts of primary and
tertiary amino groups (Fig. 1, (9,10)):

I. Primary Amine Derivatives:

$$PAA\text{-}CONH_2 + NH_2(CH_2)_nNH_2 \xrightarrow{\text{ethyleneglycol}} PAA\text{-}CONH(CH_2)_nNH_2 + NH_3$$

$$n=2,4,6,8$$

II. Tertiary Amine Derivatives:

$$PAA\text{-}CONH_2 + NH_2CH_2CH_2N(CH_2CH_3)_2 \xrightarrow{\text{ethyleneglycol}} PAA\text{-}CONHCH_2CH_2N(CH_2CH_3)_2 + NH_3$$

Fig. 1. Derivatization of PAA beads

Animal cells (anchorage dependent as well as anchorage independent)
possess a net negative charge on their surface at physiological pH (12).
These cells should therefore be electrostatically attracted to positively
charged surfaces. Preliminary experiments (not shown) have clearly
demonstrated that hybridoma cells, like anchorage dependent cells, have
the tendency to adsorb onto positively charged surfaces. Unlike
anchorage dependent cells, which spread following attachment, the
hybridoma cells maintained their round shape following attachment.

Effect of type of charged amino groups on hybridoma cell attachment: Two
series of PAA beads, charged with primary (aminoethyl) and tertiary
(DEAE) amino groups were prepared. Cell attachment on these beads was
tested. Results (Fig 2) show that in both cases cell attachment depends
on the exchange capacity of the beads, with a maximum of 80% cell
attachment. The degree of charging required for maximal cell attachment
was 0.8 meq/gram (dry PAA) in the case of primary amine and 0.5 meq/gram
in the case of DEAE. Primary amine derivatives exhibited faster kinetics
of cell attachment : 50% of maximal cell attachment was observed within 1
hour while only 25% were attached to the tertiary amine derivative.

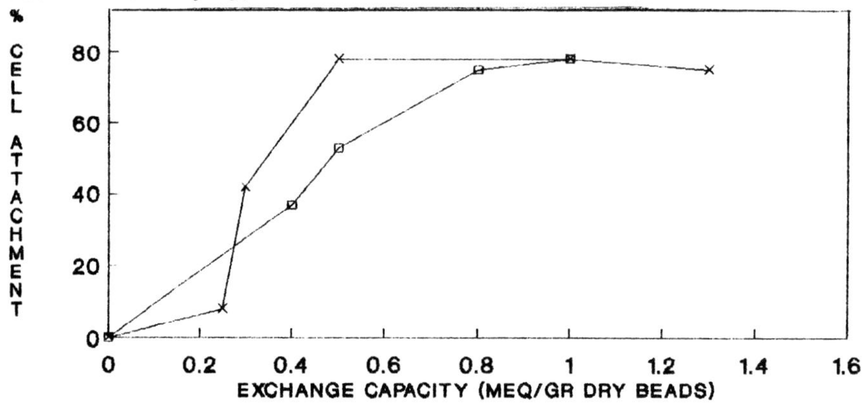

Fig. 2. F-12 hybridoma cell attachment on primary (aminoethyl (□)) and tertiary amine (DEAE (x)) derivatized beads (diameter: 80-160 μm). Cell attachment values were recorded following 4 hours of incubation.

<u>Effect of spacer hydrophobicity on hybridoma cell attachment:</u> In addition to ionic attraction, hydrophobic interactions may play an important role in cell attachment (10). This effect was studied by hybridoma cell attachment on primary amino derivatized PAA beads. Hydrophobicity was increased by gradual elongation of the hydrocarbon side chain carrying the primary amino charged group (Fig. 1). Similar to the phenomenon observed with anchorage dependent cells (10), it was found that the exchange capacity required for maximal hybridoma cell attachment is affected by the hydrophobicity. Elongation of the hydrocarbon side chain from 2 carbons to 6-8 carbons led to reduction in the exchange capacity required for maximal cell attachment from 0.8 meq/gram (dry PAA) to 0.3 meq/gram (Fig. 3).

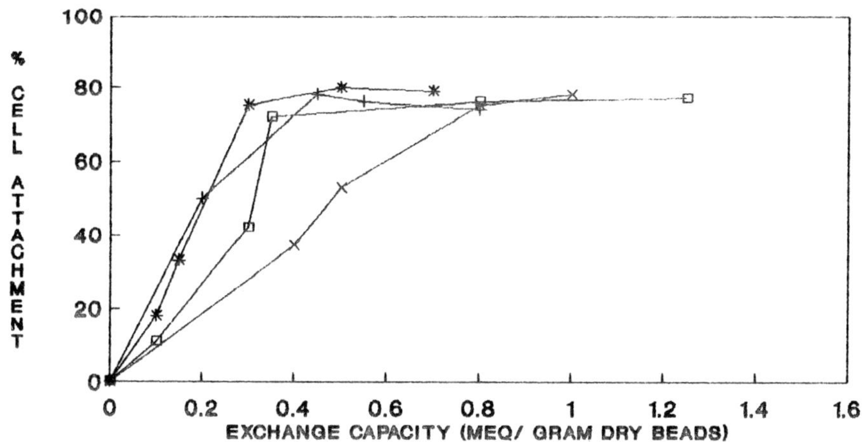

Fig. 3. F-12 hybridoma cell attachment on primary amino derivatized beads (diameter: 80-160 μm). Aminoethyl (x); aminobutyl (+); aminohexyl (*) and aminooctyl (□). Cell attachment values were recorded following 4 hours of incubation.

<u>Cell attachment on aminohexyl PAA bead derivative:</u> Diaminohexane derivatized beads having exchange capacity of 0.3 meq/gram (dry PAA) were selected as the best carrier (Fig. 3). Hybridoma cell attachment kinetics on these beads is shown in Fig. 4. About 40% of the cells attached to the beads 10 minutes after cell inoculation, while another fraction of 40% of the cells attached to the beads at a much slower rate throughout 140 minutes. As a result of cell attachment, aggregates of beads connected by cells were formed (Fig. 5 (B, C)).

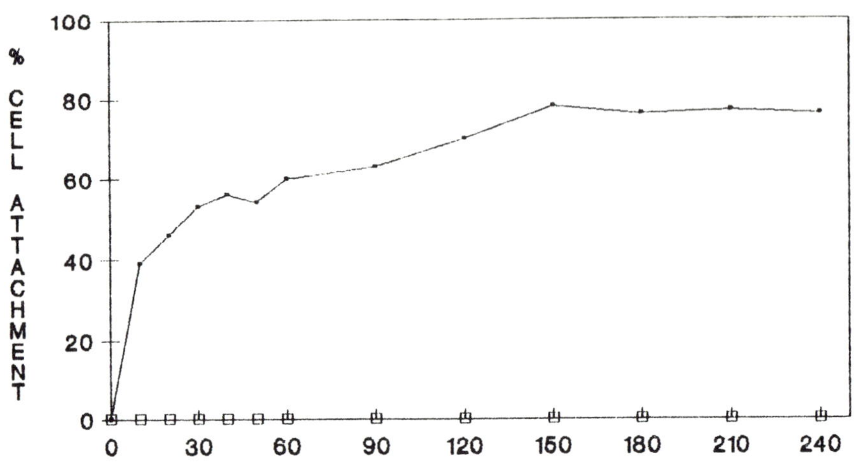

Fig. 4. Kinetics of G10G11 hybridoma cell attachment on diaminohexane derivatized beads (.) vs. control of non-derivatized beads (◻) (bead diameter : 80-160 μm).

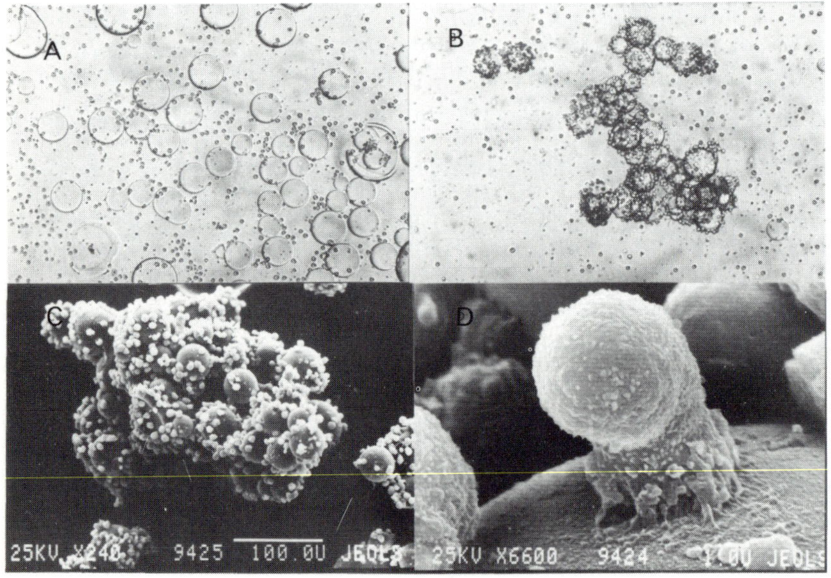

Fig. 5. Attachment of F-12 hybridoma cell line to derivatized PAA beads: (A) non-derivatized beads (control; light microscopy); (B&C) diaminohexane derivatized beads (B-light microscopy, C-scanning electron micrograph; note aggregate formation); (D) Scanning electron micrograph showing hybridoma cell attachment by small membrane extensions.

In contrast to our findings with anchorage dependent cells (13), hybridoma cell attachment to diaminohexane derivatized beads is not affected by serum (results not shown). Attachment of dead cells (as tested by the trypan blue exclusion method) to diaminohexane derivatized beads is negligible. This fact may be an advantage in perfusion cultures since dead cells will be removed in the effluent during perfusion.
Scanning electron micrographs showed that during the first hours of cell attachment the interaction between the cells and the bead is directly on the flat surface (not shown). About 24 hours after cell attachment small extensions from the cell membrane, mediating the cell adhesion, were observed (Fig. 5(D)).
Six different mouse hybridoma cell lines and two myeloma cell lines, propagated either in serum containing media or in DCCM serum free media, showed similar attachment kinetics. A level of 60-90% of cell attachment was obtained, depending on the cell line. These results indicate that the diaminohexane derivatized beads may be employed as a general carrier for lymphoid cells.
Cell attachment kinetics on diaminohexane derivatized PAA beads having diameter of 30-80 or 80-160 μm was almost the same. This finding indicates that the limiting factor preventing the achievement of 100% attachment is the unavailability of surface for attachment. In order to test this assumption a saturation experiment was conducted (Fig. 6). In this experiment, cell to bead ratio was increased from 1 to 5×10^5 cells per mg beads. This increase led to only a small decrease in percentage of cell attachment (from 80% to 60%) indicating that there is a fraction of about 20-40% of cell population which is not attached due to different surface characteristics (probably lower negative charge). In order to confirm this assumption these unattached cells were collected and reincubated with fresh diaminohexane derivatized beads. No cell attachment could be observed on these beads during the first 90 minutes after cell seeding.

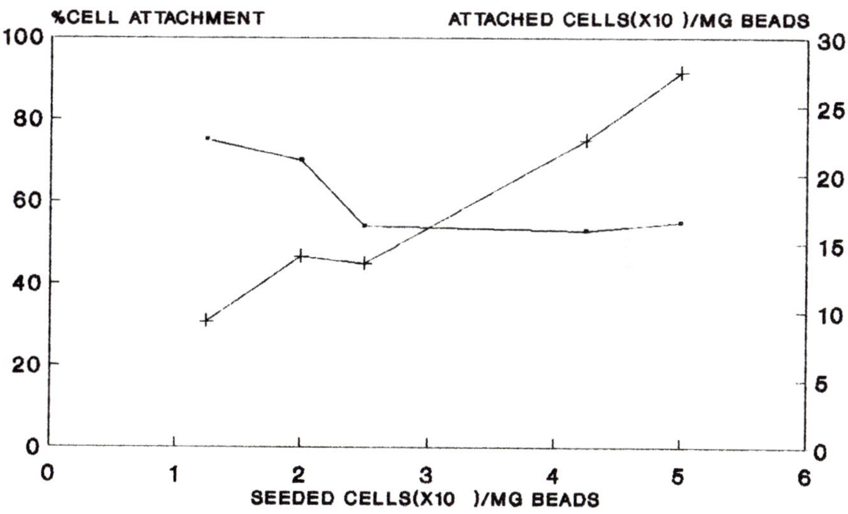

Fig. 6. Saturation of diaminohexane derivatized PAA beads (diameter 80-160 μm) with F-12 hybridoma cells. Cell attachment values were recorded following 4 hours of incubation.

<u>Cell growth on derivatized PAA beads</u>: A series of derivatized PAA beads (with diaminoethane, diaminobutane, diaminohexane, diaminooctane and DEAE), having the minimal exchange capacity required for maximal cell attachment, were tested for attached G10G11 hybridoma cell growth (Table 1). In all cases, similar levels (as with the control) of antibody and lactate re produced and similar level of glucose was consumed. These results indicate that the metabolism of the attached cells was not significantly affected by cell attachment or by the type of the charged group.

Table 1:

DERIVATIZATION	EXCHANGE CAPACITY (MEQ/GR)	GLUCOSE CONSUMED (MG/ML)	LACTATE PRODUCED (MG/ML)	ANTIBODY PRODUCED (UG/ML)
N=2	0.8	1.8	1.0	140
N=4	0.4	1.9	1.3	142
N=6	0.3	2.1	0.9	143
N=8	0.3	1.8	1.0	130
DEAE	0.5	1.7	0.8	120
CONTROL	---	2.4	1.1	140

IN CONCLUSION:

A matrix allowing for 60-90% of hybridoma cells attachment in culture was developed. The attached hybridoma cells could proliferate on its surface and monoclonal antibodies were produced. This matrix may be employed as a basis for developing homogeneous, as well as non-homogeneous, perfusion systems for the production of monoclonal antibodies.

REFERENCES

1. Reuveny, S., Velez, D., Miller, L. and Macmillan, J.D. Comparison of cell propagation methods for their effect on monoclonal antibody yield in fermentors <u>J. Immunol. Methods.</u> 1986, <u>86</u>, 61
2. Velez, D., Reuveny, S., Miller, L. and Macmillan, J.D. Effect of feeding rate on monoclonal antibody production in a modified perfusion-fed fermentor <u>J.Immunol. Methods.</u> 1987, <u>102</u>, 275
3. Marcipar, A., Henno, P., Lentwojt, E., Roserto, A. and Braun, G. Ceramic-supported hybridomas for continuous production of monoclonal antibodies <u>Ann. NY. Acad. Sci.</u> 1983, <u>413</u>, 416
4. Lydersen, B.K., Putman, J., Bognar, E., Patterson, M.N., Pugh, G.G. and Noll, L.A. In: <u>Large-Scale Mammalian Cell Culture</u> (Eds: Feder, J. and Tolbert, W.R.) Academic Press, New York, 1985. p. 39

5. Aunins, J.G. and Wang, D.I.C. Induced Flocculation of Animal Cells in Suspension Culture Biotechnol. Bioengin. 1989, 34, 629

6. Looby, D. and Griffiths, J.B. Fixed bed porous glass sphere (porosphere) bioreactor for animal cells. Cytotechnology 1988, 1, 339

7. Lazar, A., Silberstein, L., Mizrahi, A. and Reuveny, S. An immobilized hybridoma culture perfusion system for production of monoclonal antibodies. Cytotechnology 1988, 1, 331

8. Karkare, S.B., Phillips, P.G., Burke, D.H. and Dean, R.C. In: Large Scale Mammalian Cell Culture (Eds: Feder, J. and Tolbert, W.R.) Academic Press, New York, 1985, p. 127

9. Reuveny, S., Mizrahi, A., Kotler, M. and Freeman, A. Factors affecting cell attachment, spreading and growth on derivatized microcarriers. I. Establishment of working system and effect of the type of the amino-charged groups Biotech. Bioeng. 1983, 25, 469

10. Reuveny, S., Mizrahi, A., Kotler, M. and Freeman, A. Factors affecting cell attachment spreading and growth on derivatized microcarriers; II. Introduction of hydrophobic elements Biotech. Bioeng. 1983, 25, 2969

11. Velez, D., Reuveny, S., Miller, L. and Macmillan, J.D. Kinetics of monoclonal antibody production in low serum growth medium J. Immunol. Methods. 1986, 86, 45

12. Borysenko, J.Z. and Woods, W. Density, distribution and mobility of surface anions on a normal/transformed cell pair Exp. Cell. Res. 1979, 118, 215

13. Reuveny, S. Research and development of animal cell microcarrier cultures. Ph.D. Thesis, The Hebrew University, Jerusalem, Israel, 1983

Schmidt: You consistently had 80% attachment - have you an explanation for this? Is there a fraction of cells that is physically so small that there is only a limited number of interactions? Or is there a population in your cell mass that is just not able to attach?

Reuveny: We separated the 20% that did not attach and when they were incubated there was a shuffling of the negative surface charge and they attached. So it is a transient position in which 80% of the cells are negatively charged and can attach. The 20% after incubation will show 80% attachment once again.

Holtorf: Could the other 20% be mitotic cells?

Reuveny: We have no reason to believe that these cells are different from the general population in any metabolic way.

Holtorf: Do the 80% attached cells come back to the same balance of 80% plus 20% non-attachment?

Reuveny: We didn't do that experiment.

Gebert: I found your EMs of cell attachment very interesting. In particular I was interested in the cell that was coming away from the bead. How sensitive do those cells become to shear? Do they still attach in a highly stirred system?

Reuveny: They were stirred at 50 rpm for 4 hours and the rate of attachment depended upon the size of the bead. We don't have small beads in the range of 20-50 microns which would generate small aggregates which would not be affected.

Gebert: I was thinking more over several days.

Hofmann: Do you see differences in attachment if your cells are in protein-free medium? Also, you really have three populations of cells; one which attaches within 10 min (40%); one which needs a longer period (40%); and the remaining 20% which doesn't attach. Is there a difference in these two 40% populations?

Reuveny: No, we didn't differentiate between these two populations as it is hard to work on 10 minute time intervals. I do not believe that there are differences in these populations. It is only a question, I think, of negative surface charge.

Hofmann: Is there stearic hindrance?

Reuveny: No, between 50% and 80% you can flocculate. With
             regard to your first question you get the same
             results with or without protein in the RPMI medium.

Vournakis: I would like to comment. We have made microspheres
             with polyglucosamine ie chitosin, which are
             positively charged. We have found hybridoma cells
             have a greater than 95% attachment so I don't
             believe it is a question of charge.

Reuveny: We have tried different surfaces. The only general
             phenomenon is that they will attach to positive
             surfaces.

Hwang: Have you varied the charge density on your beads
             and still shown you get 80% attachment, or do
             percentages change with charge density?

Reuveny: I have shown that if you increase the exchange
             capacity there is no increase in cell attachment,
             and the same applies if you increase the cell
             number. This proportion stays constant all the
             time.

ADAPTATION OF ANCHORAGE-DEPENDENT CELLS TO GLUTAMINE-FREE MEDIUM

R.H. Thomas, H.A. Jenkins, M. Butler

Department of Biological Sciences, Manchester Polytechnic, Chester Street, Manchester, M1 5GD.

ABSTRACT

1. Glutamine was shown to have a similar regulatory effect on glutamine synthetase activity in both McCoy and MDCK cells. 2. In contrast to McCoy cells, MDCK cells were unable to grow in the absence of glutamine, with glutamate as a substitute. 3. The rates of uptake of radiolabelled glutamine were found to be similar for both cell lines. However, glutamate entered the MDCK cells at a much lower rate than the McCoy cells, which may therefore be one of the limiting factors to cell growth without glutamine.

INTRODUCTION

In addition to protein synthesis, glutamine is essential for cell proliferation as an amino group donor for purine, pyrimidine, amino sugar and asparagine biosynthsis, and as a regulatory component for DNA replication (1). Glutamine has also been recognized as a primary energy source for cultured mammalian cells (2,3,4). Glutaminolysis leads to accumulation of ammonia in the culture medium which has been shown to inhibit the growth of several cultured animal cell lines (5,6,7,8). Reduction or removal of glutamine from the growth medium could eliminate this source of ammonia production. At low glutamine concentrations, cells must be capable of synthesizing the necessary glutamine from glutamate by the action of the enzyme glutamine synthetase (GS). Glutamine has been reported to have a regulatory effect on GS activity in a variety of cell lines (9,10,11). In Chinese hamster cells (V79), the specific activity of GS was found to be inversely related to the concentration of extracellular glutamine (10). The aims of this study were primarily to investigate the effect of external glutamine concentration on glutamine synthetase (transferase) activity of two anchorage-dependent cell lines - McCoy and MDCK - in relation to their ability to grow in the absence of glutamine. Additionally, the rates of transport of radiolabelled glutamine and glutamate were studied, since this may be one of the limiting steps to cell growth without glutamine.

MATERIALS AND METHODS

Both cell lines were maintained in T-flasks (150 cm2) and grown in the Glasgow modification of Eagles medium (GMEM) (Imperial Laboratories, U.K.), which contained glucose (25 mM), supplemented with 10% newborn bovine serum (Imperial Laboratories, U.K.), sodium bicarbonate (32.7 mM) and glutamine (2 mM). The cells were incubated at 37°C with a 10%

CO_2/air overlay. McCoy cells were adapted to grow in glutamine-free
medium by harvesting cells at confluence and substituting glutamine-
containing medium (GMEM-gln) with that containing glutamate (GMEM-glu).
Glutamine concentrations of culture medium samples were determined after
conversion with glutaminase, and glutamate determined by a method using
glutamate dehydrogenase.
Assay of glutamine synthetase (transferase) activity: Cells were
harvested by trypsinization, washed twice in PBS (4°C), resuspended in
0.1 M imidazole-HCl buffer, pH 7.2, and disrupted by sonication. After
centrifugation at 6500 g for 5 min, the supernatant was assayed for
enzyme activity using the γ-glutamylhydroxamate method (1).
Amino acid uptake: Cells were subcultured into 24-well plates, and
amino acid uptake was measured (12) in complete growth medium with
either glutamine (0.1 μCi/μmol) or glutamate (0.4 μCi/μmol). Incubations
were terminated by aspiration of the medium and washing with PBS. Cells
were dissolved in 150 μl 0.5 M NaOH and assayed for radioactivity and
protein content.

RESULTS AND DISCUSSION

MDCK and McCoy cells showed similar growth characteristics in GMEM-gln.
The depletion of glutamine that occurred during growth appeared to be
associated with a 5-6 fold increase in GS activity in both cell lines.
McCoy cells readily adapted to growth in GMEM-glu, and maintained
constantly high levels of GS activity during the glutamate utilization
that occurred throughout growth.
The kinetics of degradation of GS activity upon addition of glutamine
were similar for both cell lines, as were the kinetics of induction of
activity on removal of glutamine (Figures 1a & 1b). However, in contrast
to McCoy cells, MDCK cells did not adapt to growth in glutamine-free
medium despite the induction of increased GS activity (Figures 1a &1b).

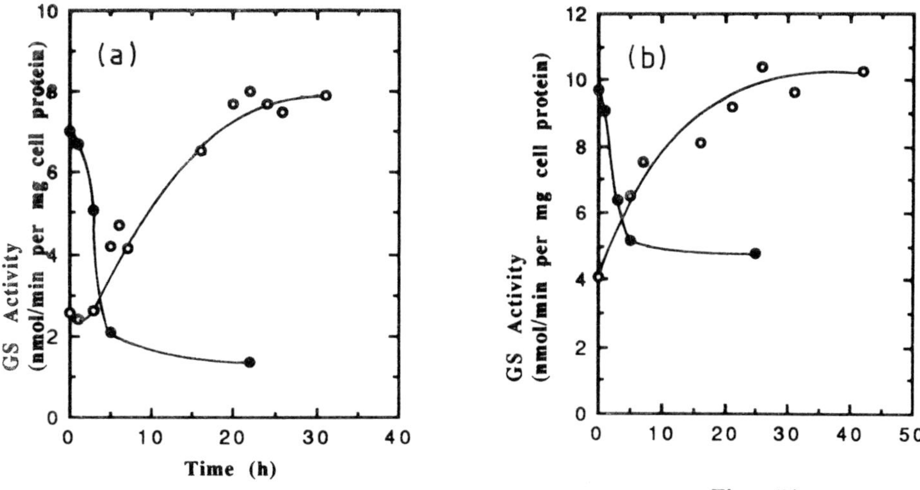

Figure 1. Effect of addition/removal of glutamine on the GS activity of
a) McCoy cells b) MDCK cells

●——● + glutamine   o——o - glutamine

MDCK cells transported glutamate into the cell at a significantly
slower rate than McCoy cells (Table 1). It was thought that this may be
one of the contributory factors to the inability of MDCK cells to grow
in the absence of glutamine.

Cell Line	Growth Medium	Uptake Rate (nmol/min per mg cell protein)	
		Glutamine	Glutamate
McCoy	GMEM-gln	5.47 ± 1.33	0.216 ± 0.078
	GMEM-glu		0.223 ± 0.133
MDCK	GMEM-gln	3.66 ± 0.71	0.043 ± 0.018

Table 1. Uptake rates of glutamine and glutamate by McCoy and MDCK cells.
(Each value represents the mean $\pm$ standard deviation of
triplicates).

ACKNOWLEDGEMENTS

This work was funded by the National Advisory Board and by Manchester
Polytechnic.

REFERENCES

1   Meister, A. Meth. Enzymol. 1985, 113, 185
2   Kovacevic, Z. and Morris, H.P. Cancer Res. 1972, 32, 326
3   Reitzer, L.J., Wice, B.M. and Kennell, D. J. Biol. Chem. 1979,
    354, 2669
4   Zielke, H.R., Zielke, C.L. and Ozand, P.T. Fedn. Proc. Fedn. Am.
    Socs. Exp. Biol. 1984, 43, 121
5   Glacken, M.W., Fleischaker, R.J. and Sinskey, A.J. Biotech. Bioeng.
    1986, 28, 1376
6   Glacken, M.W., Adema, E. and Sinskey, A.J. Biotech. Bioeng. 1988,
    32, 491
7   Butler, M. and Spier, R.E. J. Biotech. 1984, 1, 187
8   Hassell, T.E., Allen, I.C., Rowley, A.J. and Butler, M. Modern
    Approaches to Animal Cell Technology (R.E. Spier & J.B. Griffiths
    Eds.) Butterworths, London, 1987, pp 245-263
9   Paul, J. and Fottrell, P.F. Biochim. Biophys. Acta 1963, 67, 334
10 Tiemeier, D.C. and Milman, G. J. Biol. Chem. 1972, 247, 5722
11 Kulka, R.G. and Cohen, H. J. Biol. Chem. 1973, 248, 6738
12 Forster, S. and Lloyd, J.B. Biochim. Biophys. Acta 1985, 814, 398

The 2'5'oligoadenylate synthetase, a mutienzyme system involved in the growth properties and the sensitivity to viruses of mammalian cells: selection of antibodies in order to investigate their specific biological roles.

S. Lowagie[1], A. Herrera[2], E. Sexsmith[2], V. Chotteau[1], E. Ledent[1], B. Williams[2] and J. Wérenne[1].

1. Faculty of Sciences, Université Libre de Bruxelles, Brussels, Belgium.
2. Division of Infectious Diseases, Hospital for Sick Children, Toronto, Canada.

Abstract.

The interferon (IFN) induced enzyme 2'5' oligoadenylate (2-5A) synthetase has been implicated in the development of antiviral activity in animal cells. Its role in IFN-mediated growth inhibition was also proposed. More recently, other important functions of this enzyme activity involved in the control of protein synthesis and cell differentiation (related to RNA metabolism and splicing) have also been suggested.
At least 4 proteins with different molecular weights presenting a 2-5A synthetase activity can be detected. In order to elucidate the specific function of each individual 2-5A synthetase component, polyclonal antibodies raised into rabbits against the cloned 40 and 46 kDa human 2-5A synthetase expressed in E. coli were produced. The preliminary characterization of 2 such antibody preparations reported here shows that they are able to immunoprecipitate the natural human enzyme. Moreover,the antibodies do not precipitate any significant amount of bovine enzyme.
This approach appears therefore promising to further characterize the specific role of the different 2-5A synthetase entities in cell regulation.

Introduction.

A number of important biological activities including antiviral and antiproliferative effects (1,2 and for a review see ref 3) have been ascribed to 2'5' oligoadenylate synthetase (2-5Asynthetase), an enzymatic activity discovered in cells treated with interferon. By activation with double stranded RNA, the enzyme catalyzes the formation of adenosine oligomers with a novel 2'-5' linkage. This 2-5A in turn activates a latent ribonuclease which is responsible for RNA cleavage.
Other important functions involved in the control of protein synthesis (4) and cell differentiation related to RNA metabolism (5) and splicing (6) have been also suggested.
Those biological effects are certainly critical factors to control in order to obtain efficient production of biologicals from animal cell in culture.

They therefore deserve further characterization if one wish to improve the technology of animal cell culture.
We have shown previously that in bovine cells, at least two forms of 2-5Asynthetase can be induced (7). Even, in human cells, up to 4 distinct forms of the enzyme were detected (8). Among those, two enzyme entities of 40 and 46 kDa are encoded by cDNA sequences of 1.6 and 1.8 kb derived from a single gene by differential splicing (10). A specific biological activity among those reported above for each individual form of these enzymes is therefore an attractive hypotesis.
The evaluation of this assesment, of practical interest, may be carried out by an approach based on the use of antibodies raised against these two proteins. However, as the different enzymes entities are difficult to purify in sufficient amount and quite labile when purified, such a goal was not staightforward. The following strategy was proposed to solve the problems: antibodies raised directly against individual recombinant proteins expressed in E. coli containing plasmids constructed with individual genes for different 2-5A synthetase (namely the 40 and 46 kDa human enzymes) were produced in order to be characterized as described here.

Materials and methods.

A) Cell cultures and induction with Interferon :

Human T98G cells were grown in MEM medium supplemented with 10 % foetal calf serum, non essential amino acids, and penicillin/streptomycin.

Bovine MDBK cells were grown in MEM medium supplemented with 5% Newborn Calf serum (Beta propiolactone treated),non essential amino acids, and penicillin/streptomycin.

T98G cells were treated for 18 hours with 1000 international Units/ml of Human IFN α2, and MDBK cells were treated for 24 hours.

B) Cell extracts and 2-5A synthetase assay.

After IFN treatment, T98G and MDBK cells were trypsinized and washed 3 times with buffer A (140 mM NaCl; 35 mM Tris-HCl pH 7.5)
T98G cells (About 10^7 ceils) were resuspended in 0.150 ml of lysis buffer (20 mM Hepes-KOH pH 7.5 buffer; 10 mM KCl; 1.5 mM Mg Acetate; 0.5 mM DTT; 0.5 % NP40) and incubated for 30 minutes at 0°C. Cytoplasmic extracts (S10) were obtained by centrifugation (10000g for 10 min.).
MDBK cells were resuspended in 0.150 ml of buffer C (10 mM KCl; 1.5 mM Mg Acetate; 1mM DTT; 10 mM Hepes-KOH pH 7.4 buffer; 0.5 % Triton X100), incubated for 30 min. at 0°C and finally disrupted with a Dounce homogeneizer before centrifugation (S10).
The activity of 2-5A synthetase in solution was assayed in cell extracts as described before (7).

C) Immunoprecipitation and assay of immunoprecipitated 2-5A synthetase.

50 µl of crude extract (S10) from interferon treated cells were first incubated (45 min. at 4°C) with several amounts of rabbit antiserum before further incubation (3h

at 4°C) with protein A-Sepharose (15 mg/0.1ml) in buffer IP (20 mM Tris-HCL, pH 7.6; 50 mM KCl; 400 mM NaCl; 1mM DTT; 1% Triton X100;0.2 mM PMSF; and 20% glycerol V/V). The immune complexes bound to protein A-Sepharose were washed batchwise and consecutively with 3 times 1 ml buffer IP and twice with buffer C. Finally, the immune complexes bound to protein-A sepharose were resuspended in 75µl of buffer B (35 mM Mg Acetate; 2mM Fructose 1,6 diphosphate; 1mM DTT; 8 mM ATP; 15 mM Hepes-KOH pH 7.5 buffer; buffer contains also poly IC as described in ref. 7) as a reaction mixture. Incubation was overnigth at 30°C and was terminated by heating at 90°C for 3 minutes. Radioactively labelled 2-5A oligomers were treated with BAP (Bacterial alkaline phosphatase) and segregated with DEAE cellulose (DE 81 Whatman paper). Radioactivity was counted by liquid scintillation spectrophotometry.

Results and discussion.

The antibodies raised against recombinant human 2-5 A synthetase of 40 and 46 kDa (anti 1.6 and anti 1.8) produced in E. coli as schematized in Fig. 1 were characterized for their ability to recognize natural human and bovine enzymes.

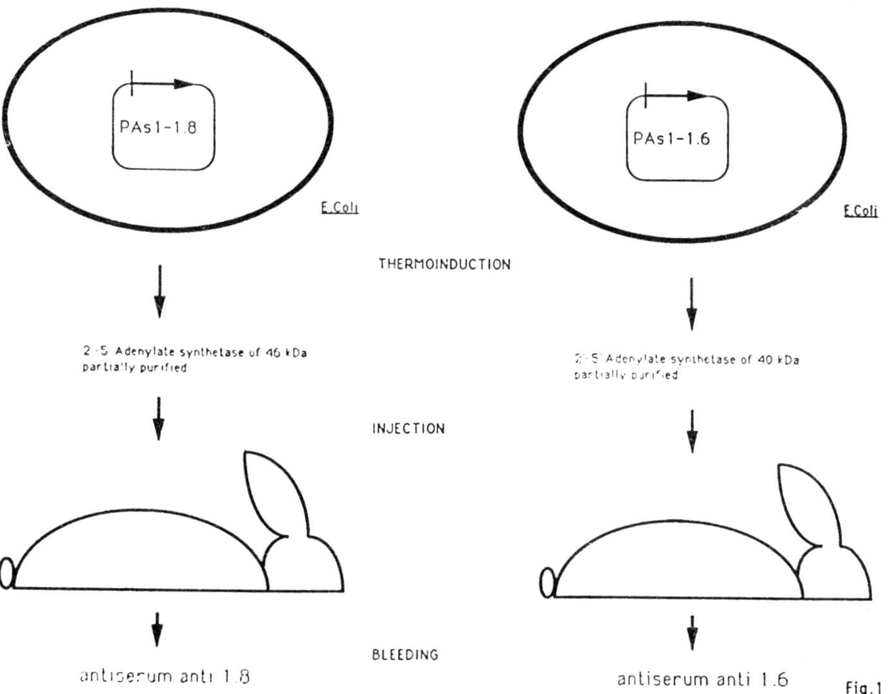

Figure 1   General strategy for anti 2-5A synthetase antibodies production in rabbits using pAs1 constructions with cDNA E1.6 and E 1.8 as source for the partially purified proteins expressed in E. coli.

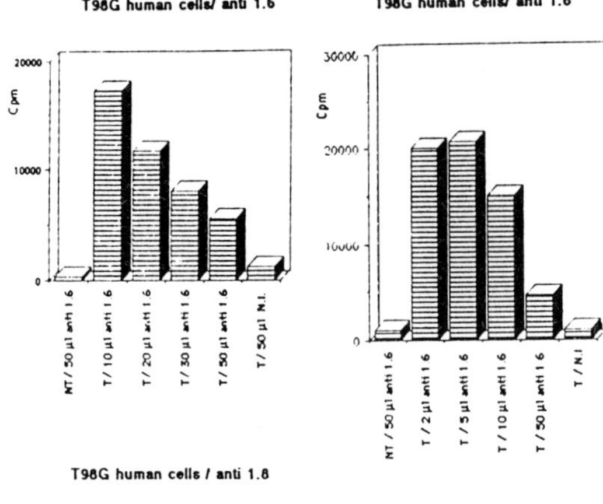

Figure 2 Immunoprecipitation of the activity of natural Human 2-5A synthetase (from T98 G cells) by 2 antisera.
The procedure is described under Material and methods; the enzyme activity reported are means of triplicate assays performed after precipitation with different volumes of serum as indicated. (N.I.: extracts treated with Non Immune serum; N.T.: extracts from control cells, Not treated with interferon; T.: extracts from cells Treated with interferon)

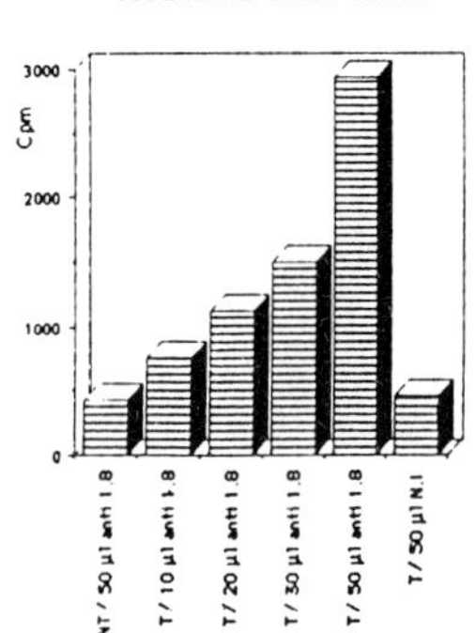

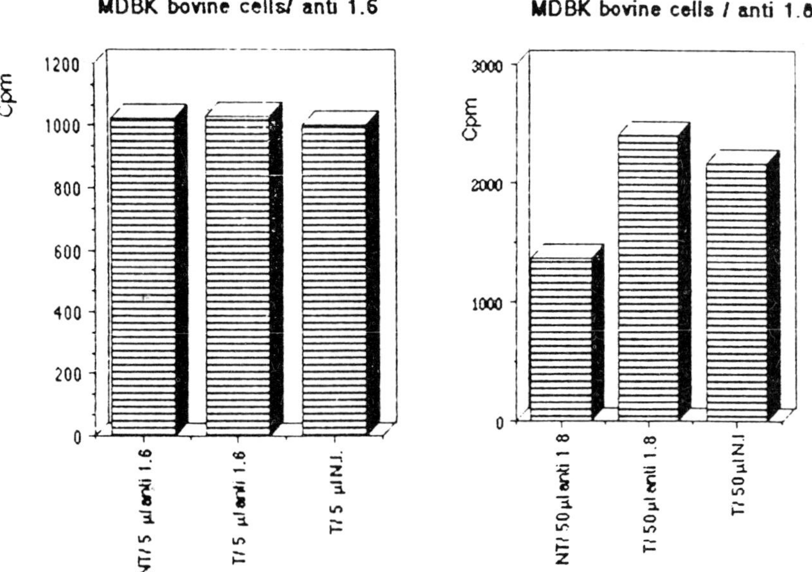

Figure 3 Immunoprecipitation tests for bovine enzyme (from MDBK cells)
The same conditions as for the Human enzyme extracts were used (cf Fig2)

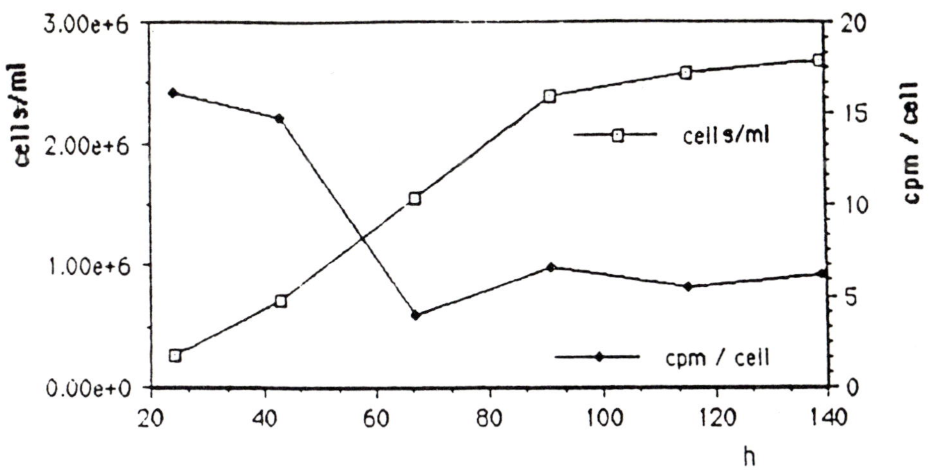

Figure 4   Activity of bovine cells (MDBK) 2-5A synthetase in function of cell growth.
The enzyme activity was measured in a "Nuclear fraction" (pellet of S10 washed by centrifugation through a sucrose cushion) after 24 h treatment of 1000U.I/ml IFN at different times after seeding.

Both of these antibodies specifically immunoprecipitate the human enzyme activity (Fig. 2). We showed also that with an anti 1.6 antibody excess, the enzyme activity can be neutralized.

No significant and specific precipitation of the bovine enzyme activity were obtained with these antibodies (Fig.3) despite existing homology between human and bovine mRNA sequences were revealed by Northern blot analysis (data not shown).

The same approach, using cloned bovine 2-5Asynthetase should therefore be undertaken to obtain antibodies specific for the bovine enzymes. This will be essential in order to define which are the enzyme entities induced in bovine cells after interferon treatment (cf Fig 4 which shows that the amount of enzyme induced is higher when cells are sparse and is reduced when they reach confluence) and if they are different to the basal activity detected in some conditions (as for exemple the basal activity detected by an immobilised assay in VERO cells and which, as shown in the accompanying paper (9), appeared to be also a function of the growth status of the cells).

Our final aim being to precipitate selectively each form of the enzyme in order to study their own properties and biological roles individually, one needs antibodies specific for each form of the 2-5A synthetase. Analysis by Western blot of the antibodies are currently undergoing and this will also establish further properties of the enzymes studied.

References.

1   Van den Broecke, C., Plasman, O., Hauzeur, K., Goossens, A., Ligongo,G., Piscitelli, S .and Wérenne, J. in "The 25A System: Molecular and Clinical Aspects of the Interferon-regulated Pathway" Eds B.R.G. Williams and R.H. Silverman (A.R. Liss, Inc. N.Y.),1985, pp 339-444

2   Rysiecki,G., Gewert, D.R. and Williams, B.R.G. <u>J. Ifn. Res.</u> 1989, <u>9</u>, 649

3   Johnston, M.I. and Torrence, F.P In <u>"Interferon 3: Mechanisms of Production and Action"</u> R.M.. Friedman, Ed., Elsevier, 1984, pp189-274

4   Williams, B.R.G. and Kerr,I.M. <u>Nature</u> 1978, <u>276</u>, 88

5   Hovanessian, A.G., Wood,J., Meurs, E. and Montagnier, L. <u>Proc. Natl. Acad. Sci. USA</u> 1979, <u>77</u>, 4479

6   Offen, D., Lehrer,R., Sperling,J.,Arad-Dann,H., Sperling,R. and Chebath, J. <u>J Ifn. Res.</u> 1989,<u>9</u>, suppl. 2, 94.

7   Severin, J.E., Chotteau,V.. Lowagie,S., Williams, B.R.G. and Wérenne, J. in <u>"Advances in Animal Cell Biology and Technology for Bioprocess"</u> R.E. Spier, S.G.Griffiths, J. Stephenne and P.J. Crooy, Eds. Butterworths, 1989,pp 136-142

8   Chebath,J., Benech,P., Hovanessian,A.G., Galabru,J. and Revel,M. <u>J. Biol. Chem.</u> 1987, <u>262</u>, 3852

9   Chotteau,V., Fabry, L., Lowagie, S. and Wérenne, J. in <u>"Production of Biologicals from Animal Cells in Culture: Research, Development and Achievements"</u> in press.

10   Benech,P.,Mory,Y.,Revel,M.,and Chebath,J. in <u>the Embo j.</u>, 1985,vol.4,n°9,p 2249-2256.

Acknowledgments

The collaboration between the laboratories in Brussels and Toronto is supported by a NATO grant (Nr 0533/88).

S.L.and V.C. hold a Belgian fellowship from the "Institut pour l'encouragement de la Recherche Scientifique dans l'Industrie et l'Agriculture" (IRSIA).

Section 5
Gene expression in animal cell systems

Recent Developments in Mammalian Expression Systems.

C. C. Hentschel
Medical Research Council, Collaborative Centre
1-3 Burtonhole Lane, Mill Hill
London NW7 1AD,England

Recombinant DNA technology provides the potential to produce
large quantities of otherwise scarce proteins. Furthermore
wholly novel "designer proteins", such as "reshaped"
monoclonal antibodies can also be synthesised using this
technology.

Although a number of expression systems are available today
the potentially greater authenticity of human proteins derived
from expression systems using mammalian cells as hosts often
makes these the systems of choice for proteins intended for
therapeutic use (Bebbington and Hentschel, 1985).

Over the last decade a variety of factors have been considered
in attempts to optimise mammalian expression systems:

Promoters

Most expression systems use strong promoter/enhancer
combination to drive transcription. The choice of these will
depend partly on the cell type, but viral promoters and
enhancers from, for example, SV40 (Mulligan and Berg 1981),
Rous Sarcoma Virus (RSV) (Gorman _et al_ 1982a) and human
cytomegalovirus (HCMV) (Boshart _et al_ 1985) have been used
widely because they work well in a variety of cell types.
When expression in a particular specialised cell type is
required, cell type specific promoters and/or enhancers may be
preferable. The immunoglobulin heavy chain enhancer (IgH
enhancer) for example directs high level expression in
lymphoid cells (Neuberger 1983). Inducible promoters may be
used when continuous high level expression of a gene product
is toxic to the cell. Examples of inducible promoters which
have been used to regulate expression of cloned genes include
heat shock protein promoters, which are responsive to
temperature shifts (Bendig _et al_ 1987), the metallothionein
promoter, which is induced by heavy metal ions and by
glucocorticoid hormones (Pavlakis and Hamer 1983), and the
glucocorticoid hormone sensitive promoter of the mouse mammary
tumour virus LTR (Lee _et al_ 1981). In addition, the E _coli_
lac repressor has been introduced into mammalian cell lines
allowing inducible expression from genes controlled by the _Lac_
promoter/operator region (Hu and Davidson 1987).

Gene source

Either genomic genes or cDNAs may be expressed in mammalian

cells. Early experiments on the expression of cDNAs in SV40
vectors indicated that the production of stable mRNA was
dependent on splicing and that this requirement could be
supplied either by a naturally occurring or a heterologous
intron (Gruss and Khoury 1980). Vectors which are suitable
for expressing cDNAs were therefore designed to include an
intron downstream from the cloning site to fulfil the splice
requirement. A series of vectors based on SV40 transcription
units are described by Berg (1981). One of these vectors,
pSV2, contains the SV40 early region promoter and enhancer,
together with the viral replication origin, upstream of the
cloning site, and the SV40 small t-antigen intron and viral
early region polyadenylation signals downstream of the cloning
site. Transcprition proceeds from the SV40 promoter, through
the cloned DNA, continuing through the intron and
polyadenylation signals thus assuring production of mature
mRNA. It has subsequently been found, however, that certain
genes can be efficiently transcribed in the absence of intron
sequences, preproinsulin is an example. (Gruss _et al_ 1981).
What determines the requirement for splicing remains unclear
but the question has been addressed recently by Neuberger and
Williams (1988) who showed that in the case of an
immunoglobulin gene the requirement for an intron is dependent
on the promoter used for transcription. When transcription of
an immunoglobulin u gene was driven by an immunoglobulin
promoter and enhancer, an intron was required for expression
of cytoplasmic immunoglobulin u mRNA. An intron was also
required when a β-globin promoter was used, but expression
from a cytomegalovirus or heat shock promoter was not
dependent on the presence of an intron. The intron requirement
was largely post-transcriptional and therefore presumably has
some effect on RNA processing or nuclear export hence
suggesting a connection between the promoter and one or both
of these processes. Since it is, in general, not possible to
predict whether or not an intron will be required for
expression, it would seem advisable to include one in the
construction of vectors when the expression of a novel cloned
gene is to be tested.

Mammalian selectable markers

Many commonly used eukaryotic vectors are derived from pSV2.
In addition to the SV40 derived sequences, pSV2 contains an
ampicillin resistance gene and the pBR322 replication origin
for selection and replication in _E. coli_. Derivatives of psV2
have been constructed containing dominant mammalian selectable
markers. These include resistance to mycophenolic acid
encoded by the _E. coli_ xanthine-guanine phosphotransferase
gene (_gpt_) (Mulligan and Berg 1981) and resistance to the
aminoglycoside antibiotic G418 encoded by the aminoglycoside
phosphotransferase gene from Tn5 (_neo_[R]) (Colbere-Garapin _et_ al
1981). Resistance to the aminocyclitol antibiotic, hygromycin
B, encoded by the hygromycin B phosphotransferase gene (_hph_)
of _E. coli_ has also been used as a dominant selectable marker
in mammalian cells (Blochlinger and Diggelmann 1984).
Recently Hartman and Mulligan (1988) described two new

dominant selectable markers based on expression of an <u>E. coli</u>
gene involved in the biosynthesis of tryptophan, <u>trpB</u>, and a
gene from <u>Salmonella typhimurium</u> involved in histidine
biosynthesis <u>hisD</u>. Expression of these genes in mammalian
cells allows growth in medium lacking either tryptophan or
histidine. Cells expressing the <u>hisD</u> gene could also be
selected on the basis of insensitivity to the enzyme
precursor, histidinol, which is otherwise toxic to animal
cells. These markers have also been incorporated into pSV2
vectors and they may provide inexpensive alternatives to the
costly antibiotics G418 and hygromycin B. The thymidine
kinase (<u>tn</u>) gene of herpes simplex virus can also be used for
selection in mammalian cells (Mantei <u>et al</u> 1979) but its use
is restricted to cell lines which are deficient in <u>tk</u> , for
example, derivatives of the mouse L cell line.

Transfection methods

Introduction of foreign DNA into mammalian cells can be
achieved in a number of ways and the choice of procedure is
generally dictated by the recipient cell line. Calcium
phosphate co-precipitation of DNA (Graham and van der Eb 1973)
was one of the first methods to be used and results in highly
efficient transfection of a variety of fibroblast cell lines
(e.g. mouse L cells, HeLa cells). Stimulation of DNA uptake
with DEAE dextran has been used for cells which are poorly
transfectable by calcium phosphate. These include a variety
of lymphoid cell lines (Sompayrac and Danna 1981). Protoplast
fusion, in which bacterial cells containing the cloned gene on
a suitable plasmid vector are converted to protoplasts and
fused directly with mammalian cells also results in efficient
transfection of cell lines which are refractory to
transfection by calcium phosphate (Schaffner 1980). Most
recently electroporation has become the method of choice for
transfection of mammalian cells because of its technical
simplicity and its application to a wide variety of different
cell types (Chu <u>et al</u> 1987).

Transient expression systems

Expression of genes in mammalian cells can either be achieved
transiently or by the generation of stable cell lines which
carry the introduced gene. Transient expression occurs during
a short period, usually between 12 and 72 hours after
introduction of DNA into cell, when the plasmid vector is
nuclear but not yet integrated into the host cell genome.
Examination of mRNA or protein produced during this time can
yield information on the contribution of regulatory elements
to gene expression. Furthermore, when relatively small
amounts of protein are required for analysis or functional
studies it may be the systems of choice for protein
production.

Transient systems are often used to study the characteristics
of a host/ vector system by incorporating a sensitive reporter

gene. The coding sequences of the bacterial enzymes
chloramphenicol acetyl-transferase (CAT) and β-galactosidase
have been used extensively as such reporter genes(Gorman _et_ _al_
1982b, Herbomel _et_ _al_ 1984). Recently the firefly liciferase
gene has been found to be a more sensitive reporter gene
(DeWet _et_ _al_ 1987) and has the added advantage of giving a
linear response over a wide range of concentrations.

Certain transient expression systems have been adapted to give
optimal protein yields, for example the SV40/cos cell system.
Cos cells are simian CV1 cells which have been transformed
with an origin defective mutant of SV40 which encodes wild
type T antigen and supports the replication of defective
viruses with deletions in the early region genes (Gluzman
1981). Genes or cDNAs cloned into vectors containing an SV40
origin accumulate to very high copy numbers in these cells,
200-400 000 per cell for a α-globin gene construct (Mellon _et_
_el_ 1981), resulting in a high level of protein expression.
The extremely high copy number of these vectors is ultimately
toxic to the cells hence it is not possible to derive stable
cell lines using this system (Rigby 1982). However, Whittle
_et_ _al_ (1987) describe the detection of 100-500 ng/ml of
chimeric antibody in the supernatant of cos cells 72 hours
after transfection with chimeric heavy and light chain
antibody genes. Another transient expression system reported
to give sufficient protein yields for preliminary analysis
utilises a vector containing the Rous sarcoma virus LTR in
HeLa cells. Browne _et_ _al_ (1988) describe the cloning of a
tissue plasminogen activator cDNA into the vector pTR312
containing the RSV LTR and SV40 intron and polyadenylation
signals. This yielded sufficient protein for estimation of
the clearance properties of wild type and mutant t-PAs in
guinea pigs. Since the RSV LTR is active in a variety of
mammalian cells the host range of this vector is not
restricted to HeLa cells (Browne _et_ _al_ 1990).

A third transient expression system has been developed using
the pox-virus vaccinia. Vaccinia virus has a long (185kb),
linear,double stranded DNA genome which encodes a complete
viral transcription system. The virus replicates in the
cytoplasm of a wide variety of mammalian cells. Because of
its large size, insertion of foreign DNA into the viral genome
is carried out by homologous recombination rather than direct
DNA manipulation (Mackett _et_ _al_ 1982). Expression of genes
from viral promoters such as the P7.5 promoter, which contains
both early and late transcription signals, results in
continuous production of foreign proteins for 1-2 days after
infection and can result in the production of 1-2mg of foreign
protein per litre of cell culture (Moss and Flexner 1987).
Fuerst _et_ _al_ (1986 and 1987) report a 15-20 fold increase in
expression levels obtainable from this system by incorporating
the gene for the highly efficient bacteriophage T7 RNA
polymerase into the vaccinia virus genome. This polymerase is
used to drive expression of a coding sequence, from a T7
promoter, located either on a plasmid or on a second vaccinia
virus in the same cell. These studies used HeLa cells but

vaccinia can be propagated on most tissue culture cell lines
(Mackett et al 1985) and it can also be used for expression in
whole animals. The most extensive use of vaccinia vectors has
been for the expression of viral proteins, (such as hepatitis
B virus surface antigen) in animals for studies on vaccine
development (reviewed by Moss and Flexner 1987). However,
vaccinia shows considerable promise as a system for high level
transient expression of foreign proteins in cultured cells.

Stable expression systems

Although transient systems are useful for the preliminary
analysis of cloned gene products, production of larger amounts
of proteins requires the development of stable cell lines
expressing the cloned gene. There are essentially two ways of
producing stable transfected cell lines. The first approach
utilises viral vectors to replicate the cloned gene
independently from the cellular genome. The viral vectors
used initially to introduce cloned DNA into mammalian cells
were derived from the genomes of SV40 and polyoma virus (for a
review see Rigby 1982). SV40 replacement vectors were
designed in which the cloned DNA replaced part of the viral
genome and recombinant viruses were used to productively
infect cultured cells in the presence of herpes virus.
Although this results in the production of large amounts of
mRNA and protein in the infected cells, viral infection also
causes cell death so stable cell lines cannot be generated.
More recently viral vectors have been derived from viruses
whose genomes are maintained episomally in the nucleus of
permissive cells. There are several potential advantages to
using episomal vectors. Firstly the copy number per genome is
generally high hence potentially increasing the yield of
protein per cell. Secondly, since, by definition, these
vectors do not normally integrate into the cellular genome
they are free, from the "position effects" which act on
integrated transfected genes as a consequence of regulatory
elements associated with DNA flanking the insert. The two
episomal vectors which have been studied most extensively are
those derived from bovine papilloma virus and Epstein Barr
virus but an episomal vector derived from the human papovirus
BK has also been described (Milanesi et al 1984).

Bovine papillomavirus is a double stranded DNA virus with a
7.95 kilobase circular genome. The virus causes epithelial
and mesenchymal tumours in vivo and transforms bovine and
rodent fibroblasts in vitro. The transforming and episomal
functions both lie on a 5.4 kb fragment known as the 69%
transforming fragment which has been used in the construction
of vectors by linkage to bacterial replicons. These are
generally derivatives of pBR222 from which the so called
poison sequences which inhibit replication of SV40 in monkey
cells (Lusky and Botchan 1981) have been deleted (Campo and
Spandidos 1983, Binetruy et al 1982, Sarver et al 1982). Such
vectors are reported to replicate as multiple copies (10-200
per cell) of unrearranged non-integrated monomers in mouse
fibroblasts (Campo and Spandidos 1983, Sarver et al 1982) and

can be rescued in E. coli by transfection with episomal DNA
isolated from transformed cells, thus providing a useful
method of shuttling DNA between bacteria and mouse cells.
Several eukaryotic genes have been successfully expressed
using BPV-1 vectors in mouse C127 cells. These include human
β-globin (Di Maio et al 1982), human growth hormone (Pavlakis
and Hamer 1983), human interferon (Zinn et al 1982 and 1983)
and human tissue plasminogen activator Bendig et al 1987). In
all cases the yields of these proteins were good, usually
between 10^6 and 10^8 molecules per cell per day (Stephens and
Hentschel 1987). Many studies, however, describe
rearrangements of BPV-1 derived vectors (Zinn et al 1982,
Pavlakis and Hamer 1983, Di Maio et al 1984, Green et al
1986). For example, Green et al describe the stable episomal
replication of a human histone gene in a BPV-1 vector in C127
cells but the episomes isolated from these cells contained a 1
kb DNA sequence of unknown origin, not present in the original
construct. Other rearrangements include deletions and
insertions as well as integrations into the cellular genome.
These variations may not be a serious disadvantage provided
that a stable derivative expressing the cloned gene can be
isolated as was the case for the human histone gene. A
further disadvantage of BPV-1 vectors, however, is their
limited host cell range. Selection of transformants by
morphological transformation can only be used in cells capable
of focus formation. Dominant eukaryotic selectable markers
have been introduced into BPV-1 vectors in an attempt to
broaden the host range. Incorporation of the HSV-tk gene
allowed transformation of tk$^-$ cell lines of mouse, hamster,
rat and human origin to the tk$^+$ phenotype (Lusky et al 1983,
Sekiguchi et al 1983, Bostock and Allshire 1986) but although
some of these clones contained a few episomes, the majority of
the exogenous DNA was incorporated in the cellular genome.
BPV-1 vectors incorporating the Tn5 neomycin resistance gene
are reported to yield mouse C127 cell transformants containing
between 20 and 200 unrearranged episomes per cell, (Law et al
1983, Matthias et al 1983, Meneguzzi et al 1984) but the same
vector always integrated into the genome in mouse L cells
(Bostock and Allshire 1986). Furthermore, Bostock and
Allshire found that the method of introduction of DNA into the
cell influences the fate of the BPV-1 vector. Microinjection
of DNA directly into nuclei appears to cause less damage to
the DNA than calcium phosphate mediated transfection and more
frequently results in BPV-1 vectors replicating autonomously
as unrearranged monomers in C127 cells.

Another series of episomal vectors have been developed based
on the genome of Epstein Barr virus (EBV) (Yates et al 1984,
Yates et al 1985). EBV is a human lymphotropic Herpes virus
with a large, 172 kilobase, double stranded DNA genome which
can infect and transform human B lymphocytes. Incorporation
of the 1.8kb origin region, termed oriP, into recombinant
plasmids is sufficient to direct episomal replication of these
plasmids in EBV transformed human lymphoid cells or in cells
expressing the EBNA-1 antigen of EBV which encodes a
transacting nuclear factor required for replication (Yates et

al 1984). Vectors have been developed which include both the
oriP region and the 2.5kb EBNA-1 gene from EBV together with a
hygromycin resistance gene. These plasmids replicate as
multiple episomal copies in lymphoid and non-lymphoid cells
from a variety of species including human, monkey, dog and
rodent (Yates et al 1985). EBV vectors would therefore appear
to represent a more versatile episomal system than the BPV-1
system. However, it was found (S. Eccles, unpublished) that
the stability of vectors containing both the EBV origin and
the EBNA-1 gene varies dramatically in different human cell
lines. Although HeLa cells could be efficiently transfected
with the vector p292 which is similar to p201 except that the
EBNA1 gene is expressed from a stronger promoter (the SV40
early promoter). However, the resulting A431 transfectants
contained a large number of rearrangements and chromosomal
integrations. The p292 vector was more stable in HeLa cell
lines but its presence had adverse effects on the growth of
both HeLa and A431 clones after prolonged culture (Vidal et al
1990). Hence, although viral vectors may provide useful
expression systems, careful choice of the combination of
vector and cell line appears to be essential for the
generation of stable episomes in recipient cells.

Amplification systems

The second approach to generating stable clones takes
advantage of the observation that, following transfection, a
small proportion of the cells which have taken up DNA stably
incorporate some of this DNA into apparently random sites in
the genome. By linking the gene of interest to one of the
selectable markers described above, such clones can be
identified and tested for expression of the co-transfected
gene. These clones contain varying numbers of copies of the
transfected gene but, in general, the level of expression of
the exogenous coding sequence does not correlate directly with
its copy number. This variable expression is believed to
result from regulatory influences of DNA flanking the
insertion site. However, expression of a transfected gene in
an individual clone can be increased by amplifying its copy
number in situ. This can be achieved by including an
amplifiable gene in the vector used for transfection. When
cells are grown in the presence of certain toxic drugs
resistant clones arise in which the gene encoding the drug
sensitive enzyme has been amplified. The first example of
this was amplification of the dihydrofolate reductase (DHFR)
gene in the presence of its inhibitor, methotrexate (reviewed
by Stark and Wahl 1984). The region of DNA amplified in these
cells was found to be much larger than the DHFR gene itself
leading to the idea that linkage of a transfected gene to
DHFR, followed by selection with increasing concentrations of
methotrexate, might result in co-amplification of the linked
gene. This was indeed the case and copy numbers as high as
2000 per cell have been generated using DHFR vectors (Crouse
et al 1983). In general the increase in copy number results
in a roughly proportional increase in gene expression
(Bebbington and Hentschel 1987). DHFR co-amplification is

most conveniently performed in cells which lack endogenous
DHFR activity and a DHFR-deficient Chinese Hamster ovary (CHO)
cell line is used frequently. In this case the DHFR gene can
also be used as a selectable marker for transfection. It is
possible to carry out DHFR co-amplification in cells which
contain active DHFR genes but because both the endogenous and
transfected DHFR genes are amplified, very high levels of
methotrexate must be used and eventually the solubility of the
drug limits the number of gene copies which can be obtained.
Examples of proteins which have been produced at high levels
in CHO cells after DHFR co-amplification include human tissue
plasminogen activator and human α-interferon (Kaufman <u>et al</u>
1985, Mory <u>et al</u> 1986). The human t-PA from CHO cells had a
similar specific activity to native t-PA but its glycosylation
pattern although similar, was not identical. The IFN-α
consisted of a mixture of glycosylated and unglycosylated
species similar to that obtained from human lymphocytes.

Other genes which have been used both as amplifiable genes and
selectable markers include the adenine deaminase (ADA) gene
(Kaufman <u>et al</u> 1986) and the glutamine synthetase (GS) gene
(Bebbington and Hentschel 1987). These genes offer potential
advantages over DHFR as they can be used as dominant
selectable markers in a variety of cell types and are not
restricted to use in cell lines which are deficient in the
respective enzymes they encode.

The major disadvantage of these gene amplification systems is
that it generally takes several months to select appropriate
cell lines with sufficiently amplified levels of expression.
Furthermore, the amplified sequences are subject to deletion
and rearrangement, both during and after amplification,
sometimes leading to loss of high level expression. Given
sufficient time, however, stable, highly expressing clones can
be selected.

Future mammalian cell expression vectors

Viral vectors and co-amplification of genes with drug
resistance markers have both been used successfully to
increase gene copy number and protein yield as can be seen
from the examples quoted above, but both systems have
disadvantages related to the stability of the multicopy genes
and the host cell specificity of the vectors. An alternative
way of achieving high level expression is to exploit the
regulatory elements associated with genes which are naturally
expressed at very high levels in particular cell types. Mouse
myeloma cells, for example, are capable of producing very high
levels of antibody protein from their endogenous rearranged
antibody genes. However, when rearranged antibody genes are
transfected into myeloma cells the production of recombinant
protein is at best generally not more than one tenth of this
level, even when the genes are linked to the strong enhancer
from the mouse (in the region of 100ug/ml) immunoglobulin
heavy chain locus. A possible explanation for this poor level

of expression is that the transfected genes integrate randomly
into the mouse genome and they may not be located in an
appropriate chromosomal environment for high level expression.
A possible way of overcoming this "position effect" is to
recombine transfected immunoglobulin genes into the endogenous
immunoglobulin loci using homologous recombination. That this
may be feasible is suggested by the results of Baker <u>et al</u>
(1988) who corrected a mutation in an endogenous
immunoglobulin u constant region gene segment (Cu) by
homologous recombination with a pSV2neo vector containing a
wild type Cu gene segment. The frequency of homologous
recombination in this experiment was estimated to be 100 to
1000 fold lower than that of random integration of the vector
(non-homologous recombination) hence this procedure is
extremely time consuming.

Dominant control regions

A promising finding which may have more general applicability
to the development of expression vectors is the identification
of sequences of DNA flanking the human β-globin locus which
confer position independent expression in erythroid cells.
Linkage of these sequences, collectively referred to as a
dominant control region (DCR), to a human β-globin gene
resulted in the transfected gene being expressed, both in
mouse erythroleukaemia (MEL) cells and in transgenic mice, at
levels equivalent to that of the endogenous mouse β-globin
gene (Grosveld <u>et al</u> 1987, Blom von Assendelft <u>et al</u> 1989).
An element with similar properties has been identified
downstream of the gene encoding the human T cell surface
protein CD2 (Greaves <u>et al</u> 1989). Both these examples involve
genes which are expressed in a tissue specific manner and, in
the case of β-globin at least, at a very high level. If
dominant control regions are found to be generally associated
with tissue specific genes which are highly expressed (e.g.
immunoglobulin genes) their identification and inclusion in
expression vectors may allow the expression of these genes at
levels which approach or even exceed the expression of the
endogenous genes.

If this approach proves generally applicable it may replace
the need for amplification of genes using viral vectors or
drug selection.

REFERENCES

Baker, M.D., Pennell, N., Bosnoyan, L. and Shulman, M.J. (1988). Homologous recombination can restore normal immunoglobulin production in a mutant hybridoma cell line. Proceedings of the National Academy of Sciences, USA. 85:6432-6436.

Bebbington, C.R. and Hentschel, C.C.G. (1985). Trends in Biotechnology Vol. 3, 314-317.

Bebbington, C.R. and Hentschel, C.C.G. (1987). The use of vectors based on gene amplification for the expression of cloned genes in mammalian cells. In **"DNA cloning Volume III"** Glover, D.M. (Ed.) pp. 163-188.

Bendig, M.M., Stephens, P.E., Crockett, M.I. and Hentschel, C.C.G. (1987). Mouse cell lines that use heat shock promoters to regulate the expression of tissue plasminogen activator. **DNA**. 6:343-352.

Berg, P., (1981). Dissections and reconstructions of genes and chromosomes. **Science**. 213:296-303.

Binetruy, B., Meneguzzi, G., Breathnach, R. and Cuzin, F. (1982). Recombinant DNA molecules comprising bovine papillomavirus type 1 DNA linked to plasmid DNA are maintained in a plasmidial state both in rodent fibroblasts and in bacterial cells. **EMBO Journal**. 1:621-628.

Blochlinger, K. and Diggelmann, H. (1984). Hygromycin B phosphotransferase as a selectable marker for DNA transfer experiments with higher eukaryotic cells. **Molecular and Cellular Biology**. 4:2929-2931.

Blom van Assendelft, G., Hanscombe, O., Grosveld, F. and Greaves, D.R. (1989). The β-globin dominant control region activates homologous and heterologous promoters in a tissue specific manner. **Cell**. 56:969-977.

Boshart, M., Weber, F., Jahn, G. **et al** (1985). A very strong enhancer is located upstream of an immediate early gene of human cytomegalovirus. **Cell**. 41:521-530.

Bostock, C.J. and Allshire, R.C. (1986). Comparison of methods for introducing vectors based on bovine papillomavirus-1 DNA into mammalian cells. **Somatic Cell and Molecular Genetics**. 12:357-366.

Browne, M.J., Carey, J.E., Chapman, C.G. **et al** (1988). A tissue-type plasminogen activator mutant with prolonged clearance **in vito**. **Journal of Biological Chemistry**. 263:1599-1602.

Browne, M.J., Carey, J.E., Chapman, C.G. **et al** (1990). The expression of tissue-type plasminogen activator and related enzymes. In **Protein Production: The Exploitation of Micro-Organisms, Cells and Animals to Make Useful Proteins** (4th Biological Council Biotechnology Symposium). Harris, T.J.R. (Ed.). Elsevier Science Publishers, London. In Press.

Campo, M.S. and Spandidos, D.A. (1983). Molecularly cloned bovine papillomavirus DNA transforms mouse fibroblasts **in vitro**. **Journal of General Virology**. 64:549-557.

Chu, G., Hayakawa, H. and Berg, P. (1987). Electroporation for the efficient transfection of mammalian cells with DNA. **Nucleic Acids Research**. 15:1311-1326.

Colbere-Garapin, G., Horodniceaunu F., Kourilsky, P. and Garapin A.C. (1981). A new dominant hybrid selective marker for higher eukaryotic cells. **Journal of Molecular Biology**. 150:1-14.

Crouse, G.F., McEwan, R.N. and Pearson, M.L. (1983). Expression and amplification of engineered mouse dihydrofolate reductase minigenes. **Molecular and Cellular Biology**. 3:257-266.

DeWet, J.R., Wood, K.V., DeLuca, M. **et al** (1987). Firefly luciferase gene structure and expression in mammalian cells. **Molecular and Cellular Biology**. 7:725-737.

Di Maio, D., Treisman, R. and Maniatis, T. (1982). Bovine papillomavirus vector that propagates as a plasmid in both mouse and bacterial cells. **Proceedings of the National Academy of Science, USA**. 79:4030-4034.

Di Maio, D., Corbin, V., Sibley, E. and Maniatis, T. (1984). High-level expression of a cloned HLA heavy chain gene introduced into mouse cells on a bovine papillomavirus vector. **Molecular and Cellular Biology**. 4:340-350.

Fuerst, T.R., Niles, E.G. Studier, F.W. and Moss, B.M. (1986). Eukaryotic transient-expression system based on recombinant vaccinia virus that synthesises bacteriophage T7 RNA polymerase. **Proceedings of the National Academy of Sciences, USA**. 83:8122-2126.

Gorman, C.M., Merlino, G.T., Willingham, M.C. **et al** (1982a). The Rous sarcoma virus long terminal repeat is a strong promoter when introduced into a variety of eukaryotic cells by DNA mediated transfection. **Proceedings of the National Academy of Sciences, USA**. 79:6777-6781.

Gorman, C.M., Moffat, L.F. and Howard, B. (1982b). Recombinant Genomes which Express Chloramphenicol Acetyltransferase in Mammalian Cells. **Molecular and Cellular Biology** 2:1044-1051.

Graham, F.L. and van der Eb, A.J. (1973). A new technique for the assay of infectivity of human adenovirus 5 DNA. **Virology**. 52:456-467.

Greaves, D.R., Wilson, F.D., Lang, G. and Kioussis, D. (1989). Human CD2 3' flanking sequence confer high-level, T cell-specific, position-independent gene expression in transgenic mice. **Cell**. 56:979-986.

Green, L., Schlaffer, I., Wright, K. **et al** (1986). Cell cycle-dependent expression of a stable episomal human histone gene in a mouse cell. **Proceedings of the National Academy of Sciences, USA**. 83:2315-2319.

Grosveld, F., Blom van Assendelft, G., Greaves, D.R., and Kollias, G. (1987). Position-independent high-level expression of the human β-globin gene in transgenic mice. **Cell**. 51:975-985.

Gruss, P. and Khoury, G. (1980). Rescue of a splicing defective mutant by insertion of an heterologous intron. **Nature**. 286:634-637.

Gruss, P., Efstratiadis, A., Karathanasis, S. **et al** (1981). Synthesis of a stable unspliced mRNA from an intronless simian virus 40-rat preproinsulin gene recombinant. **Proceedings of the National Academy of Sciences, USA**. 78:6091-6095.

Hartman, S.C. and Mulligan, R.C. (1988). Two dominant-acting selectable markers for gene transfer studies in mammalian cells. **Proceedings of the National Academy of Sciences USA**. 85:8047-8051.

Herbomel, P., Bourachot, B. and Yaniv, M. (1984). Two distinct enhancers with different cell specificities co-exist in the regulatory region of Polyoma. **Cell**. 39:653-662.

Hu M.C-T. and Davidson, N. (1987). The inducible **lac** operator-repressor system is functional in mammalian cells. **Cell**. 48:555-566.

Kaufman, R.J., Wasley, L.C., Spiliotes, A.J. **et al** (1985). Coamplification and coexpression of human tissue-type plasminogen activator and murine dihydrofolate reductase sequences in Chinese hamster ovary cells. **Molecular and Cellular Biology.** 5:1750-1759.

Kaufman, R.J., Murtha, P., Ingolia, D.E. **et al** (1986). Selection and amplification of heterologous genes encoding adenosine deaminase in mammalian cells. **Proceedings of the National Academy of Sciences USA.** 83:3136-3140

Law, M-F., Byrne, J.C. and Howley, P.M. (1983). A stable bovine papillomavirus hybrid plasmid tht expresses a dominant selective trait. Molecular and Cellular Biology. 3:2110-2115.

Lee, F., Mulligan, R., Berg, P. and Ringold, G. (1981). Glucocorticoids regulate expression of dihydrofolate reductase cDNA in mouse mammary tumour virus chimaeric plasmids. **Nature**. 294:228-232.

Lusky, M. and Botchan, M. (1981). Inhibition of SV40 replication in simian cells by specific pBR322 DNA sequences. **Nature**. 293:79-81.

Mackett, M., Smith, G.L. and Moss, B. (1982). Vaccinia virus: A selectable eukaryotic cloning and expression vector. **Proceedings of the National Academy of Sciences USA**. 79:7415-7419.

Mackett, M., Smith, G.L. and Moss, B. (1985). The construction and charcterisation of Vaccinia virus recombinants expressing foreign genes. In **DNA Cloning Volume II**. Glover, D.M. (Ed). IRL Press pp. 191-211.

Mantei, N., Boll, W. and Weissmann, C. (1979). Rabbit β-globin mRNA production in mouse L cells transformed with cloned rabbit β-globin chromosomal DNA. **Nature**. 281:40-56.

Matthias, P.D., Bernard, H.V., Scott, A. _et al_ (1983). A bovine papilloma virus vector with a dominant resistance marker replicates extrachromosomally in mouse and _E. coli_ cells. **EMBO Journal**. 2:1487-1492.

Mellon, P., Parker, V., Gluzman, Y. and Maniatis, T. (1981). Identification of DNA sequences required for transcription of the human α1-globin gene in a new SV40 host-vector system. **Cell**. 27:279-288.

Meneguzzi, G., Binetruy, B., Grisoni, M. and Cuzin, F. (1984). Plasmidial maintenance in rodent fibroblasts of a BPV1-pBR322 shuttle vector without immediately apparent oncogenic transformation of the recipient cells. **EMBO Journal**. 3:365-371.

Milanesi, G., Barbanti-Brodano, G., Negrini, M. _et_ _al_ (1984). BK virus-plasmid expression vector that persists episomally in human cells and shuttles into _Escherichia coli_. **Molecular and Cellular Biology**. 4:1551-1560.

Mory, Y., Ben-Barak, J., Seger, D. _et_ _al_ (1986). Efficient constituitive production of human IFN- in Chinese hamster ovary cells. **DNA**. 5:181-193.

Moss, B. and Flexner, C. (1987). Vaccinia virus expression vectors. **Annual Review of Immunology**. 5:305-324.

Mulligan, R.C. and Berg,P. (1981). Selection for animal cells that express the _Escherichia coli_ gene coding for Xanthine-guanine phosphoribosyltransferase. **Proceedings of the National Academy of Sciences USA**. 78:2072-2076.

Neuberger, M.S. (1983). Expression and regulation of immunoglobulin heavy chain gene transfected into lymphoid cells. **The EMBO Journal**. 2:1373-1378.

Neuberger, M. and Williams (1988). The intron requirement for immunoglobulin gene expression is dependent upon the promoter. **Nucleid Acids Research**. 16: 6713-6724.

Pavlakis, G.N. and Hamer, D.H. (1983). Regulation of a metallothionein-growth hormone hybrid gene in bovine papilloma virus. **Proceedings of the National Academy of Sciences USA** 80:397-401.

Rigby, P.W.J. (1982). Expression of cloned genes in eukaryotic cells using vector systems derived from viral replicons. In **Genetic Engineering 3**. Williamson, R. (Ed). Academic Press pp. 83-141.

Sarver, N., Byrne, J.C. and Howely, P.M. (1982). Transformation and replication in mouse cells of a bovine papillomavirus-pML2 plasmid vector that can be rescued in bacteria. **Proceedings of the National Academy of Sciences USA**. 79:7147-7151.

Schaffner, W. (1980). Direct transfer of genes from bacteria to mammalian cells. **Proceedings of the National Academy of Sciences USA**. 77:2163-2167.

Sekiguchi, T., Nishimoto, T., Kai, R. and Sekiguchi, M. (1983). Recovery of a hybrid vector, derived from bovine papilloma virus DNA, pBR322 and the HSV *tk* gene, by bacterial transformation with extrachromosomal DNA from transfected cells. **Gene**. 21:267-272.

Sompayrac, Z. and Danna, K. (1981). Efficient infection of monkey cells with DNA of Simian virus 40. **Proceedings of the National Academy of Sciences USA**. 78:7575-7578.

Stephens, P.E. and Hentschel, C.C.G. 91987). The bovine papilloma virus genome and its uses as an eukaryotic vector. **Biochemical Journal**. 248:1-11.

Vidal, M.A., Wrighton, C.J., Eccles, S.J., Burke, J.F. and F.G. Grosveld (1990). Properties of EBV-based shuttle vectors in human cells. **Biochimica et Biophysica Acta**. In press.

Whittle, N., Adair, J., Lloyd, C. *et al* (1987). Expression in cos cells of a mouse-human chimaeric B72.3 antibody. **Protein Engineering**. 1:499-505.

Yates, J., Warren, N., Reisman, D. and Sudgen, B. (1984). A cis-acting element from the Epstein-Barr viral genome that permits stable replication of recombinant plasmids in latently infected cells. **Proceedings of the National Academy of Sciences USA**. 81:3806-3810.

Yates, J., Warren, N. and Sudgen, B. (1985). Stable replication of plasmids derived from Epstein-Barr virus in various mammalian cells. **Nature**. 313:812-815.

Zinn, K., Mellon, P., Ptashne, M. and Maniatis, T. (1982). regulated expression of an extrachromosomal human β-interferon gene in mouse cells. **Proceedings of the National Academy of Sciences USA**. 79:4897-4901.

Miller: Is there some confirmation about the increase of integration of genetic material into animal cells during specific phases of the cell cycle? It has been mentioned, although I have not seen it confirmed, that DNA mediated gene transfer is more efficient during the S-phase, and that chromosomal gene transfer occurs to a higher extent during mitosis. Is this true?

Hentschel: I cannot answer that question specifically but whether you get integration or not, and where, does depend upon the method of transfer used, eg in some systems you get quite different results from micro-injection from what you get from calcium precipitation. There are many variables at work which affect integration.

Brown: With regard to cell cycle integration, this question has been addressed, and no dependency on the cell cycle with integration frequency has been found. For proteins such as truncated gp120, more attention will have to be paid to creating a more promiscuous cell line for end processing of these proteins. We have seen inefficiency in transport out of the endoplasmic reticulum with these unusual proteins. Dr Kauffmann at the Genetics Institute has done a lot of work with mutants of tPA and as you alter the structure the efficiency of secretion is reduced. It is not so much a nuclear event but a cytoplasmic event. With the use of these viral promoters we see a tremendous growth dependence on production for as replication rates go down, so does production. Would this be explained by the life cycle of the virus itself eg SV40 requiring an active nucleus for replication and expression?

Hentschel: First I would agree with your comment that the expression technology has been worked up largely by molecular biologists who don't naturally think very much about the cells. I think there is now a great need for cell biologist to develop cell lines that are more optimal for what one is trying to do. It is amazing how few cell lines are being used on any serious scale. It should theoretically be possible to engineer cell lines with very desirable characteristics eg high secretion etc.

On your question about the life cycle of the virus I cannot give a general answer. Certainly some effects do depend upon the life cycle of the virus. With transient systems, if the viruses over-replicate they can be deleterious to the cells,

even killing them. There won't be a general answer
to your question - it will depend upon each
individual system.

Mannix: In order to use the dominant control systems we
presumably either choose a region in the existing
cell, or we have to insert that region. I would
assume that it is impossible to insert both the
control region and a gene downstream. Does this
mean that we need the precise location of new genes
within existing DNA structures?

Hentschel: It is not impossible. If you can isolate the
region you can actually reduce the amount of DNA
required to a few kilobases and you can produce
vectors using those few kilobases incorporated into
standard type vectors and get dominant control in
cell lines ie you don't have to do anything fancy
like site specific integration. It does not have
to be integration into the original site on the
gene. You actually confer the same properties with
this dominant control region irrespective of where
it integrates.

Spier: I want to discuss the maximum productivity of an
animal cell for a particular protein. You said it
is good to get 10^8 molecules/cell/day. Murakami is
of the opinion that this is 1000 fold short of what
a plasma cell is capable of producing. I believe
silk glands in the silkworm have an even higher
productivity than this, though I am not sure about
that. Can you comment on these target figures?

Hentschel: For any particular cell line you will get to a
point where increasing transcription or increasing
mRNA will not improve protein production. It may
be that with some cell lines, such as the myeloma,
you will do better than with other cell lines. The
figures I gave you for that particular cell and
protein I mentioned showed that the correlation
between accumulation of mRNA with protein
production fell off apparently because the cell
line unable to produce and secrete more.

GENETIC ENGINEERING OF CELLULAR PHYSIOLOGY

S.L. Bell, C.R. Bebbington#, M.E. Bushell, P.G. Sanders*, M.F. Scott, R.E. Spier and J.N. Wardell.

Department of Microbiology, University of Surrey, Guildford, GU2 5XH, UK. #Celltech Ltd, 216 Bath Road, Slough, Berkshire, SL1 4EN,UK. *Corresponding author.

ABSTRACT

A murine hybridoma, normally dependent on glutamine in the culture media, has been transformed to glutamine independence with a gene coding for glutamine synthetase (GS). Southern blot hybridisation studies show that the gene is incorporated into the genomic DNA. Sufficient heterologous GS is expressed to enable growth in glutamine free media.

INTRODUCTION

The biotechnological application of gene transfer technology is leading to the development of cell lines producing valuable biological reagents.

Another potential aspect of this technology is to use genetic manipulation to analyse and modify cellular physiology. A programme has been initiated to modify the glutamine metabolism of animal cells in order to determine the feasibility of making specific genotypic changes to a major biochemical pathway.

Glutamine is a key metabolite for the growth of cultured mammalian cell lines (1), and is either provided in the culture medium or obtained by the intracellular activity of the enzyme glutamine synthetase. Many lymphoid cells (eg myelomas and hybridomas) cannot be grown in the absence of glutamine, possibly due to insufficient expression of the endogenous GS gene. Glutamine is also a relatively unstable amino acid and decomposes to produce ammonia, an inhibitor of cell growth (2). Consequently, it would be desirable to grow cells in the absence of glutamine. This has been achieved by replacing glutamine with glutamic acid in a number of cell lines, including human diploid cells, MCK and HeLa (3, M Butler and T Hassell, personal communication). Our alternative approach is to increase the level of GS expression in the cell by genetic engineering.

RESULTS

Transformation of the PQXB1/2 hybridoma cell line.

A glutamine dependent murine hybridoma, PQXB1/2, was transformed with the gene coding for GS (4,5) under the control of a human cytomegalovirus (HCMV) promoter. The plasmid pCMGS (Fig 1), was linearised and inserted into the PQXB1/2 cell-line using electroporation (Table 1). Glutamine independent transformants were selected using G-DMEM, a glutamine free medium (6).   Transfected colonies were expanded in culture and cloned to give the CMGS-PQXB1/2 cell-lines.

Molecular studies.

To confirm that the GS gene from pCMGS had integrated into the DNA of the transformed cells total genomic DNA was extracted. Samples were digested with Bgl 1 and Bgl 2 restriction enzymes and a Southern blot of the DNA samples was probed with a 0.5Kb GS cDNA fragment. The DNA probe cross hybridised with the endogenous GS gene in the PQXB1/2 cells.   In the transformed cells an additional band of 2Kb was also detected which is the size predicted for the Bgl1-Bgl2 GS fragment from the vector. DNA copy number analysis was carried out. On average one transfected GS gene copy was found per cell.

RNA was extracted and a Northern blot of the samples hybridised with the above GS probe. The probe hybridised to the endogenous GS mRNA of 2.8Kb and 1.4Kb but the signal was very faint. To provide a stronger control for the endogenous GS mRNA, RNA from a cell line with amplified levels of GS was also included (SPG2-E4). In the cells transfected with pCMGS an additional band of approximately 2Kb was detected.

We are currently investigating the effect of these manipulations on the physiology of the hybridoma cell line.

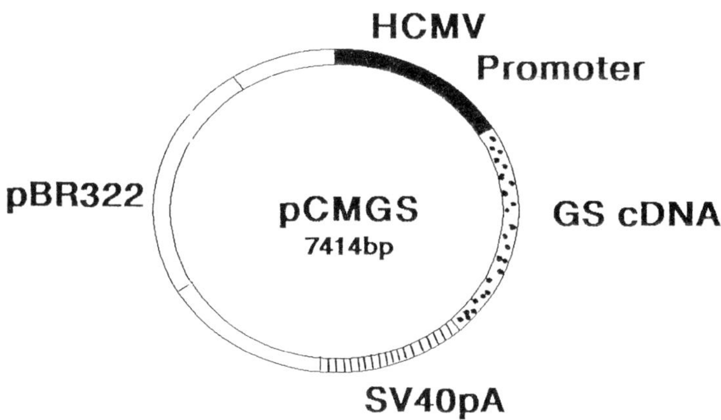

Figure 1. GS expression vector pCMGS

TABLE 1. Transformation efficiency of the PQXB1/2 hybridoma.

Vector	Transformants /10^6Cells
pCMGS	250
pEE6gpt	10
Mock	0

ACKNOWLEDGEMENTS

This work is supported by an SERC Animal Cell Biotechnology Programme Grant, GRD 96019.

REFERENCES

1   Krebs, H.A. (1980).   Glutamine: Metabolism, Enzymology & Regulation.   Eds Mora, J. & Palacios, R. pp 319-329, Academic Press, New York.

2   Reveny, S. et al. (1989). Advances in Biotechnology Processes, Volume 2. Eds Liss, A.R., Academic Press, New York.

3   Griffiths, B. (1973). Journal of Cell Science, 12, 617-629

4   Sanders P.G. and Wilson R.H. (1984) EMBO J 3:65-71

5   Hayward B.E., Hussain A., Wilson R.H., Lyons A., Woodcock V., McIntosh B. and Harris T.J.R. (1986) Nucleic Acids Res 14:999-1008.

6   Bebbington, C.R. & Yarrington, G.T. (1989).   European Patent Application EP 0 338841

Holtorf: Did you check the influence of lysine on antibody production, because you gave the impression that it was inhibiting in your rankings?

Scott: No, it is an experiment we plan to do as a mini fed-batch flask culture to see if there is a level one can demonstrate an inhibition on antibody production.

Spier: The 3-phase system is typical of what we might be seeing in bacterial systems eg streptomyces has a 3-phase system for the production of oleomycin with rapid growth, slowing growth and then stasis.

Bushell: A lot of animal cell and microbial products are event driven and I think the events are very different in each case. I suspect the events in antibiotic synthesis are very different from the events in this paper, although at the superficial level the control in the bioreactors may be according to the same principles.

Harbour: Batch systems are inherently variable so I wonder how you prepared your inocula and whether a lag phase, or absence of a lag, can affect the triphasic pattern?

Scott: What we found was that the inoculum does affect the length of the lag phase but all it does is time shift the whole tri-phasic pattern. The peak in the ammonium occurred at different time points because they were from different bioreactor runs but we always see this ammonia uptake, and other events, in the same order, but slightly time shifted.

Emborg: I am interested in factorial experimental designs and I saw that you made a long list of amino acids in a factorial design. Can you explain how you did this?

Scott: It is based on a matrix in which you try each amino acid at a high and low level, and look for an effect eg on growth or antibody production. From this you determine a response and eventually you can calculate the significance of that amino acid, and rank their importance on the degree of significance.

Emborg: How many experiments did you perform?

Scott: It is one experiment but you have 24 flasks each with different combinations of amino acids, plus controls to check for experimental error.

Schmidt: I have a problem with understanding how you get glutamine formation with the knowledge I have of metabolism. Another point to consider for the glutamine dehydration hypothesis is that I suggest you have a look at intracellular glutamate concentration to further establish if you can actually have incorporation the way you suggest from ammonium chloride.

Bell: It is a good point. The level of glutamate is something we want to look at. We see glutamine synthesis in cells; also cells transformed with the glutamine synthetase gene will grow in the absence of glutamine but still glutamine is secreted into the media ie it is definitely produced.

Gerbert: Have you done any comparisons of your analysis with CHO, or any other, cell line?

Scott: No.

Al Rubei: I want to comment on the condition of the inoculum further to Harbour's comments which I agree with. At time zero and for a few hours the cells reflect the conditions of the previous culture, not the current one. Another point concerns the death phase. All the metabolic measurements are affected by the death rate, by the number of viable cells in the fermenter.

Griffiths: With all this discussion on ammonia and glutamine relationships; which is driving the system, ammonia or glutamine - do we know?

Bushell: Our data suggest that ammonia is not only an inhibitor, which is driving the phases of our culture, but is also an essential nutrient.

Griffiths: You are then suggesting that ammonia is more important in regulation than its source, glutamine.

Bushell: All I will say is that the data is consistent with that hypothesis, but it is also probably consistent with a lot of others too!

STABILITY OF AMPLIFIED DNA IN CHINESE HAMSTER OVARY CELLS

N.H. Cossons, P.M. Hayter, M.F. Tuite and N. Jenkins

Biological Laboratory, University of Kent at Canterbury, Kent, CT2 7NJ. U.K.

ABSTRACT

A Chinese Hamster Ovary (CHO) cell line containing the human gamma interferon (IFN-γ) gene co-amplified with the gene for dihydrofolate reductase (DHFR), was continuously maintained for 120 days in serum-free medium with 0.1μM methotrexate. During this time the IFN-γ titre fell by 70% due to a reduction in the specific IFN production rate. Cell number was higher in late passage cultures and cell viability was maintained for longer periods. Chromosome studies revealed no significant difference in the overall chromosome frequency and distribution, except for a 16% increase in the modal chromosome number of 18. Southern blot analysis of DHFR showed a 45% decrease in levels over 120 days with IFN-γ decreasing by 30% over the same time period.

Keywords : CHO, stability, amplification, DHFR, interferon, methotrexate.

INTRODUCTION

In mammalian cells, resistance to the folate analogue methotrexate arises by amplification of the dihydrofolate reductase gene. During amplification flanking regions to either side of the enzyme will also be amplified. Thus, by linking a gene of interest (in this case human gamma interferon (IFN-γ)) to the original DHFR cDNA, IFN-γ will also be over-expressed. This phenomenon has been exploited for the over-production of recombinant proteins in mammalian cells (1).

The actual mechanism by which cells amplify these regions is not known although several models have been postulated (4,5,6,7). The MTX selection system itself is, however, inherently unstable and has been directly associated with many chromosomal rearrangements and abnormalities. It is not surprising then that increased resistance to MTX can arise due to mechanisms which do not involve over-production of the DHFR enzyme.

It is well characterised that levels of amplified DNA decrease in the absence of selective pressure (2,3). However, even under conditions of selective pressure, it has been found that levels of previously stable amplified DHFR enzyme can decrease to almost single copy levels after six months (4) although the mechanism by which this loss occurs is not clear. The purpose of this study was to examine physiological parameters under maintained selective pressure during long term passage and to relate these to levels of DHFR and IFN gene, as well as overall changes in chromosome frequency and distribution.

MATERIALS AND METHODS

Cell Culture

CHO cells were continuously passaged in a 500ml stirred reactor vessel (Techne, Cambridge), in serum-free medium (1) for 120 days. At 0 days (early), after 60 days (middle) and after 120 days (late) of this time period, cells were frozen and stored in liquid nitrogen. On revival, cells were transferred into 15ml of the standard selective medium containing $0.1\mu M$ MTX. Cells were passaged into 100ml medium in 250ml Erlenmeyer flasks (seeding density 1 x 10^5/ml). The headspace of the flask was purged with a mixture of 5% CO_2 in air to maintain pH and incubated at 37°C in a shaking incubator at 100rpm. Physiological studies were carried out in triplicate cultures and cells were also maintained for DNA and chromosome analysis. Cell counts were carried out daily and viability assessed using Trypan Blue dye exclusion.

Chromosome Number

Cells were grown until mid-log phase and arrested at metaphase using the addition of colchicine (Sigma) at $0.5\mu g$/ml. Chromosome spreads were carried out using standard techniques.

Southern Blots

Cells were harvested by centrifugation and DNA was extracted using standard protocols (3). Samples were run on a 1% agarose gel and blotted by capillary transfer onto GeneScreenplus. Membranes were then hybridised according to standard protocols using a DHFR probe (Wellcome Biotech) and a IFN-γ probe (obtained from Dr. H. Morris, University of Warwick). Autoradiographs were quantified using scanning densitometry.

IFN- Assay

IFN-γ was measured using a specific human IFN-γ antibody ELISA.

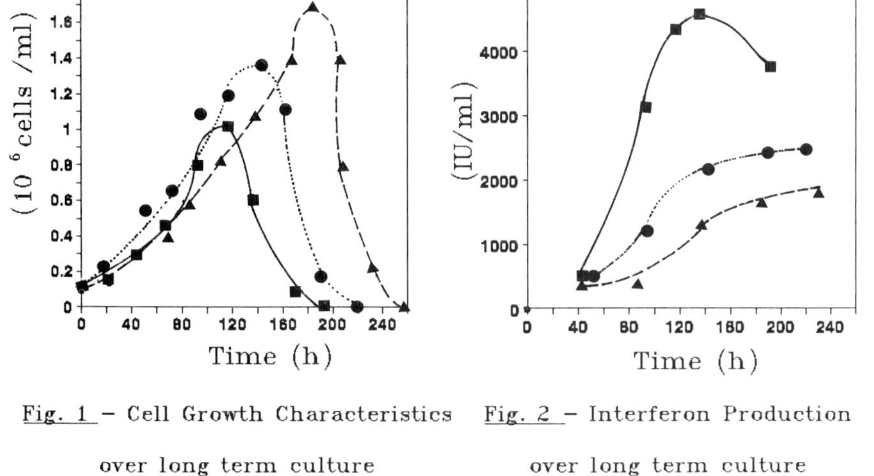

Fig. 1 – Cell Growth Characteristics Fig. 2 – Interferon Production

over long term culture   over long term culture

(Early-0 days, Middle-60 days, Late-120 days) (Early-0 days, Middle-60 days, Late-120 days)

(——■——   ⋯⋯●⋯⋯   ——▲——) (——■——   ⋯⋯●⋯⋯   ——▲——)

Table 1. Summary of Physiological and Genetic Changes.

	Early (0 days)	Middle (60 days)	Late (120 days)
Max Cell Density ($\times 10^6$ cells/ml)	1.02	1.37	1.69
Max IFN level (IU/ml)	4579	2504	1802
q(IFN) (IU/h/10^6 cells)	52.4	19.5	13.0
DHFR DNA level (%)	100	74.5	55
IFN cDNA level (%)	100	88.8	71.5

No significant variation was seen in specific growth rates,

cell viabilities or chromosome numbers.

Cell growth characteristics were compared for early (0 days), middle (60 days) and late (120 days) passage cultures (Fig. 1). Cells taken from an early passage culture, typically reached a maximum cell density of 1.02×10^6 cells/ml after 116 hours. However cells that had been derived from long term cultures grew to a higher cell density (1.69×10^6 cells/ml), a 1.5 fold greater maximum cell density than the early passage cultures with middle passage cells falling between the two (1.37×10^6 cells/ml). Cell viability in the late passage cells was maintained for longer than the early and middle passage cultures but overall there was no difference in the rate of cell death. MTX cytoxicity did not appear to change, partly reflected in the similar growth rates exhibited by the cultures (0.01-$0.02h^{-1}$). These data were consistent with previous observations which suggested that the very phenomenon of amplification gives rise to a continual generation of variability which results in cells becoming simply more efficient at survival and growth in MTX (4).

IFN-γ production in early passage cultures was up to 71% higher (at 120hrs) than the late passage cultures (Fig. 2). This correlation with the increased cell yields with passage number was corroborated by comparing the mean specific production rate (q_{IFN}) of IFN-γ for early, middle and late passage cultures (Table 1). A fall of 63% in q_{IFN} values occurred after 60 days of continuous passage and fell a further 12% during the subsequent 60 days. The majority of q_{IFN} loss therefore occurred in the first 60 days of continual passage.

In contrast to this, the level of IFN gene copy determined by DNA blot analysis (Table 1) showed a relative drop of only 11% from early to middle passage cultures but a further decrease of 17.3% from middle to late passage cultures. Although the loss of IFN-γ production was associated with a decrease in the levels of IFN DNA, this relationship was not linear.

Levels of DHFR DNA copies decreased very markedly (Table 1) by 45% overall (26% drop between early and middle passage cultures followed by a 19% drop from middle to late passage). The decrease in DHFR DNA levels coincided with a drop in the levels of IFN-γ DNA levels but not in direct proportion. The trend therefore appeared to be an overall decrease in the specific IFN-γ protein production associated with a decrease in levels of DHFR and IFN DNA. These changes were not linearly related but appeared to be associated with a concomitant rise in the maximum cell density (Table 1).

Other studies have shown that there is a good correlation between the levels of MTX resistance, DHFR enzyme production, its mRNA abundance and its gene copy number, but that this correlation declines at higher levels of amplification possibly due to other mechanisms of MTX resistance (8). Although the most common mechanism of resistance to MTX invoked is that of DHFR over-production, there are several other alterations in the cellular metabolism of the drug which could give rise to the same phenotype. These complex mechanisms include changes in the DHFR enzyme itself, possibly due to any amino acid mutation in the MTX binding sites, producing a DHFR molecule with an altered affinity for the drug. Transport mechanisms and extent of polyglutamation of the folate analogue may also be altered resulting in decreased MTX sensitivity of the cells. Alterations in the thymidylate synthetase enzyme normally inhibited by MTX would overcome the effect on DNA and RNA synthesis.

No gross changes in chromosome distribution were observed implying that any DNA losses were confined to small sub-microscopic changes, although there appeared to be a more discrete range of chromosome numbers in the late passage culture (16% increase in the modal chromosome number of 18). The significance of this observation is not clear at the present time.

In summary, there appears to be a change in the IFN-γ producing population of cells with time, under MTX selection. Cells lost some capacity to produce IFN-γ and this was associated with a loss in IFN-γ and DHFR copy number. No gross chromosomal changes were observed and no changes were seen in specific growth rate. It is possible that the cells have evolved a more complex mechanism of resistance to MTX than simply over-producing the DHFR enzyme. This could be due to any or all of the mechanisms outlined briefly above. It is also possible that as a result of this a loss of recombinant DNA from the genome occurs during selection, conferring on the cell population a reduced metabolic load on the cells and allow a higher maximum cell density to be achieved (4).

ACKNOWLEDGEMENTS

I would like to thank Ms. Lucy Gettins for carrying out the metabolite and interferon assays and also Mr. Jeremy Tong for all his help.
This work was supported by the SERC Biotechnology Directorate.

REFERENCES

1 Bebbington, C.R. & Hentschel, C.C.G. In: <u>DNA Cloning III</u> IRL Press Ltd, Oxford, 1987, pp 163-189

2 Hamlin J.L., Milbrandt J.D., Heintz N.H. and Azizkhan J.C. DNA sequence amplification in mammalian cells. <u>Int. Rev. Cytol.</u> 1984, <u>90</u>, 31

3 Kaufman R.J., Brown P.C. and Schimke R.T. Amplified dihydrofolate reductase genes in unstably methotrexate-resistant cells are associated with double minute chromosomes. <u>Proc. Natl. Acad. Sci. USA</u> 1979, <u>76</u>, 5669

4 Federspiel N.A., Beverley S.M., Schilling J.W. and Schimke R.T. Novel DNA rearrangements are associated with dihydrofolate reductase gene amplification. <u>J. Biol. Chem.</u> 1984, <u>259</u>, 9127n

5 Roberts J.M., Buck L.B. and Axel R. A structure for amplified DNA. <u>Cell</u> 1983, <u>33</u>, 53

6 Schimke R.T. Gene amplification in cultured cells. <u>J. Biol. Chem.</u> 1988, <u>263</u>, 5989

7 Stark G.R., Debatisse N., Giulotto E. and Wahl G.M. Recent progress in understanding mechanisms of mammalian DNA amplification. <u>Cell</u> 1989, <u>57</u>, 901

8 Flintoff W.F. In: <u>Drug Resistance in Mammalian Cells Vol. I : Antimetabolite and Cytotoxic Analogs</u> (Ed. Gupta R.) CRC Press, Florida, p.2-10

<u>Paper of Cassons:</u>

Sinicore:

As you know there is a considerable literature on the CHO cells exposed to methotrexate pressure; the impact of which is to adduce that cells become more stable to the expressing of heterologous protein with increased passage. Have you tried extending the time you have exposed cells to methotrexate selection pressure and as a result of that do you find that cells become more stable?

Cassons:

Not at the moment; our work was a preliminary analysis over 120 days, when we used the sustained selective pressure we observed a decrease in expression.

Wurm:

Did you clone your cell line at the 100nM methotrexate level.

Cassons:

No; this is a mixed population of cells.

Wurm:

This is an important issue as you are selecting for low producers starting from a heterogeneous situation and the presence of methotrexate is enhancing the variability in your production line.

Cassons:

The 16% increase in the modal chromosome number could be indicative of such a process.

METHOTREXATE AND CHO CELLS: PRODUCTIVITY AND GENETICS OF AMPLIFIED EXPRESSION VECTOR SEQUENCES

Florian M. Wurm, Vivek Bajaj, Wally Tanaka, Victor Fung, Amy Smiley, Adriana Johnson, Maria G. Pallavicini* and Robert Arathoon.
Genentech Inc., 460 Point San Bruno Blvd., South San Francisco, CA 94080, and *Lawrence Livermore National Lab., Livermore, CA 94550, USA.

ABSTRACT

Using fluorescence *in situ* hybridization (FISH)(1) we studied distribution, structures and statistical trends of amplified sequences in recombinant CHO cell lines. We found a high proportion of cells (40-60%) with multiple and/or unusually structured and extended chromosomal regions containing amplified sequences in the presence but not in the absence of methotrexate (MTX). Removal of MTX from culture media resulted in rapid disappearance of cells containing those amplified sequences represented by multiple and heterogeneous integrations. In cloned lines, a single, defined "master integration" became the dominant representative of amplified sequences in these cells. We studied long term genetic stability and specific productivity in the absence of MTX in uncloned, heterogeneous populations of cells representing multiple independent integration and amplification events. In order to allow for maximal growth rates and enhanced chances for selection of low producer subpopulations we used continuous high density perfusion cultures. We found no evidence for selection of subpopulations without or with significantly reduced amounts of amplified sequences. Also, specific productivity of these cell lines did not decrease over a time of about 100 days. Conclusions were: MTX is responsible for continuing rearrangements of amplified (and nonamplified) DNA sequences in recombinant CHO cells. In the absence of MTX clonal cell lines are characterized by genetically stable, single, unique, identifiable integrations of amplified sequences which can serve as identifying genetic markers.

INTRODUCTION

Mammalian cells and Chinese Hamster Ovary (CHO) cells in particular, have become very popular for large scale production of proteins for pharmaceutical applications. CHO-DUKX cells were the first mammalian host for a marketed recombinant protein (rtPA, tissue type plasminogen activator). This is due to a number of advantages these cells have over other mammalian substrates. A unique feature of these cells is the possibility of selecting subpopulations which, upon treatment with MTX, have within their chromosomes integrated and amplified transfected expression vector sequences at high copy numbers (2, 3). Such cell populations often produce the desired protein at high rates.

    The stability and identity of the producer CHO cell line are important issues for the manufacturer and regulatory agencies. Even though a particular recombinant cell line is cloned, subtle pressures applied by continuous growth in culture, cell handling and media manipulations may affect the stability of chromosomally integrated sequences. At the DNA level verification of the state of chromosomal integration and amplification of the transfected sequences may be made using Southern DNA blot analysis. This technique, however, provides little information about subpopulation heterogeneity and other characteristics, such as chromosomal location, number of sites and rearrangement of the amplified sequences.

The discussion of genetic stability of recombinant amplified sequences in CHO cells in the literature has been controversial. Two types of tools were used to investigate the chromosomal configuration of these sequences: a) radiolabelled probes in *in situ* hybridizations and b) cytogenetic analysis of HSRs (Homogeneously Staining Regions), unique chromosomal structures which have been shown to be the product of amplification processes (4,5). Although single copy and amplified sequences can be localized by using radio-labelled probes, autoradiographic development times are long (often weeks or months), statistical analysis is required, and the mapping precision is limited by the necessity of having to capture the emitted isotopic signal by an emulsion overlay. The other indicator of amplified sequences, HSRs, are defined as rather large, uniformly staining regions and are recognized as such only when they exceed a certain minimal length. Thus, the presence of cells containing fewer and less extended regions of amplified DNA may have been overlooked. Recently, however, several groups have reported the use of nonisotopically labeled probes in fluorescence *in situ* hybridizations (FISH) which offer high sensitivity with markedly improved speed and spatial resolution (1, 7, 8). We have used this method to study distribution, structures and statistical trends of amplified sequences in CHO cells in the presence and absence of methotrexate (9, 10).

RESULTS AND DISCUSSION

1. Non-amplified expression vector DNA in CHO chromosomes prior to selection in MTX.

DHFR expression vectors as selectable markers were used to establish two clonal cell lines, expressing moderate levels of rtPA and rCD4IgG (Immunoadhesin,11), respectively. These cell lines, which had not been exposed to MTX before, were grown in alpha modified medium (= medium lacking the components glycine, hypoxanthine and thymidine) without MTX and were analyzed using FISH. We did not find intense bands and/or large chromosomal regions showing fluorescent signal as observed in cell lines established after selection in MTX. Instead, in these non-amplified cell lines, the signal was only a single pair of yellow dots centered over specific chromo-somes. The paired spots were located over a chromosome in a way that they could represent one chromatid each. Similar pairs of hybridization spots have been shown by other authors for single copy genes in mammalian cells (6, 7).

Both these CD4IgG and the rtPA producing cell lines resulted from co-transfection procedures. The probe used hybridizes with sequences common to both plasmids. As we found only one pair of spots over a single chromosome in each cell it can be concluded that co-integration of the two plasmids occurred at the same chromosomal site in each case. We studied the productivity of the rCD4IgG expressing cell line for a period of almost 50 days and found it to be stable.

2. Co-amplification of co-transfected plasmids in cell lines selected in the presence of MTX.

Co-transfections are generally performed with a 5-10fold excess of the expression vector for the desired protein over the DHFR expression vector . Transfected DNA integrates into chromosomal host DNA, probably at random sites and most likely only into one site within the cell nucleus. As integration is a rare event (only 0.05% - 0.1% of cells which have taken up the DNA integrate part of it into the nucleus, 14), it is unlikely that the DHFR expression vector DNA would integrate at one site and the expression sequences for the protein of interest at a different site on the same or another chromosome. In the two cases studied above we did in fact observe only a single pair of hybridization signals per cell.

Amplification of transfected plasmid sequences is thought to occur in very large units of DNA - amplicons - which exceed the length of initially integrated DNA a hundred to a thousand fold (15, 16, 17). Thus, large regions of neighboring chromosomal DNA are amplified together with the integrated DNA. In some metaphases analyzed by FISH we observed hybridization patterns of tightly arranged bands separated by non-hybridizing regions, a cytogenetic reflection of this type of amplification. In another set of experiments we addressed the question of co-amplification of co-transfected DNA by using FISH with two, independently and distinctly (green/red) labelled probes, one representing the DHFR vector and the other the product of interest (c-myc). We found hybridization over identical chromosomal regions.

3. Patterns of amplified sequences in clonal cell lines in the absence of MTX.

FISH was used to determine the sites of integration of plasmid DNA in a number of clonal cell lines grown at various levels of methotrexate. Metaphase spreads were prepared after 4 subcultivations in medium lacking MTX. In all lines a unique integration pattern, usually on a single chromosome, was identified for the amplified DNA: 95-99% of cells contained the amplified DNA at identical chromosomal locations and length, intensity and location of the hybridization signal was found to be distinct for each cell line studied. The characteristics, reproducibility and intensity of these signals allowed us to use them as markers for the clonal nature of the respective cell lines. The characteristic hybridization pattern was found to be stable over extended periods of culture; the longest such period studied was 180 days without MTX.

4. MTX induced heterogeneity of amplified sequences.

Multiple chromosomal aberrations have been observed in mouse and human cells cultered in the presence of MTX (18-20). Goulian and coworkers (21) reported that the presence of MTX in cell culture results in an intracellular depletion of the thymidine pool thus leading to misincorporation of uridine triphoshate into replicating DNA. In a recent paper, using CHO cells expressing the mouse c-myc gene, we showed that continuous application of high concentrations of MTX during cell culture is associated with re-arrangement and variable amplification of transfected sequences in about 30-40% of cells (9). Several types of integration patterns were found: 1) chromosomes with highly extended regions of hybridizing sequences, 2) cells containing transfected DNA integrated into multiple sites on an individual chromosome or 3) into multiple chromosomes, 4) chromosomes joined at amplified regions, 5) circular chromosomes, 6) cells with small derivative chromosomes or fragments, 7) and cells containing a single "normal" integration characteristic for the particular cell line.

Interestingly, when the c-myc expressing CHO cells were grown for 5 to 10 subcultivations without MTX, a different picture emerged: those cells containing multiple and unusual hybridization patterns gradually decline in their abundance within the population and after 5-7 passages the majority of cells are characterized by a single "normal" integration (Fig 1a). We verified this type of population drift to occur with other, both cloned and uncloned, CHO cell lines carrying highly amplified plasmid sequences (Fig 1b). We conclude from these studies that the majority of multiple and unusual structures, found in cultures in the presence of MTX, are genetically unstable. Also, we found that these structures though unstable can contribute to the productivity of the respective cell lines. In the c-myc expressing cell line, c-myc protein immunofluorescence was 3.2 fold brighter with cells grown in the presence of MTX than in cells without MTX (9). Similar data showing short term declines in the productivity of CHO cell cultures in the absence of MTX had been seen earlier by other authors (13, 22) and have contributed to a generalized and oversimplified view that MTX is necessary for maintenance of selectivity and productivity in most recombinant CHO cell lines.

5. Stability of heterogeneous populations in the absence of MTX.

Most important for a cell culture based manufacturing process is a reproducible source of cells. To assure this a sufficiently large cell bank is established soon after choosing a producer line. In addition a certain qualified time limit will be set for subcultivation of the cells once they have been thawed from the bank (for example 100 days).

Recently in our lab heterogeneous cultures of cells producing chimeric CD4IgG proteins were derived by pooling about 300 colonies selected in alpha modiefied medium after transfection. This mixed population was subcultivated in increasing concentrations of MTX up to 250 nm. The population was then adapted to suspension culture over ten passages. Using FISH we established that this cell population was indeed heterogeneous having cells that differed both in sites and in degree of amplification within their genomes. Each metaphase contained most often one, two or more hybridization signals, but no overall regularity was found with respect to location, relative length and intensity amongst individual cells of the population. We transferred these cells into a 2 Liter round bottom glass vessel equipped for long term perfusion culture. The bioreactor configuration allowed the supply of up to 10 volumes of fresh medium per day while the same volume of spent medium could be removed from the vessel. The cells were grown in this system in the absence of MTX for more than 90 days and the various cultivation parameters were monitored and adjusted on a daily basis in order to allow maximal growth rates. If in these cell lines productivity is inversely correlated with growth rates, one would expect a gradual drift within the cell population to occur. This would eventually result in a new composition of the cell population having lower specific productivities, and perhaps, fewer copies of recombinant sequences per cell.

The following describes briefly the most important events and observations (fig 2a): During the first 30 days continually increased cell densities were observed, the peak density being 55×10^6 c/ml achieved when the perfusion rate was maintained at ~ 4.5 volumes per day (vvd). Following the first 30 days of culture several "crashes" were observed during which the cell density declined rapidly (within 1 - 3 days) to low values (3-5 mio cells/ml). These "crashes" were due to operator error, hardware failure and other influences exerted through medium composition and perfusion rates. Fortunately, the culture was recovered in all those instances. The highest population density observed was 103×10^6 viable cells/ml (73% viability) which corresponded to a packed cell volume of 38 %. This density was achieved by perfusing the culture vessel with ~6 volumes of fresh medium per day. The run was terminated on day 93 for technical reasons.

During the culture daily cell counts were taken and samples assayed for the presence of CD4IgG. The specific productivity (pg/cell day) of the cell population was calculated implementing assay results from both supernatants inside the reactor as well as spent perfusate. The result is shown in fig 2b, expressed in relative units throughout the run. Varying environmental conditions had profound effects on the productivity of the culture. The productivity of the cell culture was lowest at times when declining viabilities and loss of cell mass was observed. Higher values were achieved at times preceding peak densities which also correlated with logarithmic growth of the culture. In spite of the variability and noise one important conclusion can be drawn from these data: Regression analysis did not indicate any decline, rather a slight increase of specific productivity throughout the culture.

Using FISH we studied the distribution, extent and localization of recombinant sequences in this population of cells at the beginning and toward the end of the culture. Early and late samples taken revealed that 95-99% of cells showed at least one hybridizing signal. In addition, the overall intensities of the hybridizing signals did not change over this time course.

In conclusion, cytogenetic and production related data indicated stability of this mixed population of cells cultivated continuously for almost 100 days. As the population doubling time was calculated to be between 16 and 22 hours more than 140 cell generations occurred during this time.

SUMMARY

We have presented and discussed data concerning chromosomal integration and amplification of transfected DNA in CHO cells. We used FISH, the new and most sensitive method available for fast and reliable analysis of such sequences. We verified low copy integration into chromosomal DNA following transfection as well as the generation of cell lines with increased copy numbers of transfected DNA in cultures containing MTX. We found these amplified sequences to be subject to a biphasic behavior when cell cultures were shifted from media containing MTX to media lacking MTX. A subset of amplified sequences, most often characterized by multiple, sometimes unusual structures and often having increased length, was unstable and disappeared from cloned and uncloned cell populations within 10 to 20 days. The resulting populations of cells, containing various unique, often more modestly amplified sequences were stable. Stable specific productivities were also found, even with a heterogeneous population of cell cultivated for 93 days under competitive condition designed to select for faster growing subpopulations.

Note: Due to the inability to reproduce colored slides in this publication we were not able to show here the various examples of FISH slides taken. However, our recently published work regarding the CHO cells producing the mouse c-myc protein (9) shows such examples.

Fig 1: Distribution of integration patterns of amplified recombinant sequences in clonal (a and b) and heterogeneous (c) CHO cell lines (int/c = integration per cell, ext.int/c = extended integration per cell, int/chr. = integration per chromosome)

a) CHO cell line adapted to 320 μmolar methotrexate expressing the mouse c-myc gene

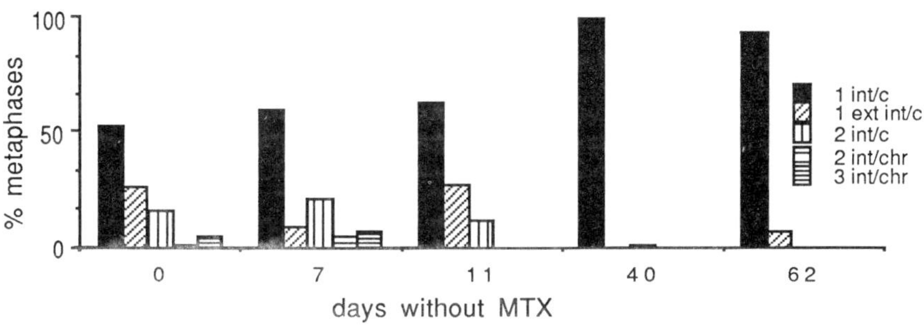

b) 2 clonal cell lines adapted to 500 nm MTX (A and B), and a heterogeneous cell line adapted to 250 nm MTX (C) expressing CD4IgG (-/+ = without and with MTX)

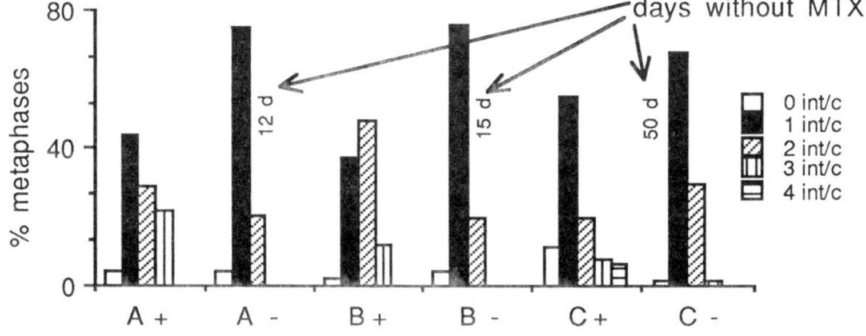

Fig 2: Perfusion cultivation of CD4IgG expressing CHO cells: a) Cell density (viable cells/ml) and perfusion rates (vvd= vessel volumes/day) b) relative specific productivities.

a)

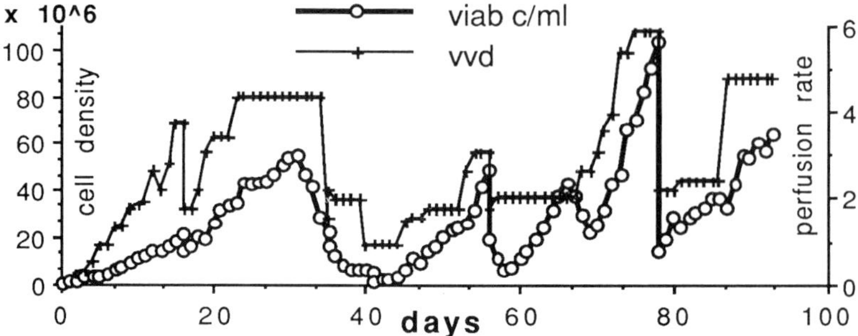

b)

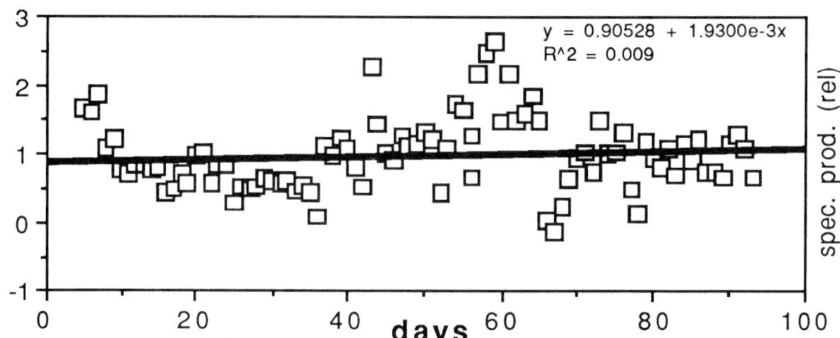

Part of this work was performed under the auspices of the U.S. Department of Energy by the Lawrence Livermore National Laboratyory under contract W-7405-ENG-48.

LITERATURE

1) Pinkel D, Straume T, and Gray J W (1986): Cytogenetic analysis using quantitative, high sensitivity fluorescence hybridization. Proc. Natl. Acad. Sci. USA 83: 2934-2938.
2) Wigler M, Perucho M, Kurtz D, Dana S, Pellicer A, Axel R, and Silverstein S (1980): Transformation of mammalian cells with an amplifiable dominant-acting gene. Proc. Natl. Acad. Sci. USA 77, 6, 3567-3570.
3) Ringold G, Dieckmann B and Lee F (1981): Co-Expression and amplification of Dihydrofolate Reductase cDNA and the Escherichia coli XGPRT gene in chinese hamster ovary cells. J. of Molecular and Applied Genetics 1, 165-175.
4) Biedler J L and Spengler B A (1976): A novel chromosome abnormality in human neuroblastoma and antifolate-resistant chinese hamster cell lines in culture. J. Natl. Cancer Inst. 57, 3, 683-689

5) Nunberg J H, Kaufman R J, Schimke R T, Urlaub G and Chasin L A (1978): Amplified dihydrofolate reductase genes are localized to a homogenously-staining region of a single chromosome in a methotrexate-resistant Chinese hamster ovary cell line. Proc. Natl. Acad. Sci. USA 75, 5553-5556.

6) Lawrence J B, Vilnave C A, and Singer R H (1988): Sensitive, high-resolution chromatin and chromosome mapping in situ: Presence and orientation of two closely integrated copies of EBV in a lymphoma line. Cell 52, 51-61

7) Lichter P, Chieh-Ju C T Call K, Hermanson G, Evans G A, Housman D and Ward D C (1990): High-resolution mapping of human chromosome 11 by in sity hybridization with cosmid clones Science 247, 64-69.

8) Lichter P, Cremer T, Chieh-Ju C T, Watkins P C, Manuelidis L. and Ward D C (1988): Rapid detection of human chromosome 21 aberrations by in sity hybridization. Proc. Natl. Acad. Sci USA 85, 9664-9668

9) Pallavicini M G, DeTeresa P S, Rosette C, Gray J W, and Wurm F M (1990): Effects of Methotrexate (MTX) on Transfected DNA Stability in Mammalian Cells. Mol. Cell. Biol.10.1, 401-404

10) Wurm F M, Gwinn K.A and Kingston R E (1986): Inducible overexpression of the mouse c-myc protein in mammalian cells. Proc. Natl. Acad. USA 83, 5414-5418

11) Capon D, Chamow S M, Mordenti J, Marsters S A, Gregory T, Mitsuya H, Byrn R A, Lucas C, Wurm F M, Groopman J E, Broder S and Smith D H (1989): Designing CD4 immnoadhesins for AIDS therapy. Nature 337, 525-531.

12) Kaufman R J and Sharp P (1982): Amplification and Expression of Sequences Cotransfected with a Modular Dihydrofolate Reductase Complementary DNA Gene. J. Mol. Biol. 159, 601-621

13) Kaufman R J, Wasley, L C, Spiliotes A J, Gossels S D, Latt S A, Larsen G R and Kay R M (1985): Coamplification and Coexpression of Human Tissue-Type Plasminogen Activator and Murine Dihydrofolate Reductase Sequences in Chinese Hamster Ovary Cells. Mol. Cell. Biol. 5,7, 1750-1759.

14) Winnacker (1987): From genes to clones. VHC Verlagsgesellschaft Weinheim, Federal Republic of Germany

15) Milbrand J D, Azizkhan J C and Hamlin J L (1983): Amplification of a cloned Chinese hamster Dihydrofolate Reductase Gene after Transfer into a Dihydrofolate Reductase-Deficient Cell Line. Mol. Cell. Biol. 3,7,1274-1282.

16) Montoya-Zavala M and Hamlin J L (1985): Similar 150-Kilobase DNA Sequences Are Amplified in Independently Derived Methotrexate Resistant Chinese Hamster Cells. Mol. Cell. Biol. 5,4, 619-627.

17) Ma C, Looney J E, Leu T-H and Hamlin J L (1988): Organization and Genesis of Dihydrofolate Reductase Amplicons in the Genome of a Methotrexate-Resistant Chinese hamster Ovary cell Line. Molec. Cell. Biol. 8,6, 2116-2317.

18) Raggetto G, Parodi S, Faggin P, and Maconi A (1979): Relationship between cytotoxicity and induction of sister-chromatid exchange in mouse foetal cells exposed to several doses of carcinogenic and non-carcinogenic chemical. Mutation research 63, 335-343.

19) Mondello C, Giorgi R and Nuzzo F(1984): Chromosomal effects of methotrexate on cultured human lymphocytes. Mutation Research 139, 67-70.

20) Vitek J A (1987): Similarity in dynamics of single and double minute chromosomes incidence and number of chromosomal aberrations during longterm treatment of a human cell line with methotrexate. Neoplasma 34, 6, 665-670

21) Goulian M, Bleile B, Tseng B Y (1980): Methotrexate-induced misincorporation of uracil into DNA. Proc. Natl. Acad. Sci. USA 77, 1956-1960

22) Weidle U H, Buckel P and Wienberg J (1988): Amplified expression constructs for human tissue-type plasminogen activator in Chinese hamster ovary cells: instability in the absence of selective pressure. Gene 66, 193-203.

Freshney: Most of the insertion and amplification sites you
             showed were chromosomal which presumably corresponded
             to HSR's within the genome.   At the longer selection
             times did you not observe the appearance of double
             minute chromosomes.

Wurm: No, never.

Freshney: Is there any evidence of the amplification of the
             endogenous DDHFR gene.

Wurm   We used the Chasin Olaf cell line which does not have
             an endogenous DHFR.

Lupker: What kind of cells do you use to make a master cell
             bank?

Wurm: The most important question concerns the productivity
             of the cell line. We make sure the cell line we store
             down is stable with respect to its productivity. There
             may be situations where the continued presence of
             methotrexate is necessary for a high level of
             expression.

Hofmann: What is the sensitivity of your detection system; can
             you see one gene copy or do you need many species?
             Also when you observe an amplified gene do you always
             get more mRNA and higher productivity.

Wurm: I have not yet verified a single copy integration but
             other people have. They are tricky and you need an
             optimised system.

             We have seen in the c-myc expressing cell line which
             was selected with high levels of methotrexate (250µm)
             that the non-master integrations do contribute to the
             productivity of those cells. In these cells the non-
             master integration accounted for one-third of the total
             productivity so we lost about one-third of the
             productivity when we reduced to the master only. But
             you should expect variation on a clone by clone basis.

Hofmann: Does your master integration take place in a particular
             chromosome or at random?

Wurm: I define a master integration as one which becomes
             dominant upon removal of methotrexate and we see
             various types of integration in both small and large
             chromosomes in short and large beads; there does not
             seem to be a rule for the master integration site.

Tolbert: You showed your master integration occurring in 50-60

days is that then stable without methotrexate for
indefinite periods of time or is there a decrease in
expression.

Wurm: We have examined the expression of cells in the absence
                of methotrexate for times of up to 180 days.

Horaud: What is the value of this method as a predictor for the
                level of expression?

Wurm: We cannot control where the DNA goes in a transfection
                and I have seen cell lines which do not seem to have
                high regions of amplified DNA which express well
                whereas others showed the opposite effect. So there is
                no general rule; you have to look at each individual
                clone.

Hentschel: When we looked at the relationship between the amount
                of DNA and expression with the glutamate synthetase
                gene we found a strict correlation between gene copy
                number and expression level. This was based on
                Southern blots on RNA and protein against standard's.
                There is a upper limit where the cell (presumably)
                can't secret more protein and the correlation fails.

                In one of your slides you showed with two dyes you get
                6 integrations when you have separate plasmids. But I
                thought I saw the two genes in separate places.

Wurm: There is some noise in the method so what you see
                outside the region I would discount as non-specific.
                I screened a lot of cells and when I found a site of
                amplification it showed that both probes had been
                integrated.

Henschel: Using the old fashioned method of Southern blotting you
                would be able to check that.

Wurm: Sure. I did not say that there was not a correlation
                between productivity and amplification within a cloned
                line. When you amplify the gene copies by going from
                50μm to 500μm methotrexate you get a correlation with
                productivity. But when you have extensive regions of
                hybridization it does not always translate into the
                maximum productivity. Another clone selected at the
                same methotrexate concentration with a short region of
                integration could have a higher productivity. It could
                be an effect of the locus of integration.

Hentschel: Position affects are well known to geneticists.

Froud: Is the site of master integration the site of initial
                integration on transfection?

Wurm: If my theory is right and you initially get only a few
          copies integrated one could assume that it could be.
          But in the selection process you could develop a sub-
          population of more stable cells which could be
          different from the original integration.

Brown: We have been increasingly concerned about the effects
          of high DHFR levels in the absence of methotrexate.
          We see some unusual patterns of serine metabolism and
          the excess DHFR might effect the change of serine to
          glycine. Do you think, therefore, that there is a
          selection of those cells which have a maximum amount of
          DHFR?

Wurm: No, we have not looked at metabolic effects.

THE STABILITY OF EXPRESSION OF HYBRIDOMA CELLS IN HOMOGENEOUS   CONTINUOUS
CULTURE SYSTEMS

C.A.M.van der Velden-de Groot, J.M.Coco Martin, D.E.Martens, J.W.Oberink,
E.C.Beuvery

Laboratory for Inactivated Viral Vaccines, National Institute for   Public
Health and Environmental Protection (RIVM), P.O.Box 1, '3720 BA Bilthoven,
The Netherlands

ABSTRACT

Several analytical techniques were applied to   obtain   information   about
stability of expression and yield and integrity of monoclonal antibodies
(Mab) produced by hybridoma cells   in   homogeneous   culture   systems.   An
immunoglobulin   specific   spot-ELISA   was   developed   to   estimate   the ratio
producing-to-non-producing cells and   the   occurance   of   isotype   switch
variants.   Flow   cytometry   (FC)   was   applied   for   determination   of
cytoplasmatic IgG content. With respect to antibody production per   cell,
data   obtained   with   spot-ELISA   and FC showed a good correlation. These
techniques proved to be worthwhile to study changes   in   productivity   of
the   hybridomas   and   integrity   of   the   Mabs   as   a   result   of culture
conditions or an extended period of culture.

INTRODUCTION

For large scale production of Mabs homogeneous continuous culture systems
are   generally applied (1, 2, 3). In such culture systems the homogeneous
environment allows a constant monitoring of the environmental conditions.
However,   to   meet   the   requirements   for   biologicals as set by control
authorities (4) special   attention   should   be   paid   to   stability   of
expression and specificity and integrity of the Mabs.
As for large scale production the cells undergo a great   number   of   cell
doublings   from   the   original   cell   bank up to the production level the
stability of the antibody production is of great   concern.   Theoretically
the   decrease   in   productivity   could   result   from a shift in the ratio
producing-to-non-producing   cells,   a   decrease   of   the   mean   antibody
production   per   cell   or   a   change   in   specificity   of the antibody as
measured in an antigen specific assay.
This   study was undertaken to develop a number of analyses, which will be
used to monitor the antibody formation in longterm homogeneous continuous
cultures.   These   analyses   include isotype ELISA, affinity ELISA and flow
cytometric analysis on cell cycle distribution,   DNA   content,   viability
and content of membrane and cytoplasmatic IgG.
In this paper data will be presented on a newly developed spot-ELISA   for
determination   of   the   ratio   producing-to-non-producing   cells   and the
incidence of   switch   variants   in   relation with   the   FC   analysis   on
cytoplasmatic   positive   cells.   Some of these data were presented at the
Symposium "From Clone to Clinic" in Amsterdam, The Netherlands (5).

MATERIALS AND METHODS

Cell lines

   Cell lines αhuIgA1/γ2b and αhuIgA1/γ1 obtained from AZU, Utrecht, The
Netherlands producing respectively mouse IgG2b and IgG1 Mabs directed
against human IgA1 were used for the spot-ELISA studies. The cells were
subcultured every second day in 150 cm^2 T-flasks (Corning Glass Works,
New York, NY, USA) in a volume of 50 ml and a cell density of 2 x 10^5
cells/ml.
   The culture medium consisted of Iscove's modified Dulbecco's medium
(Gibco Laboratories, Paisley, Scotland) supplemented with 0.25% (w/v),
Primatone RL (Sheffield Products, Norwich, NY, USA), 5% (v/v) heat
inactivated fetal bovine serum (FBS) (Flow Laboratories, Woodcock Hill,
UK) and antibiotics (35,000 U/l polymixin B, 14,000 U/l neomycin and
75,000 U/l streptomycin).
   Cell line MN12 (RIVM, Bilthoven, The Netherlands), producing IgG2a
antibodies directed against the outer membrane protein P1.16 of Neisseria
meningitidis, was cultured in a continuous culture system. This culture,
which ran for 50 days, was inoculated with 2 x 10^5 cells/ml in a 3 liter
bioreactor in the medium described above. At a cell density of about 1 x
10^6 cells/ml the medium flow through was initiated and kept at a flow
rate of 0.5 culture volume per day. The FBS concentration was gradually
reduced from 5% to 2% (v/v). The culture conditions were controled on pH:
7.3, temperature: 36.5°C, dissolved oxygen (DO): 50% air saturation and
stirrer speed: 100 rpm by means of a CF500 (Applikon Dependable
Instruments, Schiedam, The Netherlands) control unit. Cell numbers and
viability were determined by trypan blue exclusion.
   Cell line RIV6 (RIVM) producing IgG2a antibodies against the CD4
receptor on human T-lymphocytes was cultured in a continuous perfusion
system. This culture, which ran for 25 days, was inoculated with 2 x 10^5
cells/ml in a 3 liter bioreactor in Dulbecco's modified Eagle's medium
(Gibco) supplemented with 10% FBS (Bocknek, Toronto, Ont., Canada) and
antibiotics. At a cell concentration of 1 x 10^6 cells/ml the perfusion of
medium was started at a flowrate of 0.5 culture volume per day and
increased to 1 volume per day at a cell concentration of 6 x 10^6
cells/ml. During the cultivation the FBS concentration was reduced from
10 to 2.5% (v/v).

Mouse IgG isotype specific ELISA

   The materials for the mouse IgG isotype specific ELISA were as follows:
- Microtitre plates (Flow Laboratories, Woodcock Hill, UK).
- Coat: sheep anti-mouse IgG 28 μg/ml (SMuG 73, RIVM).
- Washing fluid: PBS with 0.05% Tween 20 (Merck, Darmstadt, FRG).
- Conjugate: peroxidase labeled isotype specific anti-mouse IgG (Cooper
  Biomedical, Malvern, PA, USA).
- Substrate: 300 mg 3,3',5,5'-tetramethylbenzidine (Sigma, St.Louis, MO,
  USA) in 50 ml dimethylsulfoxide.
The procedure was performed as described before (2).

Spot-ELISA

For the mouse IgG isotype specific spot-ELISA, wells of microtitre plates (Costar, Broadway, Cambridge, MA, USA) were coated for 3 hours at $37^{\circ}C$ with 30 μg/ml monoclonal rat anti-mouse kappa light chain specific antibodies (RIVM) in PBS, pH 7.3. After 3x washing with sterile PBS, a cell suspension of 750 cells/ml (100 μl per well) was added. The plates were incubated for 20 hours at $37^{\circ}C$ in a CO_2 incubator. After removal of the cells by thoroughly washing, successive incubations were performed for 1 hr at $37^{\circ}C$ with biotynilated monoclonal isotype specific rat anti-mouse IgG2b antibodies (RIVM) followed by an alkaline phosphatase-avidine (Sigma, St.Louis, MO, USA) conjugate. After the final washings enzyme substrate, 5-bromo-4-chloro-3-indolyl phosphate in 2-amino-2-methyl-1-propanol (both from Sigma, St.Louis, MO, USA) buffer was added to the wells in 0.6% agarose. The spots were either counted under a microscope (14x magnification) or analyzed by an image processing system (TIM, Difa, Breda, The Netherlands).

For the antigen specific spot-ELISA coating of the microtitre plates was performed with 50 μg/ml human IgA1 (AZU, Utrecht, The Netherlands) in PBS, pH 7.3 while respectively biotinylated goat anti-mouse total IgG, goat anti-mouse IgG2b (both from Southern Biotechnology Ass., Birmingham, AL, USA) or monoclonal isotype specific rat anti-mouse IgG2b antibodies (RIVM) were used as conjugate. The procedure was as described for the isotype specific spot-ELISA.

For the determination of isotype switch variants with the spot-ELISA mixing experiments were performed with αhuIgA1/γ2b en γ1 cells. Of the γ2b cell line 20 cells/well were added in an excess of γ1 producing cells (1 x 10^3 cells/well to 20 x 10^3 cells/well). The testprocedure was as described for the isotype specific spot-ELISA.

Determination of cytoplasmatic IgG content

Cell suspensions (10^6 cells/ml) were fixed after washing with PBS, pH 7.3 with 1 ml methanol (Merck, Darmstadt, FRG) at $-70^{\circ}C$. Fixed cells were kept at $-20^{\circ}C$ prior to analysis. After washing with PBS pH 7.3 containing 0.5% bovine serum albumin, the cells were incubated with goat anti-mouse IgG2b specific antibodies labeled with FITC (Southern Biotechnology Ass.) for 1 h at $37^{\circ}C$. After washing and resuspension in 1 ml PBS/BSA the cells were analyzed with a flow cytometer (Becton Dickinson, Mountain View, CA, USA). Dead cells, clumps and artefacts were gated out according to their forward angle and right angle scattering properties. An HP310 computer (Hewlett-Packard Corp., Pittsburgh, PA, USA) with a Consort 30 program (Becton Dickinson) was used for data processing.

RESULTS AND DISCUSSION

The first part of this study was dedicated to the development of analytical methods. For the spot-ELISA, a technique first described by Czerninsky (6) and Sedgwick (7), a comparison was made between a mouse IgG isotype specific spot-ELISA and antigen specific spot-ELISA's in which different conjugates were used.

Figure 1 shows the results of these four spot-ELISA's performed at four different passage levels (n, n + 3, n + 6, n + 9) of the αhuIgA1/γ1 cells. There appeared to be a good correlation between the IgG isotype specific and the antigen specific spot-ELISA's. Also the comparison of the spot-ELISA and the FC analysis of the cytoplasmatic IgG content (8) showed a good correlation as can be seen in Figure 2. This means that the cytoplasmatic positive cells from this cell line indeed secreted the antibodies in the culture fluid.

For the determination of the occurance of Ig isotype switch variants in a cell population mixing experiments were performed with the αhuIgA1/γ2b and αhuIgA1/γ1 cells with ratio's γ2b:γ1 from 1:50 to 1:1,000. At the same time a comparison was made between coating with antigen or subclass specific antibodies. The results of these experiments presented in Figure 3 indicate that in all experiments about 10 cells per well producing antibodies with a different isotype could be detected. As spontaneous switch variants occur at an incidence of 10^{-4} to 10^{-7}, a higher cell concentration should be used.

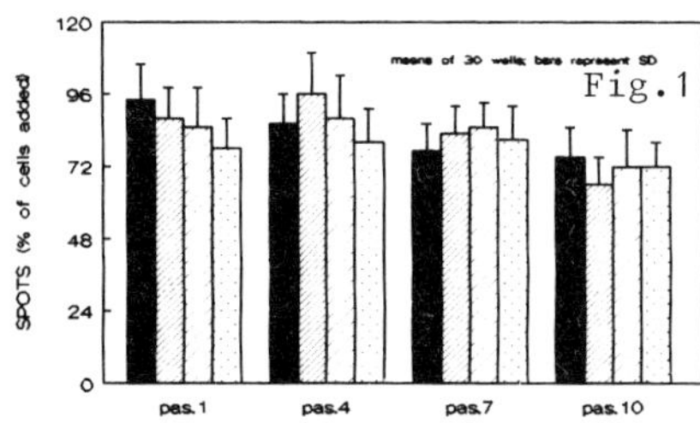
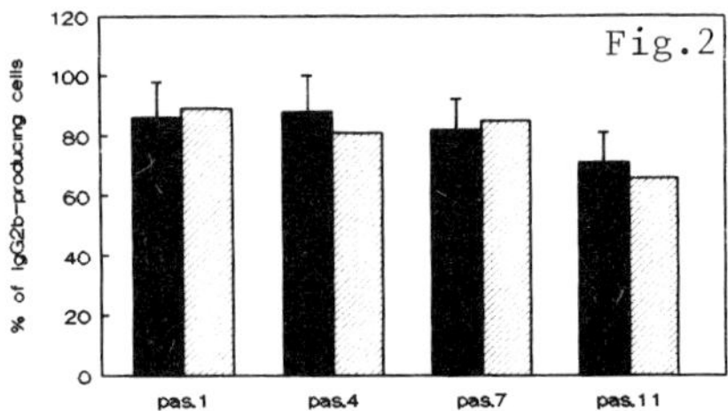

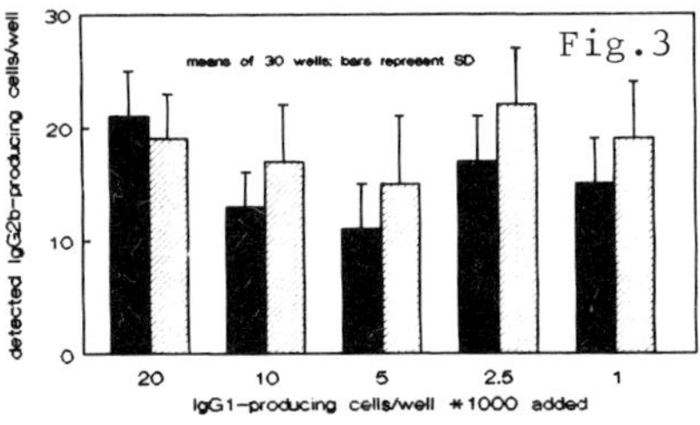

Figure 1. Comparison of four spot-ELISA systems to enumerate antibody producing cells. [■] coat isotype specific, [ ] coat antigen specific - conjugate gαm total IgG, [ ] coat antigen specific - conjugate gαm IgG2b, [ ] coat antigen specific - conjugate Mab rαm IgG2b.
Figure 2. Enumeration of antibody producing cells with spot-ELISA and FC. [■] spot-ELISA, [ ] FC.
Figure 3. Enumeration of IgG2b producing cells in an excess of IgG1 producing cells. [■] coat human IgA1, [ ] coat RαM IgG2b k.

The usefulness of the spot-ELISA and the FC analysis of cytoplasmatic positive cells was investigated by analyzing a continuous culture of MN12 cells and a continuous perfusion culture of RIV6 cells. Figure 4 shows the viable cell concentration of MN12, which reached a value of $\leq 6 \times 10^6$ cells/ml at 5% FBS and declined to 3×10^6 at 2% FBS. The viability remained about 90%. The Mab production in μg/ml reached maximum values of 120 μg/ml (Figure 5). Figure 6 shows that the percentage of antibody producing cells as determined by FC analysis was high and very stable, namely about 97% producing cells. The specific antibody production calculated as μg/10^6 viable cells and 10^6 producing cells was about 20. As the percentage of producing cells was as high as 97% these two curves are identical as can be seen in Figure 7. From these data it can be concluded that MN12 is a cell line which is very stable in antibody expression. The specificity of the antibodies was confirmed by antigen specific and anti-total IgG ELISA's which gave comparable data with the isotype specific ELISA. No change in integrity of the antibodies could be detected in isoelectric focussing (IEF) experiments (data not shown).

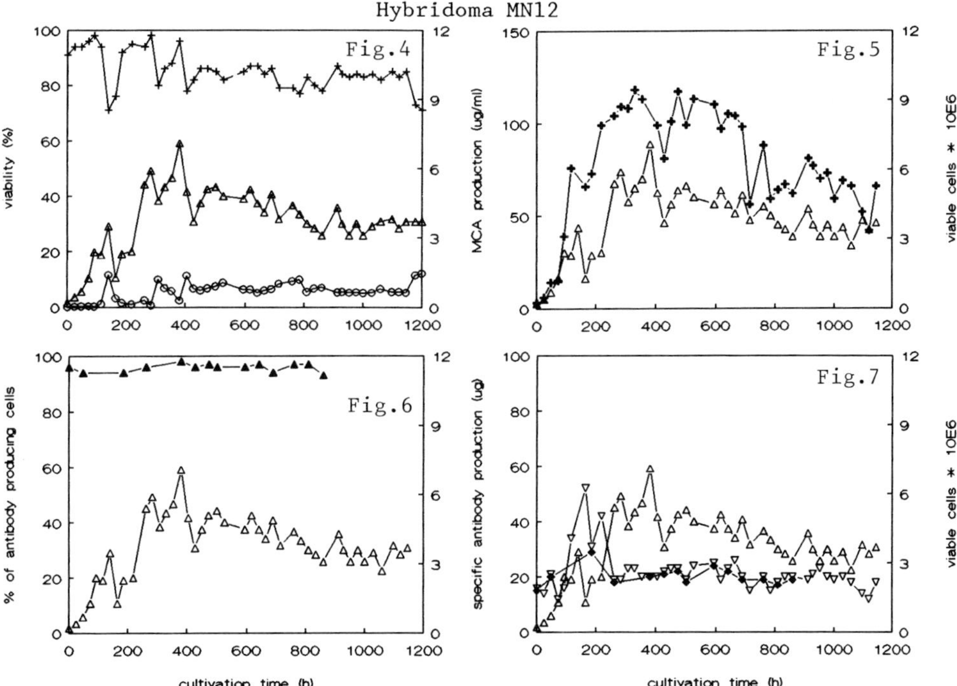

Figure 4. Growth curve and viability. Δ viable cells; o dead cells; + viability.
Figure 5. Growth curve and Mab production. Δ viable cells; + Mab.
Figure 6. Growth curve and percentage of antibody producing cells. Δ viable cells; Δ cytoplasmatic IgG positive cells.
Figure 7. Growth curve and specific antibody production. Δ viable cells; ∇ μg/10^6 viable cells; μg/10^6 producing cells (FC).

The data obtained from analyzing the continuous perfusion culture of RIV6 were, however, different. In Figure 8 it can be seen that the viable cell concentration reached values of 8 to 9 x 10^6 cells/ml with a viability of about 85%. The Mab concentration reached a value of 60 μg/ml during the logarithmic growth phase and declined rapidly to only 30 μg/ml in the steady state (Figure 9). Figure 10 shows the percentage of antibody producing cells as determined by FC analysis and spot-ELISA. Although the data from these two test-systems showed some discrepancies in number of producing cells both curves demonstrate a comparable tendency (FC, 60% → 30%, spot-ELISA, 45% → 20%). The specific productivity calculated on the basis of viable cells declined from 10 to 5 μg/ml (Figure 11) while the curve calculated on the basis of producing cells (FC analysis) was rather stable (≤ 15 μg/ml).

These results clearly indicate that no steady state of antibody production was realized and that the non-producing cells overgrew the producing ones. Our findings are confirmed by data from literature (10). The discrepancy between data from FC analysis and spot-ELISA suggests that a fraction of the cytoplasmatic IgG positive cells did not secrete antibodies. The conclusion of these experiments is that cell line RIV6, even after several clonings, is unsuitable as cell line for large scale production due to instability of expression.

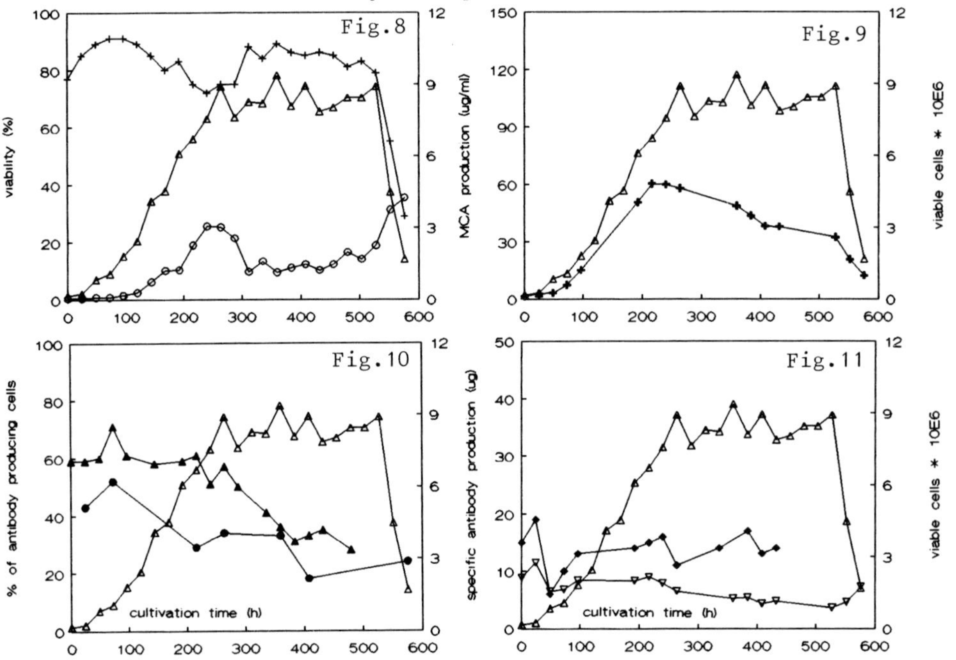

Figure 8. Growth curve and viability. Δ viable cells; o dead cells; + viability.

Figure 9. Growth curve and Mab production. Δ viable cells; + Mab.

Figure 10. Growth curve and percentage of antibody producing cells. Δ viable cells; Δ cytoplasmatic IgG positive cells; o spot-ELISA.

Figure 11. Growth curve and specific production. Δ viable cells; ▽ μg/10^6 viable cells; μg/10^6 producing cells (FC).

CONCLUSION

The results of this study indicate that the analytical methods presented (spot-ELISA and FC analysis of cytoplasmatic IgG positive cells) together with analysis of specificity (ELISA) and integrity (IEF) are suitable methods not only to follow a longterm cultivation of hybridoma cells, but also to establish whether specific cell lines meet the requirements for production purposes.
These techniques will allow us further to investigate the influence of culture conditions on yield, stability and integrity of antibody production.

REFERENCES

1. Van Wezel, A.L., van der Velden-de Groot, C.A.M., de Haan, H.H., van den Heuvel, N. and Schasfoort, R. Large scale animal cell cultivation for production of cellular biologicals. _Dev. Biol. Stand._ 1985, _60_, 229-236.
2. Van der Velden-de Groot, C.A.M., Witterland, W., Beuvery, E.C. and van Wezel, A.L. Evaluation of the continuous perfusion culture system for the production of monoclonal antibodies. _Modern Approaches to Animal Cell Technology_. Spier, R.E. & Griffiths, J.B. (eds), Butterworth & Co. Ltd., pp.513-518.
3. Van der Velden-de Groot, C.A.M., Coco Martin, J.M. and Beuvery, E.C. New developments in the cultivation of hybridoma cells in homogeneous continuous perfusion systems. _Dev. Biol. Stand._ 1990, _71_, 45-54.
4. Ad hoc Working Party on Biotechnology/Pharmacy. Notes to applicants for marketing authorizations on the production and quality control of monoclonal antibodies of murine origin intended for use in man. _J. Biol. Standard._ 1989, _17_, 213-222.
5. Coco Martin, J.M., Martens, D.E., Oberink, J.W., van der Velden-de Groot, C.A.M. and Beuvery, E.C. Development of analytical methods for monitoring the stability of antibody formation by hybridomas in continuous culture systems. _Biotherapy_, in press.
6. Czerkinsky, C.C., Nilsson, L.A., Nygren, H., Ouchterlony, O. and Tarkowski, A. A solid phase enzyme-linked immunospot (Elispot) assay for enumeration of specific antibody secreting cells. _Immunol. Methods_ 1983, _65_, 109.
7. Sedgwick, J.D. and Holt, P.G. A solid-phase immunoenzymatic technique for the enumeration of specific antibody secreting cells. _J. Immunol. Methods_ 1983, _57_, 301-309.
8. Jacobberger, J.W., Fogleman, D. and Lehman, J.M. Analysis of intracellular antigens by flow cytometry. _Cytometry_ 1986, _7_, 356-364.
9. Martens, D.E., Coco Martin, J.M., van der Velden-de Groot, C.A.M., Beuvery, E.C., de Gooijer, C.D. and Tramper, J. To an optimal design of an airlift bioreactor for the cultivation of hybridomas. _Biotherapy_, in press.
10. Frame, K.K. and Hu, W.S. The loss of antibody productivity in continuous culture of hybridoma cells. _Biotechnol. Bioeng._ 1990, _35_, 469-476.

<u>Paper of van der Gelden de Groot</u>

Bethold:

You showed data from 2 cell lines in one of which the productivity decreased. What do you do from the point of view of product in a long term run; have you continued to generate useful product.

Van der Gelden
de Groot:

We produced this cell line as a pilot scale run but if you look at the EEC requirements you should not use the product even though the product was very stable and the interpreting was good but from a production point of view it would not be useful.

Bethold:

Would you redo your process with another cell line.

Van der Gelden
de Groot:

Yes; with this cell line which we had recloned several times before we started because the production level was low; it is not a good cell line to go on with. I would search for a different cell line with better properties from a production point of view.

CLONING AND EXPRESSION OF A BOVINE ANTI-TESTOSTERONE MONOCLONAL ANTIBODY

T. Jackson, B.A. Morris# and P.G. Sanders*

Molecular Biology Group, Microbiology Department and #Heterohybridoma Antibody Group, Biochemistry Department, University of Surrey, Guildford, GU2 5XH, U.K. *Corresponding author.

ABSTRACT

We have cloned heavy and light chain cDNAs for a bovine monoclonal antibody to testosterone. Expression of the cDNAs in Cos-1 cells resulted in the production of functional antibody which binds testosterone.

INTRODUCTION

As part of a research programme to investigate the role of steroid hormones in the reproductive cycle we have developed Mouse-Bovine and Mouse-Ovine heterohybridomas which secrete specific Bovine and Ovine monoclonal antibodies to Testosterone (1). These monoclonal antibodies can now be used to replace polyclonal antibodies to immunomodulate the negative feedback effects of Testosterone on the secretion of gonadotrophins which control both follicle maturation and ovulation (2).

The work presented here is aimed at defining the molecular basis of the binding between one of our Bovine antibodies to Testosterone, and subsequently using this information to improve the immunomodulatory properties of these antibodies. This will involve a combination of computer aided molecular modelling and site directed mutagenesis.

The data will also further our understanding of the molecular requirements for production of high affinity antibodies and will allow the construction of interspecies chimaeric and bovinised antibodies of veterinary importance.

METHODS

Gene cloning and manipulation were carried out according to Maniatis et al (3). DNA sequencing was based on the method of Sanger et al (4), Cos cell transfection by the method of Cullen (5) and Elisa assays as in Groves et al (1).

RESULTS

cDNA cloning and analysis of clones.

A cDNA library was constructed using mRNA extracted from a (mouse-bovine) x bovine heterohybridoma (1), secreting a monoclonal antibody to testosterone. Screening this library with mouse immunoglobulin heavy

and light chain DNA probes and a bovine lambda light chain probe
identified putative clones for bovine heavy and light chain cDNAs.

One putative Immunoglobulin heavy chain clone, clone 8, was sequenced
and translation confirmed that it coded for a protein similar in amino
acid sequence to the partial protein data published for bovine IgG1 (6).
This clone ws not full length and a second oligonucleotide primed library
was produced to clone the missing 5' terminal sequences.

33 putative light chain cDNA clones were identified using a bovine
lambda light chain probe (7) and sequencing of one confirmed that it
contained an immunoglobulin light chain cDNA.

Expression of recombinant antibody.

The heavy and light chain cDNAs were manipulated for expression in a
eukaryotic expression vector (pEE6 gpt) under the control of the HCMV
promoter, Figure 1. Cos-1 cells were co-transfected with heavy and light
chain expression vectors and supernatant samples collected at 70 hr post
transfection. The presence of functional anti-testosterone antibody was
determined using an ELISA specific for bovine IgG1 (1), Figure 2.

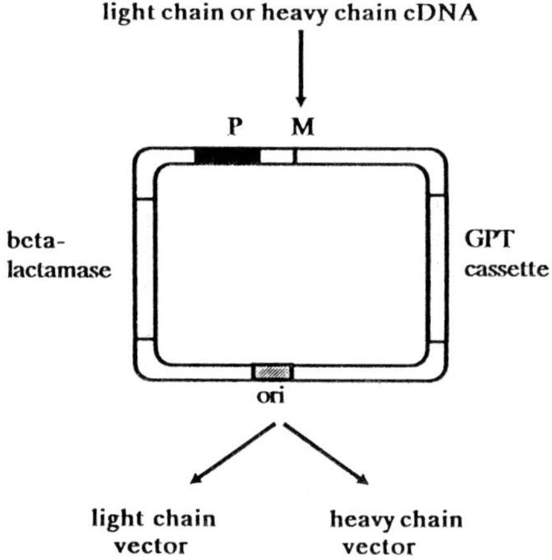

FIGURE 1.   Heavy and light chain expression vectors.

DISCUSSION

cDNAs for a bovine monoclonal antibody to testosterone have been cloned
and expressed to produce recombinant anti-testosterone antibody in animal
cells.

We are now using this antibody to define, by computer aided molecular
modelling and site directed mutagenesis, the determinants of its
specificity and affinity in order to develop techniques to design
recombinant antibodies of defined specificity and affinity.

ACKNOWLEDGEMENTS

T. Jackson was supported by a MAFF studentship. We thank Celltech for
the vector pEE6gpt, M. Neuberger for mouse immunoglobulin probes,

V.N.Ivanov for the bovine lambda probe and W. Shaffner for the HCMV promoter.

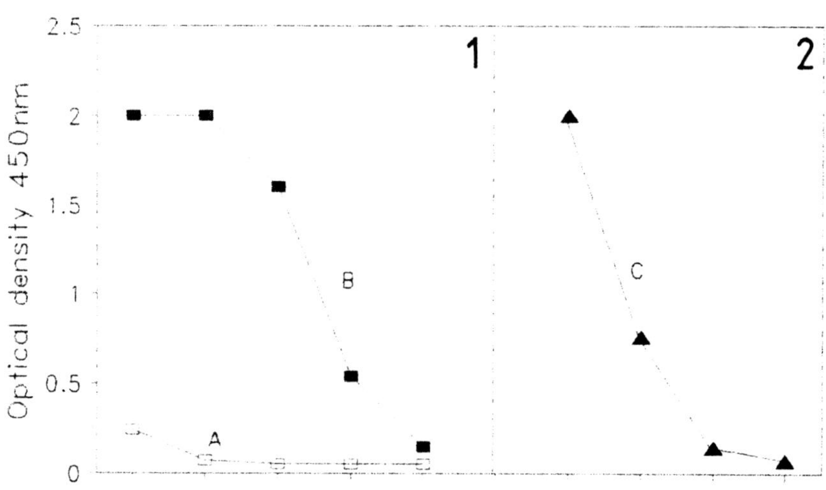

FIGURE 2. Box 1: A; control, B; Cos cell produced antibody. The dilutions are from Neat in 5-fold dilutions to 1:625.
Box 2; C, Hybridoma produced anti-testosterone antibody. The dilutions are tenfold from 10^{-2} to 10^{-5} of culture supernatant.

REFERENCES

1   Groves,D.J., Morris,B.A. and Clayton,J. (1987). Res. Vet. Sci. 43:253-256.

2   Webb,R., Land,R.B., Pathiraja,N. and Morris,B.A. (1984). In "Immunological aspects of reproduction in mammals", Ed. D.B.Crighton, pp475-499, Butterworths, London.

3   Maniatis,T., Fritsch,E.F. and SambrookJ. (1982) Molecular cloning: A laboratory manual. Cold Spring Harbor, New York.

4   Sanger,F., Nicklen,S. and Coulsen,A.R. (1977). Proc. Natl. Acad.SCi. USA. 74:5463-5467.

5   Cullen,B.R. (1987). In "Methods in enzymology:Guide to molecular cloning. Eds. S.L.Berger and A.R.Kimmel, pp 684-704, Academic Press, San Diego.

6   Milstein,C.P. and Feinstein,A.(1968). Biochem. J. 107:559-564.

7   Ivanov,V,N. Karginov,V.A., Morozov,I.V., Gorodetsky,S.I. (1988). Gene 67:41-48.

USE OF DICISTRONIC TRANSCRIPTION UNITS FOR THE CORRELATED EXPRESSION OF TWO GENES IN MAMMALIAN CELLS

Manfred Wirth, Lorin Schumacher and Hansjörg Hauser

GBF, Gesellschaft für Biotechnologische Forschung mbH, Department of Genetics and Cell Biology, D-3300 Braunschweig, FRG

ABSTRACT

Expression vectors were constructed in which translation of inserted genes occurs from dicistronic mRNAs. The first cistron could encode the cDNA for a secreted glycoprotein, the second cistron a detector gene from which expression can easily be monitored. Expression of two cistrons in stably transfected cells was compared to the respective monocistronic constructs and the influence of the nature of the intercistronic region (IR) on expression efficiency was examined. The translation of the second cistron is clearly dependent on the type of the intercistronic region. The polio virus leader allows efficient expression of the second cistron with unaltered expression from the first cistron. Expression of the first and second cistron are linked as demonstrated by the expression values found in isolated subclones. The use of these vectors should allow the expression of two different peptide chains in a correlated fashion.

KEYWORDS

Gene expression, translation, dicistronic mRNA, transfection, screening system, luciferase

INTRODUCTION

Investigations of Peabody and Berg[1,2] and the contributions of M. Kozak[3,4] showed that translation from dicistronic transcription units in mammalian cells is possible, albeit the translation of the second cistron is influenced by structural constraints of the intercistronic region in a manner different from that in bacteria. Usually, translation from cistrons preceeded by a protein encoding reading frame is comparably inefficient. The use of dicistronic vectors for isolation of high-yield expressing animal and plant cell clones has been demonstrated[5,6]. These expression plasmids show a common structure in which the first cistron represents the gene of interest and the second cistron is a selectable marker. Due to inefficient translation of the second cistron transfection efficiency with these plasmids is low. It is to be regretted that long term stability of cell clones or the ratio of deleted to intact vectors were only partially subject of investigation in these publications.

Here we present a new type of dicistronic vector for high-yield expression in mammalian cells and show coexpression of both cistrons in transfected animal cells. While the first cistron consists of the gene of interest, the second harbors a marker that can be easily screened for.

MATERIALS AND METHODS

Cell lines and bacterial strains

Plasmids were transformed into either E. coli DH1 or DH5 alpha cells by the Hanahan procedure[7]. BHK (ATCC CCL10) cells were grown in DME-medium supplemented with antibiotics and 10% fetal calf serum.

Plasmid construction

pSVIFNLUC was constructed by ligation of a cDNA fragment encoding the reading frame of the human IFN-ß gene into pLUCIL2, which contains the firefly luciferase cDNA preceeded by the 5'NTR of the human IL2-gene under control of the SV40 early promoter region. pSVIFN was created by elimination of the luciferase cDNA fragment from pSVIFNLUC. POLIO1 and 2 resulted from ligation of the 630bp MseI/BalI fragment (containing the polio type 1a 5'NTR) of pGEM3-5'Polio[8] and pSVIFNLUC after linearization with BglII.

Gene transfer

Transfections were performed by the calcium phosphate coprecipitation method by cotransfer of the respective expression plasmids and the pSV2PAC selection plasmid[9] as described[10]. Puromycin (5 μg/ml for BHK cells) was applied two days after transfection. Arising clones were counted after 8-14 days and pooled.

Detection of expressed genes

The amount of secreted human IFN-ß was determined by a specific virus protection assay[11]. For detection of luciferase activity the transfected cells were lysed by three cycles of freezing and thawing in a phospate buffer followed by the bioluminescent reaction essentially as described[12] and quantification of emitted light in a Berthold bioluminat.

RESULTS AND DISCUSSION

We have designed plasmids for expression of dicistronic mRNA. The first cistron contains the cDNA for a secreted human glycoprotein, here interferon ß. The second cistron harbors the cDNA of the firefly luciferase (Fig. 1). Expression can easily be monitored by a simple and sensitive bioluminescent assay. The luciferase gene is preceeded by the 5'-nontranslated leader of IL2-cDNA leading to an intercistronic region of 60 bp devoid of interfering AUG's. According to Kozak should such longer IR's should allow efficient translation from the second cistron.

To investigate the level of expression from the dicistronic construct
plasmids pSV-IFN-LUC and their monocistronic counterparts were stably
transfected into BHK cells. Pools of stable transfectants were tested
for expression of both cistrons (Fig. 1). Translation of the second
cistron was lower if compared to the respective monocistronic

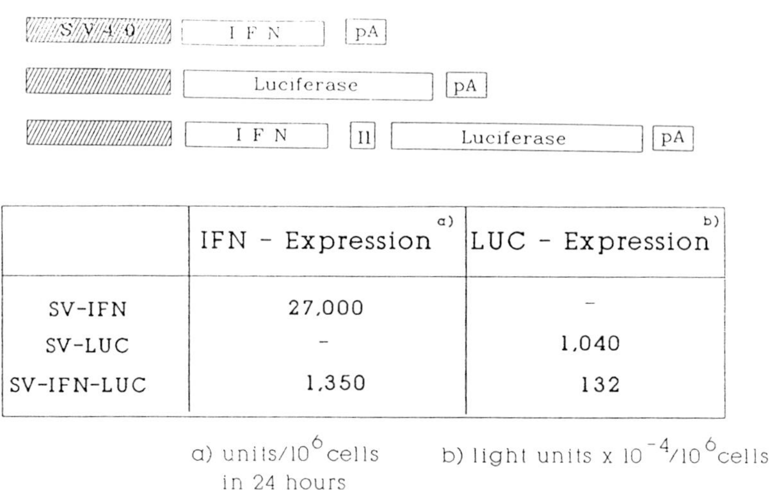

	IFN – Expression [a)	LUC – Expression [b)
SV-IFN	27,000	–
SV-LUC	–	1,040
SV-IFN-LUC	1,350	132

a) units/10^6 cells   b) light units x 10^{-4}/10^6 cells
in 24 hours

Figure 1   Expression from mono- and dicistronic transcription units.
IFN-ß and luciferase expression were determined from BHK cells stably
transfected with the indicated mono- or dicistronic expression
plasmids. Transcription is controlled by the SV40 early
promoter/enhancer (SV40) and is terminated by the polyadenylation
signal of the luciferase cDNA (pA). The intercistronic region of pSV-
IFN-LUC contains the 60 bp human IL-2 5'nontranslated region (IL).

constructs. This could be due to the structure of the intercistronic
region which is nonoptimal with respect to reinitiation of translation
at the second cistron[3]. However, expression from cistron 1 is also
reduced. A reason for this relies in the steady state level of specific
RNA in cells transfected with the dicistronic constructs which is low
compared to the monocistronic (data not shown).

To investigate coordinate expression of both cistrons we isolated
subclones. Expression values of both interferon and luciferase from
isolated subclones roughly correlate (Fig. 2). Exceptions may be due to
rearrangements of the plasmid following transfection. This correlation
allows the application of such constructs for screening expression of
the first cistron by monitoring the second. The method enables an
rapid screening of a large number of transfectants. This is
particularly of interest when simple detection methods for the protein
of interest are not available.

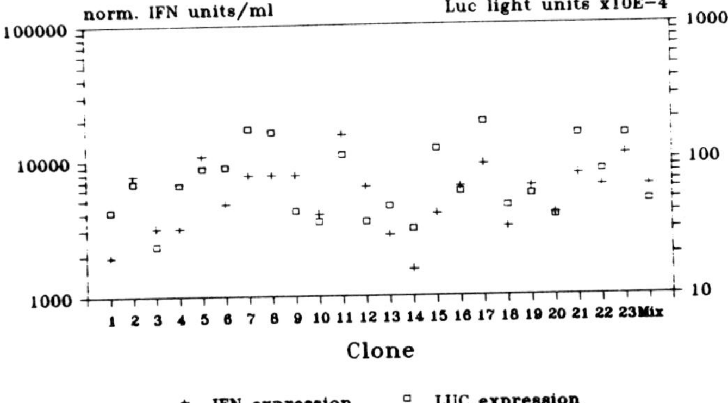

Figure 2   Correlation of expression in isolated subclones from cells transfected with the dicistronic plasmid pSV-IFN-LUC.

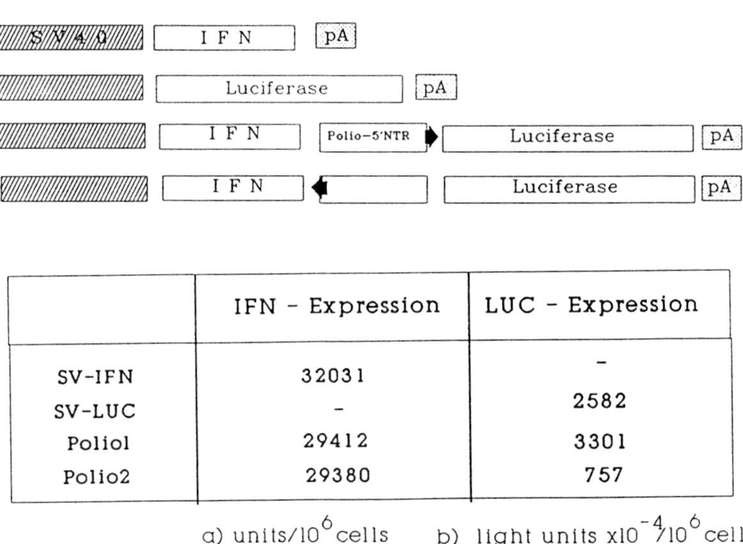

	IFN – Expression	LUC – Expression
SV-IFN	32031	–
SV-LUC	–	2582
Polio1	29412	3301
Polio2	29380	757

a) units/10^6 cells in 24 hours   b) light units x10^{-4}/10^6 cells

Figure 3   Equimolar expression of dicistronic transcription units by independent initiation of translation from the second cistron. Comparison of expression of IFN-ß and luciferase in BHK cells stably transfected with mono- and dicistronic expression plasmids.

Equimolar expression of both cistrons is optional if dicistronic expression vectors are used for expression of proteins that are composed of two subunits. Each subunit would be simultaneously synthesized in equal amounts in a spatial arrangement that favorates association. To address this approach we have constructed a plasmid in which the intercistronic region contains the 5'nontranslated leader (NTR) of poliovirus. This leader is known to mediate cap-independent, internal initiation of translation of mRNAs presumably by binding of ribosome subunits to a defined region of the 730 bp NTR[13,14]. Results are shown in Fig. 3. The data clearly demonstrate equimolar expression of both cistrons.

In conclusion we believe that it is possible to express different peptide chains from dicistronic expression vectors at desired ratios whereby expression of the second cistron is mainly dependent on the intercistronic sequence. Low expression of the second cistron facilitates screening for high-producer cell lines, whereas equimolar expression from both cistrons allow simultaneous synthesis. However, the fusion of different sequences in dicistronic constructs leads to unpredictable new half-life-times or translatabilities of the resulting mRNAs.

ACKNOWLEDGEMENT

We cordially thank Dr. Peter Sarnow for supply with pGEM3-5'Polio.

REFERENCES

1   Peabody, D. S. Termination-reinitiation occurs in the translation of mammalian cell mRNAs. <u>Mol. Cell. Biol.</u> 1986, <u>6</u>, 2695

2   Peabody, D.S., Subramani, S., Berg, P. Effect of upstream reading frames on translation efficiency in Simian virus 40 recombinants. <u>Mol. Cell. Biol.</u> 1986, <u>6</u>, 2704

3   Kozak, M. Effects of intercistronic length on the efficiency of reinitiation by eucaryotic ribosomes. <u>Mol. Cell. Biol.</u> 1987, <u>7</u>, 3438

4   Kozak, M. The scanning model for translation: an update. <u>J. Cell. Biol.</u> 1989, <u>108</u>, 229

5   Kaufman, R.J., Murtha, P.P., Davies. M.V. Translational efficiency of polycistronic mRNAs and their utilization to express heterologous genes in mammalian cells. <u>EMBO J.</u> 1987, <u>6</u>, 187

6   Balland, A., Faure, T. Carvallo, D., Cordier, P., Ulrich, P. Fournet, B., De la Salle, H., Lecocq, J.P. Characterisation of two differently processed forms of human recombinant factor IX synthesised in CHO cells transformed with a polycistronic vector.

7   Hanahan, D. Studies on transformation of Escherichia coli with plasmids. <u>J. Mol. Biol.</u> 1983, <u>166</u>, 557

8   Sarnow, P. Role of 3énd sequences in infectivity of Poliovirus transcripts made in vitro. <u>J. Viol.</u> 1989, <u>63</u>, 467

9   Vara, J., Protela, A., Ortin, J. Jimenez, A. Expression in mammalian cells of a gene from Streptomyces alboniger conferring puromycin resistance. <u>Nucl. Acids Res.</u> 1986, <u>14</u>, 4617

10   Wirth, M., Bode, J. Zettlmeißl, G, Hauser, H. Isolation of overproducing recombinant mammalian cell lines by a fast and simple selection procedure. <u>Gene</u> 1988, <u>73</u>, 419

11   Finter, N.B. Dye-uptake methods for assessing viral cytopathogenicity and their application to interferon assays.<u>J. Gen. Virol.</u> 1969, <u>5</u>, 419.

12   De Wet, J.R., Wood, K.V., DeLuca, M., Helinski, D.R., Subramani, S. Firefly luciferase gene: Structure and expression in mammalian cells. <u>Mol. Cell. Biol.</u> 1987, <u>7</u>, 725.

13   Pelletier, J., Sonenberg, N. Internal initiation of translation of eukaryotic mRNA directed by a sequence derived from polyovirus RNA. <u>Nature</u> 1988, <u>334</u>, 320

14   Meerovitch, K., Pelletier, J., Sonenberg, N. A cellular protein that binds to the 5'noncoding region of poliovirus RNA: Implications for internal translation initiation. <u>Genes Dev.</u> 1989, <u>3</u>, 1026

Pietri: How did you select the cell clones you investigated for luciferin and interleukin production.

Wirth: We co-transfected with puramycin resistance gene.

LARGE-SCALE RECOMBINANT PROTEIN PRODUCTION USING THE INSECT CELL-BACULOVIRUS EXPRESSION VECTOR SYSTEM: ANTISTASIN AND β-ADRENERGIC RECEPTOR.

D. Jain*, K. Ramasubramanyan†, S. Gould*, A. Lenny*, M. Candelore*, M. Tota*, C. Strader*, K. Alves*, G. Cuca*, J. S. Tung*, G. Hunt*, B. Junker*, B.C. Buckland* and M. Silberklang*.

* Merck Sharp and Dohme Research Laboratories, P.O. Box 2000, Rahway, N.J. 07065.

† Department of Chemical and Biochemical Engineering, Rutgers, The State University of New Jersey, PO Box 909, Piscataway, NJ 08855.

ABSTRACT

We have used the recombinant baculovirus expression vector system, based on *Autographa californica* Nuclear Polyhedrosis Virus (AcMNPV) grown in *Spodoptera frugiperda* (Sf9) insect cells, to produce three proteins: antistasin, half-antistasin, and β-adrenergic receptor. Sf9 cell growth and baculovirus infection processes were developed in gassed spinner flasks and stirred tanks (1-40 liter scale). Both serum-containing and serum-free media were evaluated. Cell growth and product accumulation were found to be adversely affected by too low (below 20% air saturation) or too high (over 100%) a level of dissolved oxygen. The post-infection increases in modal cell diameter and percent cell death were identified as useful indicators of optimum harvest time. In the case of antistasin, productivity was improved by optimizing cell density at infection, multiplicity of infection, dissolved oxygen level and harvest time. In the case of β-adrenergic receptor, protein yield was further enhanced by the addition of protease inhibitors late in the infection cycle.

Antistasin, Half-antistasin, β-adrenergic receptor, insect cell culture, recombinant protein, baculovirus, fermentation, large-scale, serum-free, protease inhibitors.

INTRODUCTION

Antistasin (ANS) is a 15 kDa anticoagulant protein found in the salivary glands of the Mexican leech *Haementaria officinalis* (1,2) which acts as a stoichiometric inhibitor of Factor Xa (3); it also exhibits antimetastatic activity in a mouse model system (3,4). ANS has no homology to Hirudin (5), another leech (*Hirudo medicinalis*) derived anticoagulant. Mature ANS has 119 amino acid residues, has no N-linked glycosylation sites and has a 17% cysteine content. There is a significant two-fold homology between the N- and C- terminal halves, with the active site residing in the N–terminal half (6). ANS purified from natural leech populations contains multiple primary sequence variants (6), two of which have been cloned and expressed in the insect baculovirus expression vector system (7). A truncated gene expressing a portion of one variant, called half-antistasin (H-ANS, J.S. Tung et. al., manuscript in preparation) has also been expressed.

β-adrenergic receptor (BAR) is a membrane glycoprotein receptor which is coupled to the G-protein Gs (8). The non-glycosylated receptor has a molecular weight of 47 kDa. Signal transduction in response to β-adrenergic agonists involves cyclic AMP production. The cloned Hamster BAR gene (9) was expressed in the baculovirus system (M. Silberklang et. al., manuscript in preparation).

In this paper we present studies on the production of ANS, H-ANS and BAR in batch suspension culture under different culture conditions.

MATERIALS AND METHODS

Cell Growth

Sf9 cells, a clonal derivative of a pupal ovary line from the Fall Army Worm, *Spodopetra frugiperda*, were obtained from the ATCC (#CRL 1711). IPL-41 basal medium (J.R. Scientific, Woodland, CA) supplemented with 2% heat-inactivated Fetal Bovine Serum (FBS, Gibco, Grand Island, NY) and 3.3 g/l each of yeastolate and lactalbumin hydrolysate (Difco, Detroit, MI) and Excell-400, a serum-free medium from J.R. Scientific were used for cell culture. Suspension cultures were supplemented with 1.0-2.0 g/l Pluronic F-68 (BASF Corporation, Parsippany, NJ). Microcarrier-type spinner flasks, 100-8000 ml (Bellco Glass, Vineland, NJ) were maintained on magnetic stir plates (Barnstead/ Thermolyne, Dubuque, Iowa) at 50-60 rpm. An 8-l "Biostat E" fermenter from B. Braun Biotech (Bethlehem, PA) utilizing a bubble-free silicone tube gassing system, an 18-l Sulzer-MBR (Woodbury, NY) "Spinferm" using a 2 μm stainless steel microsparger for direct sparging of air and oxygen and a 70-l fermenter from Chemap (S. Plainfield, NJ) equipped with hydrofoil impellers and an open pipe (5mm diameter) sparger for direct sparging of oxygen were used for larger scale processes.

Viral stock and protein production

Recombinant *Autographa californica* nuclear polyhedrosis virus (AcMNPV) clones containing the gene for either ANS, H-ANS or BAR were generated by standard procedures (10). Viral stocks were made by growing Sf9 cells in spinner flasks in Hink's TNMFH medium with 10% FBS (8; Gibco, Grand Island, NY) and infecting them with the appropriate recombinant AcMNPV at an MOI of 0.1. Viral titer was obtained by end-point dilution (10). ANS, H-ANS and BAR were produced in both large (up to 5-l working volume) gassed spinner flasks and fermenters (described above). Cells were grown to a density of 1.0-2.0 x10^6 cells/ml and infected with virus. The culture was harvested 24-36 hr after the modal cell diameter peaked or when the cell viability dropped to 50%.

Assay Methods

ANS and H-ANS activity was measured by a colorimetric Factor Xa inhibition assay using a commercial (Helena Laboratories, Beaumont, Texas) Factor Xa assay kit. The assay was performed in a 96-well micro-titer plate with a Bio-Rad (Richmond, CA) kinetic microplate reader. BAR was assayed and protein immunoblotting was performed on cell lysates as previously described (11); immunoblotting was done with an anti-peptide antibody specific for the C-terminal tail of the hamster BAR, followed by ^{125}I-Protein A. The protease inhibitors used were aprotinin 2 mg/l, soyabean trypsin inhibitor 5 mg/l, and leupeptin 3 mg/l. Viability counts were made by a trypan-blue (0.4% in 0.85% saline, Gibco) dye exclusion method using a haemacytometer. Modal cell diameter was determined with a Coulter Counter (Hialeah, FL) Model ZBI outfitted with a channeliser. On-line dissolved oxygen (DO) measurements were made with a polarographic DO probe from Ingold (Wilmington, MA).

RESULTS

Figure 1 compares cell growth in head-space gassed spinner flasks in IPL-41 medium containing 2% FBS as compared to Excell-400 medium. It is evident that cell growth rates are similiar in the two media.

Growth of cells in IPL-41 basal medium with 2% FBS was earlier found to be similiar in a head-space gassed spinner flask, silicone tube gassed fermenter and a microsparged fermenter (14). Cell growth in Excell-400 medium was scaled-up from a 500 ml head-space gassed spinner flask to the18-l microsparged fermenter and to a 70-l Chemap (open pipe sparger) pilot-scale fermenter (Figure 2). Figure 2 shows that cells grow similarily in the three systems; there is a lag in the spinner flask growth because of a lower seeding density.

In our early experiments with ANS variant 1, yield was found to be highest when the multiplicity of infection (MOI) was less than 1.0 (unpublished observation). However,

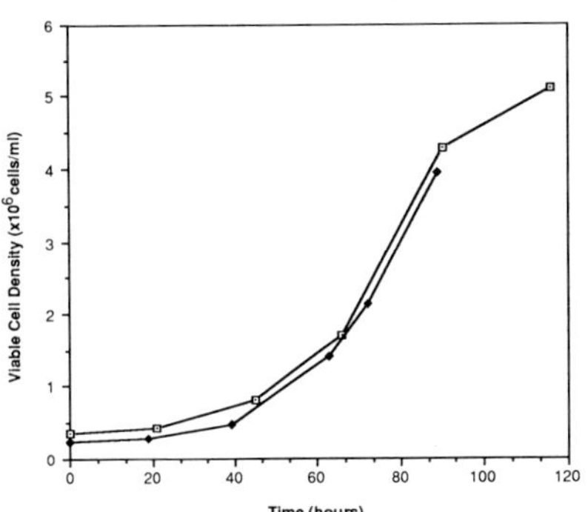

Figure 1. Cell growth in serum-containing (IPL41+2% FBS) (□) and serum-free (Excell-400) (◆) medium.

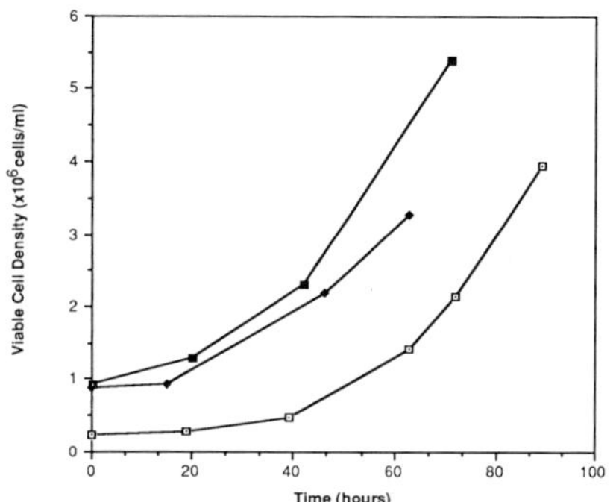

Figure 2. Cell growth in serum-free Excell-400 medium in 18-l microsparged (■), 70-l direct spraged (◆) and head-space gassed spinner flask (□).

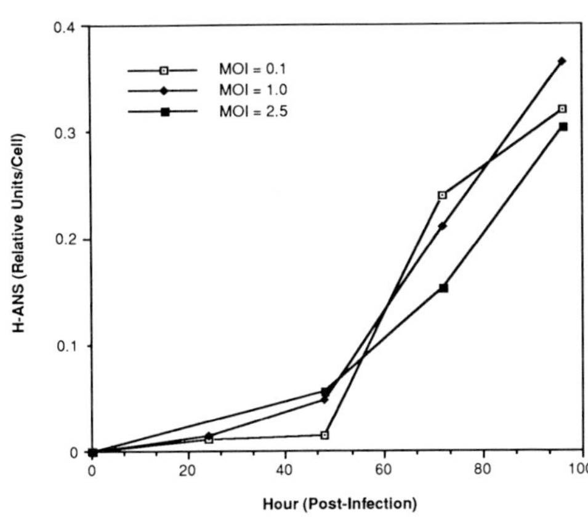

Figure 3. Effect of MOI on H-ANS production.

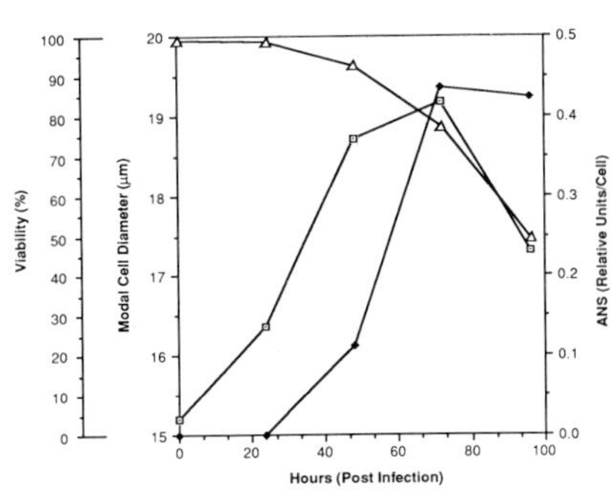

Figure 4. Modal cell diameter (□) and viability (Δ) during production of ANS (◆).

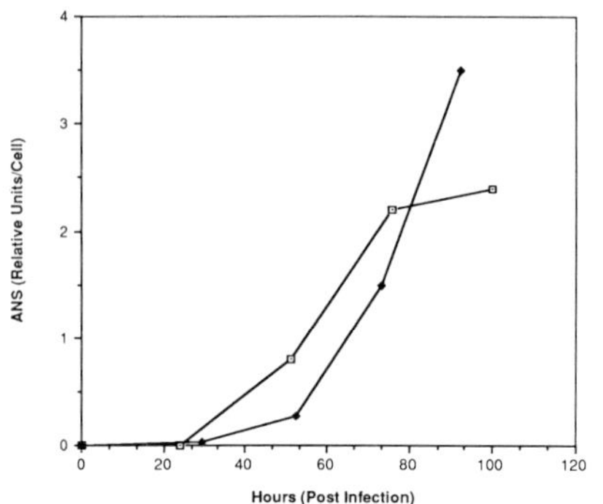

Figure 5. ANS production at the 18-1 (□) and 70-1 (♦) scale fermenters in serum-free Excell-400 medium.

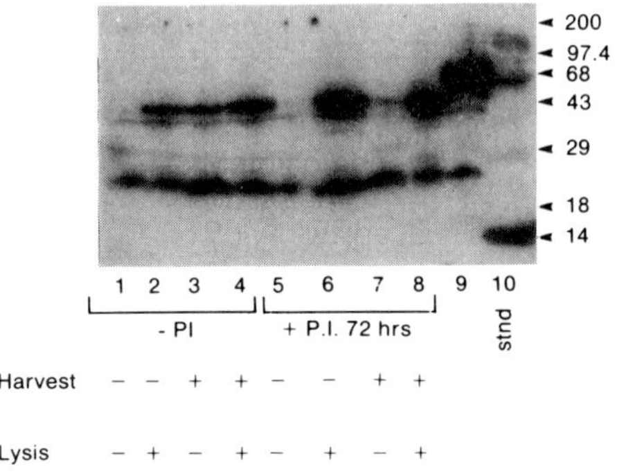

Illustration 1. Effect of the addition of protease inhibitors on ßAR production.

DO (%)	Max. Specific Growth Rate (hr^1)	Max. Specific H-ANS Production Rate (Rel. Units/ Cell/hr)	H-ANS Yield (Rel. Units/ Cell)
10	0.020	0.003	0.123
65	0.027	0.009	0.205
110	0.020	0.003	0.110

Table 1   Effect of dissolved oxygen on cell growth and H-ANS production in IPL41+2% FBS medium.

with the ANS variant 2 and H-ANS baculovirus vectors, MOI did not seem to affect production. Figure 3 shows product yields for H-ANS cultures at MOI's of 0.1, 1.0 and 2.5. In order to conserve virus all infections for production of ANS and H-ANS were therefore carried out at an MOI of 0.1. Conversely, for BAR, productivity was found to be lower at MOI's of less than 1.0 (not shown) so all infections for production of BAR were carried out at an MOI of 1.0-2.0.

A good correlation was obtained between the increase in modal cell diameter, which is a cytopathic effect of baculovirus infection, and protein production. Cell viability, though not as accurate a parameter, is much more convenient to follow; a 50% drop in viability also correlated well with peak product accumulation. Figure 4 illustrates the relation between the kinetics of ANS accumulation, modal cell diameter and cell viability in the 18-l fermenter. In a typical fermentation, modal cell diameter increases rapidly as ANS accumulates in the medium and peaks about 24 hours before maximum ANS production (which coincides with a 50% loss in viability).

ANS production in serum-free Excell-400 medium was scaled up to the 70-l direct sparged fermenter. ANS accumulation rates were found to be similar to those seen in the 8-l microsparged fermenter as shown in Figure 5. Though the peak ANS concentration was lower for the 18-l fermenter in this particular experiment, yields in the two systems were typically similar.

Table 1 shows the effect of DO concentration on cell growth and H-ANS production in IPL-41 medium with 2% FBS. Both the specific cell growth rate and specific H-ANS production rate are somewhat lower at DO levels of 10% and 110% as compared to 65% DO. The maximum H-ANS production at100 hours is almost double at 65% DO in comparison to 10% and 110% DO. Cell viabilities during growth for the three DO levels were similiar. Cell death was, however, accelerated at 110% DO during production of H–ANS (data not shown).

Illustration 1 shows the effect of protease inhibitors (PI) on production of BAR as visualized by immunoblotting. Lanes 1 through 4 are samples from culture medium harvested at 96 hr post-infection while lanes 5 through 8 are samples from culture medium at 96 hr to which PI's were added at 72 hr post-infection. PI's were also added to the harvest and lysis buffers, as shown in illustration 1. Sample 1 had no PI's added and showed very little intact BAR (52 kDa band) while there were significant lower kDa bands (degraded receptor). A good amount of intact receptor was obtained when PI's were added to the lysis buffer (sample 2). Adding PI's to the harvest buffer did not seem to improve yield (samples 3 and 4). Adding PI's to culture medium at 72 hours improves intact BAR yield but requires presence of PI's in the lysis buffer (samples 5 and 6). Again addition of PI's to harvest buffer seemed to have no effect.

DISCUSSION

We have observed that various parameters of Sf9 cell growth, infection and protein production scale up well from 500 ml spinner flasks to 70-l pilot-scale fermenters. The progress of a baculovirus infection can be monitored effectively by following the increase in cell volume and also by following the decrease in cell viability. The production of ANS and H-ANS in our study was not dependent on the multiplicity of infection (MOI) while BAR production was lower at MOI's of less than 1.0. Very low (10%) and very high (110%) DO levels adversely affect cell growth (at least up to 100 hours in culture), and H-ANS production. Good specific growth rate and H-ANS productivity were obtained at 65% DO. The effect of DO on cell growth and H-ANS production is striking. Without more data, we can only hypothesize that cells grow slowly at 10% DO because they are oxygen starved while at 110% DO they are experiencing oxygen toxicity. In both situations cell death does not seem to increase. During the infection cycle, however, cell death is accelerated at 110% DO. BAR production can be improved by addition of protease inhibitors to the culture and harvest media.

ACKNOWLEDGEMENTS

The authors wish to acknowledge the contributions of L. O'Neill with H-ANS gene
expression, C. Dunwiddie with antistasin assays, and to thank G. E. Mark and
R. W. Ellis for advice and support during the course of this work.

REFERENCES

1. Gasic, G.J., Iwakawa, A., Gasic, T.B., Viner, E.D., and Milas, L.: Leech salivary
    inhibitor of cyclophosphamide- and radiation-induced artificial metastasis
    enhancement. Cancer Res. 1984, 44, 5670-5676.

2. Murer, E.H., James, H.L., Budzynski, A.Z., Malinconico, S.M. and Gasic, G.J.:
    Protease inhibitors in *Haementaria* leech species. Thromb. Haemotasis, 1984, 51,
    24-26.

3. Dunwiddie, C., Thornberry, N.A., Bull, H.G., Sardana, M., Friedman, P.A., Jacobs,
    J.W., and Simpson, E.: Antistasin, a leech-derived inhibitor of Factor Xa. J. Biol.
    Chem. 1989, 264, 16694-16699.

4. Tuszynski, G.P., Gasic, T.B., and Gasic, G.J.: Isolation and characterization of
    antistasin, an inhibitor of metastasis and coagulation, J. Biol. Chem. (1987) 262,
    9718-9723

5. Harvey, R.P., Degryse, E., Stefani, L., Schamber, F., Cazenave, J.P., Courtney, M.,
    Tolstoshev, P. and Lecocq, J.-P.: Cloning and expression of a cDNA coding for the
    anti-coagulant hirudin from the bloodsucking leech *Hirudo medicinalis*. Proc.
    Natl. Acad. Sci. USA, 1986, 83,1084-1088.

6. Nutt, E., Gasic, T.B., Rodkey, J., Gasic, G.J., Jacobs, J.W., Friedman, P.A., and
    Simpson, E.: The amino acid sequence of antistasin, a potent inhibitor of factor Xa,
    reveals a repeated internal structure. J. Biol. Chem., 1988, 263, 10162-10167.

7. Han, J.H., Law, S.W., Keller, P.M., Kniskern, P.J., Silberklang, M., Tung, J-S., Gasic,
    T.B., Gasic, G.J., Friedman, P.A., Ellis, R.W.: Cloning and expression of cDNA
    encoding antistasin, a leech-derived protein having anti-coagulant and anti-
    metastatic properties. Gene 1989, 75, 47-57.

8. Strader, C.D., Sigal, I.S., Dixon, R.A.F.: Mapping the functional domain of the ß-
    adrenergic receptor. Am. J. Respir. Cell Biol. 1989, 1, 81-86.

9. Dixon, R.A.F., Kobilka, B.K., Strader, D.J., Benovic, J.L., Dohlman, H.G., Frielle, T.,
    Bolanowski, M.A., Bennett, C.D., Rands, E., Diehl, R.E., Mumford, R.A., Slater, E.E.,
    Sigal, I.S., Caron, M.G., Lefkowitz, R.J., Strader, C.D.: Cloning of the gene and cDNA
    for mammalian ß-adrenergic receptor and homology with rhodopsin. Nature 1986,
    321, 75-79.

10. Summers, M.D. and Smith, G.E.: A manual of Methods for Baculovirus Vectors and
    Insect cell culture Procedures, Texas Agricultural Experiment Section Bulletin, No.
    1555, 1987.

11. Dixon, R.A.F., Sigal, I.S., Strader, C.D,: Structure-function analysis of the ß-
    adrenergic receptor. Cold Spring Harbor Symposia on Quantitative Biology 1988,
    LIII, 487-495.

<u>**Paper of Jain**</u>

Bushell: I have been told that one of the advantages of
insect cells is that they grow very quickly -
almost as quickly as E. coli. You quoted maximum
specific growth rate of 0.27, which is slow even
for an animal cell. Have I misunderstood the
units, or would you like to comment?

Jain: In our hands, cells adapted to 2% serum have a
miximum doubling time of 24 hours.

QUANTITATION OF mRNA SPECIFIC FOR HEAVY AND LIGHT CHAINS OF IgG IN HYBRIDOMAS DURING DIFFERENT PHASES OF BATCH CULTURE

OTTO W MERTEN, MICHEL LENO and JEAN HACHE*

Laboratoire de Technologie Cellulaire, Institut Pasteur, 28 rue du Dr Roux, 75724 Paris cedex 15, France
*Division Génie Chimique et Biochimique, Bertin & Cie, Boîte Postale 3,78373 Plaisir cedex, France

Key words: mRNA; in situ, dot blot and northern blot hybridizations; cytoplasmic , total cell-associated and secreted IgG kinetics; murine hybridoma cells.

ABSTRACT

We have investigated the regulation of IgG synthesis in relation to the physiological state of two hybridoma cell lines during the different phases of batch culture: mRNA, specific for the gamma and kappa chains region genes, were quantitated either by dot blot, northern blot or in situ hybridization procedures. Steady-state levels of the two mRNAs correlate well with the specific growth rate ($R2= 0,72$, $R2= 0,66$) and the cytoplasmic or the total cell-associated IgG concentrations. However, no correlation was found between the levels of these mRNAs and the rate of accumulation of secreted IgG in the medium.

INTRODUCTION

Immunoglobulin molecules are multichain proteins consisting of heavy (H) and light (L) chains joined together by disulphide bonds. The H- and L- chains are synthetized on independant classes of polysomes of different sizes (1,2) and subsequently joined to form the complete antibody molecule. Control of gene expression may be effected at several different levels, including transcription of the gene, processing of the primary transcript, mRNA stability and translation of the mRNA on the polysomes (3). Early studies indicated a high turnover of H- or L- chains mRNAs during the differentiation of immunoglobulin secreting cells (4,5,6). During the synchronous and asynchronous hybridoma cultures, DNA synthetic activity peaks during the early exponential phase and declines rapidly during late exponential and dead phases (7). Previous results have attempted to explain the phenomena that govern the differential antibody biosynthesis/secretion during the culture of hybridoma cell lines by pulse and pulse-chase experiments (8,9,10). However, little is known about the mecanisms which govern the relative rate of H- and L- chains synthesis in hybridomas.
To investigate the molecular events involved in the variation of the specific productivity rate of IgG during the culture, it may be useful to study the different levels of control of the gene expression.
The purpose of this report is to determine which information concerning antibody synthesis and secretion can be obtained by measuring steady-state levels of gamma and kappa chains mRNAs and by comparing this information with the kinetics of secreted, cytoplasmic and total cell-associated IgG during hybridoma batch cultures. Correlation between these data will be postulated.

MATERIALS AND METHODS

Cell lines and culture conditions:
Two mouse hybridoma cell lines (I.13.17. and ID2C3), based on X63.653 and SP2/0 myelomas respectively, were used. I.13.17 cell line was cultured either in static batch (250 ML Roux bottles) and in agitated batch (1L rollers bottles) conditions. ID2C3 cell line was culured in agitated batch 1L rollers bottles.
All cultures were conducted using Dulbecco's modified Eagle's Medium (DMEM) supplemented with 5% fetal calf serum for I.13.17. and 5% fetal calf serum +5% new born calf serum for ID2C3. All experiments were performed in duplicates.
At daily intervals, an aliquot of the suspension was harvested; cells were counted and viability was determined using trypan blue dye exclusion procedure. After centrifugation at 1000 rpm at 4°C for 10 min. , the supernatants were frozen and kept at -20°C until subsequent analysis. Sedimentated cells were washed two times in PBS buffer, quickly chilled in liquid nitrogen and kept at -8O°C.

In situ hybridization:
Fixation of hybridoma cells to filter was done as previously described (11). Biefly, 10exp5 cells were transferred, with vacuum on, onto a Hybond extra C filter (Amersham) previously prewetted in 2xSSC in a 96-well manifold apparatus. The filter was then fixed in 3% NaCl-10 mM NaH2PO4-40 mM Na2HPO4 (pH 7.4) , 1% glutaraldehyde at 4°C for one hour and rinced three times with proteolytic buffer (50 mM EDTA, 0.1 M Tris-HCl pH 8.0). Fixed cells were digested in proteolytic buffer containing 20 ug/ml of proteinase K (Boerhinger-Mannhein) at 37°C for 30 min. The filter was rinced once in proteolytic buffer, immersed in 0,1 M triethanolamine pH 8.O at room temperature for 10 min. and in 0,1 M triethanolamine-0,25% acetic acid as described (12). The filter was rinced in 2xSSC, briefly air-dried and placed directly in prehybridization buffer.

Dot blot hybridization:
Total cellular RNA was isolated by guanidine thiocyanate phenol chloroforme (AGPC) procedure (13). Five micrograms of each RNA was incubated at 65°C for 5 min. in three volumes of the denaturing solution : 65% formamide, 22% formaldehyde (37% solution), 13% 100x MOPS buffer. One volume of 20x SSC was added and the sample was spotted onto prewetted Nitrocellulose filter (Amersham). The filter was baked at 80°C for two hours and prehybridized.

Northern blot hybridization:
Five micrograms of each AGPC extracted RNA sample were denatured as described, and separated on 1.2% agarose gels prepared in 2.2 M formaldehyde, 0.2 M MOPS buffer (pH 7.0), 52% deionized formamide (14). Gel markers (18 S and 28 S rRNA) were stained in ethidium bromide and photographed using U.V. light.
The RNA in each gel was transferred overnight to nitrocellulose paper (Amersham), prehybridized and hybridized to 32-P labelled gamma or kappa cDNA probes.

DNA probes description and preparation:
The gamma (heavy chain) region probe was a 2500 bp SAC1 fragment encompassing domains CH1-CH3 of the mouse gamma gene, subcloned into Bluescript (15).
The kappa (light chain) region probe was a 830 bp fragment encompassing the constant and the variable domains of the mouse kappa gene, subcloned by oligo(dC).oligo(dG) tailing in the Pst1 site of pBR 322 (16).
Both were kindly provided by R. Nageotte of the Institut Pasteur, Paris.
DNA restriction linearized fragments (200 ng) were labelled using an in vitro random Multiprime labelling kit (Amersham). Bound and unbound labelled DNA were separated using Sephadex G-50 columm chromatography followed by liquid scintillation count. Specific activities of labelled probes used were 2,5x10exp8 cpm/ug.

Single-stranded DNA preparation:
In order to investigate the specificity of the two probes and the sensibility of hybridization conditions, we have synthetized in vitro two single-stranted DNAs (ss-DNA) containing either the kappa or the gamma gene sequence probe described (15,16).This preparation was done using M13mp18 cloning kit (Boehringer).

Hybridization conditions:
Prehybridization and hybridization were conducted as described early (14), with some modifications. The prehydidization buffer contains 50% formamide, 5xSSPE buffer, 0,1%SDS, 10xDenhart solution, sonicated denatured salmon sperm DNA at 100 ug/ml. The RNA blots are prehybridized for 12 hrs at 65°C. The random primer labelled probes were denaturated at 100°C for 2-5 min, cooled, and added to the hybridization buffer, and the blots were hybridized overnight at 65°C. The blots were washed with two changes of 2xSSPE/0,1%SDS for 15 min at room temperature, two changes of 1xSSPE/0.1%SDS for 15min at room temperature and once in 0,1xSSPE/0.1%SDS for 15min at 60°C. The blots were exposed to X-ray film at -80°C, using a Kodak intensifying screen after the damp blots have been wrapped in Saran Wrap (Dow).

Data analysis:
After suitable exposures, the autoradiograms were quantitated by densitometric tracing or by cutting spots out of the filters and counting in a liquid scintillation counter.

Extraction of cytoplasmic IgG:
To extract cytoplasmic antibody, 2x10exp6 freezed cells were resuspended in 1 ml PBS, freezed-thawed three times and centrifugated at 10.000 rpm, at 4°C for 15 min.

IgG concentration measurement:
The IgG concentration in the culture medium, in the cytoplasmic and total cell-associated extracts was determined by using an enzyme-linked immunosorbent assay (ELISA) (9,10).

RESULTS

Growth and antibody production kinetics:
Six different batch cultures of two antibody-secreting hybridoma cell lines were performed. The development of cellular growth and antibody accumulation in the medium are shown in Fig.1. It can be seen that the results obtained for both cell lines were quantitatively the same, although medium and culture conditions were different to some extent. The growth curves show a typical profile, reported peviously (9); with a exponential growth ranging from 20 h to 70 h (Fig.1A) and from 4 h to 40 h (Fig.1B and Fig.1C) which was followed by a rapid decrease in viability (not shown).
The antibody concentration and growth profiles were similar (Fig.1). The increase of IgG in the medium was relatively rapid until the onset of dead phase with the majority having been produced during logarithmic growth.

Steady-state levels of mRNAs:
Standardisation experiments showed that there was a linear dose-reponse relationship between variable amounts of single-stranded DNAs immobilized onto nitrocellulose filter and hybridized either with gamma or kappa 32-P labelled probes (not shown). This argues for the speficity of the probes used, for the optimal conditions of hybridization, and of cause for the possibility to quantify the amounts of H- and L-chains mRNAs.
The results of the in situ hybridization are shown in Fig.2. It can be seen that the steady-state levels of kappa and gamma chains mRNAs varied significantly during the

different phases of batch culture, independently of cell line and culture conditions.
For cell line I.13.17. (static batch culture), the levels of L- chains mRNAs peaked at 48
hours during the early exponential growth phase and decreased rapidly during the late
exponential and stationary growth phases (Fig.2A); whereas the levels of H- chains
mRNA stayed relatively constant during the growth phase with a decrease tendancy
towards the stationary phase.

Using the same cell line, cultivated in agitated batch culture (Fig.1B), dot blot and
northern blot hybridization were performed using total cellular RNA. The profiles of
gamma and kappa chains mRNA obtained with dot blot studies showed two peaks, one at
the onset of the culture and the second one during stationary phase (Fig.2B). The high
amount of mRNAs detected at the beginning of the culture may be account to the
physiological stage of the inoculum in transient log-stationary growth phase. The
decrease of the viability (not shown) during the early growth phase correlates directly
with the reduction of the levels of gamma and kappa chains mRNAs. The late and
exponential phases are paralleled by an incease to maximal levels of H- and L- chains
mRNAs. These levels decreased very rapidly during the dead phase.
The death phase is associated with a 3 fold drop of the amount of both mRNAs.
These results are consistent with previous observations on DNA synthetic activity (7). It
is also interesting to note the relatively constant ratio between the levels of L- and H-
chains mRNAs during the culture. This ratio, which is ranging from 2 to 3, is in
accordance with literature data (18).

For cell line ID2C3, cultivated in agitated batch cultures, similar results were found
like for the agitated cultures of I.13.17. The difference was the direct start of the
culture without lag phase , which may be the reason that high amounts of H-and L- chain
mRNAs was found throughout the growth phase, whereby the maximal level of kappa
mRNA appeared before 45 hrs, while the gamma mRNA peaked at 48 hrs (Fig.2C).

Although Northern blot analysis is relatively difficult to quantify mRNA and only semi-
quantitative results have to be expected, this method was attemped to examine the size
distribution of molecules containing light or heavy chains IgG sequence in total cellular
RNA fractionnated on formaldehyde gel. It is evident from Fig.4 that no transcript forms
of kappa nor gamma chains IgG mRNAs was detected from total cellular RNA, during the
culture. Bands corresponding to H-mRNA (2,6 kb) and L-mRNA (0,9 kb) were discerned.
These sizes are consistent with literature data (19).

Correlations
The relationship between specific growth rate and steady-state levels of H- and L-
chains IgG mRNA is shown is Fig.5. Each of the two measures was correlated with a
regression coefficient of 0,72 and 0,66 respectively for gamma and kappa chains mRNAs.
Otherwise, cytoplasmic IgG correlate well with the levels of the two mRNAs as
summarised in Fig.6. However, there was correlation between the levels of the two
mRNAs and the specific productivity rate (Fig.7).

DISCUSSION

This work has demonstrated that the steady-state levels of gamma and kappa chains IgG
mRNA, as measured by dot blot and in situ hybridization procedures, are correlated
with the specific growth rate during hybridoma batch culture.

The high concentrations of mRNAs observed during exponential growth is consistent with the maximal metabolic activity (26,27) during this culture phase and a high specific productivity. However, the strong reduction of the amounts of H- and L- chains mRNAs and the degradation of ribosomal RNA during the dead phase argue against an increased of specific IgG synthesis. This is supported by other authors (21), who reported a decrease of the protein synthesis rate in the stationary phase of hybriboma batch cultures.

The processes which are assumed to influence the accumulation of IgG in the supernatant are: synthesis, storage and degradation of IgG within the cell; secretion of IgG into the medium and probable degradation of IgG in the medium. Actually, little is known about the influences of the physiological stages of mouse hybridoma batch culture on IgG production. It became evident that the maximum levels of H- and L- chains mRNAs showed some variations between different culture conditions.,the cell line and the physiological stage of the inoculum. It seems that the difference between the two cell lines used (both: mouse hybridomas; however based on two different myelomas) have a minor influence, whereas culture conditions and physiological state of the inoculum stronly influence the development of cellular H- and L- chains mRNAs. The last mentioned factors might be the reason for the differences, observed for the profiles of gamma and kappa chains mRNAs during the different I.13.17. batch cultures.

It was recently stated that the released IgGs are only secreted by viable cells and that the accumulated antibody is linearly related to the integral of viable cells (17,22). In view of our results, these statements are only valid to a limited extent as no real correlation was observed between secreted IgG and integral of viable cells (Fig.8), due to the physiological changes during the onset of the dead phase. In addition, no correlation was found between cell specific productivity and the steady-state levels of both mRNAs during the batch cultures. The high concentrations of gamma and kappa mRNAs, of ribosomal RNA (not shown), of ribosomal proteins involved in mRNA translation (21) during the exponential growth is consistent with the high metabolic activity observed during this phase (20,27). It seems that the cells are limited in energy and that they use a more important part of this energy for growth and biomass production than for IgG synthesis and secretion during this phase (20). In the late exponential and stationary growth phases,characterized by profound physiological changes (8,20), a minimum in the specific productivity rate was found (8,17,23), although maximal levels of mRNAs have been observed (Fig.7). At the beginning of the dead phase of mouse hybridoma cultures, the observed decrease in the immunoglobulin synthesis rate (17), may be in part related to the 20-70% drop in the levels of of kappa and gamma chains mRNAs. This suggest the hypothesis that the non correlation observed between specific productivity rate and mRNA levels may be also related to other events such as transport processes or mRNA translation rate. This hypothesis is in accordance with statements of other authors (21), who reported a 15-25% decrease in ribosome content per cell, a 2-fold decrease in the ribosome proteins involved in mRNA translation and a 5-15% decrease in the mRNA translation rate during stationary and beginning dead phase of hybridoma cultures.

A still unresolved problem is whether the increase in the antibody production during the decline phase of hybridoma growth is due to a passive release or to an active secretion of IgG. Early reports have provided sometimes controverse answers (7,10,17,23,25). Recently, we calculated by mass balance, that 14-50% of secreted IgG (pulse chase experiments) during the dead phase of hybridoma cultures was of storage origin (8). The present report has demonstrated that there was a 60-70% decrease in the steady-state levels of either gamma or kappa chain mRNA associated with the viability drop during the dead phase of hybridoma cultures, whereas the amount of secreted IgG increased slightly.

It seems probable that this IgG secreted during the dead phase may be of storage origin rather than from de novo synthesis as shown by several groups (8,20,26). Therefore, our results and literature data lead to the suggestion that, depending on cell lines used and culture conditions employed, the rate of antibody production is related in part to the steady-state levels of H-and L- chains mRNAs, but also to some post-transcriptional events during mouse hybridoma batch culture.

REFERENCES

1. Cowan NJ, DS Secher and C Milstein (1974) Mol.Biol.,90,691-701
2. Alzari PM, Lascombe MB and RJ Poljak (1988) Ann.Rev.Immnunol.,6,55-580
3. Darnell JE (1984) Nature, 297,365-371
4. Genster T, Picard D and W Schaffner (1986) Cell,45,45-52
5. Kelly DE and RP Perry (1986) Nuc.Ac.Res.;14,13,5431-5447
6. Zhou FH, Guo KZ, Tilles SA and GA Gutman (1987),Mol.Immunol. ,24,11,1151-1158
7. Al-Rubaei and   AN Emery (1989) Cytotechnol. S9 (Abstract)
8. Merten OW, H Keller, L Cabanie, M Leno and M Hardefelt(1990) Cytotechnol.(in press)
9. Merten OW, S Reiter, G Himmler, W Scheirer, H Katinger (1985),   Develop.Biol.
    Standard, 60, 219-227
10. Merten OW (1988) Cytotechnol, 1, 113-121
11. Paeratakul U, PR De Stasio and WM Taylor (1988) J.Virol, 62,   1132-1135
12. Sy-May and AM Gorosky (1986) Nucl. Acid.Res., 14, 7597-7616
13. Chomczynski P and N Sacchi (1986) Anal. Biochem.,162, 156-159
14. Maniatis T, EF Fritsch and J Sambrook (1982) Molecular Cloning: a laboratory
    Manaul, Cold Sping Harbor Laboratory, N-Y.
15. Tasuku H,M Obata and Yuriko (1979) Cell, 18, 559-568
16. Rougeon F. and B Mach (1977)Ann.Immunol.128C, 189-192
17. Meilhoc E, KD Wittrup, and JE Bailey (1989) J.Immunol.Meth.,121, 167-174
18. Reuven LMD and MD Schaff (1970) J.Exp.Med.,131, 515-541
19. Schibler U, KB Marcu, and RP Perry (1978) Cell, 15, 1495-1509
20. Al-Rubeai and Emery (1990) J.Biotechnol. (in press)
21. Morenkov OS, YA Mantsyghin and EI Leshnev (1989) Tsitologiya, 31,   324-325
22. Renard JM, R Spnagnoli, C Mazier, MF Salles and E Mandine (1988)
    Biotechnol.Lett.10, 91-96
23. Reuveny S, D Velez, L Miller and Mac Millan JD (1986)J.Immunol.Meth.,86,53-59
24. Merten OW, Palfi GE, Klement G and Steindl F (1987) in Modern approaches to animal
    cell technology,eds:Spier RE,JB Griffiths,pp 381-396, Butterworths
25. Walker AG, W Davison, CA Lambe (1987) Proc. 4th European Congress on
    Biotechnol.,eds:Neijssel OM, RR Van Der Meer, AM Luyben, Vol3, pp587, Elsevier Sc.
    publishers, Amsterdam/NL
26. Al-Rubaei M , S Rookes and AN Emery (1989) in. Advances in animal cell
    and technology for bioprocesses, eds: RE Spier, JB Griffiths, J Stephenne
    and JJ Crooy, pp. 241-245, Butterworths
27. Merten OW, Keller H, Siami, L Cabanié M Leno (1990) (This Volume)

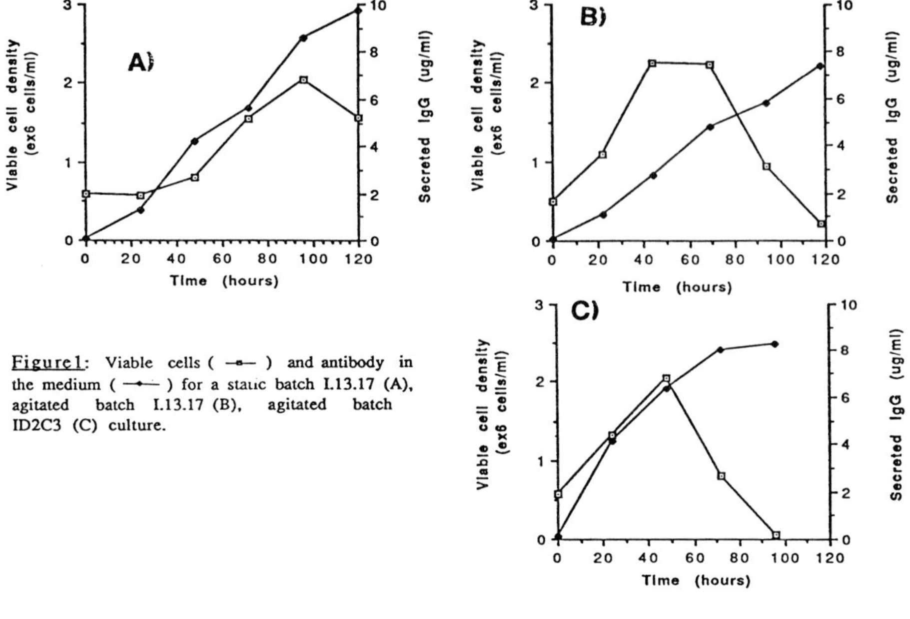

Figure1: Viable cells (—□—) and antibody in the medium (—●—) for a static batch I.13.17 (A), agitated batch I.13.17 (B), agitated batch ID2C3 (C) culture.

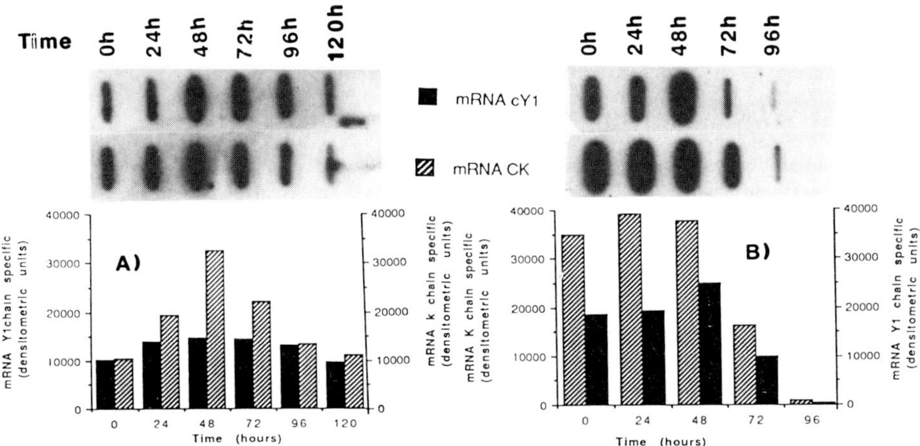

Figure 2: Steady-state levels of Y1 chain mRNA(■) and k chain mRNA(▨) quantitated by in situ hybridization during I.13.17 (A) and ID2C3 (B) batch culture

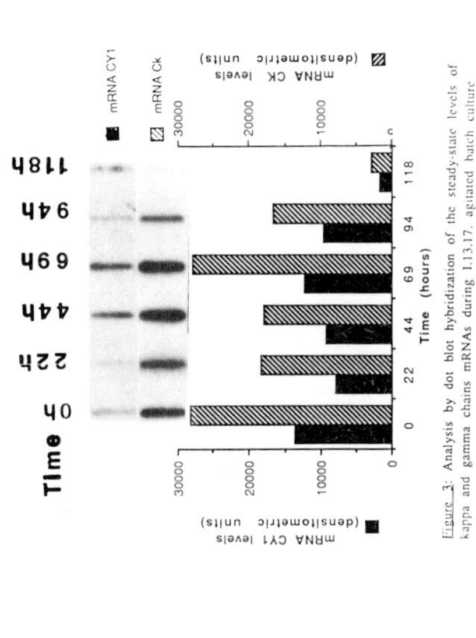

Figure 3: Analysis by dot blot hybridization of the steady-state levels of kappa and gamma chains mRNAs during I.13.17. agitated batch culture

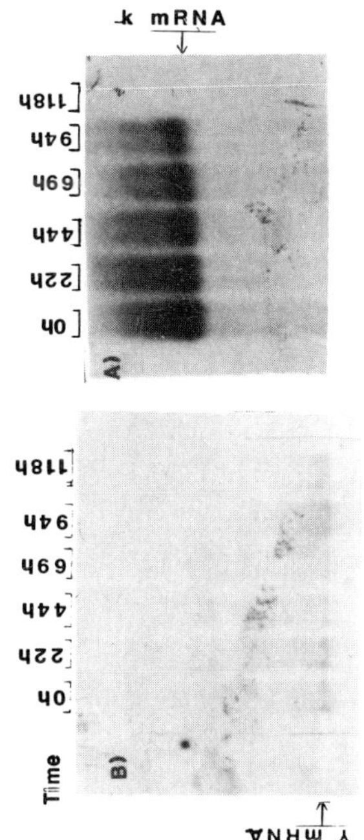

Figure 4: Northern blots analysis of total cellular RNA extracted from I.13.17. agitated batch culture (Fig.1B), separated on formaldehyde gels. Filters were hybridized separetly, either with kappa (A) or with gamma (B) specific 32-P labelled probes.

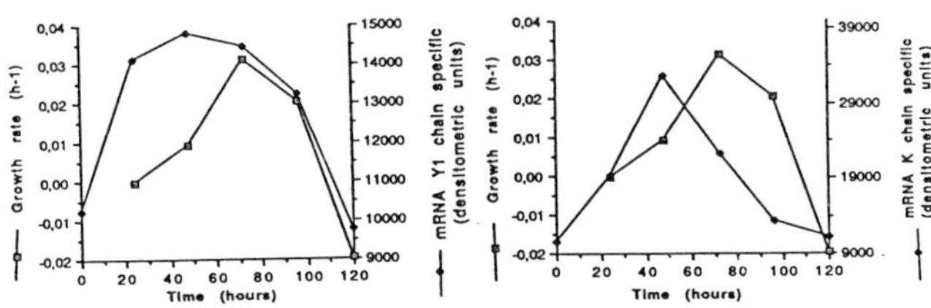

Figure 5 A: kinetics of growth rate , kappa chain mRNA and gamma chain mRNAs during I.13.17. static batch culture (Fig.1A)

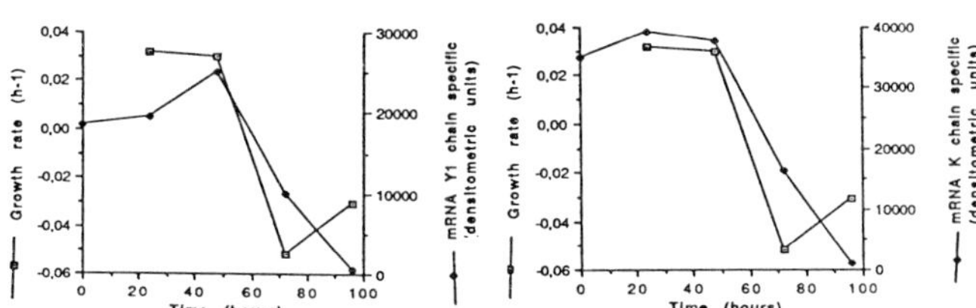

Figure 5B: Kinetics of growth rate , kappa chain mRNA and gamma chain mRNA during ID2C3 agitated batch culture (Fig.1C)

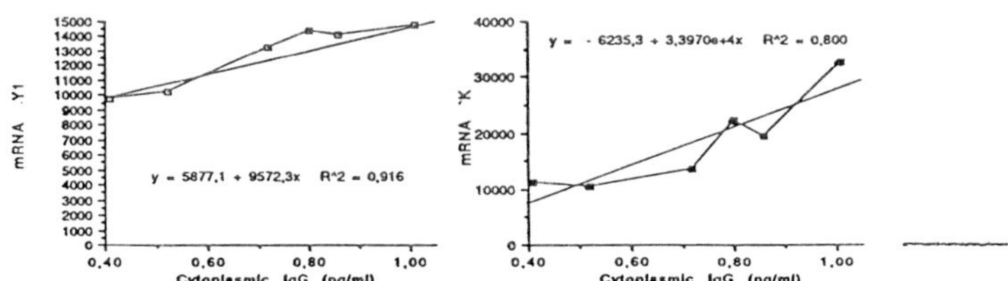

Figure 6: Correlation between cytoplasmic IgG and steady-state levels of H-chain (—□—) and L-chain (—■—) mRNAs during I.1317. culture (Fig.1A)

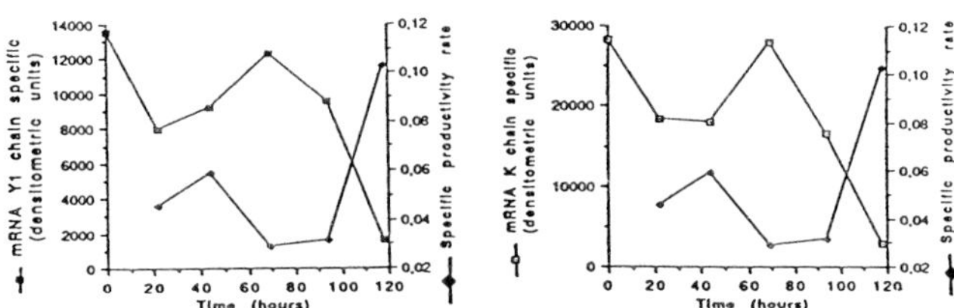

Figure 7: Profiles of specific productivity, steady-state levels of k-chain and L-chain mRNAs during I.13.17. agitated batch culture (Fig.1A)

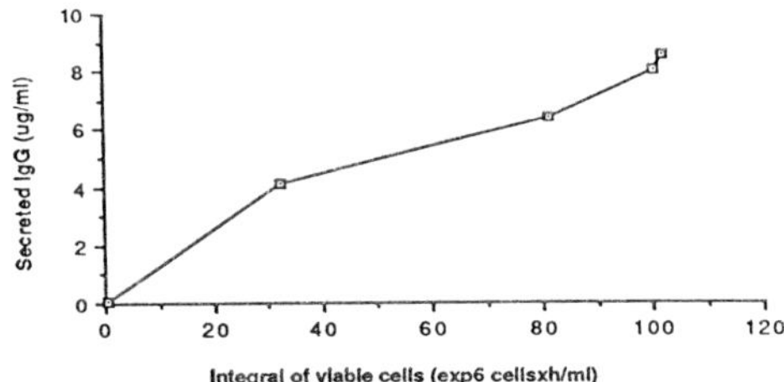

Figure 8: Relationship between integral of viable cells and accumulation of IgG in the medium during I.13.17. agitated batch culture (Fig.1A)

Section 6.1
Bioreactors: overview

DEVELOPMENT OF MAMMALIAN CELL MANUFACTURING PROCESSES

James Hope, Morris Rosenberg and <u>William Tolbert</u>

Invitron Corporation, 4649 Le Bourget Dr., St. Louis, MO 63134

ABSTRACT

Productivity of mammalian cell culture based manufacturing may be significantly enhanced by careful integration of upstream and downstream process development. A detailed process development study is necessary to maximize product recovery and overall productivity of a particular bioreactor system. This study must define and optimize media components, bioreactor control parameters and other operational variables to maximize cell specific productivity and cell density. Downstream process development should be performed in parallel with cell and bioreactor studies to ensure that conditions for maximum upstream production will be compatible with recovery of purified product with high overall yield and bioactivity. It is also important for clinical products that final specifications for the product and analytical methods be defined as early as possible to support regulatory filings.

INTRODUCTION

Biopharmaceutical products present a wide range of challenges for development of efficient manufacturing processes in compliance with US FDA requirements. Biologics produced by any means, including mammalian cell culture, are often inherently heterogeneous and represent a collection of similar molecules with various activities. This heterogeneity may result from differences in cell populations or from post-translational modifications within a single cell. The molecule may be further modified after secretion by proteolytic degradation, aggregation, oxidation, etc. The resultant biological activity may also vary. Acceptable pharmaceutical use requires that a drug be safe, pure, efficacious with specific potency and consistent in its characteristics. Particularly for biological products, it is difficult to ensure these latter requirements by analysis of the finished product itself. For this reason, regulatory agencies require development of a consistent, controlled manufacturing process.

All phases in the development of a manufacturing process are of interest to the regulator but specific requirements generally begin with the development of the cell line and subsequent Master Cell Bank. These requirements in the USA are described in a series of FDA Points-to-Consider documents and are generally defined in more detail in direct correspondence and meetings between the FDA and the company developing a specific product. While changes throughout the development of a product are expected, and even encouraged to increase process efficiency and control, it is important to define and fix a manufacturing process as early as possible during clinical investigations. Significant changes late in the program will often result in the delay of product approval, require additional patient trials and added expense.

In addition to regulatory concerns, there are ample economic reasons for the development of an efficient manufacturing process. Not only must upstream research and development, cell culture production and downstream processing be optimized individually; they must be optimized together in a coordinated fashion to result in a minimum cost of manufacturing. The selection of a cell substrate will effect the choice and efficiency of the culture production method and potential existence of viral contaminants. Nutrient medium and additives will stipulate contaminants that must be removed and ultimately the complexity of the required purification procedures. Cell viability during production will impact nucleic acid and cellular protein challenges to purification. Several fold reduction in cost is possible by careful optimization of the total manufacturing process.

INITIAL PROCESS DEVELOPMENT

The process actually begins with development of a cell line making a specific product followed by further cloning and amplification to increase specific productivity and ensure stability of expression. The discussion here will describe the steps after the cell line has been received from the internal or external research and development group and is scheduled for development of a commercial manufacturing process. The first step is to obtain as much information as possible from the cell line's developers. It is particularly important to acquire results of all biosafety or contaminant assays that have been performed, in addition to exchange of information on the cell growth characteristics, media, etc. A facility biosafety committee should review this information to determine if the cell line is acceptable for manufacturing. After this approval, the cell line must be quarantined and tested prior to production release.

If the cell has been grown with antibiotics, the cells must be passaged in antibiotic-free medium before samples are submitted for full microbiology testing including mycoplasma testing. Reverse transcriptase and transmission electron microscopy studies should be performed to detect viral contamination. If the cell is human or contains human components additional tests should be performed for HIV, EBV, Hepatitis B, CMV and HTLV-1 where appropriate. While waiting for test results, small scale experiments may be performed within the quarantine laboratory to determine or verify doubling time, product expression and to evaluate various media and additives. If the cell line grows in suspension, spinner experiments comparing candidate growth and production media formulations selected in multiwell or T-flask studies may be performed. If attachment is required or desirable, various microcarriers can be examined for growth and production. Microcarrier experiments in spinners are used for media studies. Cell expression and stability must be part of this evaluation. It is also useful to prepare a small freeze of a few vials of cells during this time unless several vials of the <u>same</u> freeze were obtained initially from the developers of the cell line.

After release from quarantine, a vial of frozen cells is recovered within the manufacturing area for preparation of Master and Manufacturer's Working Cell Banks in accordance with approved written procedures. These cell banks must be characterized as suggested in the Points-To-Consider documents or in accordance with direct FDA discussions. Different levels of testing are required for each bank and the list of tests will vary with cell type. Additional cell line testing will also be required for post-production cells, i.e. cells removed after the end of the production cycle. These tests are performed to ensure that production conditions did not induce new viral contaminants or otherwise change the cell line characteristics.

As part of the initial process development, product and other assays necessary for product characterization need to be developed and shown to correlate with those generated during research and development. Biological assays should be included that demonstrate bioactivity of the molecule. It is most important that a biological potency assay be available to evaluate the product during production, clinical trials and beyond. It is also critical at this stage to begin the development of a scaleable purification process. Most laboratory methods used by research groups will not be scaleable or will not meet the stringent requirements of pharmaceutical manufacturing. Cell conditioned medium from the small scale cell culture experiments can be used to begin this development.

PROCESS OPTIMIZATION IN MODEL BIOREACTOR SYSTEMS (NON-CLINICAL)

At this stage it is necessary to conduct experiments in a model bioreactor system that will allow direct correlation to full-scale production. A number of parameters need to be optimized with operating ranges defined for maximum production yields and wider ranges for these parameters which will allow production of acceptable product. The following is a list of many of these parameters for a perfusion bioreactor (note they are not independent): cell growth rate, cell density, specific productivity, viability, perfusion rate, cell harvest rate, pH, dissolved O_2, dissolved CO_2, NH_4 ion concentration, temperature, glucose consumption, glutamine consumption, lactate production, amino acid utilization, LDH levels, and product specific parameters, eg., single chain content for tPA.

An approach to defining these parameter ranges is operation of the reactor at several combinations of perfusion rates and cell densities. After consistent operation has been established under each set of conditions, specific productivity, metabolic parameters and other dependent variables are monitored. Dissolved gas, pH, temperature, etc., are set at known acceptable values and the medium and additive concentrations from the initial studies are employed. The experiments are iterative in nature with initial set parameters such as dissolve gas or pH varied after other ranges are determined. Metabolic information and cell utilization of medium components allow further optimization of the nutrient mix. In most circumstances a medium designed for rapid growth is used to produce cell mass in the reactor without concern for downstream processing constraints. Then a second production medium designed for high productivity and a low contaminant profile is used during the production phase. This will generally be a low or very low protein containing medium and may include additives to provide shear protection, viscosity modification, and to increase lipid and O_2 solubility. It should be noted that conditions for maximum product expression most often do not coincide with those for maximum growth and viability. Some controlled environmental stress may result in greater total production and may be acceptable during optimization of the total process. With perfusion bioreactors operated at 1 to 5 reactor volumes per day the washout period necessary to effect change from growth to production medium becomes insignificant, particularly as the production cycle for these reactors often extends to months.

It is very important to define these parameters in a perfusion mode as the rapidly changing environment of batch experiments will infer significantly different conclusions. At all stages, however, close communication between cell culture and purification groups is necessary to prevent upstream conditions unacceptable for product recovery from being established. Sufficient material is made during these experiments to allow both laboratory scale definition and intermediate scale confirmation of the purification process. It is also worthwhile at this stage to delineate the bulk formulation buffer and final product concentration. These will vary with the characteristics of the protein product and its intended use. Concerns about aggregate formation, proteolytic degradation, long-term stability and excipient acceptability should also be addressed. In addition, performance against previously established specifications may be appraised. Often the results of these experiments are critical in assigning appropriate final bulk product specifications.

PILOT PRODUCTION RUN (PRE-CLINICAL SUPPLIES)

A full-scale production run is necessary to corroborate the preceding results and further refine bioreactor operating conditions. All aspects of the process including preparation of inoculum, scale-up, reactor growth phase, production phase, purification, and bulk formulation should be evaluated against productivity, yield and specification targets.

A minimum of one or two weeks under production conditions, after washout of the growth medium, and 1000 to 3000 liters of product containing, cell conditioned medium should be provided. This material is then used in a full-scale purification run and final bulk product analyzed to ensure that it will have necessary biological activity and meet all specifications. During the pilot run it is vital that control of the process is demonstrated within the previously determined ranges for each parameter. If adjustments need to be made, their impact must be assessed carefully, and the new values incorporated into the batch records for the first clinical run.

CONTINUED PROCESS DEVELOPMENT DURING CLINICAL PRODUCTION

After batch records are issued for a clinical production run by the Quality Assurance Department, production can be initiated. The process development work is, however, not finished or complete. A data base needs to be assembled from the initial clinical runs that will support lot-to-lot production consistency and can be statistically analyzed to demonstrate control of the process for each operational parameter. The FDA expects in most cases as this additional information is accumulated, that operating ranges can be tightened and a higher level of consistent control demonstrated. If a change in a parameter setpoint or widening of a parameter range is necessary, production records should justify the need for this change. Any change or deviation from the prescribed operational plan set out in the batch records must have appropriate approvals from production and QA management.

Data on the length of the production cycle must be gathered during clinical runs, with cell and product characteristics studied at different times during the run to demonstrate process consistency. Evaluation of cell conditioned medium to determine levels of viral contamination followed by validation of the purification process for virus removal and inactivation must be performed. Similar studies for DNA challenge and removal may also be done.

The time required for clinical production means that there may be improvements or enhancements to the bioreactor or purification systems that could increase the efficiency of a production process. Table 1 illustrates process development during full-scale pilot and clinical runs displaying increase in average bioreactor productivity of over four fold. Refinement of the purification process, tighter product specifications, changes in raw material vendors or medium changes all may require adjustment of the culture and purification processes and could potentially effect the product. Changes in the latter phases of clinical evaluation

should be avoided but, if necessary, may require expansion of
the clinical program to demonstrate product equivalency.

	Cell Density (ml/liter)*	Viability (%)	Perfusion (liters/D)	Production (grams/mo)
Hybridoma				
Stage 1	6.2	85	62	48
Stage 2	16.2	74	128	84
Stage 3	14.2	79	159	93
Stage 4	23.6	87	309	207
R-CHO				
Stage 1	12.5	54	141	75
Stage 2	17.7	86	303	147
Stage 3	25.1	81	305	228
Stage 4	48.5	73	543	387

Table 1. Stages in bioreactor process development. Average
parameter values displayed from full-scale runs. * Milliliters
of wet packed cells per liter of culture suspension.

In preparation for filing a Product License Application (PLA),
three or more "qualification lots" of product are produced with
submission of detailed information to the FDA to demonstrate
lot-to-lot consistency of the manufacturing process. Data
obtained from these runs can also be used to meet process
validation requirements. These of course must be combined with
complete validation packages for the facility, equipment,
computer software, etc. that are required for the manufacturing
facility but may not be specific to a given product.

CONCLUSION

Development of a manufacturing process for biopharmaceutical
products from mammalian cells is indisputably a complex and
continuing affair with major regulatory and economic
consequences. The goal must be to produce the most efficient
and cost effective process possible meeting product
specifications and regulatory requirements. Optimization of
individual components of the operation is only the starting
point and must be combined with optimization of the total
manufacturing process and appropriate compromises as required.
Significant efforts and resources need to be committed early in
the evolution of a product to minimize later costs. Deferral
of necessary process development studies will increase later
expense and will likely cause delay in regulatory approval.

Hofmann: You need to have a high productivity over the complete run, but why is production consistency so important from a regulatory point of view.

Tolbert: One of the things you are trying to establish is consistency of production to demonstrate that you have control over the process.   If you have a process where the product decreased over time and that such a decrease was a consistent phenomenon and that the product generated was invariant then it might be possible to obtain acceptance.   But in practice you want to work with as stable a cell line as possible and define your production cycle within some bounds (a decrease of production of 10-15% for example).

A NEW LOOK AT ANIMAL CELL BIOREACTOR DEVELOPMENT

Wei—Shou Hu,[*] Matthew T. Scholz, Eric Favre and T. Craig Seamans
Department of Chemical Engineering and Materials Science, University of
Minnesota, 421 Washington Avenue SE, Minneapolis, MN 55455—0132 U.S.A.

INTRODUCTION

Bioreactors for animal cell culture processing have evolved extensively in
the past three decades. The advancement was most profound in the last ten
years. Figure 1 summarizes the evolution of animal cell bioreactors for both
anchorage—dependent and suspension cells. These developments have proceeded in
two ways, adopting either a mixing vessel or a plug—flow reactor. A general
trend of the animal cell bioreactor development is to achieve a high cell
concentration; this is usually accomplished by some mechanism of retaining cells
in the bioreactor. In a number of these bioreactors the cell concentration can
be ten times that achievable in roller bottles. To accommodate the higher
reaction rate encountered at higher cell concentrations, fed—batch replenishment
or continuous perfusion of medium has been used. Most developments listed in
Figure 1 have proven successful technologically, some even commercially.
However, in some cases the design of the bioreactor is still empirical; in
almost all cases the operation of the perfusion is arbitrary. In the following
we will describe the challenges we face in designing two types of bioreactors
and in the operation of perfusion cultures.

ROTATING WIRE-CAGE BIOREACTOR

One of the cell retention stirred—tank bioreactors which has stimulated
much interest in the last few years is the wire—cage bioreactor. It was first
reported in 1969[1] and was subsequently successfully applied to the cultivation
of hybridoma cells.[2] The configuration of a wire—cage bioreactor is shown in
Figure 2. The liquid circulates upward inside the draft tube and downward
outside the draft tube. Fresh medium is fed continuously into the bioreactor
and spent medium is withdrawn from inside the cage at the same rate to maintain
a constant volume. As fluid passes through the wire cage some cells are
retained in the outside region, thus resulting in a higher cell concentration
outside the cage. The opening of the wire cage ranges from 25 to 64 μm. The
mean diameter of the cells is in the range of 10 to 15 μm. Cell concentration

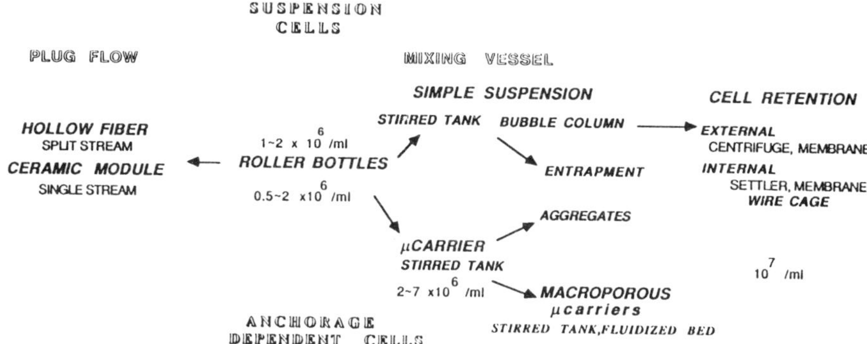

Figure 1. Historical development of animal cell bioreactors.

as high as 10^7 cells/ml has been reported.[2] Because the opening is larger than the cells, this device is not a simple filter and is not readily plugged by filter cake after a short time of operation. The mechanism of cell retention by wire cage is not well understood, thus making its scale—up difficult. Under normal operating conditions, the terminal settling velocity caused by the centrifugal field on the cells will tend to move the cells away from the cage. However, this velocity is at least one order of magnitude lower than that of liquid moving inward to the wire cage. Therefore, centrifugal force is unlikely to be the dominant mechanism responsible for cell retention. Another possible mechanism is related to hydrodynamic effect, probably one that is similar to the movement of small particles away from the wall in a Poiseuille flow.[3]

We have performed preliminary studies on the mechanism of cell retention in a wire—cage bioreactor. Instead of using cells in culture, we used latex beads with 10.2 ± 0. μm in diameter and a specific density of 1.02.[4] The

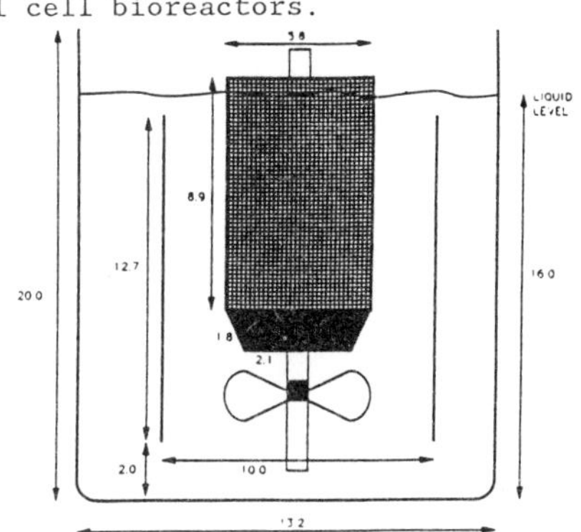

Figure 2. An experimental wire—cage bioreactor.

experiments were carried out with phosphate buffer saline (PBS) and with a
perfusion rate of 3.4 v/v/d (volume per volume per day) or without perfusion.
Two types of initial conditions were used, one with particles present only
outside the wire cage, the other with equal concentrations of particles both
inside and outside the wire cage. The ratio of particle concentration inside
the cage to that outside the cage thus changed from an initial value of 0 or 1
to a new steady–state value as the experiment proceeded. The ratio at the
steady state is defined as the discharge factor. The lower the discharge factor
is, the more efficient the system is in retaining the particles. We hypothesize
that the mechanism of particle transfer across the cage with perfusion is
different from that without perfusion. With perfusion particles are transferred
by convection, while without perfusion the particles are transferred by
diffusion. The material balances for the particles inside and that outside the
cage during perfusion can be written as

$$V_o \frac{dC_o}{dt} = - F\alpha C_o + FC_i \tag{1}$$

$$V_i \frac{dC_i}{dt} = - F\alpha C_o + FC_i \tag{2}$$

Those for the cases without perfusion are

$$V_o \frac{dC_o}{dt} = - kA(\alpha C_o - C_i) \tag{3}$$

$$V_i \frac{dC_i}{dt} = k'A(\alpha C_o - C_i) \tag{4}$$

where V is volume of the liquid; C is the concentration of particles; F is the
flow rate; subscript o and subscript i denote variables outside and inside of
the wire cage, respectively; A is the area available for transfer; k and k' are
the equivalent of mass transfer coefficient. We further assumed that the
discharge factor (α) as shown in the above equations remained constant in
transient states. The results of one set of such experiments comparing the
presence and absence of a draft with perfusion is shown in Figure 3. The ratio
of particle concentrations inside to that outside the wirecage decrease from an
initial value of 1 to approximately 0.4 and 0.8, respectively. It thus appears

that the presence of the draft tube has a beneficial effect in particle
retention. Shown in Figure 4 are the results with different agitation rates.
The experiment was carried out without perfusion. Particle retention improved
when the agitation rate was increased from 30 rpm to 100 rpm; however, when the
agitation rate was increased even further, the particle retention was decreased

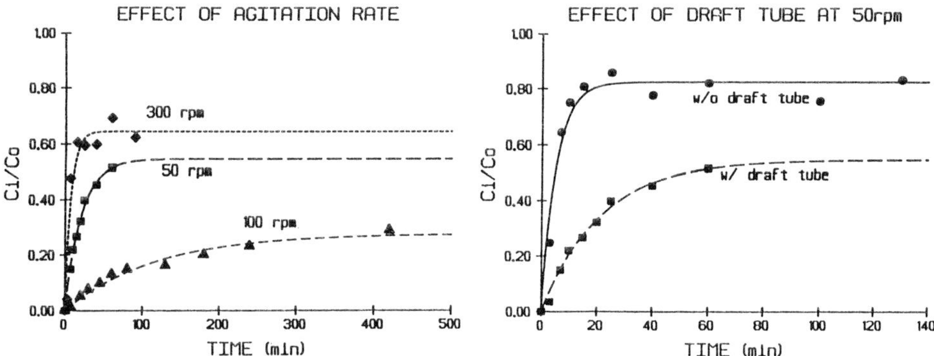

Figure 3. Effect of agitation rate
on discharge ratio.

Figure 4. Effect of draft tube on
discharge ratio.

and the discharge factor increased. Therefore there appeared to be an optimal
range of agitation rate for particle retention. The results also indicate that
the centrifugal force is not the major mechanism for cell retention. If it were
the major mechanism, one would expect that the discharge facotr decreases
monotonically with increasing agitation rate. From a series of experiments
without perfusion, we determined the value of k in Equations 3 and 4 to be in
the range of 0.02 to 0.18 cm/min. In the case with perfusion, the velocity of
fluid flow across the cage is 0.17 cm/min. The value of k is thus in the same
order of magnitude as that of fluid velocity across the cage in the case with
perfusion. If a diffusive type of mechanism is truly responsible for particle
transfer across the wire cage in the case without perfusion, one would expect a
much lower value of k due to the large particle size. Therefore, our results
suggest that the true mechanism of particle retention in the case without
perfusion is probably not a diffusive one. It is conceivable that even in the
absence of perfusion there may be fluid into and out of the cage at different
-locations of the cage; however, since there is no perfusion the net flow rate
has to be zero. We are currently performing fluid visualization studies to
examine if this hypothesis is true. This example clearly shows that even though

the wire—cage bioreactor is getting widespread applications in animal cell culture processing, our understanding of its operating mechanism is rather limited.

A NEW CELL ENTRAPMENT BIOREACTOR

Cells in a bioreactor are equivalent to the catalysts in a heterogenous chemical reactor. Ideally they should be kept in the bioreactor as long as they are metabolically or catalytically active. The holding time for cells therefore should be almost infinite. The high molecular compounds in a cell culture medium which are comprised of growth factors, serum proteins, ,etc. should be retained in the bioreactor for a long but finite period so that they can be utilized efficiently and eventually be replenished. Most cell culture products are also of high molecular weight and should be allowed to accumulate in the bioreactor to a high concentration. Therefore, the high molecular compounds should also have long but finite holding time. The small molecular weight compounds are mostly components of basal medium and metabolites excreted by cells. These compounds in general should have a short holding time so that metabolites do not accumulate to a high concentration. Therefore, an ideal bioreactor should have three different holding times for cells, high molecularand low molecular components. Such a bioreactor was achieved by combining cell entrapment and a hollow—fiber bioreactor.[5] Cells suspended in a solution of collagen or a mixture of collagen and chitosan were loaded into the lumen of hollow fibers. After the temperature was brought up to 37°C, collagen fibers began to form and cells were entrapped in the gel. Subsequently contraction occurred and the diameter of the fiber reduced to 40—60% its original value. A new zone was thus created inside the lumen of the hollow fiber which was occupied by liquid. The schematic diagram of a single fiber is shown in Figure 5. Only small molecular weight compounds diffuse through the hollow fiber membrane. The low molecular weight basal medium stream was recirculated through the extracapillary space while the high molecular weight

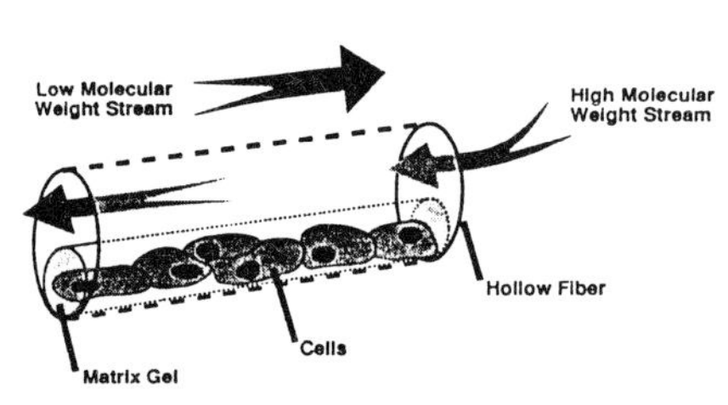

Figure 5. A two—compartment three—zone bioreactor.

species were retained inside the lumen and were harvested and replenished intermittently. Three different holding times for low molecular weight, high molecular weight compounds and cells were achieved in such a hollow fiber bioreactor.

Recombinant 293 cells producing Protein C were cultivated in this reactor. The medium used was a 3:1 mixture of DME/F12. Initially 5% FBS was used. After 15 days of cultivation DME/F12 without serum supplement was used both inside and outside the lumen. Both glucose consumption and Protein C production remained at relatively constant rate over a 60-day period (Figure 6).

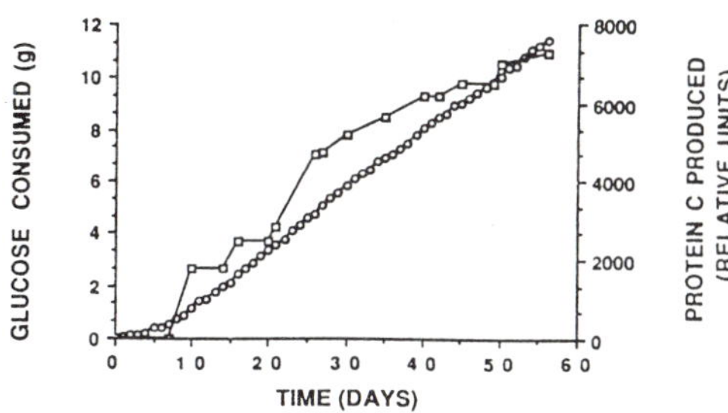

Figure 6. Cumulative glucose consumption and Protein C production in the two-compartment three-zone bioreactor.

Shown in Figure 7 is a micrograph of a thin section of 293 cells entrapped in the gel. Cells are very densely packed in the gel and the nuclei appear to be normal.

This approach of bioreactor design appears to be rational; however, its operation is still empirical. The timing of switching from serum-containing medium to protein-free medium and the selection of medium replenishment rate were largely determined by empiricism. Furthermore the mass transfer characteristics, especially those for growth factors, are poorly understood. The consumption or degradation rate of growth factors or the production rate of autocrine are unavailable. Our poor understanding of the mass transfer and reaction kinetics of the system has hindered the development

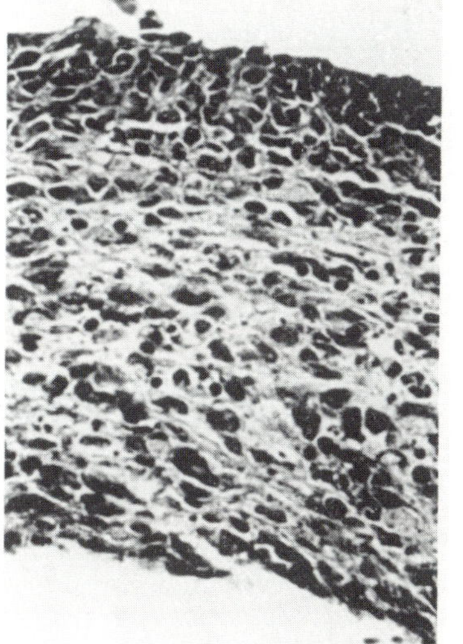

Figure 7. Micrograph of thin section of 293 cells in the gel phase.

of the operation strategy of animal cell bioreactors. Such empiricism is existent in most perfusion cultures in animal cell culture processing today.

PERFUSION RATE IN CELL RETENTION CULTURE

Shown in Figure 8 is a schematic diagram of a cell culture bioreactor equipped with a microfilter membrane for cell retention. The culture was operated in a batch fashion until the cell concentration reached approximately 10^6/ml (Figure 9). Two exhaust streams were employed: the one passing through the microfiltration membrane was cell-free, while the other carried cells at a concentration equaled to that in the reactor. The flow rates as well as the ratio of the two exhaust streams,

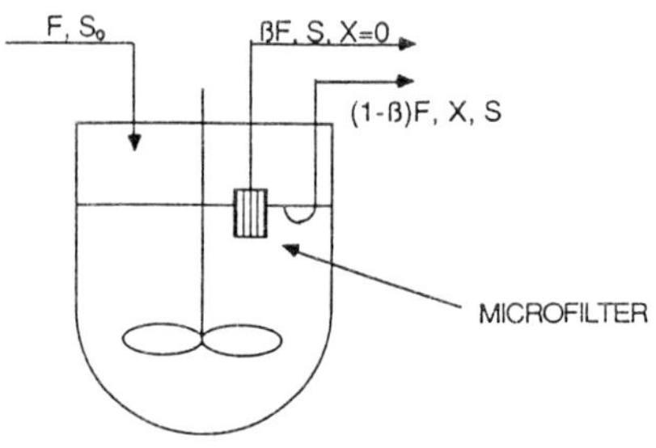

Figure 8. Schematic diagram of a cell retention bioreactor with microfilter.

defined as retention factor (β), were controlled by a computer. The total volume of the reactor was maintained constant. Balances on viable and dead cells, and substrate and product give

$$V\frac{dx_v}{dt} = V(\mu - \mu_d)x_v-(1-\beta)Fx_v \tag{5}$$

$$V\frac{dx_d}{dt} = V\mu_d\, x_v - (1-\beta)Fx_d \tag{6}$$

$$V\frac{ds}{dt} = F(s_f-s) - q_sx_vV \tag{7}$$

$$V\frac{dp}{dt} = q_px_vV-Fp \tag{8}$$

The symbols used are: x_v, x_d, viable and dead cell concentrations, respectively (cells/ml); V, volume (l); F, flow rate (l/hr); μ, μ_d, specific growth and death rate (hr^{-1}); s, substrate concentration; p, product concentration; q_p, specific product formation rate; q_s, specific substrate consumption rate; subscript f denotes concentration in the feed. It was assumed that only viable cells consume substrate and produce antibody. The initial perfusion rate was set at 5 ml/hr (corresponding to a dilution of 0.013 hr^{-1} at 400 ml working volume), with retention ratio β of 1.0 (thus no cells in the exit media flow stream). This dilution rate was maintained until the residual glucose concentration started to fall below 1 mg/ml. The specific glucose consumption rate and the specific growth rate were determined after each sampling point and used to calculate the glucose demand for the next 12–hour period assuming that the same specific growth rate and specific glucose consumption rate could be maintained. At 60 h, the retention factor, β, was changed to 0.9. As cell concentration increased further, the viability began to decrease. After 150 h the concentration of total and viable cells stabilized in 1.2–1.3 x 10^7 and 0.9–1.0 x 10^7 cells/ml, respectively, and the flow rate was not adjusted. Glucose, lactate and antibody concentrations were maintained at relatively constant levels.[6] However, even though the strategy was to maintain

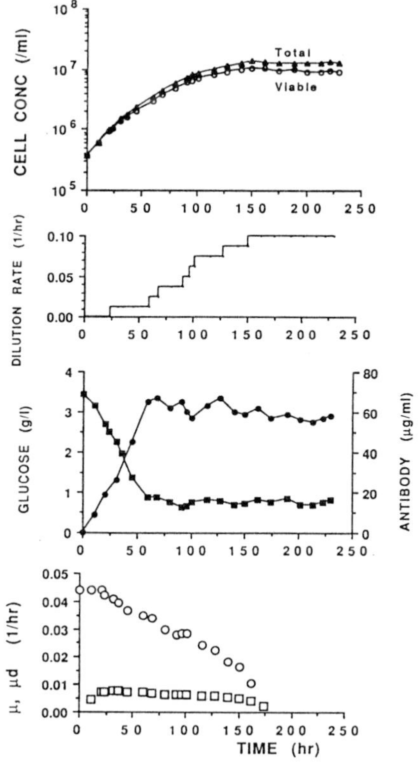

Figure 9. Growth kinetics and specific rates of AFP–27 hybridoma cells in a perfusion culture with cell retention.

a balanced growth condition by increasing the flow rate to sustain a constant glucose concentration, the specific growth rate decreased steadily after the initial stage of cultivation (Figure 9). The specific death rate increased from a very low value in the early stage to a steady level at about 40 h and remained at that value in the remaining period. Both the specific glucose consumption rate and the specific antibody production rate decreased from their peak value in the batch culture stage and reached steady level at approximately 100 h after initiation of the culture (data not shown).

Our ability to control a perfusion culture suffers from the lack of kinetic expressions for μ, μ_d, q_s, and q_p. In the results presented above, the values of these parameters were all determined from the preceding sampling period and lacked predictive power. By and large, the culture drifted to new states continuously. Ideally, we like to select the timing of the commencement of perfusion, the values of F and β as well as μ and μ_d using a predictive model which relates μ_d, q_s and q_p to a limiting substrate. Furthermore, we will also need on-line measurement of the rate-limiting substrate as well as some method of measuring cell concentration to estimate the specific rates.

CONCLUDING REMARKS

In conclusion, animal cell culture bioreactors have made great strides in the last decade; however, in a number of aspects our approach to the design and operation of the bioreactor is still relatively empirical. Shedding light on these aspects can be the new challeng and excitement for cell culture biotechnologists.

ACKNOWLEDGEMENTS

We thank the National Science Foundation (ECE-8552670), Schering Corporation, and Lilly Research Laboratories for their support.

REFERENCES

1.   Himmelfarb, P., Thayer, P.S., Martin, H.E. (1969) Spin filter culture: The propagation of mammalian cells in suspension. Science 164:555-557.

2.   Varecka, R. and Scheirer, W. (1987). Dev. Biol. Stand. 66:269-272.

3.   Brenner, H. (1966) Hydrodynamic resistance of particles. Adv. Chem. Eng. 6:377-403.

4.   Favre, E., Peringer, P., Wolden, C., Kyung, Y. S., Hu, W-S. (1990) Retention of animal cells in a rotating wire-cage bioreactor: A mechanistic study. Proceedings, Japanese Association of Animal Cell Technology, annual meeting, Tsukuba City, Japan (November 20-21, 1989).

5.   Scholz, M. and Hu, W-S. A two-compartment cell entrapment bioreactor with three different holding times for cells, high and low molecular weight compounds. Cytotechnology (accepted for publication)

6.   T. Craig Seamans (1988) Instrumentation of a cell-retention reactor for suspension culture of hybridomas. M.S. Thesis, University of Minnesota.

Hofmann: If you have a smooth surface on your spin filter by for example covering it with a micro porous membrane do you get similar results or is the microturbulence generated by your mesh important?

Shou-Hu: The mesh has an unknown effect if it is too small you get a cake; if too large a pore the cells will pass through.

Hofmann: Did you check the effect of the orientation of your mesh?

Shou-Hu: The configurations do affect the fluid flows but all of them can work.

Emery: In the case where cells liberate product when they die there is a case for growing the cells as rapidly as possible and then generating the product following cell lysis in contradistinction to other cell lines which secrete product in either the absence of cell growth or when increasing in cell mass slowly.

Shou-Hu: You are right, the type of cells I used do not require growth for product formation.

Hwang: Do you think you could lower the discharge ratio by not spinning the spin-filter but by circulating the rest of the medium?

Shou-Hu: No.

Bernard: Do you think you can achieve cell proliferation in your shrinking gel reactor?

Shou-Hu: It is cell type dependent. For the 293 cell type it appears they are not dividing and the cells appear not to be dying either as the lactate dehydrogenase concentration is very low. Hybridomas constantly divide in the gel.

Schierer: If you are using a non-homogeneous screen it is important to mount it with the correct orientation; with regard to Shou-Hu's statement that scale-up is difficult, we did a lot of experiments in scaling-up by keeping some characteristic parameters constant and we went from 22 to 250L. The scale-up parameters are similar to those of an air-lift. All the parameters seem to improve as you scale-up; the problem is when you scale-down.

Shou-Hu: You certainly are one of the most experienced people but I believe at this time you need good luck.

Bushell: Have you thought of using an empirical model reduction
                technique such as principle components analysis to make
                some sense of your cold fusion experiments.

Shou-Hu: No, we have not.

Steiner: How do the optimum conditions for retention depend on
                the perfusion rate used in the experiments?

Shou-Hu: We do not have enough experimental data but over a
                limited range of perfusion rates it does not have much
                effect on cell retention but this was over a narrow
                range.

MAMMALIAN CELL FERMENTATION:
Are specialized bioreactors a necessity?

Persson, Bo, J. Kierulff and C. Emborg
Dept. of Biotechnology, Centre for Food and Process Biotechnology, The Technical University of Denmark.

INTRODUCTION.

The expanding research in the field of mammalian cell
fermentation has carried along the entry of a lot of different fermentation equipment on the market (1). Despite all
the great efforts and hard work done so far, none of these
systems has proven to be superior. The question therefore
emerge, if such specialized bioreactors are necessary at all,
for a satisfactory research on mammalian cell fermentations.
We doubt it, at least as concerns laboratory-scale fermentation. Obviously there are some major problems with the cells
in the area of shear-sensitivity and others (2,3), but
nevertheless we believe, that taking the cells through a
gentle stepwise adaption, one can grow mammalian cells in
such simple equipments as shake-flasks, big spinnerflasks,
spin-bar devices and modified bacterial fermentors, with
allmost the same production yield, as one can get from most
of the specialized mammalian cell reactors, available on the
market today.
In this paper we report on some preliminary fermentations
made with <u>non-adapted cells</u> in several different "home-made"
reactors. The results are compared with fermentations done
under same conditions in a Biostat MC bioreactor.
Our results show, that mammalian cells not necessesarily are
so fragile and shear-sensitive as believed, and that one
might change attitude toward the basic considerations for
shear-forces etc. in mammalian cell fermentations.
Also it is interesting to see, that maximum specific production rate (i.e. max. production/cell in growth phase/hr) is
higher in the "low-technology" systems, than in the Biostat
MC.

MATERIALS & METHODS:

Cell lines: All preliminary studies was carried out with a
x63-Ag8.653-derived mouse/mouse hybridoma cell line, NUC 1-
4, a low-producer of monoclonal antibodies against the enzyme
nuclease. The cell line was established on The Technical
University of Denmark (DTH) in 1987. Further investigations
used other cell lines, e.g. NUC 1-2, STI 4C6 (mouse/mouse
hybridomas (DTH)) and BHK-21 cells (GBF, W.-Germany)).
Media: Standard DMEM (Biochrom) with 10% fetal calf serum was
used in all experiments. There was no antibiotics added to
the media.
Fermentation parameters: Batch fermentations carried out
under following standard conditions: Temperature: 37°C; pH:
7,2 - 7,4; DO: 40% with regard to atm. air; CO_2: 5% and
agitation was varied in the range: 60 - 180 rpm.
Equipment: As reference system we used a Biostat MC (B.Braun,

Melsungen, W.-Germany), and results from other systems (**fig. 1**, made at DTH) has been compared to the values optained from the Biostat MC. The working volume was in all cases 300-600 ml (i.e. small scale systems).

Equipment	Vessel	Temp.contr.	Stirring	speed (rpm)	Aeration
Biostat MC	round bottom	water jacket	marine impeller	80	silicone tubing
Blue-cap bottle	flat bottom	incubator	spin-bar	180	small bubbles
Plastic jar	flat bottom	incubator	spin-bar device	80	surface
Ordinary shakeflask	flat bottom	incubator	orbital shaker	100	surface
Bacterial fermentor	flat bottom	incubator	turbine impeller	80	silicone tubing

Fig. 1: *Different kind of equipment used*

<u>RESULTS</u>:
For the clearness of this report, only results from fermentations with the cell line NUC 1-4 is shown. It is clear from **fig. 2** that while the cells in the "low-technology" systems need quite a lag fase, before they begin to grow, the Biostat MC very fast brings the cells into growth phase. Also we see, that the amount of (viable) cells obtained in the specialized reactor are several fold higher than even the best home-made system. The high cell number brings along a relative good amount of product (**fig. 3**), but both the cell number and the yield (IgG) decreases rapidly after about 144 hours of fermentation. In contrast to this, we find, that despite the extended lag phase in the simple systems, they do support cell growth and a fairly good antibody production. Also it looks as if the product-degradation rate is slower in most of the simple systems, than in the Biostat MC.
Looking behind the figures in the graphs in figs. 1 & 2, and calculating the maximum specific production rate (i.e. max. production/cell in growth fase/hr), the situation is as pictured in **table 1**. From this table it is obvious that cells grown in socalled "low-technology"-systems -(with one exeption)- have a much higher maximum specific production rate, than found in the specialized Biostat MC. Even the blue-cap bottle, which has a quite simple stirring device that runs with a relatively high speed shows better figures than the Biostat MC.

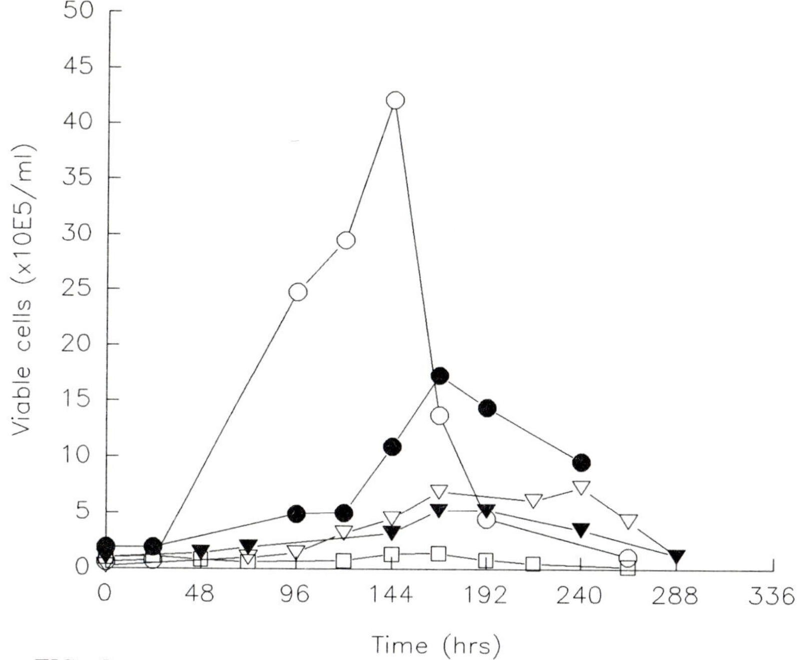

FIG. 2:

○ Biostat MC
● Bluecap−bottle with bubble−aeration & spinbar
▽ Plastic−jar with surface−aeration & spinbar−device
▼ Traditional shakeflask
□ Bacterial fermentor with bubble−free aeration

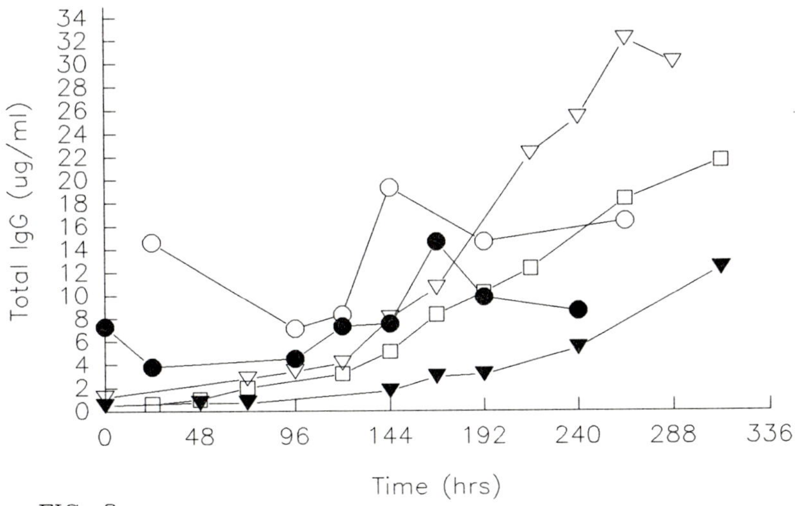

FIG. 3:

DISCUSSION:

Our results support the general assumption that specialized bioreactors for mammalian cell fermentations improve cell growth and production yields (4). In our case it is obvious, that the Biostat MC support cell growth and antibody-production perceptibly, compared to the "low-technology"-systems tested. A guess is that this is due to a better pH- and DO- control in the Biostat MC, since high-speed stirring (>200 rpm) in the Biostat MC (data not shown) do not influence considerably on these figures. However, in case of maximum specific production rate, the situation is totally different: Here we find, that allmost all the simple systems show significant better figures, than the Biostat MC. Thus even if the cells grow rather slow with a long lag period (adaption?), they are completely capable of producing good amounts of antibodies. Since we must assume to find inferior growth conditions in the "home-made" equipment, compared to the specialized systems, this means, that the cells presumably are more resistant to conditions such as high shear, pH- and/or DO-fluctuations etc., than formerly assumed. This again means that a slow and gentle adaption of the cells might improve cell growth and product formation even in rather simple fermentation equipment. Therefore we believe, that at least in laboratory-scale, one can reach very far by concentrating on cell adaption instead of making huge investments in specialized fermentation systems. On the other hand: Because of the superior monitoring- and control abilities build into most specialized reactors today, we certainly need such systems, when it comes to continuous fermentation, pilot- and production-scale fermentations and similar arrangements. However, also in this area we believe, that cell adaption might solve some up-scaling problems (e.g. shear, in-homogenious medias etc.) in large-scale mammalian cell fermentation today.

Table 1:

Equipment	Max. Spec. Prod. Rate (grams/cell/hr)
Biostat MC	1.60 x10E-13
Blue-cap bottle	2.75 x10E-13
Plastic jar	5.08 x10E-13
Ordinary shakeflask	1.56 x10E-13
Bacterial fermentor (modified)	10.90 x10E-13

REFERENCES:
1. Van Brunt,J. et al. <u>Bio/Technology</u>, 1987, <u>5</u>, 1134-1138
2. Cherry,RS. et al. <u>Bioprocess Engineering</u>, 1986, <u>1</u>, 29-41
3. Marquis,CP. et al. <u>Cytotechnology</u>, <u>2</u>, 163-170
4. Feder/Tolbert:<u>"Large Scale Mammalian Cell Culture"</u>, (1985)

Section 6.2
Bioreactors: hardware

ENGINEERING FOR STERILITY AND CONTAINMENT:
DESIGN OF A 225L "POLYMODAL" FERMENTER FOR THE CONTAINMENT OF P3
PATHOGENS

Ross Cameron*Bryan Griffiths+ and Peter Hambleton+.

* European Collection of Animal Cell Cultures, PHLS CAMR, Porton Down,
Salisbury, SP4 OJG, UK. +Biologics Division, PHLS CAMR, Porton
Down, Salisbury, SP4 OJG, UK.

ABSTRACT

The design approaches to the maintenance of sterility and containment
in large scale fermentation plants desccribed together with the
solutions arrived at in the design and fabrication of a multi-purpose
225 dm³ fermentation pilot plant capable of being used for the
growth of animal cells or bacteria under P3 containment conditions
as defined by the UK government Advisory Commiittee on Dangerous
Pathogens.

INTRODUCTION

In the planning and design of fermentation equipment for
pharmaceuticals development and production applications there
is, in the main, an absolute requirement for sterility to be
maintained during operation. Provisions must also be made to
contain the process if hazardous. It is inevitable that the design
of equipment which meets pharamaceutical production standards
for high integrity in terms of maintenance of sterility and providing
containment will lead to increased complexity and thus greater
expense. Avoiding contamination and maintaining a contained
environment are essentially compatible and form the basis of a
common solution to design problems.

DESIGN CONSIDERATIONS

The technology required for the reliable and long-term maintainance
of sterility of fermentation equipment has long been available
and is applicable to vessels ranging in volume from laboratory
scale to industrial production plants.
The methods of containing biohazardous processes have traditionally
been based on the isolation of the process from the environment
by the use of microbiological safety cabinets. This approach
becomes impractical as processes are scaled-up due to the increasing
size of process equipment. We have considered the reactor itself
as the primary containment barrier and in this context Figure
1 shows the "microbial transport pathways" on a fermenter which
require protection.

DESGIN SOLUTIONS

Steam Barrier Isolation

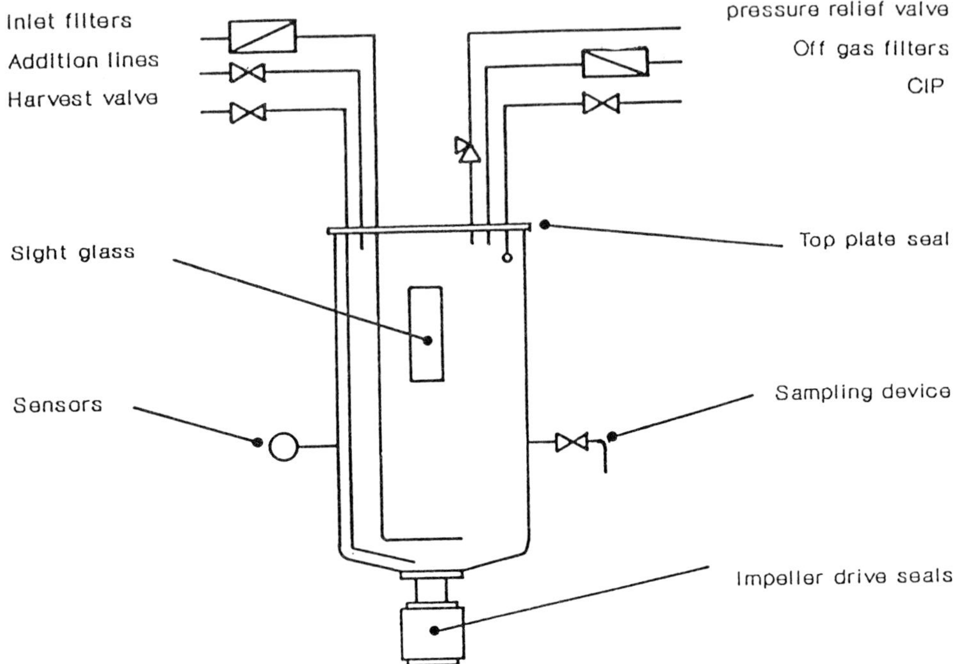

Figure 1. Components on a conventional stirred tank reactor which
could present a safety hazard if component failure occurs.

All addition and process lines which enter the main reactor and
harvest vessels can be blocked with steam when not in use.

Impeller Drive Shaft Seals

Double mechanical seals are deployed when the reactor has either
the high speed bottm drive assembly (bacterial cultures) or the
low speed top drive assembly (animal cell cultures) fitted. The
seals are lubricated and leakage protection achieved by the use
of live steam lubrication of the seal housing. A low power
magnetically coupled drive option is also available.

Static Seals

When sealing large diameter orifices such as the lid seal and
air filter housings double "O"- rings with a steam trace have
been used. This sealing method was not considerd to be suitable
for small orifices such as sensor ports and in such cases triple
"O"-ring seals have been used.

Gas Filters

The inlet filters and off-gas lines are fitted with double HEPA filters
and steam tracing as described above. Should filter binding occur
an over-pressure sensor on the fermenter head plate will shut down
the gas feed to the fermenter. Double addition
vessel pressurisation filters are fitted.All filters can be replaced
whilst a fermentation is on-going and can be fully validated by
the PALL Forward Flow method.

Sampling and Sensor Ports

The lack of a validated high containment sampling device has resulted
in a need to isolate the sample and sensor port area. This has
been achieved by the innovative use of a flexible isolator (Isotec
Ltd., Bicester, UK) fitted to a flange welded to the reactor and
providing localised Class III secondary containment.

Harvest Line

To avoid the use of a submerged bottom mounted harves valve an
internal dip tupe has been used.

Steam Condensate

All steam traps are of a hermetically sealed design welded into
a common manifold leading to the effluent treatment tank.

Pipework

All process lines are continuously welded, with short pipe runs
designed to be self-draining.

Valves

Conventional diaphragm valves have been fitted throughout the
plant and are subject to a regime of routine maintenance including
diaphragm replacement and pressure testing.

Pressure relief system

The use of a common effluent manifold system precluded the use
of bursting discs. As an alternative a high containment spring-
loaded relief valve (Leser GmbH, FRG) has been employed.

Effluent treatment

All condensate drain lines and pressure relief valve lines lead
directly into a high containment kill tank which may be steam
sterilised. The tank is vented to atmosphere via high flow
hydrophobic filters which may be sterilised and validated in situ.

MONOCLONAL ANTIBODY PRODUCTION USING AN AIRLIFT FERMENTERSYSTEM CONSISTING OF A CONTINUOUS SEED FERMENTER AND A FED BATCH PRODUCTION FERMENTER

Kurt Konopitzky, Otto Kanzler, Katharina Windhab

BENDER VIENNA, PRODUCTION AND ENGINEERING, BIO PILOT PLANT
Dr.Boehringergasse 5-11, 1120 Vienna, Austria

INTRODUCTION

In the production of monoclonal antibodies there are available a multitude of fermentation methods. The most commonly used fermentation method is that of Batch-Fermentation; the reason being that the ''Batch-Definition'' presents conditions preferable for the quality control of an antibody batch. It also presents the least problems in maintaining sterility. The continuous fermentation method is by far the more efficient but is not as commonly used as it lacks these advantages. We have been looking for a method which combines the advantages of both fermentation methods, while minimising the disadvantages.

MATERIALS AND METHODS

Systemspecification:
The production unit consists of two Airlift-Fermenters which can have a volume of 5 l and 30 l or depending on the scale of the fermentation, 30 l and 80 l.

The fermenters are equipped with pumps which supply the media, and transport the cell-suspension from the smaller to the larger fermenter.

Specification of the cell line: Mouse-Mouse Hybridoma P3 X 63
Ag 8.653

Media specification: RPMI 1640, Gibco;
20% Tryptose Phosphate Broth, Difco;
1% FCS, free of IgG, PAA;
0,1% Pluronic F68, Serva;
$NaHCO_3$, Merck;

RESULTS

The combined advantages of the continuous and batch system were used in the following way:

The seed culture fermenter is run as a continuous system. In doing so one can achieve high cell density with an excellent viability. The production fermenter is run by the Fed-Batch method, satisfying the Batch Definition, and allowing the extraction of the cells at the end of a production. The IgG production can be dramatically improved at the end of the culture operation by reducing the viability to 40%. (Fig.1)

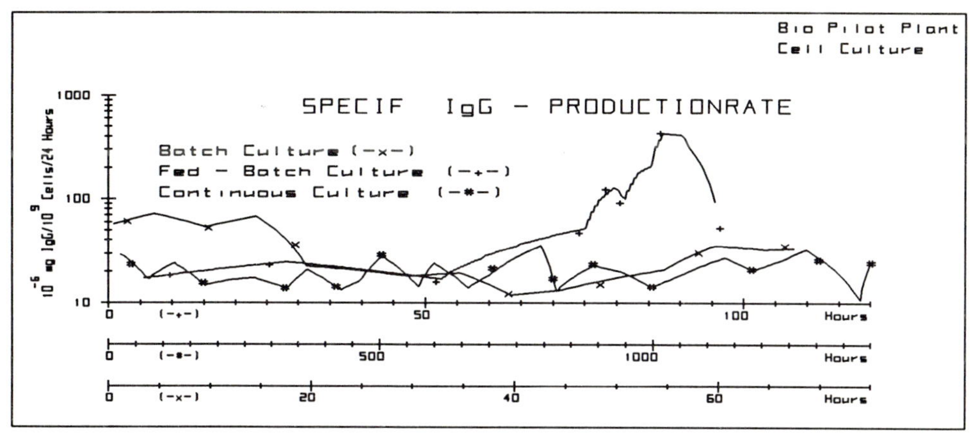

Fig. 1

Culture operation

<u>Seed culture fermenter:</u> The seed culture fermenter is inoculated at a cell density of 5×10^5 cells/ml (culture density). From the time of inoculation we used a diluton rate of 0.03 h^{-1} with a generation time of approx. 20 hours. The dilution rate is dependent on the generation time and is calculated using the following equation:

$$D_s = \frac{\ln 2 \quad x \quad 0{,}9}{T}$$

D_s = Dilutionrate Seed Fermenter

T = Generationtime

With this system we achieve a cell density of up to 4×10^6 cells/ml with a viability of 90%. (Fig.2 + 3)

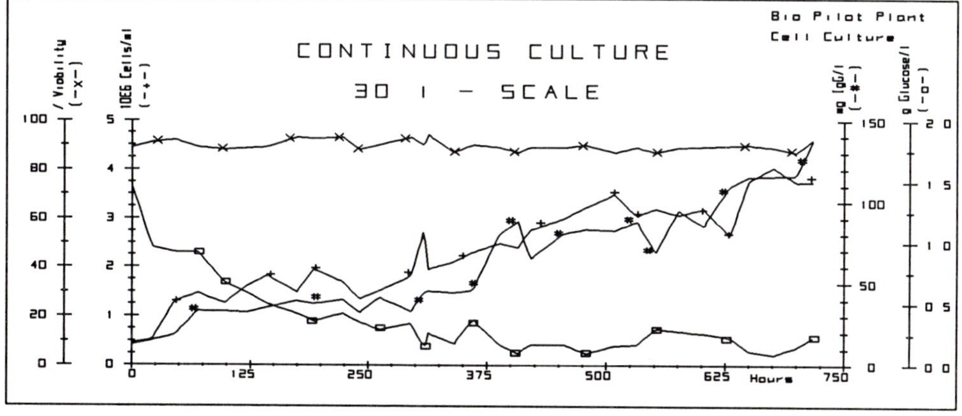

Fig. 2

391

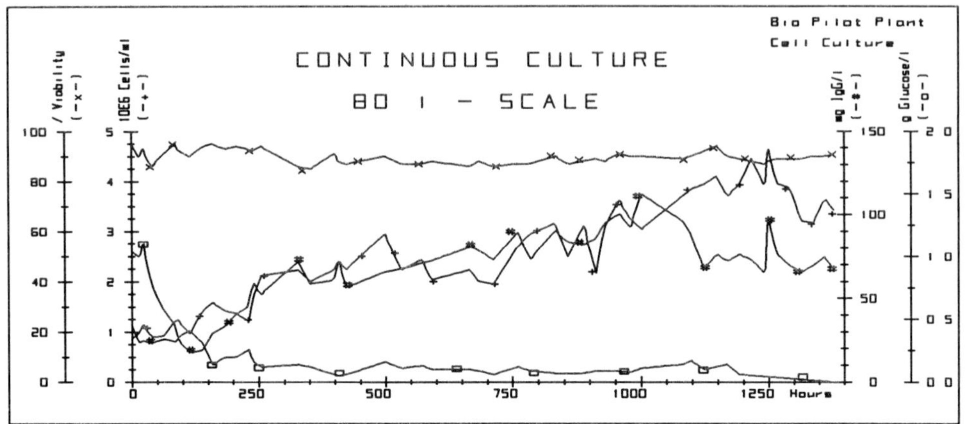

Fig. 3

<u>Production fermenter:</u> Reaching a cell density of approx. $1,5 \times 10^6$ cells/ml in the seed culture fermenter (after a period of 5 days on average) the production fermenter is charged with the cell suspension which has accumulated through the continuous operation of the seed culture fermenter. Approx. 20% of media is introduced into the Fed-Batch fermenter - the exact ammount being determined by the location of probe inlets in the fermenter design. To achieve optimum nutrition of the cells in the production fermenter further medium is fed through a second line from the beginning, according to following equation:

$$D_P = \frac{D_S \times F_{Dilution}}{3 \times F_{Vessel}}$$

$$F_{Dilution} = \frac{V_{End}}{V_{Start}}$$

$$F_{Vessel} = \frac{V_{Prod.Ferm.}}{V_{Seed\ Ferm.}}$$

D_P = Dilutionrate Prod. Fermenter
D_S = Dilutionrate Seed Fermenter
$F_{Dilution}$ = Factor Medium Dilution
V_{End} = End Volume Prod. Fermenter
V_{Start} = Start Volume Prod. Fermenter
$V_{Prod.Ferm.}$ = Volume Prod. Fermenter
$V_{Seed\ Ferm.}$ = Volume Seed Fermenter

After about 2 days, depending on cell growth, the production fermenter reaches it's fill-volume. From this point onwards, further supply of medium and cell suspension is discontinued. The seed culture fermenter continues to operate, and can either be used for feeding a second Fed Batch fermenter, or can be operated on standby until the production cycle is completed. The production fermenter is operated until a cell viability of 40-50% has been reached. During this time - that is the time of decreasing viability - the highest antibody production can be observed (Fig.4 + 5). By harvesting the fermenter using the Batch method a ''batch'' is easily defined. The whole cycle can then be repeated.

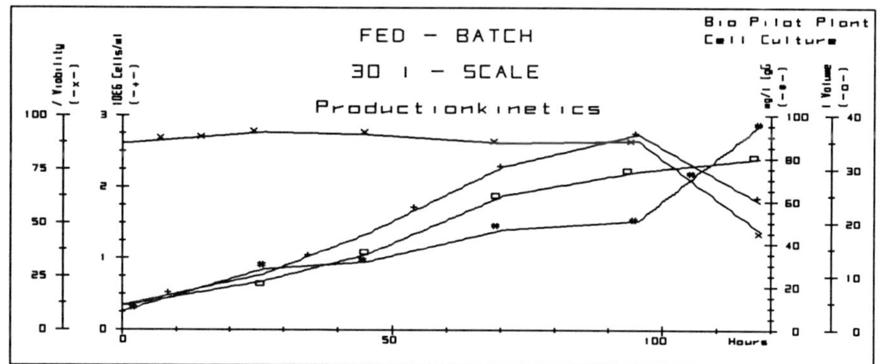

Fig. 4

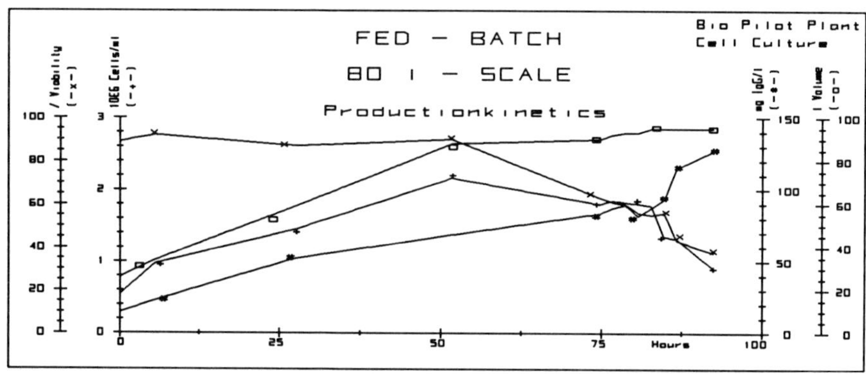

Fig. 5

CONCLUSION

Throughout the continual seed culture operation a high cell
density plus a high viability are achieved. Consequently, the
cells can be fermented over a period of months without any
problem. The advantages of the Fed Batch production are two fold.
Firstly, it is possible to harvest semi-continuous which leads
to a continual operation of the biochemical purification to
follow. Secondly, the cells can be monitored to give a high
production rate. Additionally, the requirements of the regulatory agencies are fully met.

REFERENCES

1. CONTINUOUS CULTURE: A TOOL FOR RESEARCH, DEVELOPMENT AND   PRODUCTION; C.L.Cooney; Perspectives
in Biotechnology and Applied   Microbiology; 271-285
2. A STUDY OF HYBRIDOMA CELL GROWTH AND ANTIBODY PRODUCTION KINETICS IN CONTINUOUS CULTURE; K.S.Low,
C.Harbour and J.P.Barford; Biotechnology Techniques Vol 1; No 4; 239-244; 1987/9
3. SCALE-UP ENGINEERING IN ANIMAL CELL TECHNOLOGY: PART I.; Rudolf Bliem and Hermann Katinger;
Tibtech Vol 6; 190-195; 1988/8
4. PRODUCTION OF mAb TO HUMAN IFN-_ AND THEIR USE FOR ANALYSIS OF THE ANTIGENIC COMPOSITION OF
VARIOUS NATURAL INTERFERONS; G.Adolf, G.Bodo, P.Swetly; J.of Cell.Phys.Suppl.2; 61-68; 1982
5. BATCH PRODUCTION OF MONOCLONAL ANTIBODY BY LARGE-SCALE SUSPENSION CULTURE; William B.Lebherz III;
Biopharm; 22-32; 1988/2
6. PRODUCTION KINETICS OF MONOCLONAL ANTIBODIES; O.W.Merten, S.Reiter, G.Himmler, W.Scheirer, and
H.Katinger; Develop.biol.Standard Vol 60; 219-227; 1985

BLEEDING OUT DEAD CELLS FROM FERMENTATION SYSTEMS

Torsten Björling and Ulf Malmström
Alfa-Laval Centritech AB, S-147 80 TUMBA, Sweden

ABSTRACT

In all fermentation systems some cells die as a natural part of the process. If they are allowed to remain in the fermenter, they will hamper the growth and productivity of the live cells, and in continuous and fed batch systems this may seriously reduce yield.

Experiments have shown that dead cells settle slightly slower than live cells, and this opens up the possibility to bleed out dead cells in a continuous centrifuge. Tests in a mammalian cell separator prove that this is feasible, and although complete fractionation will not be achieved, a significant portion of the dead cells can be removed from the system.

Keywords: Dead cells; bleed; centrifuge; perfusion; continuous.

INTRODUCTION

Animal cell perfusion cultures contain cells in various growth phases. Invariably, a fraction of the cell population in a perfusion culture will be non-viable. Dead cells lyse and release proteolytic enzymes that can be detrimental to the yield and quality of the (protein) product. Therefore, a continuous bleed of dead cells and cell debris out of the system should result in a better product yield and quality.

Normally dead cells sediment slightly slower than live cells in a gravitational or centrifugal field. This property opens up the possibility to fractionate live cells from dead cells (and cell debris) in a centrifugal separator. It has been observed in field trials with centrifugal cell separation (not shown here) that dead cells from various cell lines are enriched in the supernatant.

The purpose of this investigation has been to measure the bleed of dead cells from a cell culture using a continuous centrifugal separator.

MATERIALS AND METHODS

The device used was a Centritech® Cell continuous cell centrifuge (Alfa-Laval Centritech AB, Tumba, Sweden), connected to a 150 l cell reactor (Electrolux, Sweden) containing HeLa S3 cells (5×10^5 cells/ml) grown on fDMEM with 2 % serum. The cell suspension was run through the centrifuge using 6 different settings of feed rate and rotor speed. Samples were taken from feed, effluent and concentrate at each setting. Cell number and viability were counted and evaluated with Bürker chamber under the microscope using Trypan blue exclusion.

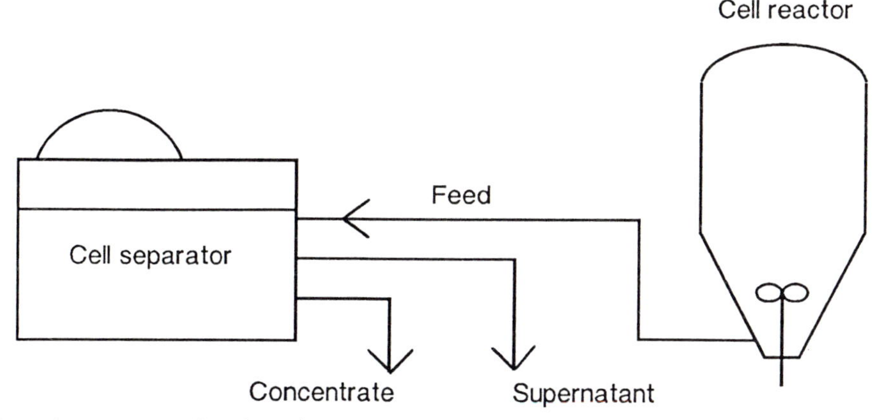

Figure 1   Experimental set-up.

RESULTS

Bleed of cells to supernatant.

The relative loss of dead and live cells from the feed to the supernatant is shown in Figure 2.

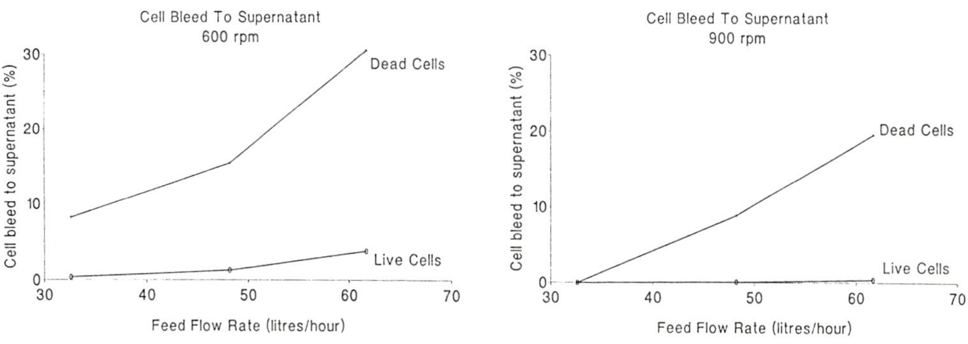

Figure 2   Effect of feed flow rate and rotor speed on the relative loss of HeLa S3 cells to supernatant.

It is evident that the proportional loss of cells to the supernatant is considerably higher for dead cells than for live cells, reflecting a slower settling rate for dead cells. High feed rate or low rotor speed increases cell numbers in the supernatant. Generally the loss of viable cells is very small.

Viability increases in concentrate.

A consequence of bleeding out dead cells to the supernatant should be a corresponding increase in viable count in the concentrate. The data shown in Figure 3 support this assumption. Again, high flow rate or low rotor speed increases viability count in the concentrate.

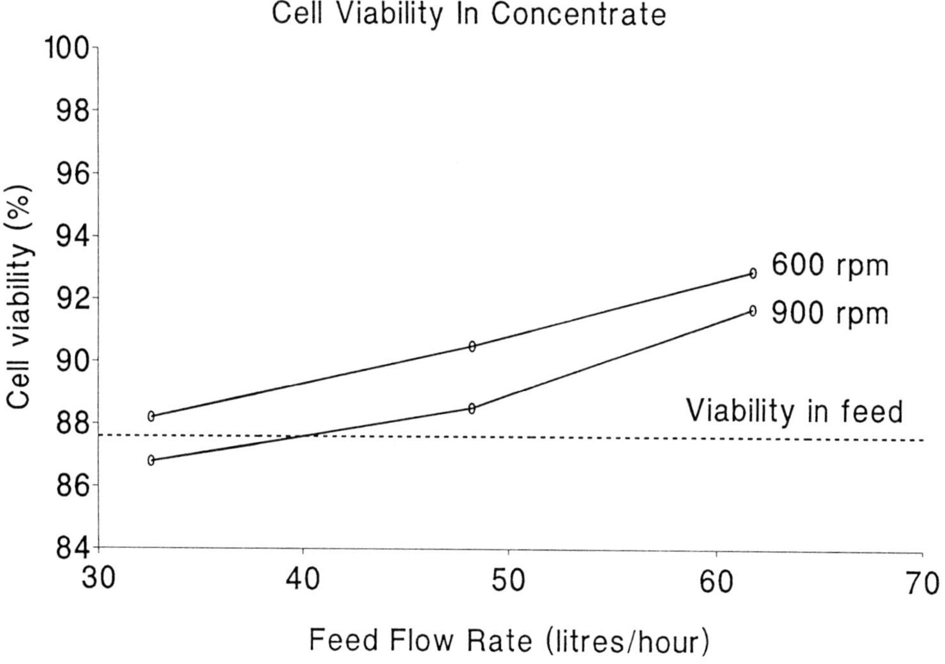

Figure 3:   Effect of feed flow rate and rotor speed on HeLa S3 cell viability in concentrate.

<u>DISCUSSION</u>

When suspension cells are cultivated in a perfusion
system they can be recycled with a continuous centrifuge.
The results of this investigation show that it is possible
to set the separation parameters so as to obtain a deliberate loss of mainly dead cells and debris to the supernatant, thus removing some potentially harmful substances
such as proteases and inert material from the culture.
This purge of the cell culture should lead to improved
oxygen and nutrient transfer, and less proteolytic activity in the cell medium, resulting in an overall improved performance of the perfusion system.

<u>ACKNOWLEDGEMENT</u>

The experimental work has kindly been carried out by
Hans Frieberg, SVA, Uppsala, Sweden.

<u>**Paper of Bjorling**</u>

Emery: It worries me that the results as presented could
               be the perfect self-fulfilling experiment. Could
               I present the hypothesis that the actual bleeding
               process kills cells?

Bjorling: We did material balances of what went in and came
               out of the centrifuge and although there is always
               a big variation, we didn't kill the cells (within
               the accuracy of the measurements). Our experience
               with long term perfusion experiments is very
               encouraging.

Brown: Using gravity sedimentation in an inclined
               sedimentation chamber we also see a selective
               removal of non-viable cells from the culture.

Bjorling: I have not tried this but it must work.

Griffiths: What density difference do you get between live and
               dead cells?

Bjorling: We have not measured this - it could be density
               difference or it could be size difference that
               makes them sediment more slowly.

Merten: Cells in batch cultures vary in diameter, between
               logarithmically growing and stationary cells. In
               a late culture you often have the same size of
               living and dead cells. Is it possible to use your
               method for stationary phase cultures?

Bjorling: I do not know for sure. We can bleed out dead
               cells in both perfusion and harvest a late batch
               culture.

Handa-Corrigan:
               How significant do you think the problem is of dead
               cells accumulating in a perfusion culture? If you
               are getting a large number of dead cells I would
               suggest that you haven't optimised your perfusion
               system or bioreactor. One should maintain over 90%
               viability so how can you justify a cell bleed
               system when it might be better to improve your
               whole process?

Bjorling: We haven't done the experiment to see what effect
               it has on a perfusion culture by trying to
               manipulate the percentage viability with this
               centrifuge.

Noe: When performing a perfusion culture you normally
              need a lot of time to perform these long term
              processes. Could you give us more information on
              the long term stability of your device? To what
              range of fermenter volumes would you recommend such
              a device?

Bjorling: The normal lifetime of the plastic separation
              insert is between 2-4 weeks, depending on the rotor
              speed. You can aseptically change these inserts.
              The ideal culture medium is less than 1000 litres
              and more than 5 litres.

HIGH INTENSITY GROWTH OF ADHERENT CELLS ON A POROUS CERAMIC MATRIX

D. W. Lee, J.R. Grace, P. Allardyce and D.G. Kilburn
Biotechnology Laboratory, University of British Columbia
Vancouver, B.C., Canada V6T 1W5

ABSTRACT

A perfusion culture system has been developed which utilizes a porous ceramic foam for the cultivation of adherence–dependent cells. The cells grow within the interconnected pores of a rigid, reticulated, alumina foam matrix. Concentrations of BHK cells in excess of 10^8 per ml of matrix volume have been achieved. Stable expression of human transferrin in these cells was maintained at high levels (2.4 μg 10^6 cell^{-1} day^{-1}) for a period of greater than 4 weeks. Vero cells grown in the matrix could be recovered readily by trypsinization making this system suitable for the large–scale preparation of inocula for other cultivation systems such as conventional or porous microcarrier cultures. The matrix can be installed in stirred tank or air lift reactors and is amenable to scale–up.

INTRODUCTION

A variety of systems are used for large–scale animal cell growth at high cell concentration. These include microcarriers, hollow fibers, encapsulation, packed beds, and porous matrices. Those in which medium is continuously perfused through immobilized cells offer the potential for growing cells in an environment that mimics their in–vivo existence. Cell densities in perfusion systems far exceed those reached in traditional suspension cultures (e.g. 10^8–10^9 cell/ml as opposed to a maximum of 5×10^6 cell/ml[1]). These methods also allow more efficient utilization of medium, the possibility of production phases with reduced serum[2], and faster, simpler purification of a cell–free, low serum, concentrated product. Perfusion of high density, immobilized cells offers a relatively cheap and efficient method for production of proteins.

This paper describes the use of a rigid, ceramic matrix as a substrate for adhesion and growth of animal cells to high densities in a recirculating perfusion system. The system combines the advantages of immobilization with the use of a supporting matrix that is cheap, reusable, has variable pore sizes and volumes, and is suitable for the growth of a variety of adherent cell types.

MATERIALS AND METHODS

Cell Lines

Vero cells and transformed BHK 21 cells producing human transferrin[3] were maintained in flasks or roller bottles in DMEM supplemented with 5% FCS. The recombinant BHK cell expresses transferrin under the control of the MT–1 metallothionein promoter. A dihydrofolate reductase gene coding for a mutant form of the enzyme with low affinity for methotrexate (MTX) allows for the selection of transformants in high concentrations of MTX (0.5mM). The medium used for transferrin production was a mixture of DMEM and F12 (50:50) containing 5% FCS and gentamycin (0.1mg L^{-1}). MTX (0.5mM) was included only during the preparation of inocula and the first 3 days of large-scale cultures.

Culture system

The perfusion system (Figure 1) provides a continuous supply of aerated medium from the equilibration vessel to the ceramic support. The matrix (manufactured by Selee Corporation, Hendersonville, N.C., Figure 2) consists of a reticulated lattice of sintered alumina with a sponge-like structure. In the present work, a 40 ml cylindrical matrix with a pore size rated as 30 pores per inch was used. Oxygen probes in the equilibration vessel and in-line directly after the growth vessel allowed oxygen uptake rates to be monitored continuously.

Assays

Total immobilized cell counts were determined at the end of each run by nuclei counts following prolonged recirculation of citric acid/crystal violet mixture (1:10) through the matrix. Glucose and lactate concentrations were analysed using enzyme-based electrode. Recombinant human transferrin concentration was determined by ELISA.

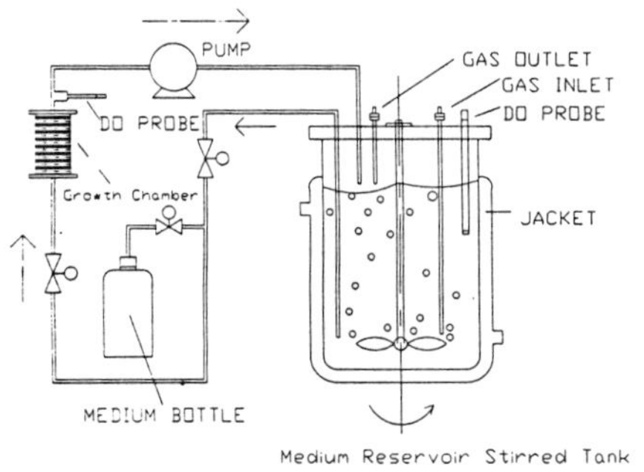

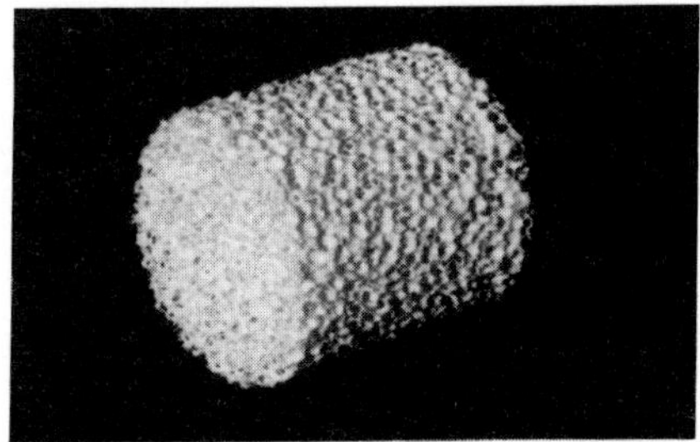

Figure 1–Culture system. The ceramic matrix and equilibration vessel were maintained at 37ºC. A mixture of air, 5% CO_2 was sparged into the equilibration vessel, controlled on the basis of pO2

Figure 2–Ceramic cylinderical matrix with a 3.5 cm diameter. The void space of the matrix is about 80%.

RESULTS

Cell growth on the ceramic surface

A series of scanning electron micrographs were taken to show the progressive stages of cell growth on the ceramic surface. The initial attachment and spread of cells onto the surface of the ceramic matrix were very similar to what was seen in flasks. The cells flattened and extended following attachment and grew to confluence (Figure 3A). Continued growth ultimately resulted in a multilayered tissue about 10 cells deep (Figure 3B).

Estimation of total cell number

Total cell concentration on the ceramic support was estimated on the basis of glucose uptake rate and oxygen uptake rate (OUR). Figure 4 shows the glucose uptake rate during the course of a culture of BHK cells. This reached steady state after about 20 days. Based on a specific glucose uptake rate of 0.46 g day^{-1} per 10^9 cells[4] for BHK cells, the final cell count was estimated to be 5 x 10^9 total cells, equivalent to 1.2 x 10^8 cells ml^{-1} of matrix or 1.6 x 10^{11} cells m^{-2} of ceramic surface. Cell recovery of cell nuclei from the matrix was about 70% of this value. Figure 5 shows the cumulative glucose consumption and lactate production for Vero cells grown in this system. The estimated final cell concentration was 1.3 x 10^8 cells ml^{-1}.

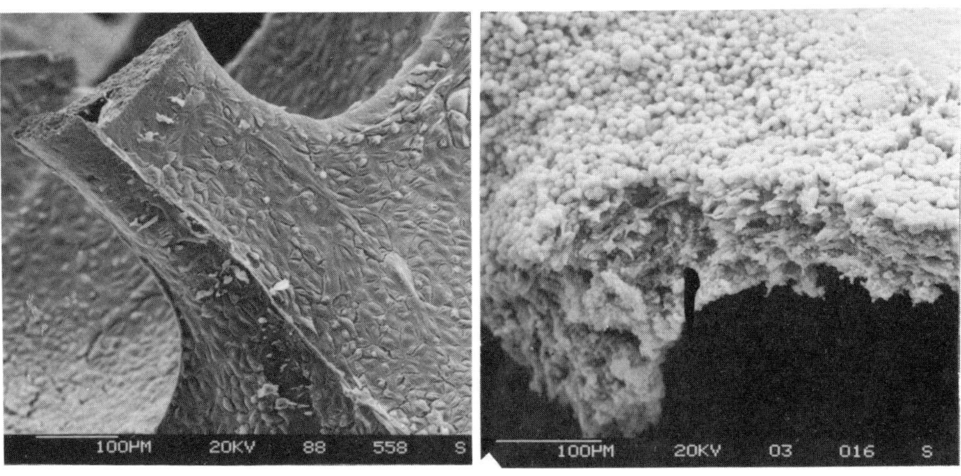

(A)   (B)

Figure 3–SEM photographs of BHK cells grown on ceramic surface. A: confluent monolayer 8 days after seeding. B: multilayer tissue after 20 days of culture.

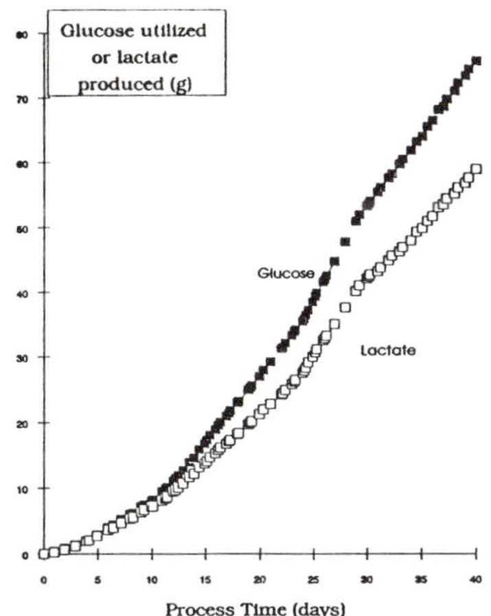

Figure 4–Glucose consumption and lactate production, BHK cells.

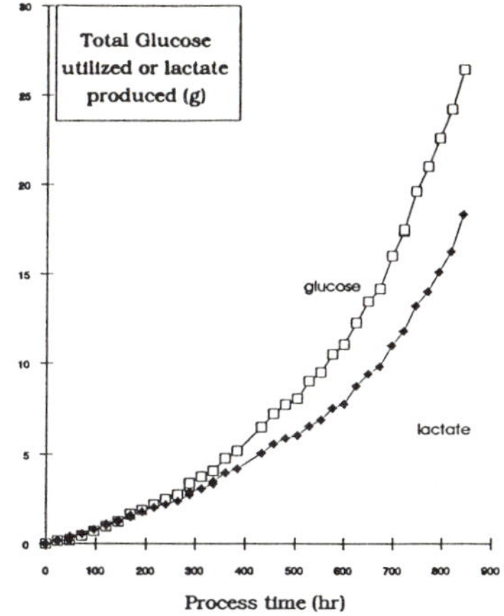

Figure 5–Glucose consumption and lactate production, Vero cells.

Transferrin production

Figure 6 shows the cumulative production of transferrin for cells grown in DMEM or in DMEM/F12. Zinc present in F12 acts as an inducer of the metallothionien promoter. Under induced conditions at steady–state the culture produce up to 30 mg day^{-1} (6 mg per 10^9 cells^{-1} day^{-1}).

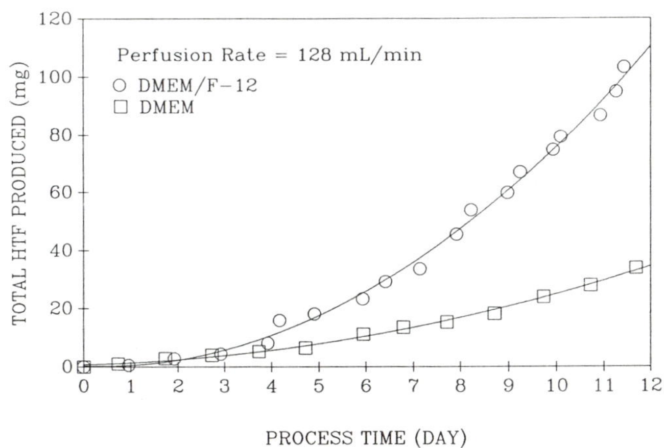

Figure 6–Induction of transferrin production. At time zero medium containing Zn was added to DMEM/F–12. Control culture in DMEM without Zn.

DISCUSSION

The ceramic substrate used in these experiments provides a large surface for growth within a cartridge of relatively small volume. The ceramic is cheap, reusable, available in many pore sizes and volumes, requires no special pretreatment for adhesion, and is able to support growth of a variety of adherent cell lines. Blockage of pores and subsequent cell death does not appear to be a problem as the pore system is irregular and media flow can reach all areas. Estimation of the minimum pore size requires further experimentation. The irregular pore system also appears to allow cell colonization throughout the ceramic. SEM of samples taken from different areas showed similar confluent growth.

The advantages of cell immobilization within the ceramic are common to other large scale immobilization techniques. These include: 1. Aeration and agitation of medium is external to the cells, thus protecting the cells from disruptive forces. 2. Medium may be changed without the need of a cell separation step, thus providing the possibility of continuous feed and harvest. 3. High cell densities are achieved, thus allowing higher product concentrations, easier recovery and reduced serum requirements.

Comparison of this system with the analogous Opticell system[5] indicates that similar cell densities are reached. The primary differences between the two systems appear to be the increased complexity of the Opticell system, (requiring a gas permeator and on-line pH and oxygen probes) and the use of a ceramic with continuous, regular pores. The ceramic core used in Opticell has several disadvantages; it is non-reusable and subject to pore blockage.

To compete with the use of microcarriers, the system described above must be scaled up without the creation of diffusion gradients. If a fixed bed system is used, a radial flow scheme or multiple cylinders in parallel would be feasible alternatives to increasing the size of the cartridge. Fluidization of the ceramic material is likely to be the most practical alternative for large scale applications. This would decrease diffusional resistance, and facilitate cell recovery.

ACKNOWLEDGEMENTS

This work was supported by grants from the British Columbia Science and Technology Development Fund and the British Columbia Foundation for Non-animal Research.

REFERENCES

(1) Adamson, S.R., Industrial Mammalian Cell Culture <u>Can. J. Chem. Eng.</u>, 1986, <u>64</u>, 531

(2) Reuveny, S., and Thoma, R.W., Apparatus and Methodology for Microcarrier Cell Culture <u>Adv. Appl. Microbiol.</u> 1986, <u>31</u>, 139.

(3) Funk, W.D., MacGillivray, T.A., Mason, A.B., Brown, S.A., and Woodworth, R.C., Expression of the Amino-Terminal Half-Molecule of

Human Serum Transferrin in Culture Cells and Characterization of the Recombinant Protein, <u>Biochemistry</u> 1990, <u>29</u>, 1654.

(4) Bognar, E.A., Pugh, G.G., and Lydersen, B.K., Large Scale Propagation of BHK$_{21}$ Cells using the Opticell Culture System, <u>J. Tissue Cul. Methods</u>, 1983, <u>8</u>, 147.

(5) Lydersen, B.K., In: <u>Large Scale Cell Culture Technology</u> (Ed. Lydersen, B.K.) Hanser, New York, 1987, p.169–192

Paper of Kilburn

Steiner: What is the exact material of the matrix, is it comparable to that used in the Opticell system, and was the ceramic surface modified?

Kilburn: The surface was not modified. The material is fused alumina, which is different to Opticell (cordurite).

Noe: Is the ceramic material commercially available?

Kilburn: Yes, it is used as a standard material for filtering molten metal.

Lehmann: In your last EM I saw particles totally empty of cells - am I right?

Kilburn: There are blobs of some sort there with empty spaces.

Lehmann: Do you have an explanation?

Kilburn: No.

Berthold: How do you reconcile the ever changing nature between viable and necrotic cells in packed cell bioreactors as a source material for pharmaceutical and regulated material? These high cell densities (described by you as hamster meat) must have a cost on controllability. Can you comment on these concerns?

Kilburn: There is a mystique that if you use high cell densities you can have a simpler medium because cells feed one another. We find that we can reduce serum concentrations. In terms of production rates of recombinant proteins it is relatively stable over 20 days of steady state conditions. The viability is in the order of 90% so we don't know if there are changes taking place.

CONSIDERATIONS IN THE DESIGN, DEVELOPMENT AND SCALE-UP OF
GLASS BEAD PACKED REACTORS

R. Bliem*, R. Oakley, V. Taiariol, K. Matsuoka, J. Long

Bio-Response Inc., Hayward, CA, USA
* Bristol-Myers Squibb Company, Syracuse, NY, USA

Keywords: animal cell culture, packed bed bioreactor, scale-
-up, continuous culture;

The propagation of animal cells on glass bead packed bed
reactors (PBRs) was first demonstrated over 26 years ago by
Earle and co-workers (1). However, their technical development was discontinued until the the 1970s (2). Our particular
development interest in the packed bed reactor arose from a
need for a system, which would support the mass propagation
of anchorage-dependent cells, and would offer an alternative
to microcarriers.

It had already been well established that solid glass beads
would support cell adhesion and multiplication - the problems
we encountered were associated with the industrial scale-up
of the continuous PBR process. We required reactors, with
demonstrated scalability that would supply approximately 1500
liters of medium per week in continuous operation. Figure 1
presents a schematic of the principle reactor elements: an
oxygenator, a recirculation pump and the cell reactor itself;
not shown are optional on-line sensors. The scale-up difficulties affected all 4 reactor elements and broadly encom-
passed: the fouling of oxygenator and sensor membranes, pumping damage to cells, biomass and medium gradients and dispersion across the reactor bed, and the finally scale-up performance of the individual elements.

Much of the industrial work to-date has been conducted on
homogeneous reactor systems, such as air-lift and stirred
reactors. Medium gradient and dispersion effects together
constitute a design aspect, which most clearly distinguishes
the design requirements of homogeneous from heterogeneous
reactors, such as packed bed systems. This aspect also represents one of the critical design components of packed systems.

Therefore the following brief discussion of the disign criterion serves as a means of presenting some of the considerations particular to packed bed systems, such as as those
pertaining to medium gradients and matrix characterization.

In contrast to homogeneous reactors, medium dispersion should
be low in PBRs, whereas the recirculation rate should be
high. Therefore, we began to investigate the effect of vari-

ous design and operating parameters on reactor dispersion. For this purpose we employed a stimulus-response technique (see e.g. 3). This involved the injection of a tracer pulse into the fluid entering the reactor bed and then measuring the tracer leaving the reactor.

The tracer eluate at the outlet presents a distribution profile, which is a measure of the overall dispersion coefficient of the reactor bed and also reflects the extent of localized medium hold-up and channeling. Dispersion is a function of the reactor dispersion coefficient, as well as the liquid velocity and the reactor length; reactor dispersion is therefore commonly expressed in dimensionless form, such as the reactor Peclet Number (Pe); the numbers used in the presented data are calculated as: Pe=(reactor length * liquid velocity)/axial dispersion coefficient. The liquid velocity is based on the residence time in the reactor.

The rate of medium dispersion throughout a reactor must at least equal the rate of maximum medium and\or oxygen consumption. Based on anticipated cell mass, the substrate concentration and the relevant consumption rates we may estimate an allowable hold-up time for the medium throughout the reactor. For example, we may want no more than 5% of the cells to be in contact with the medium for longer than twice the mean residence time. From this requirement we may in turn calculate a minimum Peclet Number, which provides us with a scalable design parameter.

For PBRs the spread of the dispersion profile should be narrow, symmetric and, based on the above considerations should preferably yield a Peclet Number above 20.

The choice of an appropriate bead size is dependent on the culture, as well as metabolic characteristics of the cell line, and may be selected on the basis of the dispersion coefficient measured with and without cells. Although the dispersion of 5 mm beads (cell-free) is relatively high with a Peclet Number of around 20, they are still useable (see figure 2). However, dispersion and channelling may increase with cell packing, particularly with large beads due to the large interstitial void space and the greater variance in possible aggregate size. Figure 2 shows that the cell-free 2 mm beads showed the most lowest level of dispersion. However, these beads also exhibited the highest degree of sensitivity to cell packing (comparable cell packing of approximately 10% total void space, using Bowes melanoma; table 1). This indicates that when using the 2 mm beads for this cell line (Bowes melanoma) we may also expect to see the highest degree of change in the axial dispersion over the cultivation period, which is also undesirable. On the other hand the the dispersion in the 5 mm beads had reached unacceptably low level (Pe< 20), so that the 3 mm beads were chosen for this operation. By minimising the medium dispersion across we minimise the any medium channeling and hold-up. However we also want to minimise the non-dispersion gradient across the reactor, by maximising the recirculation rate. Fortunately, the Peclet Number generally increases with the recirculation rate under the conditions we normally employ for cell cultivation (0.1 - 1 cm/s bulk velocity).

These and similar considerations may be reduced to a series of reference parameters, which can serve as a first guide in the development of a prototype system (table 2). This table also represents a condensed list of the considerations, which we applied in our scale-up work and which supported the development a new reactor configuration (figure 3). In this configuration the bed height is simply held constant by using a multiple of stacked baskets filled with packing matrix (beads). This design principle alleviates the problem of scale-dependent gradient and dispersion effects, as the bed height remains constant irrespective of reactor size. Scale-up is then achieved by increasing the radius and/ or the number of baskets. This glass bead PBR configuration has been scaled up and operated continuously at a volumetric capacity of over 1500 liters per week (see table 3). In addition to supporting the propagation of anchorage-dependent cells we have also demonstrated that GB-PBRs are able to support the propagation of suspension cells as illustrated in the production of monoclonal antibody (figure 4; Cytotechnology, in press).

The utility of such a PBR system for industrial applications is now firmly established. Our recent experience with suspension cells presents PBRs not only as an interesting alternative to microcarriers for anchorage-dependent cells, but also offer practical possibilities for some aggregate and suspension cells. The extent to which PBRs may be applied to suspension cells remains to be determined by future work.

REFERENCES

1.   W. R. Earle, J.C. Bryant, E.L. Schilling (1953/54). Certain factors limiting the size of the tissue culture and the development of massive cultures. Ann. N.Y. Acad. Sci. Vol. 58, pp. 1000-1011.

2.   R.E. Spier, J.P. Whiteside (1976) The production of Foot- and Mouth disease virus from BHK 21 C13 cells grown on the surface of glass spheres. Biotech. Bioeng. 18, 649 -657

3.   J. M. Coulson, J.F. Richardson (Eds.) Chemical Engineering, Volume 3, Second Edition, Pergamon Press, Oxford. pp. 85 - 94.

PACKED BED REACTOR SCHEMATIC

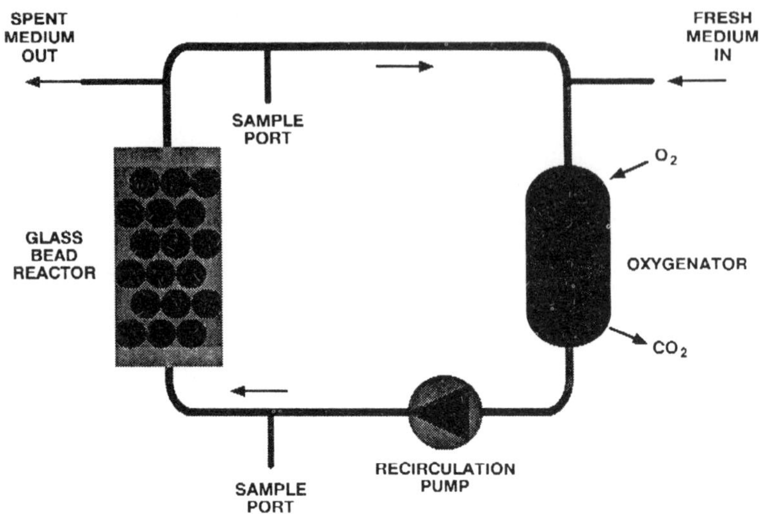

FIGURE 1

EFFECT OF BEAD SIZE ON MEDIUM DISPERSION
(CELL-FREE DISPERSION TESTS)

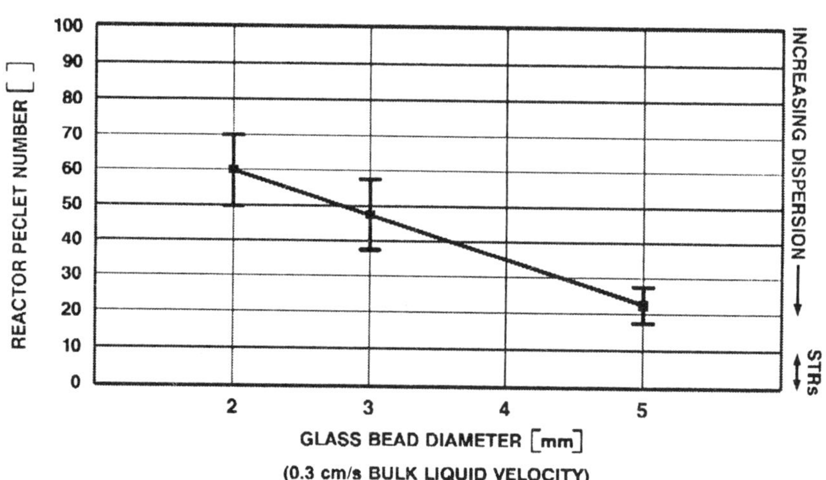

FIGURE 2

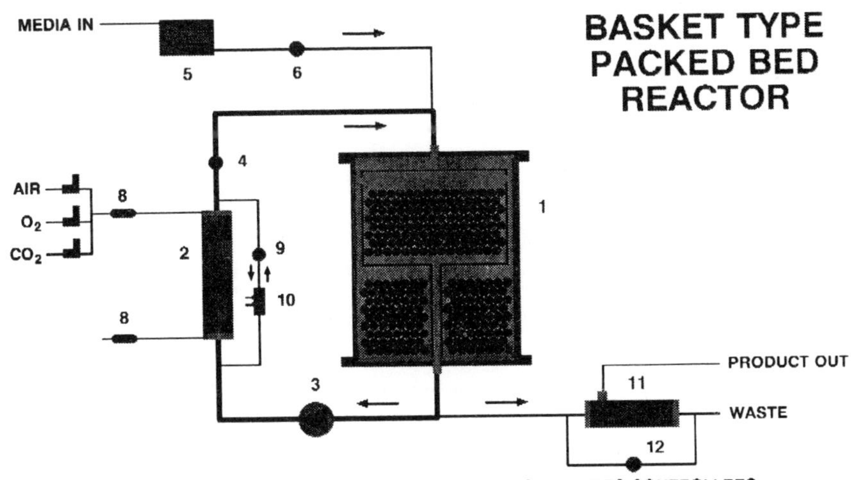

FIGURE 3

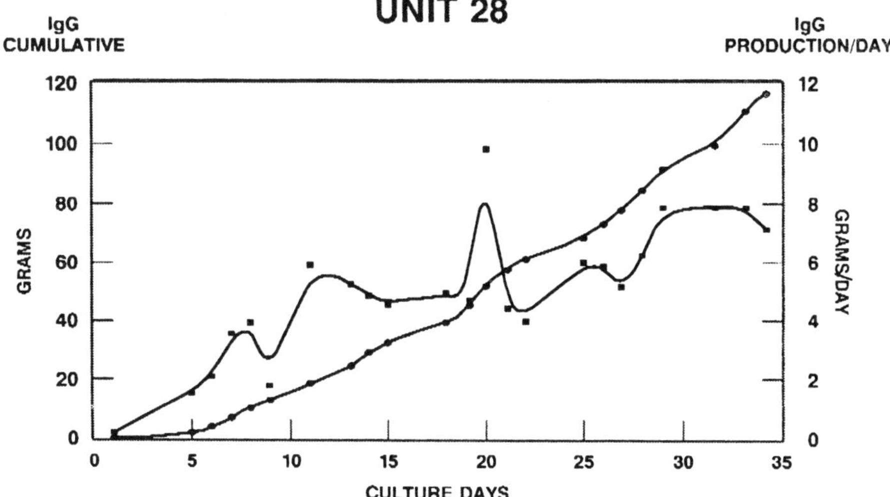

FIGURE 4

411

EXAMPLES OF CHANGES IN REACTOR PECLET NUMBER (N_{Pe}) AS EFFECTED BY CELL PACKING

BEAD DIAMETER [mm]	N_{Pe} [ ]		
	WITHOUT CELLS		WITH CELLS (~ 10% PACKING DENSITY, v/v)
2	70	$\longrightarrow$	27
3	52	$\longrightarrow$	22
5	27	$\longrightarrow$	14

TABLE 1

REACTOR DESIGN PARAMETERS
EXAMPLES OF FIRST REFERENCE VALUES

- OXYGEN TRANSFER COEFFICIENT
  (PREFERABLY BUBBLE-FREE): $K_L a$ > 10^{-4} [s^{-1}]

  or K_L > 10^{-3} [cm/s]

- LIQUID MIXING RATE: > 10^{-4} [s^{-1}]

- DISPERSION FOR HETEROGENEOUS REACTORS:
  REACTOR PECLET NUMBER (Pe)   > 20 [ ]

- HYDRODYNAMIC SHEAR STRESS: < 1 [N/m^2]

- POWER INPUT: < 100 [W/m^3]

- DIFFUSIVITY THROUGH CELL AGGREGATES:
  EFFECTIVE THIELE MODULUS, ϕ < 1 [ ]

TABLE 2

SCALE-UP COMPARISON OF
tPA PRODUCTION IN PBR SYSTEM

ACTUAL		NOMINAL	
PERFUSION RATE (LITERS/DAY)	tPA PRODUCTION (RELATIVE UNITS/DAY)	PERFUSION RATE [ ]	tPA PRODUCTION [ ]
0.55	21	1	1
6.90	200	12	9
51	2200	93	105
220	9500	400	452

TABLE 3

Figueroa: Do you think you would have better cell distribution if your packed bed culture had initially been operated at higher velocities?

Bliem: The packed bed is very velocity dependent and initial conditions do affect the dispersion.

Noe: What is your inoculation system to inoculate a 200 litre glass bead bed reactor?

Bliem: Anchorage-dependent cells settle on the glass surface and propagate relatively easily. For suspension cells it is a question of settling the cells out, waiting until they have formed small nuclei/aggregates capped on the glass bead, and then increasing the re-circulation rate. These are the two basic approaches but it is largely trial and error depending upon cell type and amount of protein in the medium.

Hofmann: Can you give us your flow rates so that one can get an idea of what the oxygenation situation is? If you grow hybridomas I would think you get some cell entrainment, and the possibility of measuring cell viability.

Bliem: The cell density is between 5×10^9 and 10^{10} per litre packed bed. Cells are generally held in a substrate limited mode, otherwise they can overpack. Cells are nearly always present in the re-circulation loop with a very variable viability (30%-70% in the bed, 60%-70% in the loop).

Hofmann What substrate do you limit, and what is the flow rate?

Bliem: 5-6 litres/litre reactor/day feed rate at a re-circulation rate of 0.5 cm/sec (bulk velocity). The culture is usually glucose limited.

Emery: Have you considered geometries other than spheres? Industrial catalysts use cylindrical supports because they are more easily made and have better process properties.

Bliem: The reason we use spheres is for developmental purposes where their uniformity is important to calculate dispersion characteristics.

Handa-Corrigan:

Sedimentation rates in packed bioreactors (beds, fibres etc.)are very important during inoculation and determine the bioreactor performance. One needs to know the fluid velocities that can be used during inoculation.

ON-LINE REMOVAL OF CELLS FROM CONTINUOUS SUSPENSION CULTURES

Peter C. Brown, John C. Lane, Mark T. Wininger, and Robert Chow

Chiron Corporation, Emeryville, California 94608, USA

ABSTRACT

Prototype inclined sedimentation chambers have been incorporated downstream of 40-liter continuous suspension cultures of CHO cells in order to remove cell aggregates and a majority of single cells prior to medium collection and storage. For these prototype chambers, operating limits have been established and provide an experimental basis for design improvements.

INTRODUCTION

The on-line removal of particulates from conditioned medium produced in continuous mammalian cell production systems that do not employ some form of membrane filtration[1-3] would be advantageous by simplifying processing downstream of the bioreactor. A theoretical benefit of continuous on-line cell removal could be a reduction of cell-associated proteolytic activity towards secreted proteins contained in conditioned medium during product collection and storage prior to recovery. Finally, on-line clarification of bioreactor effluents would either be required by or greatly simplify the design of continuous recovery system coupled to these continuous production systems.

Existing technologies that might be adopted in achieving on-line clarification include filtration (dead end or tangential flow), continuous centrifugation[4], and spin filter devices with or without Taylor vortex formation[5,6]. All of these approaches have significant limitations for long term, continuous sterile operations (limited service life, complexity, expense, etc.).

We have pursued on-line clarification by taking advantage of the enhanced sedimentation characteristics of CHO cell aggregates and the widely recognized ability of highly asymmetric inclined chambers, lamella settlers, to remove particulates from continuous effluent streams[7-9].

MATERIALS AND METHODS

The cells were CHO cells expressing a truncated HSV gB2 glycoprotein[10]. Medium used during production was modified DME/F-12 (JRH Biosciences) with insulin (5 μg/ml, Waitaki), human transferrin (5 μg/ml, Miles), Excyte VLE (17 μg cholesterol, Miles), and 0.5% heat inactivated FCS (Hyclone). The bioreactors were modified Bellco 36 liter vessels (40 liter working volume) with overhead drives. Conditioned media exiting the bioreactor initially passes through one of two in-dwelling 1 cm x 45 cm inclined settling tubes arranged to allow for the partial recycling of cells within the bioreactor. Oxygenation was by sparging and headspace overlay. The sedimentation chambers were machined from polycarbonate. The chamber dimensions were 25 cm x 7.6 cm x 0.63 cm (L x W x H). The length does not include a tapered cell/debris reservoir extending beyond the inlet port and distal to the outlet ports. Medium was introduced into the chamber through 2 mm stainless tubes penetrating the bottom plane and extending approximately 4 mm into the chamber. Fluid flow was in an upward direction. Cells and debris were periodically removed from the tapered reservoir through a three-way valve attached to a syringe and vented collection bottle. To maintain non-turbulent flow in the chamber, a bubble trap was installed in the effluent stream downstream of the bioreactor. All components were sterilized by autoclaving. For the determination of packed cell volume (PCV), samples were spun (1000g for five minutes), pellets transferred to calibrated microfuge tubes, and spun again.

RESULTS

General description

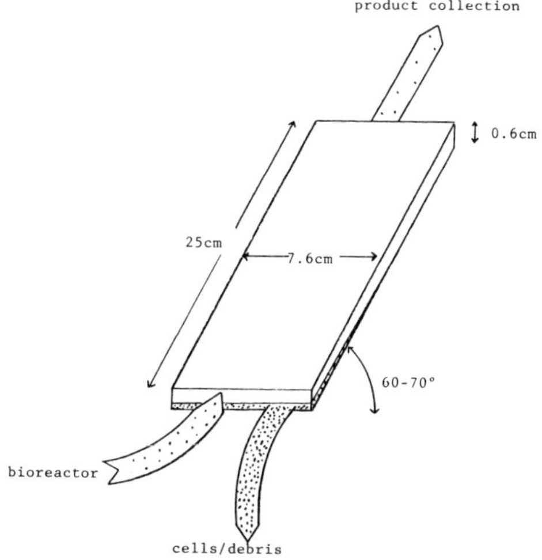

Figure 1. Schematic of the inclined sedimentation chamber.

A schematic of the sedimentation chamber is shown in Figure 1. Conditioned medium from the bioreactor enters at the bottom of the inclined chamber. Because of the arrangement of the inlet ports, this incoming medium initially contacts the top panel and progresses upwards leaving the bottom panel relatively undisturbed. As the conditioned medium progresses toward the outlet, cells and debris accumulate on the bottom panel at a rate determined by individual sedimentation values. If the surface of the bottom panel prohibits adherence, the angle of inclination is sufficiently steep, and upward flow not excessive, then countercurrent (downward) migration of the debris results in the accumulation of the debris in the bottom most portion of the chamber. This downward convective flow is termed the Boycott Effect and is thought to result from localized apparent density increases associated with the concentration of particulates. Accumulated cells and debris are then easily removed by intermittent pumping resulting in very small losses of secreted products. Critical factors for effective particulate removal include height of the chamber, residence time, surface area, angle of inclination, and flow rate.

Angle of inclination

The effect of inclination angle on cell removal (but not downward convective flow) is summarized in Table 1. With the settler placed vertically, greater than 50% of the incoming particulate material was removed; progressive decreases in inclination through 40° led to a 5-fold reduction in the amount of cells/debris exiting the settler.

	PCV (ml/L)		
Inclination	Pre-settler	Post-settler	% reduction
90°	0.56	0.25	55
80°	0.74[2]	0.17	77
70°	1.06	0.13	88
60°	0.74[2]	0.10	86
50°	0.74[2]	0.07	90
40°	0.62	0.05	92

Table 1. Effect of inclination angle[1].

[1] flow rate: 4.8 ml/min
[2] not determined, average of three pre-settler values

Flow rate

In a similar experiment, the effect of different flow rates at fixed inclination (60°) is summarized in Table 2. Pre-settler PCVs varied significantly over the range of flows tested. This variation resulted from progressively ineffective cell recycle by in-dwelling inclined sedimentation tubes within the bioreactor at higher flow rates.

	PCV (ml/L)		
Flow rate (ml/min)	Pre-settler	Post-settler	% reduction
28	1.68	0.86	48
21	1.42	0.54	62
14	1.14	0.29	74
7	1.30	0.14	89
3	0.32	0.09	71

Table 2. Effect of flow rate[1].

[1] angle of inclination: 60° from horizontal

Overall performance

In Figure 2, photographs of representative samples taken from the bioreactor, pre-settler and post-settler are shown. PCVs were determined from each sample: bioreactor, 1.85 ml/L; pre-settler, 0.54 ml/L; post-settler, 0.06 ml/L. Thus, at a flow (i.e., perfusion) rate of 8.3 ml/min, the total reduction in particulates was about 30-fold with a 9-fold reduction resulting from the external settler above. As the photographs show, only single cells and debris are found in the post-settler sample.

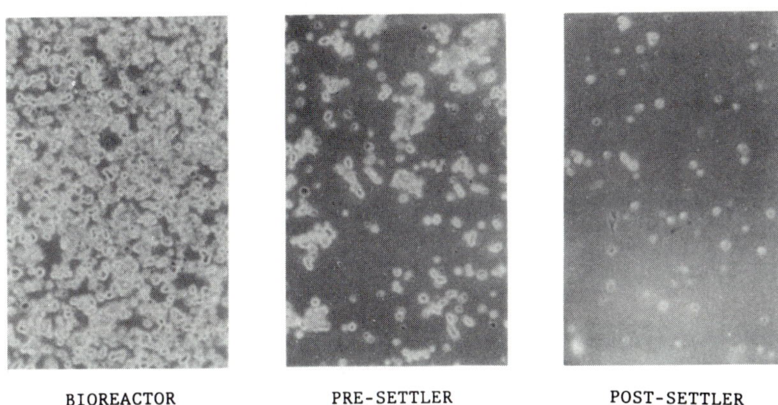

Figure 2. A 40 liter bioreactor and inclined sedimentation chamber (60° from horizontal) was perfused at 8.3 ml/min. Samples (5 ml) were taken directly from the bioreactor, before the downstream settler (but downstream of the in-dwelling settling tubes), and after the downstream settler. Each sample was transferred to a 25 cm^2 flask and immediately photographed. Companion samples were processed for PCV determinations.

DISCUSSION

For cells that grow as aggregates in suspension such as CHO, the inclined sedimentation chamber appears to be a worthwhile addition to production systems that generate a continuous stream of conditioned medium containing cells and cell aggregates. Previous applications of various multi-lamella settlers focused on cell and biomass recycle rather than on mere removal[7,11,12]. The angle of inclination clearly influences the extent of cell removal through we were surprised by the effectiveness of a vertically oriented chamber that relied on sedimentation alone without the wall effect of the inclined chamber. From our experience, an angle of not less than 60° appears to be the best compromise between cell removal and downward convective flow of cells and debris. An alternate strategy is to collect cells/debris in horizontally oriented chambers and periodically increase the angle of inclination to allow for settling and subsequent removal of material. Further, unconfirmed studies indicated that intermittent flow, rather than continuous, provided somewhat superior cell removal at roughly equivalent daily rates.

Under the conditions described in Figure 2, approximately 3-6% of the total cell mass of the bioreactor was not removed by the inclined chamber if one disregards the effect of the less efficient in-dwelling sedimentation tubes. Further, most of this mass consisted of single cells and essentially no aggregates were observed. Independent estimates of the extent of aggregation in comparable cultures suggest that 20-30% of all cells exist as single cells (unpublished). Therefore, at least 75% of these single cells are removed along with virtually all of the aggregates. Therefore, the applicability of this method to less aggregating culture systems, such as hybridomas, seems likely with more highly engineered and larger surface area systems.

REFERENCES

1   Knazek, R.A. and Gullino, P.M. Artificial capillaries: an approach to tissue growth in vitro. Tissue Culture: methods and applications, Kruse, P.F. and Patterson, M.K. eds, Academic Press, 1973, 321

2   Conversion of bioreactors to continuous perfusion using hollow fiber cell separators. Microgon, Inc. technical manual, 1989

3   Avgerinos, G.C., Drapeau, D., Socolow, J.S., Mao, J., Hsaio, K. and Broeze, R. Spin filter perfusion system for high density cell culture: production of recombinant urinary type plasminogen activator in CHO cells. Bio/Technology 1990, 8, 54

4   Alpha Laval promotional literature

5   Sulzer Biotech promotional literature

6   Membrex Inc. promotional literature

7   Tabera, J. and Iznaola, M. Design of a lamella settler for biomass recycling in continuous ethanol fermentation process. Biotech. Bioeng. 1989, 33, 1296

8   Leung, W-F and Probstein, R.F. Lamella and tube settlers. 1. Model and operations. Ind. Eng. Chem. Process Des. Dev. 1983, 22, 58

9   Hill, W.D., Rothfuss, R.R. and Kun, L. Boundary-enhanced sedimentation due to settling convection. Int. J. Multiphase Flow 1977, 3, 561

10   Stuve, L.L., Brown-Shimer, S., Pachl, C., Najarian, R., Dina, D. and Burke, R.L. Structure and expression of herpes simplex virus type 2 glycoprotein gB gene. J. Virol. 1987, 61, 326

11   Tyo, M.A. and Thilly, W.G. Novel high density perfusion system for suspension culture metabolic studies. AIChE annual meeting 1989

12   Batt, B.C., Davis, R.H. and Kompala, D.S. Inclined sedimentation for enhancing viable hybridoma concentration in continuous suspension bioreactors. AIChE annual meeting 1989

Section 6.3
Bioreactors: particles

MICROSPHERE-INDUCED AGGREGATE CULTURE OF ANIMAL CELLS

Stephane Goetghebeur and Wei-Shou Hu

Department of Chemical Engineering and Materials Science, University of
Minnesota, 421 Washington Avenue SE, Minneapolis, MN 55455-0132 U.S.A.

ABSTRACT

Microspheres were used to induce aggregate formation for CHO cells which
grow either as aggregates or in suspension, as well as Vero and ST cells
which are strictly anchorage-dependent. In the case of Vero and ST
cells, they do not spread out after attachment to the microsphere as they
typically do when cultivated on conventional microcarriers or tissue
culture flasks. Instead, they grow in a more spherical form and
eventually form a tightly packed cell mass. In all cases cells grew as
aggregates and a very high cell concentration was reached. To achieve a
similar cell concentration using conventional microcarrier culture
technology a large amount of microcarrier would have to be used. The
viability observed in our microsphere-induced aggregates are very high,
as determined by FDA/EtBr stain.

INTRODUCTION

A variety of microcarriers, including those based on dextran,[1]
polystyrene[2,3] or cellulose,[4] collagen[5] or gelatin-based macroporous
beads,[6] are often used for the cultivation of anchorage-dependent cells.
The mean diameter of microcarriers is in the range of 130 μm to 200
μm,[7,8,9,10] even though a range as wide as from 100 to 400 μm has been
said to be suitable for growth.[11]   A major advantage of microcarrier
technology is the large amount of growth area in a reactor vessel. A
drawback of microcarrier technology is the large amount of settled bead
volume per unit volume of the reactor. Virtually all these volume is
inert except for providing the surface for cell growth. This large
amount of settled bead volume increases the degree of sophistication
required for the design of agitation system to suspend the beads without
damaging the cells.[12]

To circumvent the drawback of microcarriers some have opted to use cells
which are adaptable to grow in suspension, an example is the use of
Chinese hamster ovary (CHO) cells.[13]   However, the use of suspension
cells suffers another shortcoming: the maximum cell concentration
achievable in a conventional stirred-tank bioreactor is only in the
vicinity of 2 x 10^6/ml.

An approach recently adopted is to cultivate some transformed cells as
cell aggregates.[14] Different methods have been used to induce the
aggregate formation for cells which normally grow on surface or prefer to
grow on surface. This usually involves the use of medium containing a
low concentration of calcium in conjunction with a moderately high
agitation rate. This method of cell cultivation allows for an easier

cell retention due to the larger size of the particles. Thus, a high cell concentration can potentially be achieved. The agitation conditions required for an aggregate culture resembles that of a simple suspension culture. The size of cell aggregates span widely from single cells to very large aggregates of hundreds of μm in diameter.

Here we report the use of microspheres to induce aggregate formation for anchorage-dependent cells, or cells which grow in either suspension or on surface. This methodology is analogous to the seeding of crystals in a crystallization process to induce crystal growth. The microspheres added to the cell suspension allow cells to attach to the surface preferentially than to each other. Thus, the process of "aggregate induction" is fast. The aggregate is formed by the outgrowth of cells on the microspheres and/or by agglomeration of a number of beads. Many types of material, essentially any one which allows a rapid cell attachment, can be used to prepare the microspheres.

MATERIALS AND METHODS

Sephadex G25-50 was purchased from Sigma Chemical Co., MO. The beads were derivatized with Diethylaminoethylchloride-hydroxychloride (DEAE·Cl·HCl) (Sigma) as described previously, except the reaction time was 30 min.[7,15] After the reaction, the beads were resuspended in 100 ml PBS, autoclaved, and stored until use.

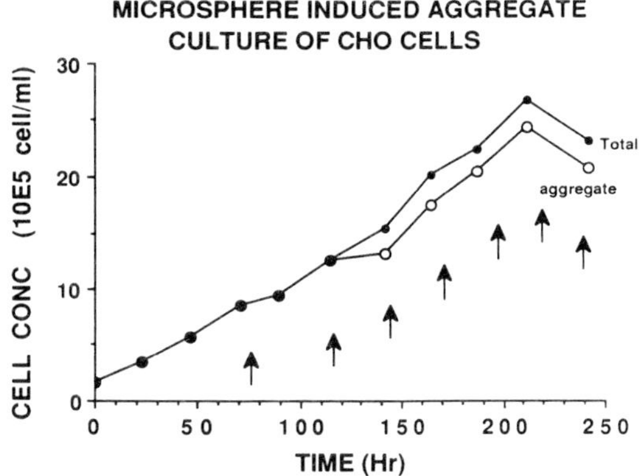

Figure 1. Growth kinetics of CHO cells in microsphere-induced aggregate culture.

The cell growth experiments were carried out in 250 ml spinner flasks with a suspended magnetic stirring bar (Wilbur Scientific Co., Boston, MA). The working volume was 100 ml and the concentration of microspheres was 0.5 g/l. The agitation rate was adjusted to be as low as possible without causing the microspheres or the aggregates to settle down. The cell concentration was determined by nuclei count using crystal violet in citric acid.

The size distribution of the microsphere induced aggregates was determined by taking micrographs of the aggregates at a constant magnification. The longest diameter of each aggregate was measured on the prints. Beads of 86.81 μm in diameter were used as a reference to estimate the size of the aggregates.

RESULTS AND DISCUSSION

The growth kinetics of CHO cells cultivated on microspheres are shown in Figure 1. The arrows indicate the medium changes. Both the total cell concentration and the concentration of cells adhere to microspheres are

shown. The difference between
total cell concentration and
adherent cell concentration is
the amount of cells growing in
the suspension. Cells grew
exponentially after inoculation
with a doubling time of
approximately one day. The
concentration of the cells
reached 2.7 x 10^6 cells/ml at
210 h.

After inoculation, the
formation of aggregates of
cells and microspheres was
observed. The microspheres
were bridged by one or two
cells. 72 h after inoculation
all the cells grew in aggregate
form with varying numbers of
microspheres per aggregate.
However, after 114 h some
single cells and small
aggregates (without the

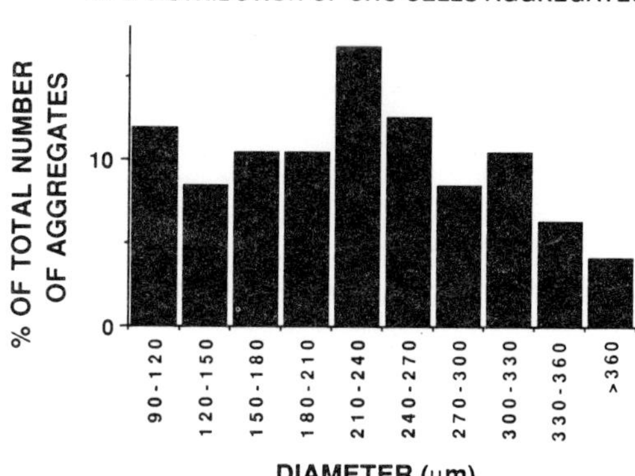

Figure 2. Size distribution of
microsphere-induced aggregate culture of
CHO cells at 250 h.

presence of microspheres) as well as empty microspheres begin to appear
in the suspension. A sample at 250 h was taken for particle size
distribution determination. The histogram of the diameter distribution
of the microsphere-induced aggregates is shown in Figure 2. As can be
seen, the diameter ranged from 90 μm to more than 360 μm.

To determine the viability of
the cells in the aggregates,
samples were taken from the 250
h culture and were stained with
Fluorescein Diacetate (FDA)
(Sigma) and Ethydium Bromide
(EtBr) (Polysciences, Inc.,
Warrington, PA). The FDA
stains the cytoplasm of the
living cells in green and EtBr
the nuclei of the dead cells in
red. Most of the cells in the
culture appeared to be viable
even in the relatively large
aggregates (data not shown).

Swine testicular cells (ST)
were cultivated in a similar
fashion. After inoculation,
cells readily attached to the
microsphere, and aggregates of
microspheres bridged by cells
were formed. The cell
concentration increased
steadily to a final cell

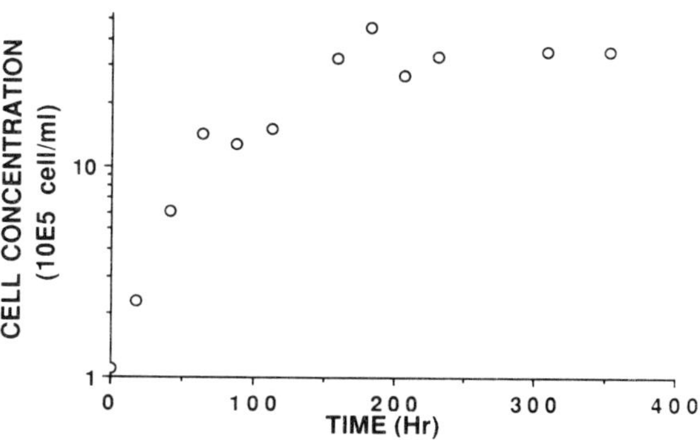

Figure 3. Growth kinetics of ST cells
in microsphere-induced aggregate
culture. (O): cell concentration;
($\bullet$): glucose concentration.

concentration at 230 h of approximately 3.3 x 10^6 cells/ml (Figure 3).
Figure 4 shows the morphology of cells grown as aggregates on

425

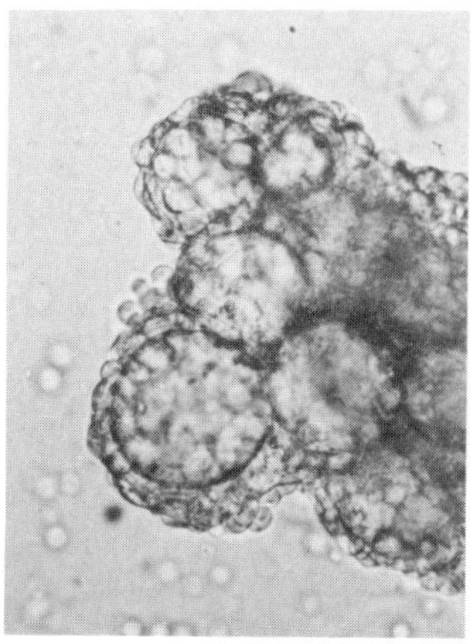

Figure 4. Micrograph of ST cells grown as aggregates.

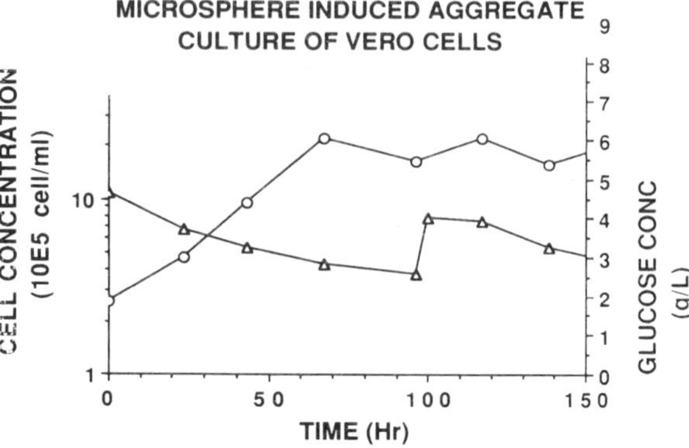

Figure 5. Growth kinetics of Vero cells in microsphere-induced aggregate culture. (O): cell concentration; (Δ): glucose concentration.

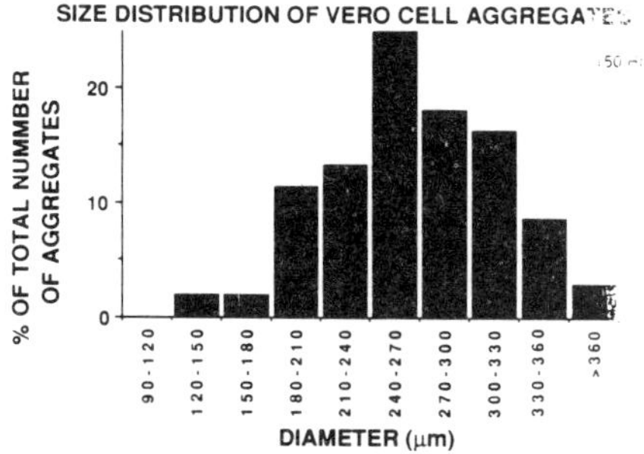

Figure 6. Size distribution of Vero cells grown as aggregates.

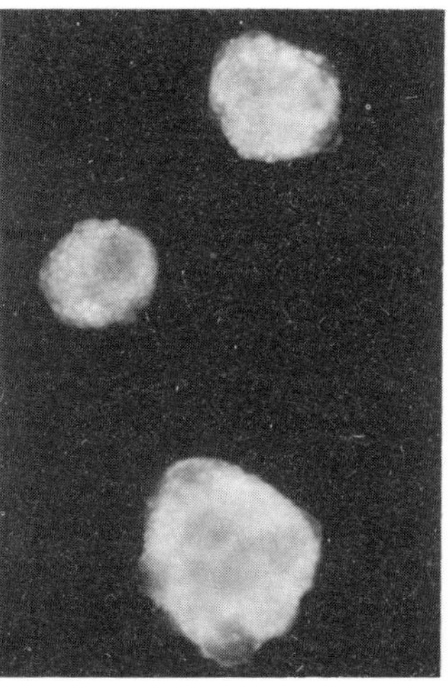

Figure 7. Micrograph of Vero cells cultivated on microspheres.

microspheres. The size of the ST cell aggregates varies from 60 to 540 μm, with a peak between 300 and 420 μm. The growth kinetics of Vero cells on these microspheres are shown in Figure 5. Cell concentration reached approximately 2×10^6 cells after approximately 100 h of cultivation. After 43 h, many empty microspheres were observed in the culture. The microspheres used constituted less than 1% of the volume of the culture. Using conventional microcarriers, such as Cytodex 1 or polystyrene beads from commercial sources, an equivalent of approximately 6–8% settled volume of beads are required to achieve the same level of cell concentration. A histogram of size distribution of these aggregates

are shown in Figure 6. The median diameter is approximately 250 μm.
Shown in Figure 7 is a micrograph of the aggregate obtained at the end of
cultivation. A very high extent of viability was attained, as indicated
by the FDA/EtBr stain.

ACKNOWLEDGEMENT

This work was supported in part by a grant from the National Science
Foundation (ECE–8552670).

REFERENCES

1   van Wezel, A.L. (1967). Nature 216:64-65.

2   Johansson, A. and Nielsen, V. (1980). Dev. Biol. Stand. 46:125-
        129.

3   Kuo, M.J., Lewis, C. Jr., Martin, R.A., Miller, R.E., Schoenfeld,
        R.A., Scheck, J.M. and Wildi, B.S. (1981). In Vitro 17:901-906.

4   Reuveny, S., Silberstein, L., Shahar, A., Freeman, E. and Mizrahi,
        A. (1982). Dev. Biol. Stand. 50:115-123.

5   R.C. Dean et al. (1985). In <u>Large Scale Mammalian Cell Culture
        Technology</u>. Ed. A.S. Lubineicky, Marcel Dekker, Inc., New York,
        NY, pp. 145-167.

6   Cultisphere, Technical Bulletin, Percell Biolytica AB.

7   Hu, W-S., Meier, J. and Wang, D.I.C. (1985) Biotechnol. Bioeng.
        27, 585-595.

8   Varani, J., Dame, M., Fediske, J., Beals, T.F. and Hillegas, W.
        (1985). J. Biol. Stand. 13:67-76.

9   Microcarrier Culture, Pharmacia Fine Chemicals Technical Bulletin

10   Blasey, H.D., Grossebueter, W., Lehman, J., Giehring, H. and
        Schwengers, D. (1988). Presentation at the Engineering Foundation
        on Cell Culture Engineering, Palm Coast, FL, U.S.A., January 31-
        February 5, 1988.

11   Butler, M. (1987). Adv. Biochemical Engineering/Biotechnology
        34:57-84.

12   Hu, W-S. and Wang, D.I.C. (1986) In <u>Mammalian Cell Technology</u>, Ed.
        W.G. Thilly, Butterworths Publishing Company.

13   Murata, M., Eto, Y. and Shibai, H. (1988). J. Ferment. Technol.
        66:501-507.

14   Tolbert, W., Hitt, and Feder, J. (1980). In Vitro 16:486-490.

15   Levine, D.W., Wang, D.I.C. and Thilly, W.G. (1979). Biotechnol.
        Bioeng. 21:821-845.

<u>**Paper of Hu**</u>

Sinacore: What is the influence of serum concentration in your cell aggregation system, and have you tried protein producing cells in this aggregated format and, if so, what was the impact on cellular productivity of aggregated cells?

Hu: Serum had some effect but was variable with cell type - in fact the attachment in aggregates is similar to that on microcarriers. We do have data on virus infection of Vero cells and protein production in 293 cells, but I have not carried out a kinetic analysis to compare productivity. I can only say they produce at a reasonably good rate.

Miller: Without using microcarriers you can have cell aggregation by spinning at low speeds (eg 25 rpm).

Hu: Yes I agree, it varies with cell type but many cells will form aggregates without microcarriers. However, the rate of formation is different and it will induce aggregates in cells that don't normally produce aggregates.

Miller: The advantage of your approach of revolving at relatively high speeds (50-100 rpm) is that you don't normally get aggregates, but these aggregates with 30 micron spheres can be used directly in flow cytometry - you can analyse the cell in situ on the microsphere without clogging the hydrodynamic focusing system. This has been used with beating muscle cells.

Figueroa: How did you measure your aggregates size distribution?

Hu: By measuring micrographs.

THE GROWTH OF CHO AND BHK CELLS AS SUSPENDED AGGREGATES IN SERUM-FREE
MEDIUM

Jack Litwin

State Bacteriology Lab., 105 21 Stockholm, Sweden.

ABSTRACT

CHO and BHK cells were grown in similar serum-free medium containing
transferrin and an undefined serum replacement concentrate. In both cases
transferrin could be replaced with 1 uM $Fe_2(SO_4)_3$. The cells grew in
suspension cultures as densely packed aggregates to about $3x10^6$ cells/ml.

KEY WORDS

CHO, BHK, Serum-free medium, Suspension cultures.

INTRODUCTION

Chinese Hamster Overy (CHO) and Baby Hamster Kidney (BHK) cells have
become of commercial interest because of their use as host for transfected
genes programed to produce biologicals of importance. The adaptation of
these cells to growth in serum-free media (SFM) allows one better control
over growth and the production of the biologicals of interest, and
facilitates down-stream processing. The growth of these cells in suspension culture without the use of microcarriers has the advantage of
simplicity and reduced costs.

MATERIAL AND METHODS

Cell lines: The BHK-K1 cell line was obtained from the State Bact. Lab.,
Stockholm, Sweden. A CHO-49 cell line genetically engineered to produce
parathyroid hormone was obtained from Karo-Bio, Huddinge, Sweden. The
cells were routinely grown as monolayer cultures in MEM + 10% calf serum
(CS). The medium for the transfected CHO cell line contained 1 mM extra
proline and dialyzed serum.

Media: The SFM had the following composition:

                    Base medium (MEM, Iscove's, F-12, etc.)
            4 mM Glutamine (final concentration)
            1 mM Na pyruvate
            25 mM HEPES, pH 7.1
            0.2 % Galactose
    Either 10 ug/ml Human transferrin
        or   1 uM $Fe_2(SO_4)_3$
            0.1 % Na bicarbonate
    1:20 dilution Serum Replacement Concentrate

The Serum Replacement Concentrate (Med. & Vet. Supplies Ltd., Botolph
Claydon, Buckingham, U.K.) is an undefined concentrate which had been
ultra-filtered to remove all substances above a mol. wt. of 3000. The
same material was used previously for the growth of hybridoma cells in
SFM (2, 3).

The base media were prepared from powder form (Sigma). The human transferrin was purified by the State Bact. Lab. as a partially iron saturated
preparation. Ferric sulfate was prepared as a 1 mM solution in ethanol
and diluted 1:1000 in the medium when used.

Trypsinization: The cells were suspended from monolayer cultures with 100
ug/ml crystalline trypsin in phosphate buffered saline without Ca^{++} and
Mg^{++}.

Cell Counting: Because the cells in suspension culture grew in relatively
large aggregates they could not be counted directly. A two ml alequate
was taken from the spinner. The cells were centrifuged and resuspended in
two ml (or a multiple thereof) in a citric acid – crystal violet (42 g/l
and 0.5 g/l, respectively) solution. After 30 min. at room temp. and with
occassional aggitation the cell nuclei were counted in a Bürker chamber.
Only nuclei containing a well defined internal structure were counted.

Culture system: Monolayer cultures were made in plastic Roux bottles
(Costar) containing 100 ml medium.

Suspension cultures were made in 1 liter spinner bottles. The impeller,
a magnet bar with a teflon paddle mounted at right angles, was rotated
at about 60 – 100 RPM.

Neither BHK nor CHO cells grew as monolayers in SFM; the cells did not
attach, although both cell strains attached and grew well as monolayers
in SFM + 1% CS. The cells used to start the suspension cultures were
trypsinized from monolayer cultures with MEM + 10% CS. The suspension
cultures were started with 100 ml SFM + 1% CS. After 5 – 7 days 100 ml
SFM without serum was added. Thereafter, half the medium was changed
with retention every 4 days by allowing the impeller to stop rotating
and after 20 – 30 min., when most of the cells had settled to the bottom,
the top half of the medium was sucked-off and replaced with fresh SFM.
Very few cells were lost during this procedure. Thus, the volume in these
experiments was kept constant at 200 ml and the serum concentration was
reduced by half with each medium change.

RESULTS AND DISCUSSION

The growth of BHK cells in suspension
(fig. 1 & 2) eventually reached a level
of 2 – 3x10^6 cells per ml in several
different base media. Although most of
the media contained transferrin, this
protein could be replaced with 1 uM
$Fe_2(SO_4)_3$ (fig. 2). In this case the
SFM was completely protein free. The
cells grew as densely packed aggregates (fig. 3) which grew to as large
as several hundred microns in diameter.

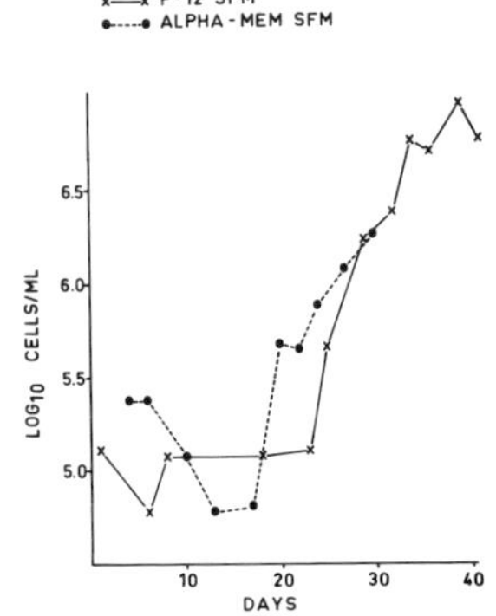

Fig. 1 – Growth of BHK cells
in suspension culture with
SFM.

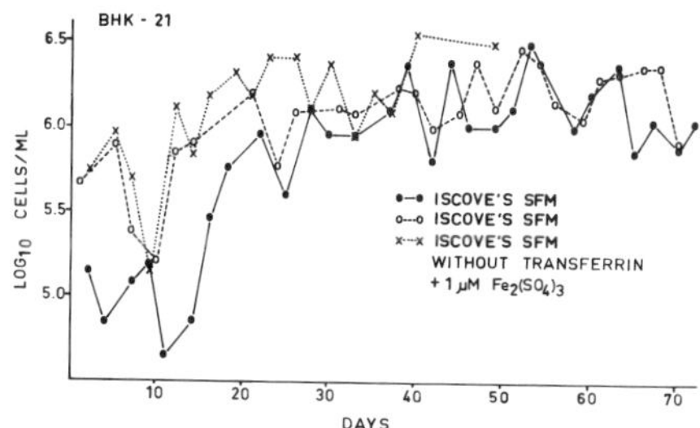

Fig. 2 – Growth of BHK cells in suspension culture with SFM.

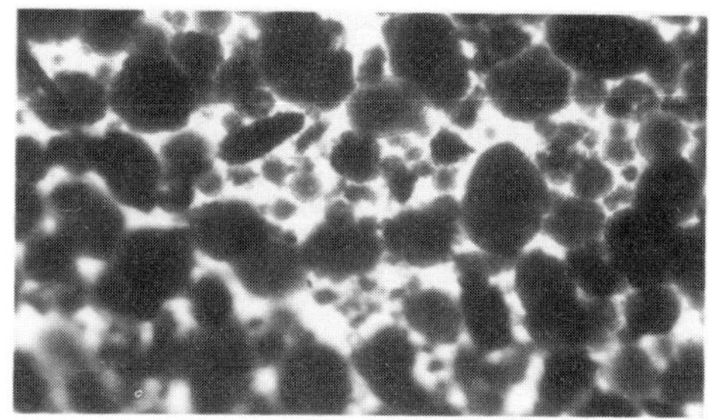

Fig. 3 – BHK cells growing as aggregates in suspension culture. Mag. 30X.

The CHO cell line was transfected to produce parathyroid hormone. The growth of these cells in different base media (fig. 4) demonstrate that transferrin can be replaced with 1 uM $Fe_2(SO_4)_3$. To facilitate genetic amplification (4) the cells were grown in the presence of 5 uM methotrexate (MTX) and compared with growth in SFM without MTX. Good growth was obtained with base medium MCDB 302 (fig. 5), Iscove's (fig. 6) and MEM (fig. 7). The MEM contained the non-essential amino acids and 1 mM extra proline was added. The final cell concentration obtained was the same with or without MTX, although the initial growth was slower in the presence of MTX. The cells were able to produce micro-gram quantities per ml of parathyroid hormone (assay performed by Karo-Bio), however, MTX had no inhancing effect on hormone production.

CHO cells also grew as aggregates in suspension culture (fig. 8), although the aggregates were not as dense as those formed by BHK cells.

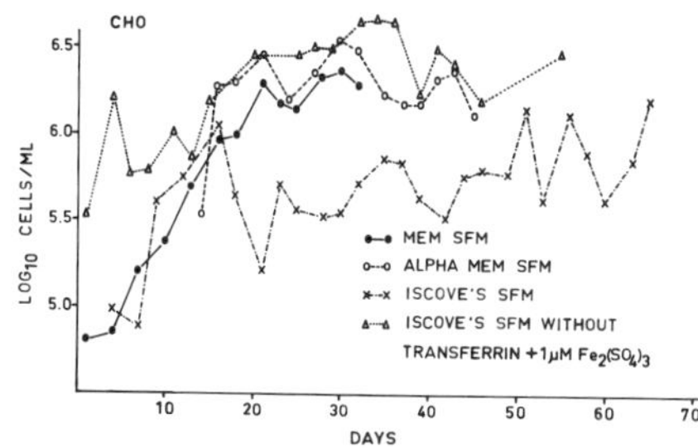

Fig. 4 – Growth of CHO in suspension culture in SFM with different base media.

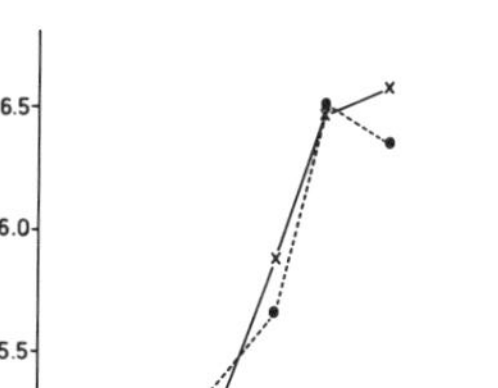

Fig. 5 – Growth of CHO in suspension culture in SFM with MCDB 302 as base medium.

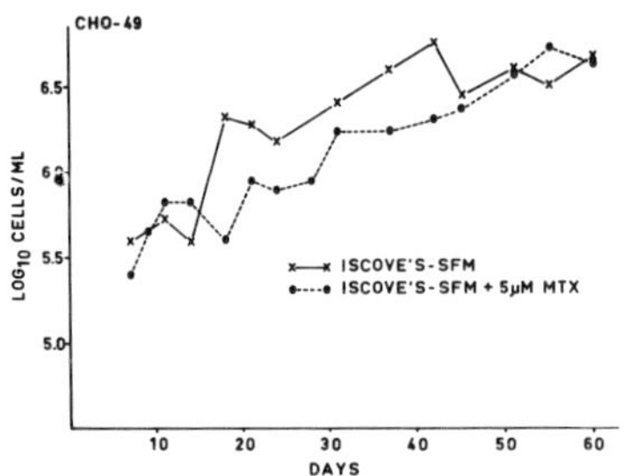

Fig. 6 - Growth of CHO in suspension culture in SFM with Iscove´s as base medium.

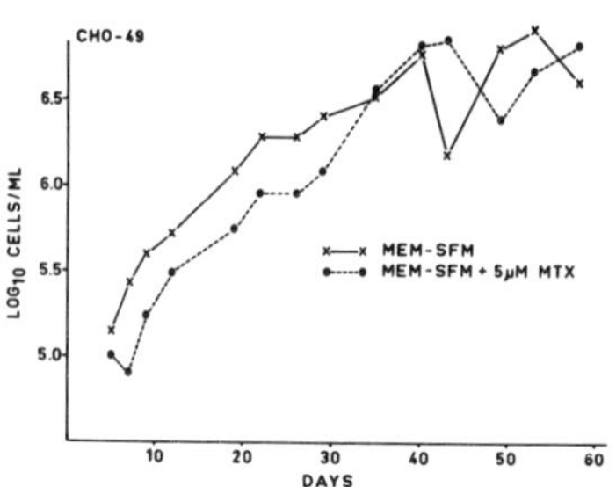

Fig. 7 - Growth of CHO in suspension culture in SFM with MEM as base medium.

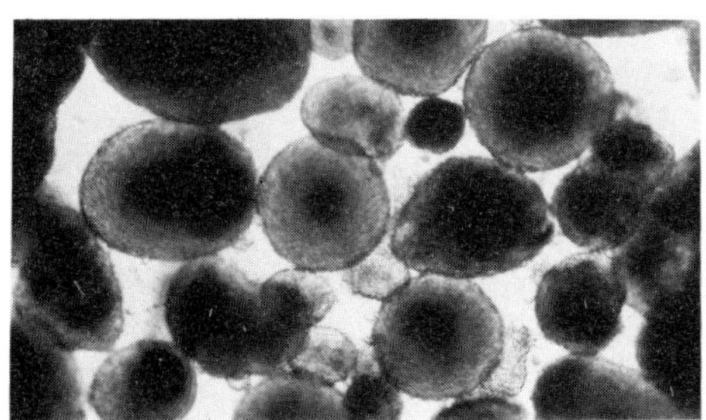

Fig. 8 - CHO cells growing as aggregates in suspension culture. Mag. 30X.

The growth of cells as suspended aggregates have two main advantages: (1) the aggregates settle out very quickly and, thus, it is easy to change medium with retention, and (2) the cell concentration within the aggregates are at tissue-like density without the need of encapsulation techniques (5) or special microcarriers (1). The disadvantage with these aggregates is that when they become too large there occurs cell death within their center and it is difficult to accurately enumerate the cell concentration.

The serum replacement concentrate appears to support cell growth of strains other than CHO and BHK. With a similar type of media composition hybridomas (2, 3), Namalwa (unpublished data) and Vero (unpublished data) may also be grown in SFM. Thus, with a simple technique and a highly adaptable, inexpensive serum and protein free medium both BHK and CHO cells can be grown in a system which is easy to scale-up.

ACKNOWLEDGEMENTS

The author wishes to acknowledge the excellent technical help of Mrs. Ann Björk.

REFERENCES

1 Butler, M. A comparative review of microcarriers available for the growth of anchorage-dependent animal cells. In: Animal Cell Biotechnology (Eds. Spier, R.E. & Griffiths, J.B.) Academic Press 1988 pp. 283 - 303.

2 Litwin, J. The growth of hybridoma cells in a serum- and protein-free medium. In: <u>Advances in Animal Cell Biology and Technology for Bioprocesses</u> (Eds. Spier, R.E., Griffiths, J.B., Stephenne, J. & Crooy, P.J.) Butterworth & Co. 1989 pp. 273 - 276.

3 Merten, O.-W., Keller, H., Cabanie, L., Litwin, J. & Flamand, R. Development of a serum-free medium for hybridoma fermentor cultures. In: <u>Advances in Animal Cell Biology and Technology for Bioprocesses</u> (Eds. Spier, R.E., Griffiths, J.B., Stephenne, J. & Crooy, P.J.) Butterworth & Co. 1989 pp. 263 - 269.

4 Schimke, R.T. Gene amplification in cultured cells. J.B.C. 1988 <u>263</u>, 5989 - 5992.

5 Shirai, Y., Hashimoto, K., Kawahara, H., Sasaki, R., Hitomi, K. & Chiba, H. Production of erythropoietin by BHK cells growing on the microcarriers trapped in alginate gel beads. Cytotech. 1989 <u>2</u>, 141 - 145.

CULTISPHER - MACROPOROUS GELATIN MICROCARRIER - NEW APPLICATIONS

Joakim Almgren, Charlotte Nilsson, Ann-Christin Petersson and Kjell Nilsson.

Percell Biolytica and HyClone AB, S-223 70 LUND, Sweden

ABSTRACT

A macroporous gelatin microcarrier reduces some of the problems associated with utilization of solid microcarriers during cultivation of surface dependent cells. New types of porous microcarriers have been developed with diverse applications in the cell technology. Their charcateristics and the use of them for cultivation of 1. Cells with larger size, 2. Cells in perfused systems as the fluidized bed bio reactor, and 3. Hybridoma cell lines, is described.

INTRODUCTION

CultiSpher - General properties

A porous microcarrier will reduce some of the problems associated with cultivation of anchorage dependent cells on solid microcarriers;

1. Mechanical stress imposed to surface grown cells.
2. High concentrations of microcarriers are necessery in order to obtain dense cultures
3. Large inoculum size is needed,
4. Small increases in total cellmass reflected by a low growth span,
5. Cell harvest procedure is complicated by the separation of cells from the carriers
6. Not optimal recovery of cells after harvesting.

The porous structure provides protection against mechanical stress generated by the agitation system and bead-to-bead collisions. The growth of cells inside the gelatin matrix leads to a more efficient utilization of the microcarrier. A larger surface area is made available for cell to grow on and compared to a solid microcarrier of the same size, the cell yield is at least 5-fold higher pro g dry weight microcarrier.

The inoculum size can be reduced to as low as 4 cells pro
bead, due to the protected environment, and the fact that
less numbers of carriers is needed in order to obtain the
same area as with a solid carrier. The low inoculum size has
no negative effect on the final cell yield and a growth span
(final cell yield/inoculum size) of 390 times is obtained in
spinnerflasks without any especially designed oxygen supply
system.

The higher growth span is a matter of importance during
the procedure of scaling up as fewer steps is required
compared to a scale-up with a solid carrier. Thereby, the
risk of microorganism infection will be minimized during the
critical passage of cells to a new fermentor and fewer
reactors are required.

The problem of separating the cells from the carriers
after the harvesting procedure is avoided by the
enzymatically degradable gelatin matrix. The specific
enzymes utilized, Dispase and collagenases, will dissolve
the beads at 37°C in ½ hour and results in a high recovery
of viable cells. Trypsin can also be used to dissolve the
beads, obtaining up to 98% viable cells.

A continuing research & development program has resulted
in new types of macroporous gelatin microcarriers with
diverse applications for cell cultivation. Their
characteristics and the use of them for cultivation of;

    1. Cells with a larger cell size,
    2. Cells in a perfused system as the fluidized bed bio
       reactor,
    3. Hybridoma cell lines, will be outlined here.

CultiSpher-G

CultiSpher-G is the standard type with a pore size
optimized for cells similar to CHO cells. The physical
characteristics of CultiSpher-G is shown in table I.

Tab.I Physical characterstics -G

Matrix:	100% gelatin
Density:	1.04 g/ml
Size in PBS d_{50}	220 um
d_{5-95}	170-270 um
Swelling in PBS:	14-18 ml/g
Approx.no.of Microcarriers:	$2\text{-}3 \times 10^{6}$/g
Sedimentation velocity:	0.16 cm/s
Pore size in PBS:	10-20 um

CultiSpher-G has been used in fermentors up to 320 L.
Production of recombinant van Willenbrand factor, the
physiologic stabilizing molecule of Factor VIII, has been
described (1). The production was constant during 30-45 days
while the cell densities remained between 10^7 and 2×10^7
cells / ml. The microcarrier concentration used was 4g/L and
after 4 days, the serum supplemented medium was replaced by
serum free medium containing protein at a concentration
lower than 10 mg/L. Allthough oxygen transfer were improved
by a high agitation rate, cell detachment was neglible as
the cells were protected by the porous structure. Some of
the cell lines tested for growth on CultiSpher-G a given in
Tab.II.

Tab.II Cells grown on CultiSpher-G	
Name	Species / Tissue
CHO-K1	Chinese hamster ovary fibroblast
r-CHO	Recombinant CHO
BHK-21	Syrian hamster kidney fibroblast
L929	Mouse areolar & adipose tissue fibroblast
Vero	African green monkey kidney fibroblast
MDCK	Canine kidney epithelial
V79	Hamster lung fibroblast
F9	Mouse teratocarcinom
HeLa	Epitheloid carcinoma,
GMK	Green monkey kidney
HU549	Urine bladder carcinoma
HN5	Head and neck tumor
A72	canine tumor
G7	Mouse myoblast tumorgenic
3T3	Embryo mouse
?	Human breast cancer

CultiSpher-GL

As certain cell lines are larger than the pores of
CultiSpher-G (10-20 um), a carrier with larger poresizewas
developed in order to accomodate such cells. CultiSpher-GL
has a pore diameter about twice or three times that of the
-G type. The physical characteristics are given in Tab.III.

Tab.III Physical characteristics of -GL	
Matrix:	100% gelatin
Density:	1.04 g/ml
Size in PBS: d_{50}	220 um
d_{5-95}	170-270 um
Swelling in PBS:	14-18 ml/g
Approx.no.of microcarriers:	$2\text{-}3 \times 10^6$/g
Sedimentation velocity:	0.16 cm/s
Pore size in PBS:	50-70 um

Cells that have been cultivated on the -GL type include;
C127 (Mouse mammary tumor) and Endothelial cells. All the
cell types described under -G, can also be cultivated on the
-GL, but as the pores are larger the available surface area
will be smaller pro gram.

In order to compensate the decreased area, a higher
concentration of beads must be used. In spinner flasks
with recommended oxygen supply, 1.5-2 g dry weight pro L is

CultiSpher-GD and -GLD

CultiSpher-GD & GLD are macroporous microcarriers with an
increased density. They are designed to fullfill the
criterias for a microcarrier used in perfusion system, such
as the fluidized bed bioreactor system.

In order to obtain a proper fluidized bed system with a
linear fluid velocity high enough to provide the cells with
an adequate supply of oxygen and nutrients, the
microcarriers have to be tailormade for the system used.

The density is increased through inclusion of a
propriatory titanium compound into the gelatin matrix.
Depending on the flow rate in the reactor, the sedimentation
velocity and the bead size have to be optimized.

The characteristics of a bead consisting of gelatin and
71% (w/w) titanium compound, having a large pore size (-GLD)
and a diameter of 300-500 um (dry size) are given in Tab.IV.
The amount of included weightening material have been varied
in the range of 38 - 80 % (w/w) in order to obtain other
sedimentation velocities.

<u>Tab.IV Ex. of physical characteristics GLD</u>

Matrix:	gelatin + titanium comp.
Size in PBS: d_{50}	510 um
d_{5-95}	430-560 um
Swelling in PBS:	3.9 ml/g
Approx.no.of microcarriers:	3.45×10^6/ g
Sedimentaion velocity:	2.0 cm / s
Pore size in PBS:	50-100 µm
Approx. surface area:	2500 cm^2/g

The volumetric cell densities (Vero & CHO-K1) achieved in
the first report describing the use of these type of beads
were one order of magnitude higher compared to conventional
techniques using spherical microcarriers (2).

CultiSpher-GH

The latest type of microcarrier is the -GH which is a
product under development. It was designed for the
cultivation of hybridoma cells and is at the moment under
going trials at different companies and institutes.

The major physical difference is the bead diameter which
is about twice to that of CultiSpher-G. The basic hypothesis
is that the hybridoma cells will attach loosly to the
surface or will be entrapped in the gelatin matrix. The
three dimensional substrate will have a beneficial effect on
the behavior of the cells which will be translated into
increased product formation and cell stability of the cells.

The results so far indicates that for tested hybridoma
cell lines, the prescence of CultiSpher-GH increases maximal
cell densities and generation times. The matrix appeared to
increase the time, duration and intensity of cellular
diffrentiative phenotypic expression by four McAbs clones
tested with reference to their ability to produce and
secrete immunoglobulin (3).

REFERENCES

(1)   Abstract; Cell culture Eng.II, Santa Barbara, USA,
        Dec.3-8, 1989, G.Mignot, V.Ganne, T.Faure, H.van de
        Pol, CNTS, France

(2)   "The use of macroporous gelatin microcarriers for the
        cultivation of mammalian cells in fluidized bed bio
        reactors", M.Reiter, O.Hohenwarter, T.Gaida, N.Zach,
        C.Schmatz, G.Bluml, K.Nilsson, H.Katinger, Submitted
        for publication.

(3)   Dr.P.Mann, Univ.of New Mexico, US, personal
        communication.

CULTIVATION OF CHO-CELLS ON MICROCARRIERS DORMACELL

M. Jacobs, G. Gummich, I. Keller, D. Schwengers

Pfeifer & Langen, Frankenstraße 25, D-4047 Dormagen,
West-Germany

ABSTRACT

Four standard types of DORMACELL have been studied concerning
their acceptability for the cultivation of CHO-cells.
DORMACELL 2.9 proved to be the best carrier type for rapid
cell growth whereas during the stationary phase the cells were
more firmly attached to DORMACELL 2.0. Additional experiments
showed that CHO-cell cultures can easily be enlarged by adding
fresh DORMACELL plus medium.

KEYWORDS : CHO-cells, microcarrier, DORMACELL,

INTRODUCTION

The chinese hamster ovary cell line CHO-K1 (ATCC CCL 61) is
the parental strain of some very important technical cell
lines. Recombinant CHO-cell lines are used for the production
of Factor VIII, t-PA, gamma interferon, and other pharmaceutical products [1]. The application of microcarriers in cultures
allows growing and maintaining these anchorage-dependent cells
in stirred vessels even on large scale where the environment
is homogenous, and observations and control can occur within
the culture vessel. Frequently when working on large scale the
only reasonable source for inoculum are cells in microcarrier
culture. Normally the cells have to be harvested by trypsinization and separation from the used microcarriers. An alternative to this trypsinization procedure is the bead-to-bead
transfer technique reported by Crespi and Thilly [2].
Herewith we present DORMACELL as a suitable microcarrier for
the cultivation of CHO-K1 cells in stirred vessels.
Furthermore the culture volumes were enlarged by simply adding
fresh microcarriers to the growing cultures.

RESULTS AND DISCUSSION

Cultivation of CHO-cells on different DORMACELL types

The experiments were performed in 250ml Techne Spinner flasks
filled with 100ml Ham's F12 medium supplemented with 10% FBS.
To each flask 0.3g of the different types of DORMACELL, which
were prepared according to the manufacturers directions [3], and

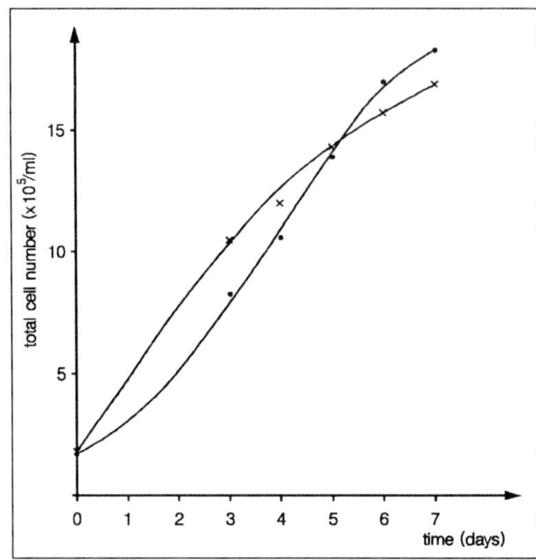

Figure 1 Cell growth on DORMACELL 2.0 (-o-) and DORMACELL 2.9 (-x-)

10^7 CHO-K1 cells were added. A daily medium exchange was necessary to prevent nutrient deficiency.
In Figure 1 the results of two DORMACELL types are shown. During the first four days after inoculation the cells on type 2.9 showed better propagation than on type 2.0. Later on the cell number in the DORMACELL 2.0 cultures increased more rapidly.

Scale-up by bead-to-bead transfer

DORMACELL 2.0 was chosen for these experiments because the CHO-cells were more firmly attached to this carrier type even after a longer period of cultivation. A series of four 250ml Techne Spinner flasks containing 100ml Ham's F12 (+10% FBS) and 0.5g DORMACELL 2.0 were inoculated with 1.5×10^7 cells. Another four flasks containing instead of 0.5g only 0.1g DORMACELL 2.0 were inoculated with 5×10^6 cells. Here DORMACELL was added step by step up to 0.5g whereby the cell to carrier ratio was kept on the level of 3 to 5×10^8 cells per gramm carrier. Each addition of new material is marked with an arrow in Figure 2.After 6 days of cultivation the cell numbers were nearly the same no matter whether the cultures had been started with 0.1g or 0.5g DORMACELL 2.0 per 100 ml.
After reaching the state of confluence the cultures were splitted in the ratio of 1:3 by adding fresh medium containing 0.5g carrier per 100 ml. Again the cell number rapidly increased showing nearly no lag-phase.
So it is possible to start a CHO-culture with a relatively low carrier quantity and cell inoculum and to enlarge the culture volume by at least factor 3.

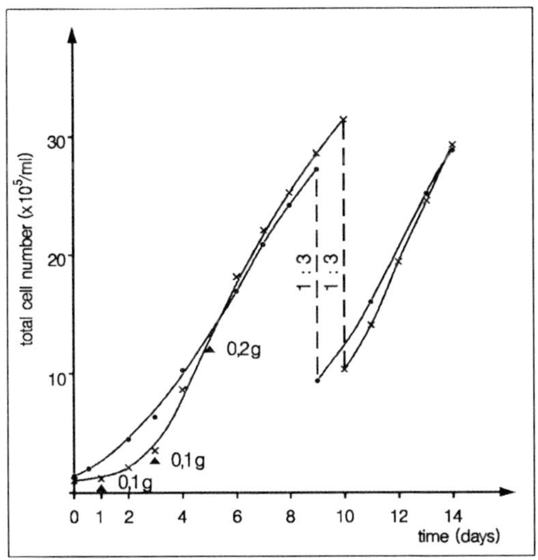

Figure 2 Cell culture with 0.5g DORMACELL 2.0 per 100ml (-o-)and with step by step increasing concentrations of DORMACELL 2.0 (-x-)

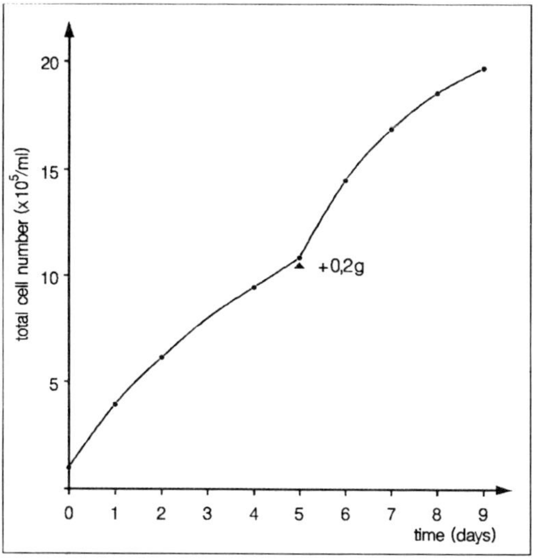

Figure 3 Vero-cells on DORMACELL 2.0 in Ham's F12 (10% FBS); carrier concentration of 0.3g/100ml was increased up to 0.5g/100ml

441

CONCLUSION

The microcarrier DORMACELL 2.0 has proved to facilitate the
scale-up of CHO-cell cultures by simple bead-to-bead transfer.
For the cultivation of other cell lines the user first will
have to find out the optimal carrier type before starting the
scale-up procedure.
We ourselves have just started to optimize the cultivation and
the scale-up of Vero-cultures on DORMACELL 2.0. The first
results are shown in Figure 3. New added beads were accepted
without a lag-phase.

REFERENCES

1 Spier, R.E., Griffiths, J.B.; Stephenne, J.; Crooy, P.J.
   Advances in animal cell biology and technology for
   bioprocesses, ESACT , 9th meeting, Butterworths 1989

2 Crespi, C.L.; Thilly, W.G. Continuous cell propagation
   using low-charge microcarriers. Biotechnology and
   Bioengineering 1981, 28, 983-993

3 DORMACELL microcarriers for cell cultures.
   Pfeifer & Langen Dormagen

Section 6.4
Bioreactors: membranes and perfusion

FERMENTATION OF AT III PRODUCING BHK CELLS IN A DOUBLE MEMBRANE PERFUSION BIOREAKTOR
some aspects about fermentation strategy and process optimization

Shu-ying Li, Bettina Röder, Manfred Wirth

Arbeitsgruppe Zellkulturtechnik, GBF - Gesellschaft für Biotechnologische Forschung mbH., D-3300 Braunschweig, FRG.

Abstract

A perfusion bioreactor based on a double-membrane agitator was used for the continuous fermentation of Antithrombin III (AT III) producing BHK cells. In this system, which totally retains the cells, a maximal cell density of more than 1 x 10^7 cells per ml can be obtained. The self-conditioning effect accompanied with high-cell density facilitated the adaptation process of the cells to serum-free condition.

Recombinant BHK cells with cell specific AT III productivity of 1.2 mg/10^9 cells*24h were cultivated in serum-free medium in this fermentation system. Their growth and production behavior in suspension and on microcarriers was compared. Comparable results concerning maximun cell density, productivity (qp) and product yield were obtained in both kinds of cultivation. Western blot analysis suggests that AT-III preserves its protein integrity better in serum-free condition.

Keywords:　antithrombin III (AT III), baby hamster kidney cell line (BHK), continuous fermentation, perfusion system, microcarrier vs. suspension culture, serum-free cultivation, protein integrity, cell specific productivity (q_p)

Introduction

For the optimization of recombinant protein production which sucessfully integrates and connects up-stream and down-stream processing, many criteria have to be taken into consideration. Firstly, the production process must be able to support a satisfactory cell specific productivity (q_p) which remains constant over a long peroid of time. Secondly, for production purposes, maximum productivity must be achieved, i.e. maximum rate of product formation with regard to the volumetric unit of the fermentor (Q_p) and maximum total yield. Thirdly, in order to facilitate isolation and purification , maximum product concentration in the medium containing low concentration of foreign proteins should be attained. Finally, the fermentation process should be able to preserve the integrity and quality of the desired protein product.

AT III (antithrombin III) is one of the most important protease inhibitors in plasma (1). It is also considered to be a potential therapeutic agent for the treatment of several acquired or inherited hypercoagulation diseases resulting from AT III deficiency(2). AT III is an α_2-glycoprotein of M_r 60000 to 64000 containing three to four polysaccaride chains attached by N-glycosidic linkage to asparagine residues(3,4).

Using fermentation of an AT III producing BHK cell line in a double membrane perfusion bioreactor as a model, this paper intend to elucidate how the four parameters concerning product yield described above can be optimized.

Material and Methods

Reactor system
The reactor system contains a hydrophobic membrane for bubble-free aeration and a hydrophilic membrane for cell retention (microfiltration) and medium exchange (5). The rate of medium exchange through perfusion was adjusted as a function of glucose consumption rate in order to meet the basic requirements of the cells.

Cell line
The recombinant AT III producing cell line BHK 21 G9 has been previously described (6). Briefly, BHK21 cells were transfected with a plasmid harboring a cDNA gene encoding human AT III, together with selectable genes conferring G418 and Methrotexate resistance to the cells. Cells were simultaniously selected by G418 and Methrotexate. The AT III gene is under the control of a SV40 early promotor. The recombinant cells constitutively secrete glycosylated human AT III.

Culture conditions
The cells were routinely cultured in DMEM-F12 (1:1 mixture) containing 5% FCS. Fermentations were carried out in a serum-free medium (DME-F12 1:1 mixture supplemented with 10mg/l insulin, 10mg/l transferrin, oleic acid, cholesterol)(7). Cytodex 3 microcarrier (Pharmacia, Uppsala) was used for microcarrier cultivation.

Analysis of fermentation samples
Total cell number was determined using crystal violet staining of cell nuclei. Viable cell counts were determined by the trypan blue dye exclusion method with a haemocytometer. Glucose and lactate concentrations in the fermentation broth were determed either off-line using glucose and lactate analyzers, respectively (YSI, Yellow Springs, OH), or on-line using FIA-Biosensors. AT-III titers were measured using a double sandwich ELISA method (8). Sodium dodecylsulfate-polyacrylamide gel electrophoresis (SDS-PAGE) was performed according to Laemmli (9). For western blot analysis, an immunological method based on the same principle as the ELISA test using rabbit-anti AT III serum was employed (10). Bradford's method was used for the measurement of total protein content (11).

Results and Discussion

Results from two fermentations (A: suspension culture, B: microcarrier culture) in a 1.2 l fermentor are shown in Figure 1. The same cell line was used for both fermentations. Both fermentations were started by inoculating the fermentor in medium containing 5% fetal calf serum (FCS) and then perfusing the culture with serum free medium. In this way, after perfusion of the culture with 2-3 reactor

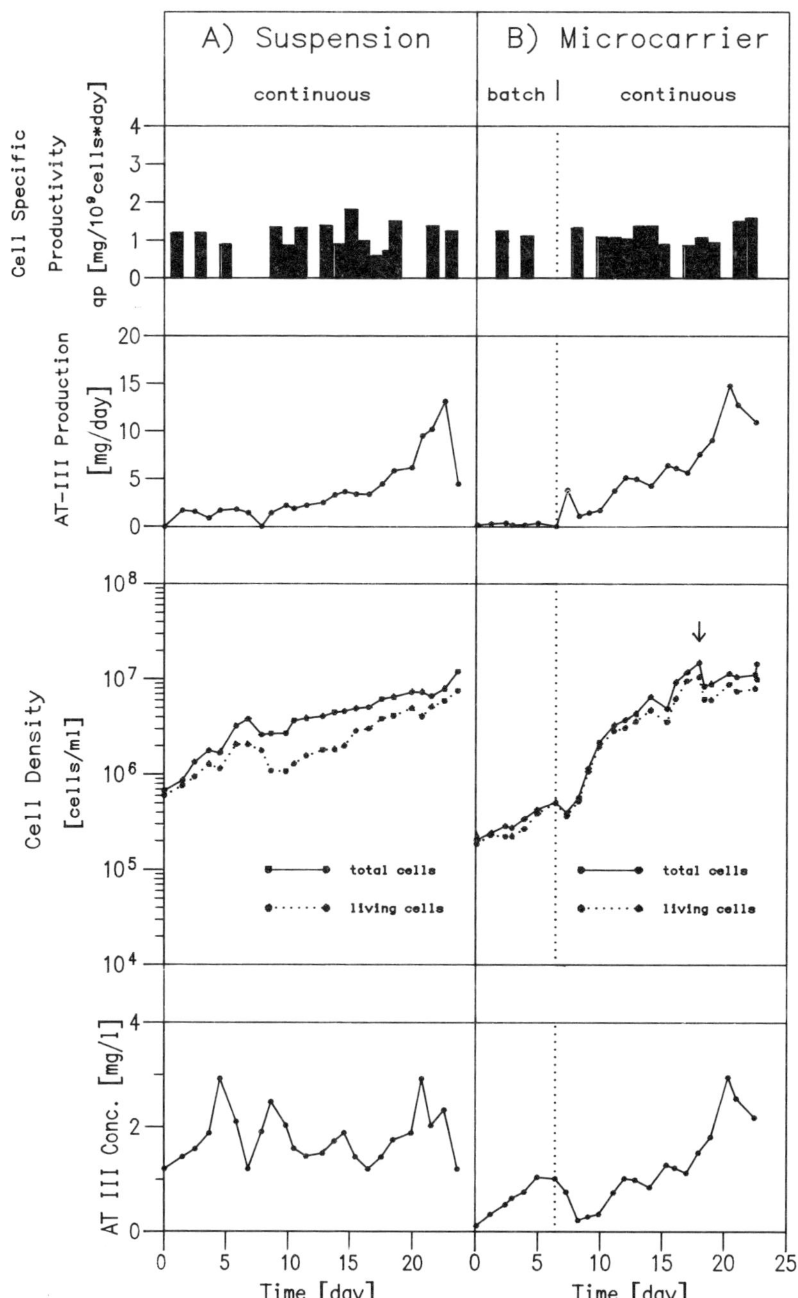

Fig.1. Comparison of the growth and production behavior of AT III producing BHK cells in suspension (A) and microcarrier (B) culture with respect to cell specific AT III productivity (q_p), AT III production, cell density and AT III concentration.

volumes of medium, the serum concentration was below 0.1% , which is also substantiated by the Bradford test of total protein concentration (less than 0.8 mg/ml, data not shown).

In fermentation A, cells were cultivated on microcarriers. Cells were inoculated at a density of 6.6 x 10^5 cells/ml. Medium perfusion was started immediatly after inoculation. At day 23, a maximal cell density of 1.2 x 10^7 cells/ml was reached. The cell specific productivity was about 1.2 mg/10^9cells*24h. During the fermentation period, 87 mg of crude AT III was harvested.

For comparison purpose, the same cell line were cultivated in suspension, namely, without a microcarrier (fermentation B). The initial cell density was 2.0 x 10^5 cells/ml. The cell had grown to 5.0 x 10^5 by the sixth day, at which time the perfusion was started by a continuous feeding in fresh serum-free medium and simultanuous removal of the conditioned medium. In fermentation A, medium supply was insufficient to meet cell requirements, especially at the higher density stage. Both cell growth and AT III production were limited at higher cell densities. This result prompted us to increase the medium exchange rate in fermentation B. Accordingly, higher growth rates and higher AT III yields were achieved. The AT-III productivity remained constant (approximately 1.2mg/10^9-cells*24h) throughout the fermentation. A total amout of 108 mg of crude AT-III was produced and harvested in 24 days.

Both fermentations were not inoculated synchronously and the medium exchange rates of both were not the same, which preclude a direct comparison. However, irrespective the kind of cultivation, a maximal cell density of 1.2 x 10^7 cells/ml and 1.4 x 10^7 was achieved in suspension (A) and microcarrier (B) culture, respectively. In both cultures, at high cell density under optimal medium supply, comparable amount of maximun AT III production was attained (suspension: 13.1 mg/day, microcarrier: 14.8 mg/day). Moreover, the cell specific productivity (q_p; mg/10^9 cells*24h) was indistinguishable in both cultures and remained constant throughout the fermentation period. Similar results were also obtained employing a BHK cell line with higher productivity (about 30 mg/10^9 cells*24h). The cell specific productivities in both suspension and microcarrier culture are almost the same and remain constant throughout the fermentation period (data not shown).

Total protein components in supernatant of fermentation samples were analysed using SDS-PAGE. As revealed in Figure 2, foreign proteins were much reduced under serum free and BSA free conditions, respectively. This proves to be especially advantageous for protein purification. Preliminary results of protein quality investigation through western blot suggest that AT III preserves its integrity under serum-free cultivation condition better (Figure 3). Under cultivation conditions containing serum, AT III fragments seem to exist, whereas under serum free conditions no AT III fragment were observed. More intensive understanding of this phenomenon, will require however further investigation(12).

Furthermore, in order to obtain an optimal process control, important physiolog-ical parameters, such as glucose and lactate concentration were continuously determined. Biosensors in combination with FIA (flow injection analysis) were used for the on-line determination of these parameters. The utilization of biosensor for continuous on-line measurement of glucose and lactate enable us to make more reliable judgment of cell metabolism at smaller interval as be-fore(14,15).

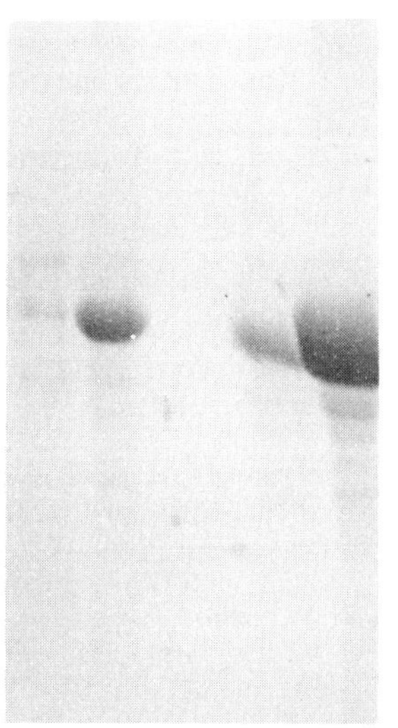

Fig.2. SDS-PAGE analysis of protein components of fermentation supernatants in

A : serum-free, BSA-free
medium

B : serum-free medium

C : medium containing 1.25% FCS

D : medium containing 2.5% FCS.

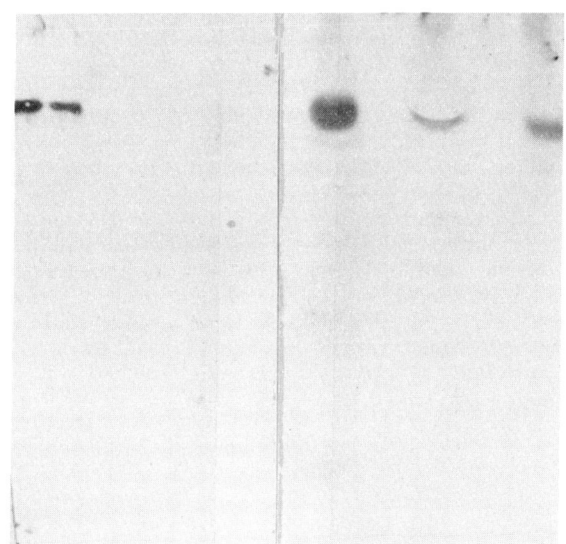

Fig.3. Westernblot analysis of fermentation supernatants for AT III integrity using rabbit-antiserum against AT III

A,B : plasma AT III

C,D : FCS & NCS control,resp.

E : supernatant containing 2.5% FCS

F : supernatant without serum

G : supernatant without serum and BSA

References

1. Travis, J. and Salvesen, G.S. Human plasma proteinase inhibitors. Annu. Rev. Biochem. 1983, 52, 655
2. Vinazzer, H. Clinical use of Antithrombin III Concentrates. Vox Sang. 1987, 53, 193
3. Peterson, C.B. and Blackburn, M.N. J. Biol. Chem. 1985, Isolation and characterization of an Antithrombin III Variant with reduced carbohydrate content and enhanced heparin binding. 260, 610
4. Franzén, L.-E., Svensson, S. and Larm, O. Structural studies on the carbohydrate portion of human antithrombin III. J. Biol. Chem. 1980, 255, 5090
5. Lehmann, J., Vorlop, J. and Büntemeyer, H. Bubble-free reactors and their development for continous culture with cell recycle. In: Animal Cell Biotechnology Vol. 3, (Eds. Spier, R. E. and Griffiths, J. B.) 1988, p.221-237
6. Wirth, M., Li, S. Y., Schumacher, L. Lehmann, J., Zettlmeißl, G. and Hauser, H. Screening for and fermentation of high producer cell clones from recombinant BHK cells. In: Advances in animal cell biology and technology for bioprocesses (Eds. Spier, R. E., Griffiths, J. B., Stephenne, J. and Crooy, P. J.) Butterworths, 1989, p.44-51
7. Bödeker, B. G. D., Berg, G. J., Hewlett, G. and Schlumberger, H.D. Screening-method to develop serum-free culture medium for adherent cell lines. Develop. biol. Standard 1984, 60, 93
8. Zettlmeissl, G., Ragg, H. and Karges, H. Expression of biologically active human antithrombin III in chinese Hamster Ovary cells. Bio/technology 1987, 5, 720
9. Laemmli, U. K. Cleavage of structural proteins during the assembly of the head of bacteriophage T4. Nature 1970, 227, 680
10. Burnette, W.N. "Western Blotting": Electrophoretic transfer of proteins from sodium dodecylsulfate-polyacrylamide gels to unmodified nitro-cellulose and radiographic detection with antibody and radionated protein A. Anal. Biochem. 1981, 112, 195
11. Bradford, M. A rapid and sensitive method for the quantitation of microgram quantities of protein utilizing the principle of protein-dye binding. Anal. Biochem. 1976, 72, 248
12. Vournakis, J. N. and Runstadler, P. W. Microenvironment: The key to improve cell culture products. Bio/Technology 1989, 7, 143
13. Dremel, B. A. A., Li, S.-Y. and Schmid, D. On-line glucose and lactate monitoring of an animal cell culture with a fibre optic detection system in combination with flow injection analysis (FIA). presented in The First World Congress on Biosensor, Singapore, 1990.
14. Huang, Y. L., Li, S. Y., Dremel, B. A. A., Bilitewski, U. and Schmid, R. D. On-line determination of glucose concentration in animal cell cultures based on chemiluminescent detection of hydrogen peroxide coupled with flow-injection analysis. submitted.

OXYGEN TRANSFER CHARACTERISTICS IN CELL CULTURE FERMENTERS: DIRECT SPARGING – MEMBRANE OXYGENATION – BUBBLE-FREE AERATION THROUGH A ROTATING SIEVE.

Thomas Thaler[#] and Jan Vanàk[*]

[#]MBR Bio Reactor AG, Werkstrasse 4, CH-8620 Wetzikon, Switzerland

[*]Inst. of Sera and Vaccines, Allendova 52, CS-77900 Olomouc, Czechoslovakia

ABSTRACT

The oxygen transfer characteristics were determined both in an airlift and in a stirred tank configuration using direct sparging, membrane oxygenation or bubble-free aeration through a rotating sieve. Very good oxygen transfer rates were achieved in airlift configuration. In a stirred tank with membrane oxygenation, a relationship between agitation speed, liquid flow pattern and oxygen transfer rates were observed. Using the bubble-free aeration through a rotating sieve, the volumetric oxygen transfer coefficient can be significantly improved without direct sparging.

KEYWORDS

Cell culture fermenter-oxygen transfer-airlift-stirred tank-direct sparging-membrane oxygenation-aeration through rotating sieve

INTRODUCTION

To sustain optimum cell growth, the rate of oxygen supply must meet the oxygen consumption rate of the cells. In addition, the dissolved oxygen concentration must be maintained above a critical value. Since animal cells are sensitive to shear stress, the aeration of the culture medium must be carried out creating minimal forces on the fragile cells. Some aeration methods are limited in large-scale operations; therefore the method used has to be adapted to the scale of the process.

MATERIALS AND METHODS

Measurments of oxygen transfer characteristics were performed in fermenters (MBR Bio Reactor AG, Switzerland) with working volumes in the range 11, 30, 140 and 270 liters using either airlift or stirred tank configuration, both equipped with draught-tubes. All studies were carried out in water at 37 Degrees Celcius. The concentration of dissolved oxygen was determined using a polarographic electrode (Ingold AG, Switzerland). Oxygen transfer rates (OTR) were measured according to the dynamic method. K_La-values were calculated as described by de Bruyne[1].

RESULTS AND DISCUSSION

Airlift Configuration

Very good oxygen transfer rates were achieved in the airlift configuration using air flow rates ranging from 0.02 to 0.05 vvm. Oxygen transfer rates observed in fermenters with different working volumes (11 l up to 140 l) were similar (Table 1).

| WORKING VOLUME | OXYGEN TRANSFER RATE [mMole/liter x hour] | | | |
[liter]	0.02 vvm	0.03 vvm	0.04 vvm	0.05 vvm
11	0.8	1.1	1.4	1.7
30	0.7	0.9	1.2	1.4
140	0.8	0.9	1.0	1.3

Table 1: Effect of the airflow rate on the oxygen transfer rate: Airlift configuration

Stirred Tank Configuration with Membrane Oxygenation System

In a stirred tank configuration (11 l working volume) with a membrane oxygenation system (silicon rubber tubing) a relationship between agitation speed of the marine impeller and the

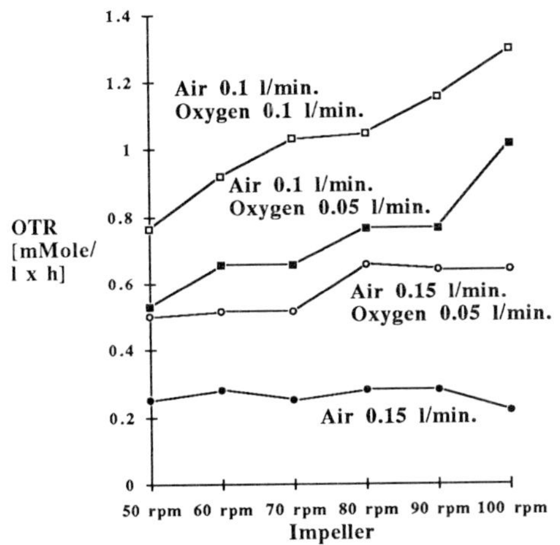

Figure 1:

Effect of the rotation speed of the marine impeller on the oxygen transfer rate:

Stirred tank (11 liter working volume) equipped with a membrane oxygenation system.

oxygen transfer rate was determined mainly at higher oxygen
concentrations in the gas mixture (Figure 1).In comparison
with the conventional airlift flow pattern, up to 25% higher
oxygen transfer rates were demonstrated in stirred fermenters
operating with an inverse liquid flow.

Bubble-free Aeration through a Rotating Sieve

Because gas-permeable-membrane tubing applications are limited
in large-scale operations by the length of the tubing, a
bubble-free aeration system allowing reliable scale-up has
been developed. This new system is based on the Spinferm® design incorporating a rotating sieve with additional sparging
of a gas-mixture in the cell-free zone within the rotating
sieve itself. Using this bubble-free aeration method in 140 l
and 270 l fermenters, the volumetric oxygen transfer coefficient can be significantly improved without direct sparging.
At given air flow rates per unit reactor volume, the $k_L a$
achieved with this system was roughly 2/3 of the values observed by direct sparging in the cell-containing space.

Reactor-working volume [l]	Airflow rate [vvm]	$k_L a$ with bubble-free aeration [h-1]	$k_L a$ with direct sparging [h-1]
140	0.02	1.9	3.2
	0.04	3.0	4.3
270	0.02	1.3	2.8

Table 2:

Effect of airflow rate on the oxygen transfer rate using bubble-free aeration through the rotating sieve (mesh size 100μm,
surface velocity 0.4 m/sec) or direct sparging in the cell-
containing space in 140 and 270 l fermenters.

REFERENCES

1 De Bruyne, N. A.,*Animal Cell Biotechnology Vol. 3*, R.E.
  Spier and J. B. Griffiths, Eds., (Academic Press, NY,1988),
  p.141-176.

HYBRIDOMA CULTURE IN A MEMBRANE SYSTEM: THE INFLUENCE OF OXYGEN ON A REACTOR'S PERFORMANCE AND ON THE EVALUATION OF CELLULAR DENSITY.

GEAUGEY V.[1], PASCAL F.[2], MARC A.[2], ENGASSER J.M.[2] and DUVAL D.[1]

1: Bertin et Cie; Div. Génie Chimique et Biochimique; B.P. n° 3; 78373 Plaisir; FRANCE.
2: Laboratoire des Sciences du Génie Chimique; CNRS - ENSIC; 1 rue Grandville;
   B.P. 451; 54000 Nancy; FRANCE.

ABSTRACT

In order to investigate the importance of oxygen in membrane reactors, mouse hybridoma cells have been grown in a deep-end filtration system. Oxygen and other nutrients are fed in by direct irrigation of the cell chamber. Thus, contrary to classical membrane reactors, the design of this apparatus clearly depicts operating conditions. We show that oxygen availability is the main factor limiting growth and MAb production. Using a constant feeding rate, we also demonstrate an inhibitory effect of lactate on cell proliferation, and a decrease in the specific production rate of MAb occuring approximatively 300 hours after seeding. In membrane reactors, viable cell density is generally assessed by measuring glucose and/or oxygen consumption rates. However, we show in stirred tank reactor experiments that specific oxygen or glucose consumption rates, and therefore the cell densities estimated from such data, are directly dependant upon oxygen concentration in the culture medium.

INTRODUCTION

The use of continuously perfused reactors is an attractive way for the production of protein by mammalian cells. However, the performance of these reactors are not yet satisfactory, and industrial production strategy is still based on discontinuous processes. It is generally assumed from both theoretical (1) and experimental (2) studies that the poor results often observed in hollow fiber cartridges are a consequence of oxygen limitation. In the present paper, we have thus determined using an appropriate experimental design whether or not the cells were limited when O2 supply is only realised by a flow of air saturated medium. We have also measured in these experiments the evolution of cell proliferation, the stability of monoclonal antibody (MAb) secretion, and the toxicity of lactate ions.
Determination of the density and viability of cells entrapped in hollow fiber reactors is not directly feasible. Usually, these data are assessed by comparing the glucose or oxygen consumption rates to those determined in stirred tank reactors (3) (4). We investigate in this report the influence of oxygenation conditions on the glucose (Sr Gluc) and the oxygen (Sr O2) specific consumption rates determined in stirred tank reactors. Consequences for the use of these evaluation methods in the case of hollow fiber runs are discussed.

MATERIAL AND METHODS

Cell Line, Media and Analysis: VO 208 mouse hybridoma cells secreting IgG 2a were grown in RPMI 1640 supplemented with 5% fetal calf serum, 2% MEM amino acids, glucose (4 g.l $^{-1}$) and glutamine (4 mM). Cell count and viability were determined using the trypan blue exclusion procedure. Glucose and lactic acid were assayed by enzymatic methods. Peroxydase conjugated goat anti-mouse IgG was used to detect the antibodies released into the culture medium in an ELISA assay.
Suspension Cultures: experiments were carried out in a 2 l stirred tank reactors (SGI and Biolafitte, France) seeded at 2 10 ^{5} cells .ml $^{-1}$. The dissolved oxygen tension (DOT) was regulated at 30% of air saturation (control experiments) or maintained below 1% by the use of constant surface aeration (oxygen limitation experiments).
Membrane Reactor: we used the deep-end filtration systems Minikap 500 (Microgon, USA) seeded with 5.10 ^{7} viable cells. Hybridomas, kept in the extracapillary space of approx. 20 ml, were directly irrigated by

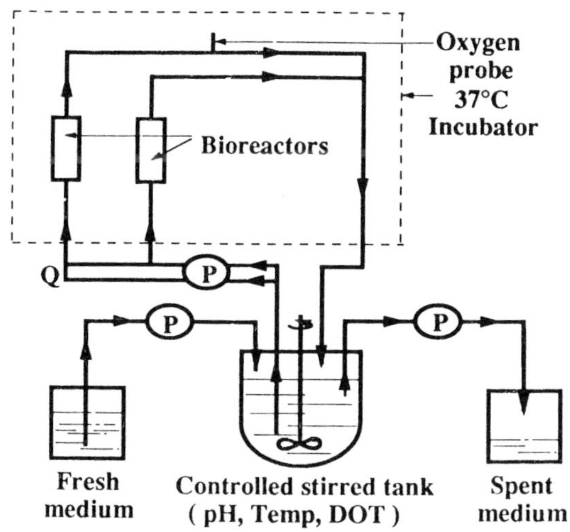

Fig. 1 - Schematic diagram of the experimental design

medium entering the reactor. DOT of the medium leaving the reactor was measured by a polarographic probe. Operating conditions (perfusion rate, nutrients and toxic wastes concentrations in the culture medium) were therefore determined more easily in this reactor as compared to the commonly used cross-flow filtration systems. Since experimental determination of cellular density and viability requires an arrest of reactor's operation, 2 cartridges working in parallel were used (see fig. 1), the first one being stopped at the end of the first operating conditions in order to provide intermediate values and the other one arrested at the end of the experiment (second operating conditions). Each reactor was perfused at the same flow rate Q with medium maintained at a constant temperature (37°C), pH (7,1) and O2 (air saturation) within a 2 l stirred tank. This reservoir was continuously renewed by fresh medium with a constant flow rate of 0,25 l.day $^{-1}$ per cartridge (i. e. a total value of 0,5 l.day $^{-1}$ during the first operating conditions and 0,25 l.day $^{-1}$ during the second one).

RESULTS AND DISCUSSION

Two separate experiments were performed with the membrane system under the conditions summarized in table 1. For a few hours after seeding and up to the end of the culture, the oxygen fed in the cartridge was entirely consumed by the cells since the DOT of the medium issued was 0. A doubling of the perfusion rate

Operating conditions			Experiment n°		Results			
Q (l.d^{1})	Lact. init (mM)	Duration (h)			Viable cells	Lact. (mM)	rMAb	Sr MAb
1	0	0-230	1	a	1,45	16	0,24	1,65
2	0	230-660		b	2,5	25	0,31	1,25
2	0	0-265	2	a	2,7	27	0,53	1,95
2	40	265-620		b	1,65	56	0,21	1,25

Table 1 - Operating conditions of membrane reactors and results obtained at cartridge arrest. "Lact. Init" represents the lactate concentration in the fresh medium. Viable cells are expressed as 10^8 per cartridge, rMAb in mg . day -1 and SrMAb in mg . (day . 10^9 viable cells) $^{-1}$

Q, and thus of the oxygen feeding rate was responsible in the experiment 1 for a 70% enhancement of viable cell population, but for a lower increase in MAb production rate (see 1a and 1b, table 1). Increasing the lactate concentration (addition of 40mM in fresh medium) in the experiment 2 led to a strong reduction of viable cell population and to a dramatic decrease in MAb secretion rate (see 2a and 2b, table 1). These data suggest that oxygen availability and lactate concentration in the 25 - 55 mM range are important factors limiting cell proliferation and MAb secretion. When considering experiments 1b and 2a which have been carried out under similar experimental conditions, it also appears that the MAb specific production rate (Sr MAb) is lower at the end of the culture (1b) than at the beginning (2a). This is confirmed by the comparison of the values of Sr MAb determined for 1a and 1b. This decrease in the MAb specific production rate, occuring between 300 and 600 h, has also been described recently (5) and should be taken into account for the evaluation of perfused reactors.

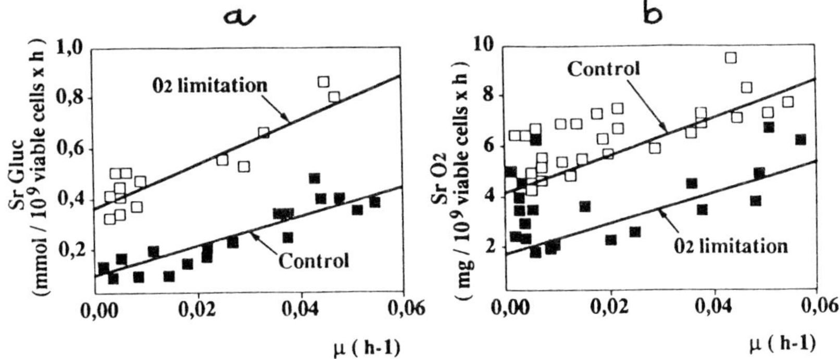

Fig. 2 - Effect of oxygenation conditions on specific metabolic rates
a) glucose specific consumption rate v.s specific growth rate
b) Oxygen specific consumption rate v.s specific growth rate

From the results obtained in stirred reactors under controlled or limited oxygenation conditions, we have plotted the glucose (Sr Gluc, see fig. 2a) and the oxygen (Sr O2, see fig. 2b) specific consumption rates against the specific growth rate (μ). Sr Gluc and Sr O2 appear highly dependant upon μ and oxygenation conditions. Since μ is generally low in perfused experiments (6), small variations of this parameter are expected during the culture, with slight consequences on Sr Gluc and Sr O2. In the other hand, oxygenation conditions of cells entrapped in a reactor are not easily measurable, which induce possible variations in a 1-4 range for Sr Gluc and 1-2,5 for Sr O2. Therefore, the accurate use of the glucose and O2 consumtion rates for the assessment of viable cell density is not possible as long as oxygenation conditions are not known.

REFERENCES

1: Geahel I., Duval D., Geaugey V., Hache J., Dufau A.F., Marc A. and Engasser J.M. Proc. Intern. Conf. on Bioreactors and Biotransformations, 9 - 12 Nov. 1987, Gleneagles, Scottland.
2: Schönherr O.T. and Van Gelder P.J.T.A. In: "Animal Cell Biotechnology Vol. 3" (Ed: Spier R.E. and Griffiths J.B.) Academic Press, London, 1988, 337.
3: Tharakan J.P. and Chau P.C. Biotechnol. Bioeng. 1986, 18, 329.
4: Chresand T.J., Gillies R.J. and Dale B.E. Biotechnol. Bioeng. 1988, 9, 983.
5: Frame K.K. and Hu W.-S. Biotechnol. Bioeng. 1990, 35, 469.
6: Wagner A., Villermaux S., Marc A., Engasser J.M., Kleuser B. and Einsele A. Advances in Animal Cell Biology and Technology for Bioprocesses (Ed: Spier R.E., Griffiths J.B., Stephenne J. and Crooy P.J.) Butterworths, 1989, 238.

HYBRIDOMA, ANTIBODY AND GROWTH FACTOR DISTRIBUTIONS IN THE
SHELL-SIDE OF ULTRAFILTRATION HOLLOW FIBER BIOREACTORS

J. M. Piret* and C.L. Cooney

Biotechnology Process Engineering Center, Department of
Chemical Engineering, Massachusetts Institute of Technology,
Cambridge MA, 02139 U.S.A.
*Address correspondence to: Biotechnology Laboratory and
Department of Chemical Engineering, University of British
Columbia, Vancouver BC, V6T 1W5 Canada.

ABSTRACT

This work has studied the spatially heterogeneous nature of
ultrafiltration hollow fiber bioreactors used for immobilized
mammalian cell culture. In reactors operated with
unidirectional medium recycle flow, downstream concentration
of high molecular weight proteins and cells in the immobilized
phase have been measured. Mechanisms responsible for these
phenomena have been investigated, and their implications in
process design and operation considered. The heterogeneous
protein and cell distributions in ultrafiltration hollow fiber
bioreactors were reduced by periodic alternation of recycle
flow direction and the reactor productivity was doubled.

INTRODUCTION

A range of mammalian cell types have been cultured in the
extracapillary (shell-side) region of hollow fiber bioreactors
(HFBR's). Ultrafiltration membrane HFBR's also concentrate
high molecular weight proteins in the immobilized phase. Thin
sections of these reactors have revealed tissue-like cell
densities in the extracapillary space (1).

MATERIALS AND METHODS

Approximately 10^8 hybridoma CRL-1606 cells (2) with 90%
viability were inoculated into Vitafiber II/PLUS HFBR's
(Amicon, Danvers MA) at the upstream extracapillary port.
Results from 6 day, 8 day and 1 month experiments are
presented where the medium was recycled through the hollow
fibers with unidirectional flow at 100 ml/min. A two week
experiment was performed in which the recycle flow direction
was inverted every 5 min in order to better distribute cell
growth. The HFBR's were run batch for about 1 week and then
perfused continuously with from 1 to 3 ml/min of fresh medium.

At the end of each experiment the medium recycle streams were
replace by air and the cartridges were place in liquid
nitrogen. After storage at -40°C, the central 13.5 cm of the
cartridges were sawed into 7 or 8 axial sections in a 4°C
room. Each section was thawed in 5 or 10 ml Dulbecco's
Phosphate Buffered Salt Solution with Ca and Mg and 1 mM
phenyl methyl fluoride (a protease inhibitor) at 4°C for 2 to
3 h. To evaluate the cell distributions, aliquotes of the
samples were diluted one hundred-fold in 0.4% Trypan blue,
0.9% NaCl (Sigma, St. Louis MO) and hemacytometer counted.
Viable cell counts were based on the recovery of dark stained,
ghost cells recently lysed by the freeze-thaw treatment (3).
Anti-fibronectin monoclonal antibody and transferrin titers
were analyzed by enzyme-linked-immunosorption-assays (ELISA).

RESULTS

A downstream polarization of high molecular weight proteins
was measured in the extracapillary space of HFBR's operated
with unidirectional recycle flow (Figure 1). This
distribution results from convective transport by a secondary
(Starling) flow (4) in the extracapillary space. This flow
causes a concentration polarization (5) of the proteins
retained by the ultrafiltration membranes (nominal 30,000 D
molecular weight cutoff). An additional vertical

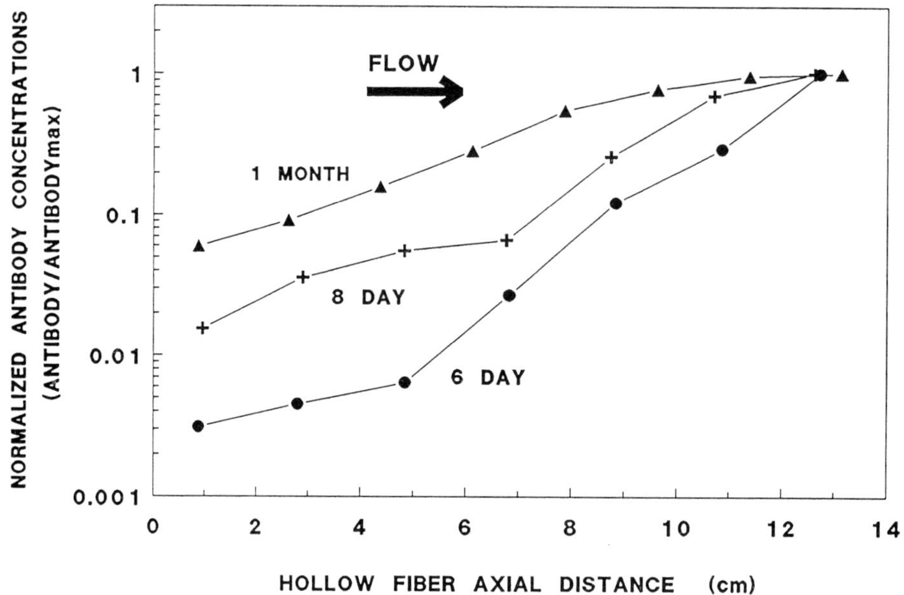

Figure 1 Axial extracapillary antibody distributions
normalized by the maximum concentration in each HFBR.

sedimentation of the concentration polarized proteins has been
observed. The protein polarization and sedimentation have
been used to maximize recovery concentrations of monoclonal
antibody from ultrafiltration HFBR's (3).

Parallel measurements of the axial distributions of cells also
revealed downstream polarization of cells. These
distributions where confirmed by the recovery of intracellular
enzymes and radial gradients resulting from metabolic activity
(i.e. lactate accumulation). The downstream skewing of the
viable cell distribution is believed to result from Starling
flow and its influence on the inoculum and high molecular
weight growth factor distributions. A downstream polarization
of transferrin was measured in the extracapillary space.

The heterogeneous distribution of hybridoma cells results in
reduced overall cell numbers and reactor productivities. By
inverting the direction of recycle flow every 5 min, both the
cell and high molecular weight protein distributions were made
more uniform. The cell loading was increased and the reactor
antibody productivity was doubled.

DISCUSSION

Ultrafiltration membranes in HFBR's retain growth factors and
selectively concentrate protein products. Extracapillary
concentration polarization and gravity sedimentation phenomena
can increase the product concentrations even further. However,
to maximize cell loading the downstream polarization of high
molecular weight growth factors should be reduced during the
growth phase. A strategy has been developed and tested to
increase cell growth and reactor antibody productivity.

ACKNOWLEDGEMENTS

This work was supported by Amicon Co., W.R. Grace and the
M.I.T. Biotechnology Process Engineering Center (BPEC).

REFERENCES

1.Knazek, R.A., Gullino, P.M., Kohler, P. and Dedrick, R.L.
   Science 1972, 178, 65
2.Schoen, R.C., Bentley, K.L. and Klebe, R.J. Monoclonal
   antibody against human fibronectin which inhibits cell
   attachment Hybridoma 1982, 1, 99
3.Piret, J.M. and Cooney, C.L. Mammalian cell and protein
   distributions in ultrafiltration hollow fiber bioreactors
   Biotechnol. Bioeng. (in press)
4.Schratter, P. In: Methods in Cell Biology 1976, 14, 95
5.Vilker, V.L., Colton, C.K. and Smith, K.A. Concentration
   polarization in protein ultrafiltration AIChE J. 1981, 27,
   632

CULTIVATION OF INSECT CELL LINES IN STIRRED

MEMBRANE REACTORS

C. Schütz[1], V. Jäger[2], A.J. Driesel[1], R. Wagner[2]
1) *Dechema-Institute, Dept. Biotechnology, D-6000 Frankfurt 97, FRG;*
2) *Gesellschaft für Biotechnologische Forschung, D-3300 Braunschweig, FRG;*

ABSTRACT

Two insect cell lines Schneider-2 and Kc, derived from *Drosophila melanogaster*, were cultivated in suspension by using stirred tank perfusion bioreactors with bubble-free aeration. To test the influence of self-produced proteins on Schneider-2 cells high molecular weight fractions were retained by using an ultrafiltration unit and led back into the bioreactor. The cell lines showed different growth behaviour. While Kc cells grew in a batch up to $6 \cdot 10^6$ viable cells/ml and with a perfusion-system to $1.7 \cdot 10^7$ cells, Schneider-2 cells reached cell densities of $1 \cdot 10^7$ viable cells/ml in batchwise mode and $3.4 \cdot 10^7$ cells/ml with continuous medium exchange.

KEYWORDS
insect cell lines, high cell density, growth characteristics, perfusion bioreactor

INTRODUCTION

During the last years insect cell tissue cultures became more important as an alternative to the various established mammalian cell culture systems. An advantage of insect cells is the easy handling of cultures, so that large-scale processes could be simplified. No CO_2 environment is required, because media are not buffered with carbonate/CO_2. Some cell lines require only small amounts of oxygen and appear to be more resistant to shear forces. Media often contain very high levels of amino acids, increasing media costs, but no supplementation with expensive agents like insulin and transferrin is needed.

Cell lines were derived from different insect species such as *Spodoptera frugiperda, Aedes albopictus, Bombyx mori* or *Drosophila melanogaster*. For some cell lines serum-free media are already established (10, 14). There are two different procedures to produce recombinant proteins in insect cells. Using coprecipitation methods cells can integrate plasmid vector DNA. Another completely different system to transfect insect cells is the infection of *Spodoptera frugiperda* cells with a recombinant baculovirus AcNPV (6). With both systems insect cells show high level expression rates (8, 13). *Spodoptera frugiperda* cells were usually grown in a batchwise mode, because of their lytic expression system with virus. In contrast to this method it is interesting to use perfusion reactor systems for cell lines that are transfected with a plasmid vector. Optimized growth can be reached combined with cell retention.

Cultivation of Schneider-2 cells in comparison with Kc cells in a stirred bioreactor under different conditions is described here. Experiments were carried out with regard to the cultivation of a Schneider-2 cell line, transfected with the vector pcopneoHAAT, that codes for the production of human α_1-anti-trypsin (2). The transfected cell line did not show any difference in growth behaviour to the wild-type Schneider-2 cell line, so that in this work the wild-type was used. Kc cells were chosen to compare two different cell lines. The suitability of the Kc cell line for further transforming experiments should be tested.

MATERIAL AND METHODS

Schneider-2 cells derived from a late embryonic state of Drosophila melano-gaster (11) were cultured in M3 Medium (12) supplemented with 5 % FCS at a temperature of 27° C. To optimize growth the medium was modified by adding lipoprotein Pentex Excyte I (Bayer Diagnostic, München) 1:500 and 2 g/l BSA complexed with cholesterin according to (7). The concentration of asparagine was increased to 4 mM, glucose content was reduced from 10 g/l to 8 g/l, the concentration of alanine was decreased to 5 mM, whereas ß-alanine could be eliminated. Kc cells derived from *Drosophila melanogaster* embryos not older than 12 h (4) were cultured in protein-free D20 Medium (5) without any supplements. Kc cells grew best at 24° C.

All experiments were carried out in bioreactors containing a moving microporous membrane as a bubble free aeration system. In continuous cultures a hydro-philized membrane was added for medium perfusion, while cells were totally retained (9). In batch cultures the volume of the bioreactor was 2.2 l, in cultures with continuous medium exchange a 1.4 l reactor was used. The oxygen was adjusted to a level of 40 % air saturation. To retain proteins a hollow fiber module (Hemoflow, E4, Fresenius, Bad Homburg, FRG) was installed between reactor and harvest bottle (3) (see fig. 1). Peristaltic pumps were used for medium perfusion. To get a cross-flow effect inside the module a gear-type pump (no 4.) was installed and adjusted to a flowrate of 240 ml/min. The flow-rates of pump no 1. was 6.1 ml/min, the maximum rate for pump no 2. was 1.26 ml/min, whereas the rates of pump no 3. did never exceed 0.195 ml/min.

Cell numbers were determined by using a hemocytometer. Viability was tested by trypan blue exclusion. Amino acid concentration was analyzed by HPLC after derivatization by orthophthaldialdehyde. Glucose and lactate concentrations in supernatants were determined using glucose and lactate analyzers (YSI, Yellow Springs, OH). Protein determinations were done according to the method of Bradford (1).

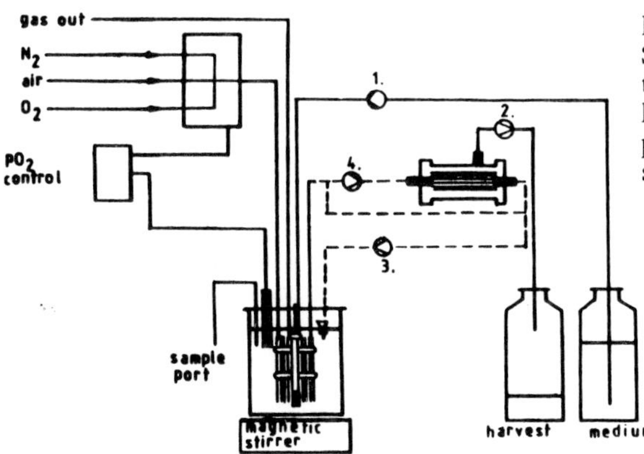

Fig. 1:
Schematic diagram of the stirred tank bioreactor system, the dash-lined part was used only for data presented in fig. 3. Explanation see text.

RESULTS AND DISCUSSION

The minimum inoculum of the Schneider-2 cell line is very high. Preliminary studies showed, that the culture did not grow at cell densities lower than $8 \cdot 10^5$ viable cells/ml. It was also important, to inoculate with 20-50 % of conditioned medium for successful propagation of cells. Schneider-2 cells could be grown as a batch culture over 14 days to a density of $1 \cdot 10^7$ cells/ml. With a perfusion-system an increase of the cell density up to $3 \cdot 10^7$ viable cells/ml was possible. These data could be achieved with perfusion rates of 1.5-2 reactor volumes/d. When applicating lower perfusion rates cells went into a stationary phase. Analysis of glucose, lactate and amino acids showed, that a limitation did not occur (data not shown). To test whether high molecular weight conditioning factors, which are necessary at the beginning of the culture, were diluted by medium exchange, these proteins had to be retained within the bioreactor. Molecules with a molecular weight more than 10.000 Dalton were recycled by using a hollow fiber cartridge. Cells were grown to $1 \cdot 10^7$ cells/ml in batchwise mode. When high molecular weight proteins were recycled cells did not grow further. The highest cell density did not exceed $3.4 \cdot 10^7$ viable cells/ml, which could be also reached in a perfusion mode without protein recycling, indicating that the lack of growth was not caused by a dilution of conditioning proteins. However, this phenomenon could be also a result of the production of inhibiting factors of high molecular weight. With the hollow fiber system inhibiting factors with a molecular weight higher than 10.000 Dalton were concentrated as well as conditioning proteins of this size. To distinguish between conditioning and inhibiting proteins an exact knowledge of those proteins would be necessary. Another possibility to explain the growth behaviour is a substrate limitation. This substrate was available at high perfusion rates and must have a molecular weight lower then 10.000 Dalton. Glucose and amino acids could be excluded as limiting agents, because concentration of this compounds were monitored during the experiment. Therefore further work will be necessary to test whether cell density can be increased by using higher perfusion rates and to identify the limiting substrate. In contrast to mammalian cells the insect cells tested here did not die immediatly, but rested for over one week on maximum cell density without any increase of dead cells, when medium exchange was stopped.

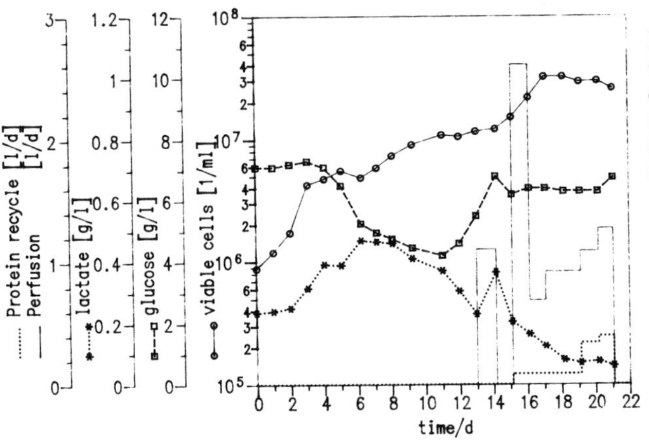

Fig. 2:
Cultivation of Schneider-2 cells with medium perfusion and protein retention in a stirred tank 1.4 l bioreactor.

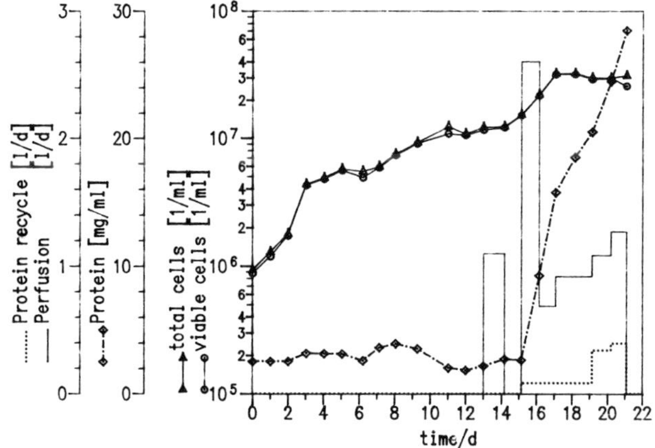

Fig. 3:
Protein recycling rates and protein concentration during cultivation of Schneider-2 cells in a perfusion bioreactor.

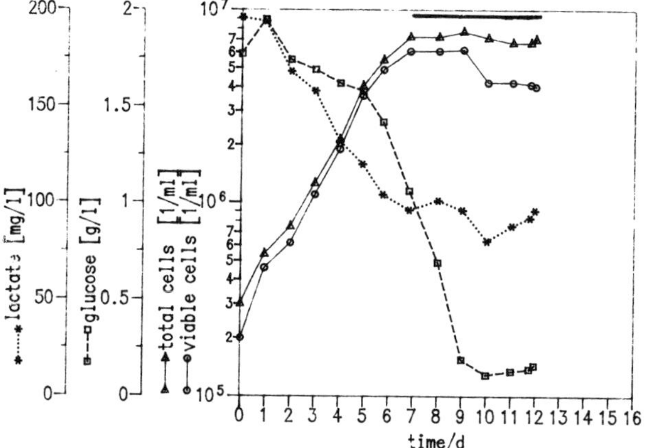

Fig. 5:
Batch culture of Kc cells in a 2 l bioreactor using batchwise mode; from day 7, as indicated by the bar, oxygen supply was limited.

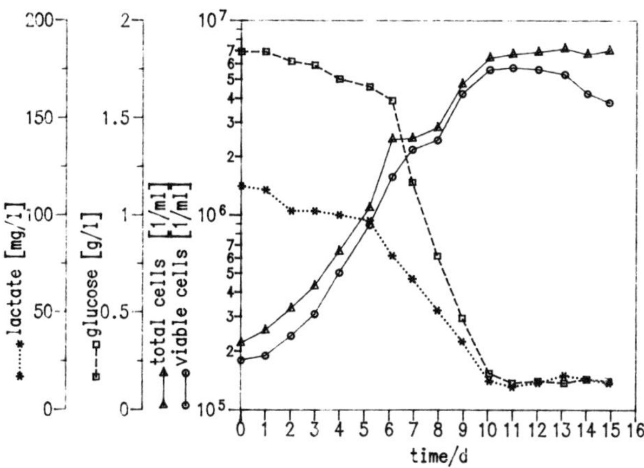

Fig. 4:
Batch culture of Kc cells in a 2 l bioreactor.

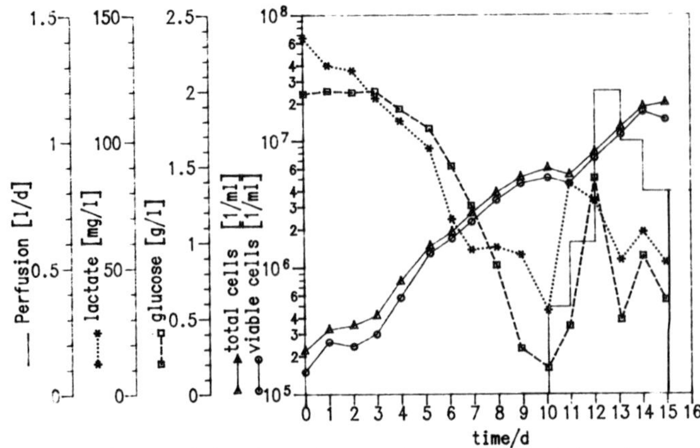

Fig. 6:
Cultivation of Kc cells in a 1.4 l bioreactor with continuous medium exchange.

Kc cells could be inoculated with $2 \cdot 10^5$ cells/ml in completely fresh medium and appeared to be independent from conditioning factors in contrast to Schneider-2 cells. During 10 days of culture cells grew in batchwise mode up to $6 \cdot 10^6$ viable cells/ml. At the initial phase of the culture Kc cells consumed 100 μmol/$10^9 \cdot$h of oxygen, twice as much than Schneider-2 cells. The final cell density which could be reached in batch culture was not affected by limited oxygen supply as shown in figures 3 and 4. The medium was supplemented with lactalbumin hydrolysate and contained significant amounts of lactate. In contrast to Schneider-2 cells, lactate was not produced but consumed permanently by Kc cells, as long as no oxygen limitation occured. An increase to $1.7 \cdot 10^7$ viable cells/ml could be reached by exchanging medium in rates between 0.5-1 reactor volumes/d. Medium exchange was necessary because of glucose limitation. Further analysis showed, that the concentration of available amino acids was not limited. As in the case of Schneider-2 cells it appeared, that at lower perfusion rates then 1 reactor volume/d a substrate limitation occured.

Both cell lines reached relative high cell densities with low perfusion rates. When using higher perfusion rates, a further increase should be possible. Schneider-2 and Kc cell lines were derived from the same organism and varied only in the age of the tissue, from which they were isolated. Their growth behaviour at low perfusion rates was similar. Schneider-2 cells reached higher cell densities as did Kc cells, but had different demands on media composition.

ACKNOWLEDGEMENTS

This work was supported by a grant from the Federal Ministry of Research and Technology, FRG.

REFERENCES

1) Bradford M. (1976) A rapid and sensitive method for the quantitation of microgram quantities of protein utilizing the principle of protein-dye binding. Anal. Biochem. **72**, 248-254

2) Bräutigam S., Driesel A.J. (1990) Gene transfer of a human α_1-Antitrypsin cDNA into cultured *Drosophila melanogaster* cells. J. Insect. Physiol., submitted

3) Büntemeyer H. (1987) Entwicklung eines Perfusionssystems zur kontinuier lichen Kultivierung tierischer Zellen in Suspension. Dissertation Universität Hannover 1987

4)   Echalier G., Ohanessian A. (1969) Isolement, en cultures *in vitro*, de lignées cellulaires diploides de *Drosophila melanogaster*. C. R. Acad. Sc. Paris **268**, 1771-1773

5)   Echalier G., Ohanessian A.   In vitro culture of *Drosophila melanogaster* embryonic cells. In Vitro **6**, 162-172

6)   Fraser M.J. (1989) Expression of eucaryotic genes in insect cell cultures. In Vitro, **25** 225-235

7)   Jäger V., Lehmann J., Friedl P. (1988) Serum-free growth medium for the cultivation of a wide spectrum of mammalian cells in stirred bioreactors. Cytotechnology **1**, 319-329

8)   Johansen H., van der Straten A., Sweet R., Otto E., Maroni G., Rosenberg M. (1989) Regulated expression at high copy number allows production of a growth inhibitory oncogene product in *Drosophila* Schneider cells. Genes and Develop. **3**, 882-889

9)   Lehmann J., Vorlop J., Büntemeyer H. (1988) Bubble-free Reactors and Their Development for Continuous Culture with Cell Recycle. In: R.E. Spier, J.B. Griffiths (eds.) Animal Cell Biotechnology Vol 3, Acad. Press London, pp. 221-237

10) Maiorella B., Inlow D., Shauger A., Harano D. (1988) Large-scale insect cell - culture for recombinant protein production. Biotechnology **6**, 1406-1410

11) Schneider I. (1972) Cell lines derived from late embryonic stages of *Drosophila melanogaster*. J. Embryol. exp. Morph. **27**, 353-365

12) Shields G., Sang J.H. (1977) Improved medium for culture of Drosophila embryonic cells. Dros. Inf. Serv. **52**, 161

13) Sissom J., Ellis L. (1989) Secretion of the extracellular domain of the human insulin receptor from insect cells by use of a baculovirus vector. Biochem. J. **261**, 119-126

14) Vaughn J.L., Fan F. (1989) Use of commercial serum replacements for the culture of insect cells. In Vitro **25**, 143-145

<u>**Paper of Schutz**</u>

Caulcott: Your slides, and what you said, imply that your insect cells were actually using lactate as a carbon source. Is this right?

Schutz: Yes, but not under oxygen limiting conditions.

Caulcott: Do you add lactate to your medium?

Schutz: Not yet, but I am considering doing this.

Bliem: We have also observed that insect cells both consume and produce lactate.

High Density Culture of Hybridoma Cells using a Perfusion Culture Apparatus with Multi-settling Zones

Michiyuki Tokashiki and Takami Arai

Biotechnology Research Laboratory, Tokyo Research Center,
Teijin Limited, 4-3-2, Asahigaoka, Hino-shi, Tokyo 191 Japan

ABSTRACT

Mouse-human hybridoma X32 cells were cultivated using a perfusion culture apparatus provided with three settling zones where the cells were separated from the culture medium by gravitational settling, as oxygen was supplied using a perfluorocarbon.

Viable cell density reached about 2×10^7 cells$\cdot$ml^{-1} at 2.0 vol$\cdot$vol$^{-1}\cdot$d^{-1} specific perfusion rate, and the monoclonal antibody was continuously produced. This viable cell density was significantly higher than in the perfusion culture of a gravitational settling type provided with one settling zone, as oxygen was directly sparged (about 1×10^7 cell$\cdot$ml^{-1}).

INTRODUCTION

It has been recognized that culture systems should be developed for high cell density and long-term culture and a variety of proposals have been made. Since mammalian cells have generally a low ability to produce target substances, perfusion culture using a large volume tank which can continue for a long period of time is thought to be advantageous for economical mass production. The authors developed a gravitational settling type perfusion culture vessel and obtained good results[1]. In scale-up, the settling area must be enlarged in proportion to the culture volume, but the enlargement becomes more difficult, as the volume increases. Thereupon, the authors have devised a new column type of perfusion vessel equipped with a plurality of settling zones and conducted high-density culture of a hybridoma[2]. At this time, high density culture of hybridoma was tried using a perfluorocarbon as a medium for supplying oxygen in a perfusion culture system[3] equipped with a plurality of settling zones.

MATERIALS AND METHODS

Experimental apparatus

The culture vessel is a column equipped with a plurality of vertically arranged settling zones and the culture medium, separated from the cells by gravitation, is taken out of each settling zone by individual pumps. The perfluorocarbon distributes in the bottom of the culture vessel and the oxygen absorber. Oxygen is always blown into the bottom of the oxygen absorber, and the perfluorocarbon sent from the culture vessel absorbs oxygen by coming into contact with the oxygen, overflows the absorber and goes back to the culture vessel.

Cells

The mouse-human hybridoma X32 line, which was obtained by fusion of mouse myeloma P3/x63-Ag8.U1 cells with human spleen cells, was used in the experiment. The line produces a human IgG1.

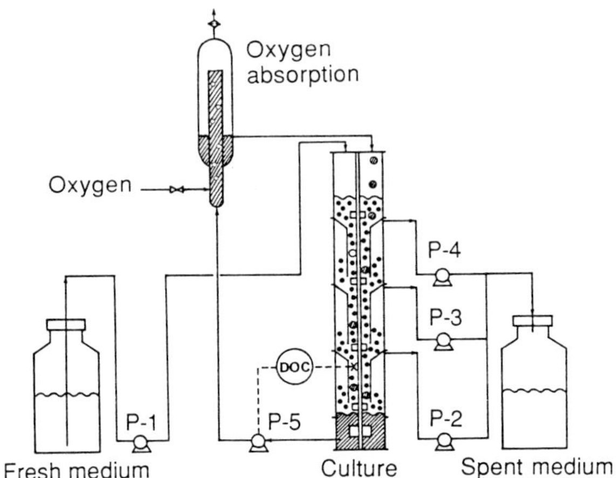

Fig.1 Perfusion culture system with multi-settling zones. In this culture system fluorocarbon are used for oxygen supply.

Culture medium

Serum-free eRDF[4] containing 9 μg·ml^{-1} of insulin, 10 μg·ml^{-1} of human transferrin, 10 μM of ethanolamine and 20 nM of sodium selenite was used as the medium.

Perfluorocarbon

Fluorinert FC-40 (3-M, USA) was used.

Assay of immunoglobulin

The antibody secreted by the hybridoma in the medium was determined by the single radial immunodiffusion assay (SRID).

RESULTS AND DISCUSSION

The cells were sterilely taken out of the perfusion culture tank of a gravitational settling type in which high density culture was continued and inoculated. The vial cell density was 1.02×10^6 cell·ml^{-1} immediately after inoculation and the net culture volume was 850 ml. Perfusion was started at once at a specific rate of 1.0 vol·vol^{-1}·d^{-1}. The viable cell density was found to be 1.8×10^6 cell·ml^{-1} 2 days later. At this point, the perfusion rate was increased to 2.0 vol·vol^{-1}·d^{-1}. The cells proliferated with the passage of time, and went over 1×10^7 cell·ml^{-1} on the 8th day. Thereafter, the density was at a level of 1×10^7 cell·ml^{-1} until the 11th day, but increased to 1.35×10^7 cell·ml^{-1} on the 12th day. It continued gradually increasing and was a level of 2×10^7 cell·ml^{-1} on and after the 18th day.

The concentration of the antibody in the supernatant was found to be 30 to 60 μg·ml^{-1}, while the viable cell density was more than 1×10^7 cells·ml^{-1}, and the IgG specific productivity was constantly about 5 μg(10^6 cells)$^{-1}$·d^{-1}. The cultivation was continued for 27 days without significant trouble with excellent operation stability.

Further, the results in this study were compared with those in the culture vessel equipped with one gravitational settling zone[1]. Fig. 3 gives the course of IgG concentration, IgG specific productivity and viable cell density with passage of time, with the X32 line cultured in a vessel of 22 l net volume with one gravitational settling zone. In the experiment, the viable cell density reached about 1.1×10^7 cell·ml^{-1} and IgG specific productivity was about 5 $\mu g(10^6$ cells$)^{-1}$·d^{-1}.

Fig. 2 and Fig. 3 are compared. Under the conditions of the same specific perfusion rate, the viable cell density and IgG concentration in supernatant are about twice higher in Fig. 2 than in Fig. 3. No difference can be observed in IgG specific productivity. The causes of the different viable cell density between them were not elucidated, but the main reason is presumably the difference in oxygen feeding.

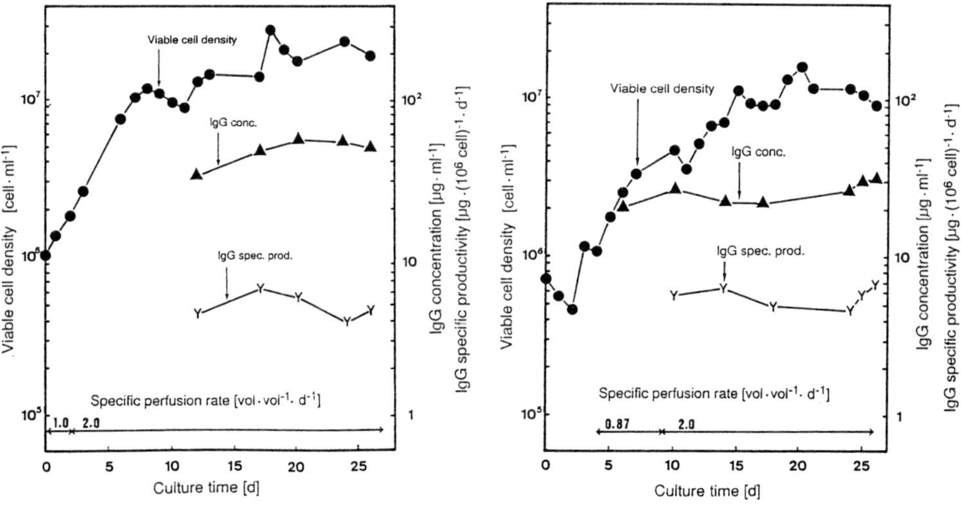

Fig.2 Perfusion culture of mouse-human hybridoma X32 cells using a culture system with three settling zone and supplying oxygen by fluorocarbon. (Net culture volume : 850 ml. Medium : ITES + eRDF

Fig. 3 Perfusion culture of mouse-human hybridoma X32 cells. (Net culture volume : 22 L, Medium : ITES + eRDF)

Thus, it has been proved that the continuous production of monoclonal antibodies by a hybridoma is possible by using a perfusion culture vessel equipped with a plurality of gravitational settling zones and using a perfluorocarbon to supply oxygen.

References

1) M. Tokashiki, K. Hamamoto, Y. Takazawa and Y. Ichikawa, KAGAKUKO-GAKU RONBUNSHU, **14**, 337 (1988).
2) M. Tokashiki and T. Arai, Cytotechnology, **2**, 5 (1989).
3) K. Hamamoto, M. Tokashiki, Y. Ichikawa and H. Murakami, Agric. Biol. Chem., **51**, 3415 (1987).
4) H. Murakami, T. Shimomura, T. Nakamura, H, Ohashi, K. Shinohara and H. Omura, J. Agric. Chem. Soc. Japan, **58**, 575 (1984).

HIGH CELL DENSITY PERFUSION CULTURE OF INSECT CELLS FOR PRODUCTION OF BACULOVIRUS AND RECOMBINANT PROTEIN

Martina Klöppinger, Georg Fertig, Elisabeth Fraune* and Herbert G. Miltenburger

Technical University, Institute of Zoology, Schnittspahn-str. 3, D-6100 Darmstadt, FRG
*B.Braun Diessel Biotech GmbH, P.O.-Box 120, D-3508 Melsungen, FRG

ABSTRACT

A method for efficient in vitro baculovirus production is described. Wildtype and recombinant Autographa californica nuclear polyhedrosis virus were propagated in the insect cell line Sf9. The cells were cultured in a 1.5 liter stirred tank bioreactor equipped with an internal micro-porous filtration module for medium perfusion. Using perfusion technology we were able to grow cells to a density of 1x10⁷/ml and to compensate the high nutrient demand of cells for virus production. In low cell density batch cultures medium perfusion during the virus production phase yielded about 50% more virus. In high cell density perfusion cultures medium perfusion was found to be necessary for effectively producing virus, resulting in 7.5 time higher yields of virus as compared to conventional batch cultivation.

INTRODUCTION

Insect pathogenic baculoviruses (BV) gain increasing interest as expression vectors for production of recombinant proteins. The BV expression system is an ideal tool for the production of proteins of medical and pharmaceutical interest due to high level protein expression, post translational modification capacity and safety (1). For commercial purposes effective large scale production systems are required.
In our studies we used the Autographa californica nuclear polyhedrosis virus (Ac-NPV). After replication in the nuclei of infected cells, wildtype viruses are embedded in inclusion bodies, the socalled polyhedra. The major structural component of the polyhedra is the 29 kDa protein polyhedrin. In recombinant viruses the DNA region encoding for this protein is replaced by a foreign gene, the product of which is then expressed at high levels instead of poly-hedrin. 3-4 days post infection (p.i.) the number of poly-

hedra and the concentration of recombinant protein reach a
maximum level, followed by lysis of the infected cells.
As in large scale mammalian cell systems, insect cells also
need efficient nutrient and oxygen supply during cell and
virus propagation. Therefore, a perfusion technique was
tested for its efficacy to enhance cell proliferation as
well as virus production.

MATERIALS AND METHODS

Cell culture and viruses

The Spodoptera frugiperda cell line Sf9 was grown in TC 100
medium (Gibco) supplemented with 5% FCS and 1 mg/ml Neomy-
cinsulfat in the 1.5 liter stirred tank bioreactor Biostat
MC (B.Braun Diessel Biotech). In the bioreactor oxygen was
supplied via a silicone tubing system. The pO_2 was kept
constant at 40%, cultivation temperature at 27°C and the
stirring speed at 50 rpm. The pH was maintained stable at
6.3. For perfusion cultivation the bioreactor was equipped
with a microporous filtration module (B.Braun Diessel Biotech) with a cell retaining pore size of 1μm (figure 1).
The medium for perfusion was supplemented with 5% or 2.5%
FCS.
In several experiments medium was changed via tangential
flow filtration by connecting a hollow fibre module (Microgon, 0.2μm pore size) to the bioreactor. Cells were pumped
through this system and 90% of spent medium was removed via
the module. The cells were then resuspended in fresh
medium.
Cells were infected with wildtype Autographa californica
nuclear polyhedrosis virus (Ac-NPV). In all experiments a
minimum of 1 MOI (multiplicity of infection) was applied.
Cells were infected synchronously and virus synthesis was
usually accomplished within 3-4 days. For recombinant
protein production we used a genetically engineered Ac-NPV
expressing Escherichia coli β-galactosidase.

Sample analysis

Cell counts were performed using a hemocytometer and viability was determined by trypan blue dye exclusion. The
percentage of infected cells and the number of polyhedra
per cell was counted by light microscopy. For the quantification of β-galactosidase cells were lysed by treatment
with 0.1% (w/v) SDS. Serial log2 dilutions of supernatant
were performed in 96 well microtiter plates in a volume of
100 μl of assay buffer (0.06 M Na_2HPO_4, 0.04 M NaH_2PO_4,
0.01 M KCl, 0.001 M $MgSO_4$, pH 7). For reference, β-galactosidase with a known concentration was tested in parallel on
each plate. To start the enzyme reaction 20 μl of 4 mg ONPG
(o-nitrophenyl-β-D-galactopyranoside) per ml assay buffer
were added to each well. The reaction was stopped by adding

50 µl of 1M Na_2CO_3. The absorbance of the yellow product was measured with an automated ELISA reader (SLT-Labinstruments) at a wavelength of 405 nm. One unit of β-galactosidase hydrolizes 1 nmol ONPG per minute at pH 7.3 and 37°C.

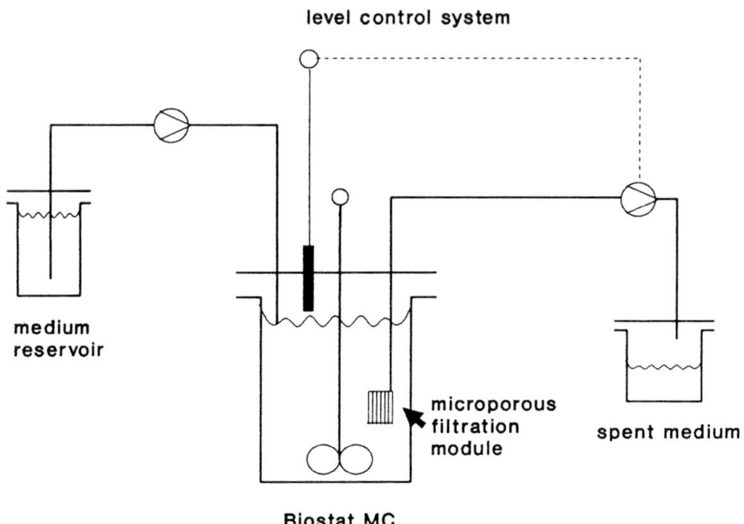

<u>Figure 1</u>: Design of the perfusion bioreactor used for cultivation of cells and virus

RESULTS

Wildtype BV-production in low cell density batch cultures

Batch cultures were started in the bioreactor with seeding densities of $1-2x10^5$ cells/ml and grown to a density of $1.5x10^6$cells/ml. The cultures were then inoculated with wildtype Ac-NPV. 4 days post infection $9x10^6$ polyhedra/ml were produced (see table 1). In order to improve the production rate, fresh medium was provided prior to virus infection: About 90% of spent medium was removed by tangential flow filtration, and cells were infected after resuspension in fresh medium. The medium replacement enhanced the production of polyhedra to $1.3x10^7$/ml (see table 1). A further increase in the yield of polyhedra was achieved when medium perfusion (with TC100 + 5% FCS) was carried out during the whole production period by using the microporous filtration module. In this case $1.7x10^7$ polyhedra/ml were produced (table 1).

Wildtype BV-production in high cell density ⌐rfusion cultures

In a next step polyhedra yield was enhanced by increasing the concentration of cells to be infected. Cells were cultivated under perfusion conditions. Medium perfusion (with TC100+2.5%FCS) was started when the cells had reached a density of $1.5x10^6$/ml. By adjusting appropriate medium flow rates the glucose concentration was maintained above 0.3 mg/ml. At a density of $1x10^7$ cells/ml medium was changed via tangential flow filtration and then viral infection was performed. 4 days p.i. only $1.1x10^7$ poly- hedra/ml were produced, a yield being lower than that obtained by batch cultivation (table 1). In a subsequent experiment medium perfusion was continued during viral propagation. To allow effective viral attachment and infection medium perfusion was interrupted for 3 hours directly after addition of the viral inoculum. Perfusion during viral replication resulted in a marked increase of virus yield: $6.9x10^7$ polyhedra/ml were produced (table 1).

Virus pro- duction condi- tions / Cell growth conditions	medium change prior to infection	perfusion	polyhedra per ml (x10^7)
BATCH $1.5x10^6$cells/ml*	-	-	0.9
	+	-	1.3
	+	+	1.7
PERFUSION $1x10^7$cells/ml*	+	-	1.1
	-	+	6.9

<u>Table 1:</u> Production of wildtype virus under different culture conditions. * Cell concentration at time of infection

Production of recombinant β-galactosidase

In a similar set up as described above for the production of wildtype virus the production of recombinant protein was studied. In a batch culture containing $1.5x10^6$ cells/ml medium was changed by tangential flow filtration and the cells were infected with recombinant Ac-NPV producing β- galactosidase. $0.52x10^6$ units of β-galactosidase per ml

were found 4 days p.i. (table 2). Infection of a high cell density perfusion culture with continuous perfusion during the production phase resulted in 1.3x10^6 units of β-galactosidase per ml (figure 3).
These results indicate, that the production of recombinant protein can be improved in a similar way as the production of wildtype virus. However, under comparable culture conditions the increase in product yield was not as significant as in the case of wildtype virus (table 1 and 2). This difference may be due to inadequate perfusion rates in the described experiment. Therefore, establishing optimal culture conditions for the production of recombinant protein is under investigation in our laboratory at present.

Cell growth conditions \ Virus production conditions	medium change prior to infection	perfusion	units of β-galactosidase (x10^6)
BATCH 1.5x10^{6}cells/ml*	+	−	0.52
PERFUSION 1x10^{7}cells/ml*	−	+	1.28

Table 2: Production of β-galactosidase using recombinant Ac-NPV under different cultivation conditions. * Cell concentration at time of infection

DISCUSSION

In studies reported earlier insect cells and BV were successfully propagated by batch cultivation in stirred tank bioreactors (2,3,4) or in airlift fermenters (4,5). The data presented in this paper inform on the application of a perfusion system during cell growth as well as during virus production. This system allows to establish high cell density perfusion cultures and to improve the virus production process. From the economical point of view perfusion technology is more effective, since under conventional batch culture conditions the polyhedra production rate per day was nearly 5 times lower than under optimized perfusion culture conditions (1.3x10^6 compared to 6.3x10^6 polyhedra per ml and day). However, higher medium consumption must be taken into account when using perfusion culture systems. Recent publications (6) and results from our laboratory with stationary cultures in flasks (data not shown)

indicate that fetal calf serum, one of the most expensive
medium ingredients, can be omitted during the virus production phase. Thus, we presently study whether FCS can be
omitted during virus replication in the described perfusion
culture system.

ACKNOWLEDGEMENT

We wish to thank Dr. M.D. Summers for providing the
recombinant Ac-NPV producing E.coli β-galactosidase. We
would also thank P. Czech and B. Vogt for technical
assistance. This work has been supported by the federal
ministry for research and technology (Bonn) and performed
in cooperation with B.Braun Diessel Biotech.

REFERENCES

1 Luckow V.A. and Summers M.D. Trends in the development
   of baculovirus expression vectors. Bio/Technology 1988,
   6, 47-55

2 Hink W.F. Production of Autographa californica nuclear
   polyhedrosis virus in cells from large scale suspension.
   In: Kurstak E. (ed) Microbial and viral pesticides 1982,
   Marcel Dekker, New York, 493-506

3 Miltenburger H.G. and David P. Mass production of insect
   cells in suspension. Develop. biol. standard. 1980, 46,
   183-186

4 Murhammer D.W. and Goochee C.F. Scale up of insect cell
   cultures: Protective effects of pluronic F-68.
   Bio/Technology 1988, 6, 1411-1418

5 Maiorella B., Inlow D., Shaugher A. and Harano D. Large
   scale insect cell culture for recombinant protein
   production. Bio/Technology 1988, 6, 1406-1410

6 Broussard D.R. and Summers M.D. Effects of serum
   concentration and media compositions on the level of
   polyhedrin and foreign gene expression by baculovirus
   vectors. Journal of Invertebrate Pathology 1989, 54,
   144-150

<u>**Paper of Kloppinger**</u>

Petrowiski:
> Did you in all cases infect the cells in suspension
> or when static; did you remove the virus containing
> medium after infection or leave it; and finally
> what was your multiplicity of infection?

Kloppinger:
> We infect at 5-10 MOI and we put the virus in and
> leave it - it is not necessary to remove the
> inoculum.

Section 6.5
Bioreactors: optimization via metabolism

METABOLITE PARAMETERS MODULATING MONOCLONAL ANTIBODY
PRODUCTION BY HYBRIDOMA CELLS IN FLASK AND MACROPOROUS GLASS
SPHERE CULTURE

AJ Racher, D Looby and JB Griffiths

Division of Biologics, PHLS Centre for Microbiology and
Research, Porton Down, Salisbury, Wiltshire SP4 OJG, UK.

ABSTRACT

The relationship of Mab production by the murine hybridoma
C1E3 to various physiological parameters was compared in
fixed bed and flask cultures. In the fixed bed culture, there
was a significant relationship between oxygen uptake and Mab
production. In contrast, in the flask culture, glutamine
metabolism was the important parameter. The nature of the
relationship varies depending upon whether the glutamine
concentration post-medium change is kept at a set level or
allowed to vary.

KEYWORDS: Hybridoma; macroporous glass sphere; metabolism;
monoclonal antibody.

INTRODUCTION

Solid glass spheres are not suitable for immobilising
suspension cells due to excessive cell washout, and are
essentially low process intensity systems. These limitations
have been overcome by substituting macroporous glass spheres
(porospheres) for solid ones. As part of our studies looking
at the potential of porospheres as a production process for
animal cell products, we examined the relationship of product
expression and metabolism to improve our understanding of the
biological processes occurring in such systems.

MATERIALS AND METHODS

Cell line and medium

The cell line used was the mouse-mouse hybridoma C1E3 (1).
Cells were tested for mycoplasma infection and found to be
negative by the Hoescht stain.
The medium was glutamine-free RPMI + 5% heat inactivated
FCS (Imperial Laboratories, Andover, UK). Glucose and
glutamine were added to the concentrations indicated in the
text.

Cell culture

The fixed bed and flask culture systems and their operation have been described in detail elsewhere (2).

Briefly, the fixed bed system consisted of a 1 l packed bed volume reactor and a 15 l reservoir for medium conditioning. The support consisted of 5 mm diam. Siran porospheres (Schott Glaswerke, Mainz, FRG), with pores of 60-300μm diam.

Both the fixed bed and flask systems were operated in a similar manner. They were inoculated with mid-exponential growth phase cells and the culture grown to early stationary phase (approx. 72 h). At 72 h, and subsequently at 24 h intervals, the conditioned medium was completely replaced with an equal volume of fresh medium.

Assays

The assays used in this study have been described elsewhere (2).

Calculations

Sample means were compared using an ANOVA test. Regression analyses were done using the Statgraphics statistical package (Statistical Graphics Corp., USA).

Methods for the calculation of rates of oxygen uptake and production of ATP by oxidative phosphorylation have been described elsewhere (2).

RESULTS

Parallel fixed bed and flask cultures (termed I2 and F2 respectively) of C1E3 cells were set up. The monoclonal antibody (Mab) production profiles of both cultures are shown in Figure 1.

In culture F2, the Mab production rate increased during the exponential growth phase (Figure 1). During the pseudo-steady state (approx. 72-320 h) following the growth phase, a cyclical pattern of increase/decrease in Mab production was observed. This cyclic pattern cannot be explained simply in terms of fluctuation in cell density, as in the pseudo-steady state period the viable cell density remained relatively constant.

The fixed bed culture I2 exhibited a different pattern of product expression to culture F2 (Figure 1). Both during the growth phase (from inoculation to approx. 72 h) and in the first half of the pseudo-steady state phase (which started at approx. 72 h and continued until the culture was terminated), the Mab production rate increased. By about 220 h, an event had occurred which caused the production rate to decrease (although later it recovered). We have no evidence that the decrease in rate corresponded to a fall in viable cell density (1).

In each system, the relationship in the pseudo-steady state of Mab production rate to a range of physiological parameters was analysed by stepwise linear regression analysis.

In culture I2, none of the relationships were significant at the 5% level, although several were significant just above this level. The most significant relationships are shown in Table 1.

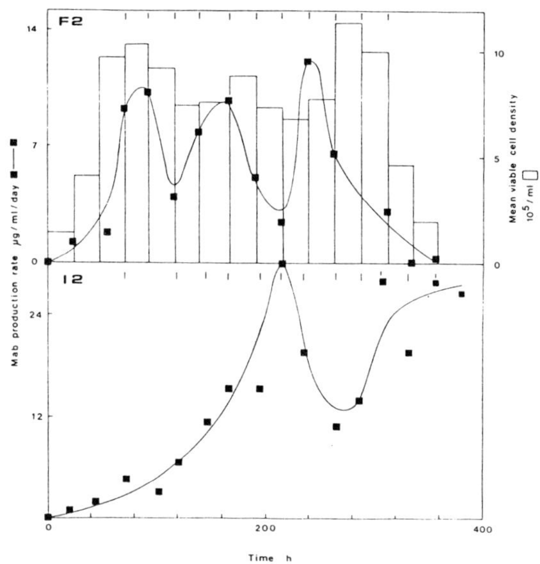

Figure 1. Mab production profiles of fixed bed (I2) and flask (F2) cultures of C1E3. The times of the medium changes are shown by the vertical lines.

Table 1. Expressions with most significant relationship to Mab production in culture I2.

	Model		P
I	QMab = $0.13P_{ATPox}$	$- 4.35$	0.0742
II	QMab = $0.50Q_{oxy}$	$- 4.35$	0.0742
III	QMab = $0.70Q_{oxy}$*	$- 4.44$	0.0743
IV	QMab = $0.50Q_{oxy}$*	$- 0.09Qoxy - 14.32$	0.0946

Q production/ uptake rate per day; * rate pre-medium change; oxy oxygen; ATPox ATP produced by oxidative phosphorylation

The models giving the best agreement between the observed and predicted rates are I and II, where the variables are the daily rates of production of ATP by oxidative phosphorylation and oxygen uptake respectively.

The models in Table 1 show that Mab production in the fixed bed system is dependent upon the oxygen uptake rate of the cells.

We have no evidence of gradients within the bed of either cell density or viability (2). This indicates that gradients of nutrients or waste metabolites were not adversely affecting bioreactor performance in the fixed bed system. However, models for I2 suggest that Mab production is dependent upon oxygen uptake. Oxygen was maintained at 10% air saturation at the top of the bed. Therefore it is possible that oxygen transfer into the porosphere became limiting - maybe due to cell growth occluding the pores.

In the parallel flask experiment F2, the most significant (P<0.01) linear relationship (eqn 1) was found with the volumetric glutamine uptake rate and the apparent yield coefficient $Y'_{NH4+,Gln}$. Comparison of the observed and predicted rates shows very good agreement.

$$(1) \qquad Q_{Mab} = 22.06 - 5.58Y'_{NH4+,Gln} - 4.08Q_{Gln}$$

When this model was tested with the data from culture I2, no significant relationship was found. As culture F2 was an un-gassed flask culture, the relationships observed in culture I2 could not be tested.

The data for cultures F2 and I2 showed that:

$$C_{Gln} \propto Q_{Gln} \qquad C_{Gln} \propto 1/Y'_{NH4+,Gln}$$

where C_{Gln} was the glutamine concentration post-medium change. Therefore the two independent variables in eqn 1 can be modulated by varying the glutamine concentration post-medium change. It should then be possible to modulate Mab production in the flask culture system by varying the post-medium change glutamine concentration.

The model of Mab production in eqn 1, plus the relationship of the two independent variables to the glutamine concentration post-medium change, predicts no Mab production at high (9 mmol/l) glutamine concentrations, but high production rates for glutamine in the range 1-3 mmol/l.

In cultures F2 and I2, the post-medium change glutamine concentration varied between 1-5 mmol/l - with glucose varying between 12-21 mmol/l. The effect on Mab production of maintaining the post-medium change glutamine concentration at set levels (1, 3 and 9 mmol/l) with a constant glucose concentration was investigated. The results are shown in Figure 2.

The mean Mab production rates at 3 and 9 mmol/l were greater than the mean rate at 1 mmol/l, although there was no significant difference between the three rates. These results show that maintenance of the post-medium change glutamine concentration at 9 mmol/l has no effect upon Mab production compared to 1 and 3 mmol/l. The results did not agree with those predicted from the model, suggesting that the model was only valid for cultures where the glucose and glutamine concentrations were allowed to vary.

The relationship of stationary phase Mab production by the cultures in Figure 2 to various physiological parameters was analysed by stepwise linear regression analysis. The results are summarised in Table 2.

These results show that at high glutamine concentrations, the relationship of glucose metabolism to Mab production is

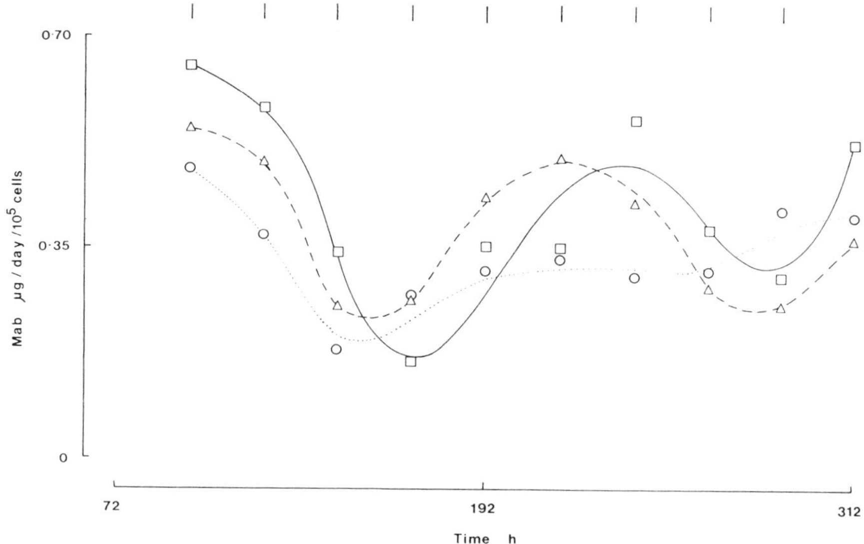

Figure 2. Stationary growth phase Mab production rates of repeated-feed-and-harvest cultures of C1E3 cells grown with 22 mmol/l glucose and different glutamine concentrations (□———□ 9; △- - - -△ 3; ○········○ 1). Times of medium changes are indicated by the vertical lines.

Table 2. Expressions showing a significant linear relationship (P<0.05) to Mab production in flask cultures grown with set glutamine concentrations

CGln mmol/l	using specific rates	using volumetric rates
9	$f(C_{glc}, Q_{lac})$	$f(C_{glc})$
3	No significant relationships found	
1	$f(C_{glc}, Q_{glc})$	$f(C_{glc})$
	$f(Q_{Gln}, C_{NH4+}, Y'_{NH4+,Gln})$	$f(C_{NH4+}, Q_{NH4+})$

C concentration; Y' apparent yield coefficient

important. Yet in cultures grown with 1 mmol/l glutamine, the metabolism of both glucose and glutamine is important. This contrasts with 3 mmol/l glutamine where none of the parameters tested exhibited a significant relationship to Mab production. Comparison of eqn 1 with Table 2 shows that different physiological parameters are important for Mab production depending upon whether the post-medium change glutamine concentration is set or allowed to vary.

The relationship of glucose and glutamine metabolism to Mab production was examined further by investigating the effect of different combinations of glucose (10 and 22 mmol/l) and glutamine (1, 3 and 9 mmol/l) levels.

The results showed that at any of the glutamine concentrations tested, there was no significant difference between the two glucose levels (data not shown). This contrasts with the effect of glutamine (Figure 3).

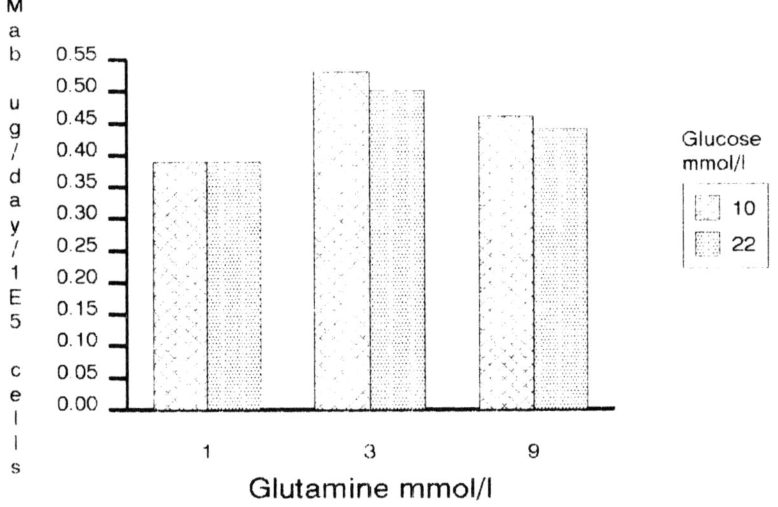

Figure 3. The effect of different glutamine concentrations on the mean stationary phase Mab production at two set glucose concentrations.

These results show a significant (P<0.05) increase in Mab production when the glutamine concentration was increased from 1 to 3 mmol/l (glucose at 10 mmol/l). In cultures grown with 22 mmol/l glucose, the same increase in glutamine concentration caused a marked increase in Mab production, although this was not as significant as at the lower glucose level (P<0.05 cf. P<0.10 for 10 cf. 22 mmol/l glucose). There was no significant difference in the Mab rates at 3 and 9 mmol/l glutamine for either of the glucose levels. At both glucose level, the Mab production rate fell as the glutamine concentration increased from 3 to 9 mmol/l.

DISCUSSION

The results in Figure 1 show that fixed bed and flask culture systems operated in repeated-feed-and-harvest mode had markedly different profiles of Mab production. Analysis of the relationship of Mab production to various physiological parameters shows that the parameters exhibiting the most significant relationship were different for the two systems. In the flask system, the relationship of glutamine metabolism was important but in the fixed bed system, oxygen uptake was the important variable.

These results were obtained in a system where the glutamine concentration post-medium change varied. The significance of the post-medium change glutamine concentration to Mab production in flask cultures of C1E3 was confirmed using cultures grown with fixed feed glutamine concentrations.

The results presented in Figure 3 explain the lack of a significant relationship observed in Figure 2. The results in Figure 2 were obtained using 21 mmol/l glucose, whereas the data in Figure 3 show that the relationship is significant at 10 but not 22 mmol/l glucose.

The data show that the nature of the relationship between glutamine metabolism and Mab production varies depending upon whether the glutamine concentration post-medium change was allowed to vary or kept constant. The reasons for this are unclear to us.

The data reported in this study show that the relationship between glutamine metabolism and Mab production by hybridomas is important. Glutamine concentrations below 3 mmol/l cause marked reductions in the Mab production rate, possibly because of the inability of the cell to generate sufficient ATP to satisfy the requirements of both maintenance energy and Mab production. At glutamine concentrations between 3 and 9 mmol/l, there appears to be a downward trend in Mab production. This suggests that for optimal Mab production, glutamine must be kept in a narrow window (3-6(?) mmol/l).

ACKNOWLEDGEMENTS

We would like to thank Mrs. D Fellows for expert technical assistance. Siran porospheres were obtained from Mr. M Radke, Schott Glaswerke, Mainz. This work was supported by the Biotechnology Group, Department of Trade and Industry.

REFERENCES

1   Wright, J.P. and Balfor, A.H. Monoclonal antibodies to Toxoplasma gondii. Parasitol. 1983, 87, LXVI

2   Racher, A.J., Looby, D. and Griffiths, J.B. Studies on monoclonal antibody production by a hybridoma cell line (C1E3) immobilised in a fixed bed, porosphere culture system. J. Biotechnol. 1990, in the press.

OPTIMIZATION OF OKT3 HYBRIDOMA CULTURES IN A PERFUSION STIRRED REACTOR

H. PINTON[1], J.N. RABAUD[1], J.M. ENGASSER[2] and A. MARC[2]

1- SGI, 15 Allées de bellefontaine, 31100 TOULOUSE, France
2- Laboratoire des Sciences du Génie Chimique, CNRS, INPL,
   BP451, 54001 NANCY Cedex, France

ABSTRACT

A new type of perfusion reactor, based on a homogeneous reactor equipped with a microfiltration module on an external loop, yields significant increase in culture performances with OKT3 hybridoma: $1.5x10^7$ cells/ml, 100 mg MAb/day.L and 2.5 g MAb/L of spent serum, compared to $2x10^6$ cells/ml, 12 mg MAb/day.L and 0.9 g MAb/L of spent serum in a batch reactor. At 1 day^{-1}, perfusion cultures can be maintained for more than two months with cell viability above 70 %. Both in batch and perfusion mode the specific rate of antibody production is found independent of the cell growth rate between 0.3 and 1.5 day^{-1}.

KEY WORDS

Perfusion reactor, hollow-fiber, microfiltration, kinetics, OKT3, high density

INTRODUCTION

Perfusion reactors are increasingly used for the continuous culture of adherent and suspension animal cells [1,2,3]. In these systems cells are confined or retained inside the reactors by different configurations of membranes or filters. In this study a new type of perfusion system based on a stirred reactor and a hollow-fiber microfiltration module on an external loop has been developped. The performance of the reactor is evaluated with respect to increased cell density, reduced serum utilization, increased productivity and prolonged culture duration using an OKT3 hybridoma. Cell kinetics in the perfusion system is also characterized.

MATERIAL AND METHODS

Cells: OKT3, a murine hybridoma were obtained from the European Collection of Animal Cells, (PHLS CAMR, Porton Down, U.K.)

Culture media: A mixture of 75% DMEM, 25% HAM's F12 with variable FCS (7.5% to 1% V:V) and with 22mM glucose, 4mM glutamine and essential and non-essential amino-acids supplementation (all products from Intermed, France).

Perfusion reactor: A 2 liters SGI stirred reactor with 1 liter working volume was used (37°C, 35 rpm, pH=7.2 and pO2=40% air saturation). The perfusion system was composed with an external hollow fiber cross-flow microfiltration module. Fresh medium and depleted cell-free medium were continuously feeding and harvesting respectively.

Assays: Cells were counted by the Trypan Blue exclusion method. Monoclonal Antibodies were determined according to the ELISA method. The others tests were purchased from Boehringer (France).

RESULTS AND DISCUSSION

When the OKT3 hybridoma is cultured batchwise with an initial 5 % foetal calf serum level two consecutive growth and death phases are observed with an intermediate maximal cell density of 2×10^6 cells per mL. The main kinetic results of the culture are given in Table 1: 50 mg/L antibody concentration and 12 mg/day.L antibody productivity.

The perfusion reactor was first operated batchwise until achieving a cell density near 2×10^6 cells/mL. The continuous medium feed flow rate is then progressively increased to reach a stationary dilution rate of 2 day^{-1} (Fig.1). The level of serum, which is at 7.5 % during the initial batch, is decreased to 1% with continuous operation. Medium perfusion allows an further increase in cell concentration up to 1.5×10^7 cells/mL while maintaining a good cellular viability around 70 % all along the 300 hours of culture. The average antibody level collected in the outlet stream is 55 mg/L, which amounts to a daily productivity of 105 mg/day.L (Table 1). This represents a 9 fold increase with respect to the batch reactor productivity.

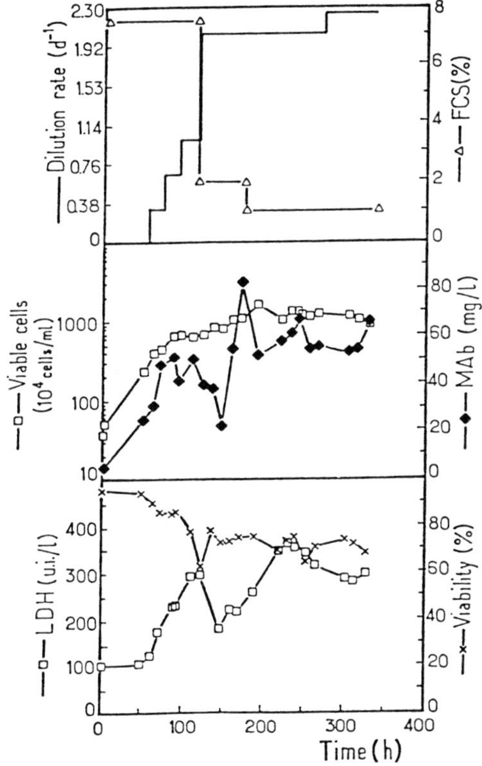

Fig. 1: *Evolution of cell density and viability, FCS level, dilution rate, LDH activity and MAb concentration in the perfusion reactor.*

When the perfusion culture is operated at a lower dilution rate of 1 day^{-1}, lower cell densities (9×10^6 cells/ml) and antibody production (40 mg/day.L) are obtained (Table 1). This indicates the presence of significant nutrients limitations at this dilution rate. For this experiment, the perfused culture   has been maintained for more than 60 days without any change of the module.

When comparing the performances of batch and perfusion cultures an additional important criterion is the utilization of medium and serum. Whereas in the batch mode 0.9 g of antibodies are produced per liter of spent serum, with the perfusion system 1.2 and 2.5 g antibodies are produced per liter of spent serum at dilution rates of 1 and 2 day^{-1}, respectively.

	Process time	Medium used	Total MAb quantity	Average MAb concentration	Average MAb production rate	Average MAb production per liter FCS
B A T C H	120 h	1,2 l	0,06 g	50 mg/l	12 mg/d	0,9 g/l
PERFUSION 1 d^{-1}	295 h	12,5 l	0,5 g	40 mg/l	40 mg/d	1,2 g/l
PERFUSION 2 d^{-1}	316 h	25,5 l	1,4 g	55 mg/l	106 mg/d	2,5 g/l

Table 1: Performances comparison between batch and perfusion cultures.

Kinetic analysis of the data and of additional measurements of LDH release [4] show that in the perfusion mode the observed stationnary phase actually results from a balance between the rates of cell growth and cell death which both amount to about 0.3 day^{-1}. Moreover the specific rate of antibody production is found similar (Fig. 2) in batch and perfusion operation, independent of the specific growth rate, at least above 0.3 day^{-1}.

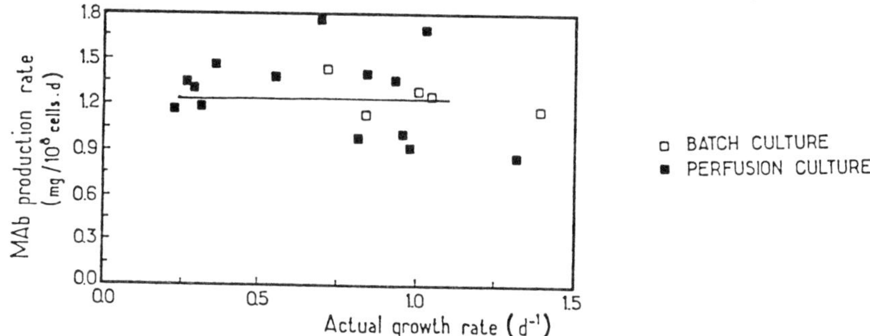

Fig. 2: Evolution of the MAb specific production rate with the actual growth rate for batch and perfused cultures.

REFERENCES

1-Takazawa, Y. and Tokashaki, M. (1989). High cell density perfusion culture of mouse-human hybridomas. Appl. Microbiol. Biotechnol., **32**, 280-284.
2-Velez, D., Miller, L. and Macmillan, J.D. (1989). Use of tangential flow filtration in perfusion propagation of hybridoma cells for production of monoclonal antibodies. Biotechnol. Bioeng., **33**, 938-940.
3-Murakami, H. (1990). What should be focused in the study of cell culture technology for production of bioactive proteins?. Cytotechnology, **3**, 3-7.
4-Marc, A.,Wagner, A., Martial, A., Goergen, J.L., Engasser, J.M., Geaugey, V. Pinton, H. (1990). Potential and pitfalls of using LDH release for the evaluation of cellular death kinetics. Proceeding of 10th ESACT Meeting. Avignon.

BIOCHEMICAL CONTROL OF MONOCLONAL ANTIBODY SECRETION IN HOLLOW FIBRE
BIOREACTORS

A. Handa-Corrigan, S. Nikolay and R.E. Spier

The Wolfson Cytotechnology Laboratory, (c/o The Department of
Microbiology), University of Surrey, Guildford, GU2 5XH, U.K.

ABSTRACT

We have recently found that the rates of monoclonal antibody production
in optimised hollow fibre bioreactors is highest for those hybridoma cell
lines that have especially high uptake rates of both glucose and
glutamine. In addition, the monoclonal antibody production rates in
these optimised systems increase linearly with the uptake rates of both
glucose and glutamine. A molar conversion of glutamine to ammonia was
seen to occur for all the cell lines cultivated. The optimisation
conditions that we have successfully implemented are:

(1) a culture pH of 7.1 and temperature of 37°C,
(2) a dissolved oxygen concentration >80 mm Hg,
(3) glucose and glutamine concentrations >150 mg/dl and 2.5 mM,
     respectively,
(4) lactate and ammonia concentrations <150 mg/dl and 2.5 mM,
     respectively,
(5) continuous harvesting of product.

In unoptimised systems the relationships between antibody production
rates and substrate uptake rates were not apparent.

INTRODUCTION

In vitro Monoclonal antibody (MCA) production is currently carried out in
a diverse range of bioreactor designs ranging from batch air lift and
stirred tank reactors to perfusion systems such as Hollow Fibre
bioreactors. The choice of bioreactor to be used for MCA production is
influenced by many factors, and has been discussed previously[1]. With
respect to hybridoma growth and MCA productivity, there are only a few
common findings that may be applied to any type of cultivation system:

(a) MCA production occurs as long as the cells remain in a viable state
     and the precursors for MCA synthesis are available.

(b) Optimum cell growth can be achieved by controlling three basic
     physical parameters: pH (7.0-7.2); Temperature (36-37°C) and
     Dissolved Oxygen Tension (20-80%). Increased specific MCA
     production may be achieved by slowing the growth rate of the cells
     by lowering any of the above parameters[2,3].

(c) Cell viability and MCA production is influenced by the availability
     of glucose and glutamine[2,4] and the subsequent accumulation of
     lactate and ammonia[5] in the culture medium.

(d) Serum or defined serum substitutes are essential for maintaining
     cell viability and MCA production.

It is common practice in batch cultivation to relate the MCA
productivity to viable cell numbers under defined physical parameters.
Based on this information, it is theoretically possible to predict (but
not always possible to achieve!) the productivity of a particular cell
line at different scales of operation.

The cultivation of hybridoma cells in hollow fibre bioreactors makes a
similar type of prediction very difficult. This is mainly because cell
growth cannot be monitored directly, and because the nutrient/serum
requirements of cells held at high densities are not clearly understood.

In this study we aim to show that MCA production in hollow fibre
bioreactors (Acusyst, Endotronics) can be closely controlled and
predicted by rigorous monitoring and control of both physical and
biochemical parameters. The principle of operation of the Acusyst Junior
hollow fibre bioreactor is summarized in Figure 1.

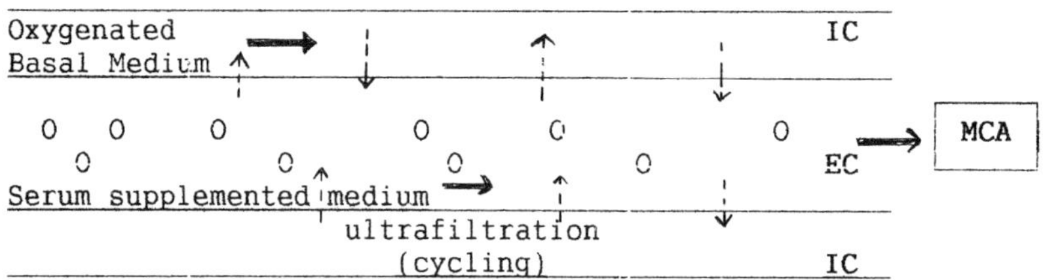

IC: Intracapillary space; EC: Extra capillary space; O: Cells

Fig 1:   Principles of Operation of the Acusyst Hollow Fibre Bioreactor

MATERIALS AND METHODS

Cell lines: Two mouse x mouse hybridoma cell lines designated AFP27 and
LX1 (both producing IgG$_1$) were utilised in this study.

Cell cultivation and Hollow Fibre perfusion media: Cells were maintained
and expanded in RPMI 1640 supplemented with 450 mg/dl glucose, 5 mM
glutamine and 5% New Born Calf Serum (NBCS). In the Hollow Fibre
bioreactor, the IC was perfused with RPMI 1640 basal medium supplemented
with 450 mg/dl glucose and 5 mM glutamine. The EC was perfused with the
same serum supplemented medium formulation described above. All media
were deviod of antibiotics.

Hollow Fibre Bioreactor set-up procedures: Two Acusyst Junior Hollow
Fibre Bioreactors were used. Full assembly and set-up procedures were
provided by Endotronics. Briefly, each ethylene oxide pre-sterilized
Hollow Fibre cartridge was washed with 10L sterile, deionized water and
10L basal medium. 24 hr prior to inoculation, the EC was flushed with
serum supplemented medium. Each hybridoma cell line was expanded in 2L,

surface aerated, stirred cultures.   Each Hollow Fibre Bioreactor was
inoculated with a total of 2 x 10^8 viable cells (>95% viability), in 50
ml of fresh serum supplemented medium.

Metabolic Assays: Glucose concentrations were determined using Glucose
HK Uni-Kit III (Roche) and a Cobas-Bio automated analyser (Roche
Diagnostics).   Lactate concentrations were determined using a Lactate
Reagent Kit (Sigma, 826-uv) and the Cobas-Bio automated analyser.
Ammonia concentrations were determined with an ammonia probe (Kent
Industrial). Glutamine was enzymatically converted to free ammonia with
Glutaminase (Sigma) and its concentration determined from the following
equation:

[Glutamine] = [Total Ammonia] - [Background Ammonia]

Monoclonal Antibody concentrations were determined by specific ELISA
techniques for each cell line.

Optimisation strategy: The method of controlling and optimising MCA
production is described in Table 1:

Factors affecting MCA production	Operating set-points and optimisation strategy
1. Supply of oxygen	Maintained above 80 mm Hg by increased recirculation of oxygenated medium and cycling (ultrafiltration)
2. pH	Maintained at 7.1 by CO_2/Air gassing initially Increased basal medium through-put or NaOH addition later on during cultivation.
3. Supply of glucose and glutamine	Maintained above 150 mg/dl and 2.5 mM, respectively, by increased medium through-put.
4. Removal of toxic and waste products (lactate & ammonia)	Increased basal medium addition, waste removal and cycling to maintain concentrations of lactate and ammonia below 150 mg/dl and 2.5 mM, respectively.
5. Supply of serum or serum supplements	Increased input to EC <u>only</u> when MCA concentration is increasing.

TABLE I   Optimisation and Control of MCA production in Hollow Fibres

RESULTS

Our experience with a number of hybridoma cell lines has shown us that
high MCA production rates can be expected in Hollow Fibre Bioreactors for
those cell lines that also have high MCA production rates in static
cultures.   Fig. 2. shows the differences between MCA production in
optimised hollow fibre bioreactors of a high secretor (AFP 27) and a low
secreting (LX1) cell line. For both cell lines, linear increases in MCA
production with time were achieved by using the optimisation strategy
discussed previously.   The high secretor (AFP-27) also had higher uptake

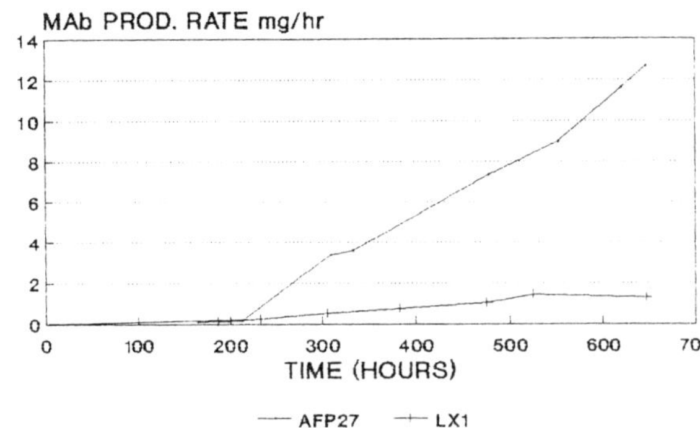

Fig 2: MCA production rates of two mouse x mouse hybridoma cell lines (AFP27 and LX 1) in optimised Acusyst Junior Hollow Fibre Bioreactors.
Continuous harvesting of product was initiated at 225 hrs.

RESULTS (continued)

rates of glucose and glutamine, and production rates of lactate and ammonia, than the low secretor (LX1), Figs 3 and 4.

The MCA production rates for both cell lines were directly proportional to the uptake rates of glucose and glutamine and to the production rates of ammonia (Figs 3 and 4). Molar conversion of glutamine to ammonia was always observed only when samples were not frozen and thawed prior to analysis. A linear relationship between MCA production rate and lactate production rate was only apparent for the AFP27 cell line, and not for any others that have been studied in our laboratory to date.

DISCUSSION AND CONCLUSIONS

Data has been presented which shows that MCA production rates are directly proportional to the uptake rates of glucose and glutamine, and the production rate of ammonia. These relationships are only apparent when the optimisation strategy discussed here has been followed closely by rigorous sampling and monitoring. We are currently using our optimisation strategy for predicting MCA production from high and low secreting hybridoma cell lines in different perfusion culture systems.

REFERENCES

1   Handa-Corrigan, A. Large-scale _in-vitro_ hybridoma culture: current status. Bio/Technology 1988, 6, 784.
2   Miller, W.M., Blanch, H.W. and Wilke, C.R. A kinetic analysis of hybridoma growth and metabolism in batch and continuous suspension culture: Effect of nutrient concentration, dilution rate and pH. Biotech. Bioeng. 1988, 32, 947.
3   Phillips, H.A., Scharer, J.M., Bol, N.C. and Moo-Young, M. Effect of oxygen on antibody productivity in hybridoma cultures. Biotech. Lett. 1987, 9, 745.
4   Luan, Y.T., Mutharasan, R. and Magee, W.E. Effect of various glucose/glutamine ratios on hybridoma growth, viability and monoclonal antibody formation. Biotech. Lett. 1987, 9, 535.
5   Dodge, T.C., Ji, G-Y. and Hu, W.S. Loss of viability in hybridoma cell culture: A Kinetic Study. Enzyme Microb. Tech. Pro. 1987, 390.

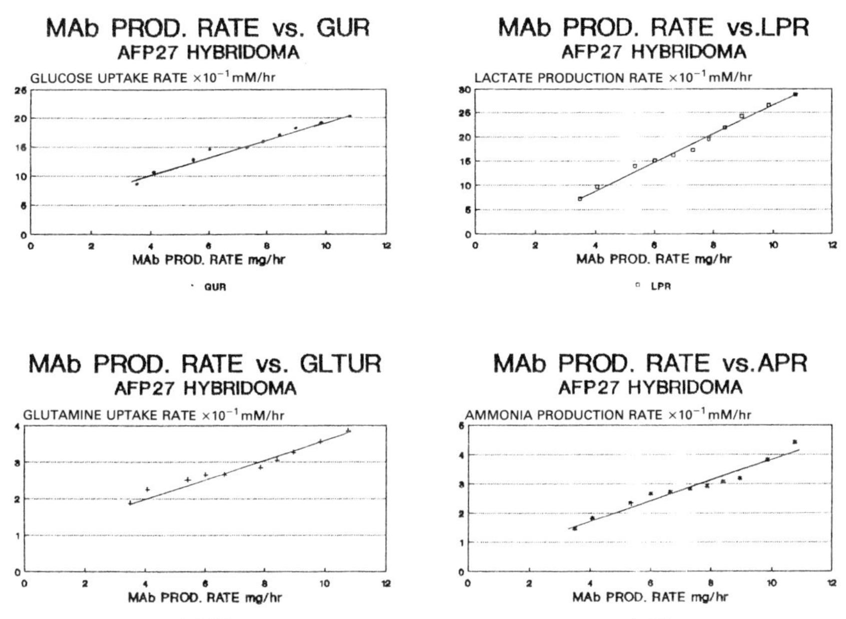

Fig 3: MCA production rates vs glucose & glutamine uptake rates (GUR & GLTUR) and lactate & ammonia production rates (LPR & APR) for AFP27 Hybridoma

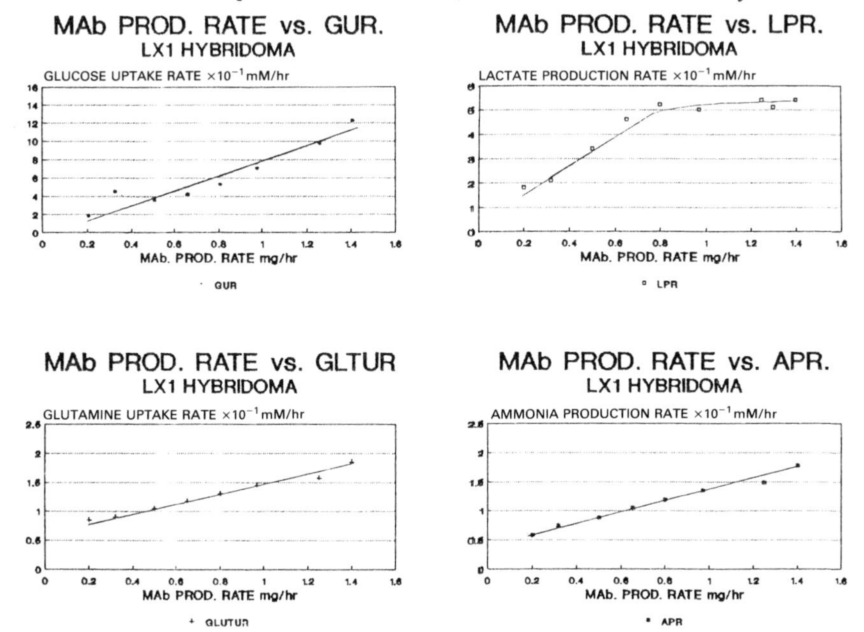

Fig 4: MCA production rates vs glucose & glutamine uptake rates (GUR & GLTUR) and lactase & ammonia production rates (LPR & APR) for LX1 Hybridoma.

Paper of Handa-Corrigan

Lehmann: The more you can measure, the more results you get.
               Sometimes you find differences between cells eg
               serine uptake or production. It is dangerous to
               generalise. The more analytical methods that are
               available, and the more data we can gather, the
               better, for we must have more detailed analytical
               work.

Handa-Corrigan:
               I agree you have to do intensive assaying in order
               to understand the process. The point I want to put
               across is that if you want to be able to control
               and predict antibody production with the minimum
               number of assays for economic reasons, then a few
               parameters are enough to predict productivity.

Lehmann: I agree, but at the end of the day you have to make
               money and yields are very important. If you just
               want to produce some antibody - fine. However if
               you want to optimise the process you have to look
               carefully at the yield. Then it is really
               necessary to do this detailed analytical work.

Handa-Corrigan:
               You can optimise for ever but you have to draw the
               line somewhere.

Hofmann: I want to make a general comment on optimisation
               of cell culture. I think there is merit to both
               sides and it depends upon what you are doing. If
               it is contract production and you want to rapidly
               get some product then Handa-Corrigan is correct.
               On the other hand Lehmann is right if you have the
               time to study and develop systems.

OPTIMIZATION OF HUMAN ANTI RHESUS IgG PRODUCTION

USING HOLLOW FIBER TECHNOLOGY

F. DHAINAUT., L. POUGET., M.J. RICHER-HERS and G. MIGNOT
TM Innovation, 3, avenue des Tropiques, BP 100 91943 LES ULIS FRANCE

ABSTRACT

The human lymphoblastoïd cell line H2D5D2F5 has been cultivated in the hollow fiber
system (ENDOTRONICS JUNIOR) using serum free medium. In order to optimize anti-rhesus
IgG production, the influence of medium feed rate, the presence of human serum albumin
(HSA) in the intracapillary space and the effect of addition of INTRALIPIDE in the
extracapillary space have been tested in 3 separate experiments.
High medium feed rate and presence of HSA improve both cell growth and IgG production.
The benefical effect of HSA may be partially replaced by INTRALIPIDE.

INTRODUCTION

Hollow fiber technology promises many advantages for large scale mammalian cell cultures
such as high cell density, the ability to perform long-term continuous cultures, and the
possibility of purchasing complete culture systems which can be upscaled.
Compact and easy to use systems are now available, such as the ENDOTRONICS systems
(JUNIOR and P/3X) but little data concerning the optimization of IgG production has been
discussed.
IgG production by lymphoblastoïd cell line (H2D5D2F5) has been optimized using the
ENDOTRONICS JUNIOR as culture system.

MATERIALS AND METHODS

Cells and media

After thawing out H2D5D2F5 cell line from the working cell bank, the cells were grown in
IMDM basal medium supplemented with 20 % FCS. Then the cells were washed twice in SA3P
medium (2) consisting of a mixture of IMDM, chemically defined supplements, and human
serum albumin (HSA) (350 mg/ml). Cells (0.8 x 10^9) were seeded in a hollow fiber cartridge
previously washed first with basal medium and then with SA3P. After 3 or 6 days, the SA3P
medium was switched to SA3S medium (2). Media were antibiotic-free.

Methods

Three experiments were performed in the ENDOTRONICS JUNIOR system using different
conditions.

Experiment 1 :   Using low medium feed rate :
                  The medium feed rate was increased from 15 ml to 90 ml/hour in 45 days and
                  then it was maintained at 90 ml/hour for 33 days.

Experiment 2 :   Using high medium feed rate :
                  The medium feed rate was increased from 15 ml/hour to 240 ml/hour in 12
                  days and then it was maintained at 240 ml/hour for 52 days.

Experiment 3 :   As experiment 2 without HSA in the intracapillary space :
                  After 25 days, medium circulating in the extracapillary space containing
                  HSA was supplemented with INTRALIPIDE (KABI) 0.1 % (V/V), which a
                  mixture of soya oil, eggs lecithins and glycerol.

Evaluation of the IgG secretion

The IgG secretion was evaluated using an autoanalyser by the method of LALEZARI (3),
which measure the anti-rhesus activity. Samples from the extracapillary harvest were
centrifugated (1800 g, 10 minutes, 4° C) and supernatants were diluted with NaCl 0.9 % +
bovine serum albumin 0.5 % to obtain a concentration of 5 to 10 µg/ml.

RESULTS AND DISCUSSION

Figure 1 and 2 represent the IgG cumulative production from the 3 experiments performed
with the ENDOTRONICS JUNIOR system.

Figure 1: cumulative production of IgG (experiment 1)

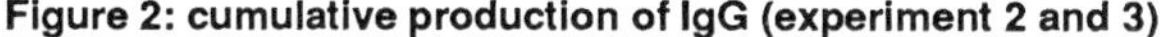

Figure 2: cumulative production of IgG (experiment 2 and 3)

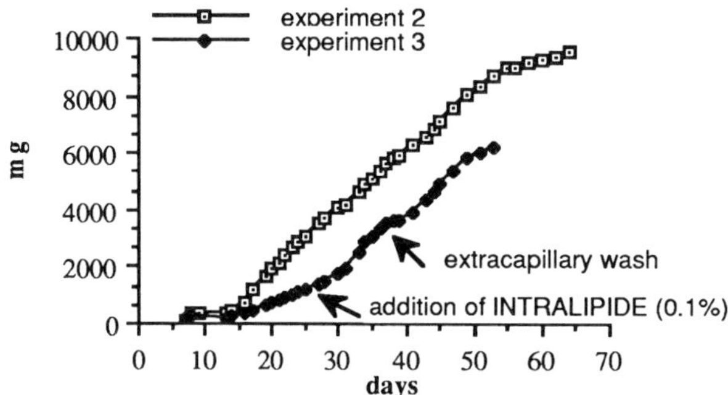

496

With high medium feed rate, the lag phase before the beginning of the IgG secretion is reduced if HSA is present in the intracapillary space (experiment 2). To produce the first two grams of anti-Rhesus IgG, the system must operate for 30 days for experiments 1 and 3, and 20 days for the experiment 2 largely due to a higher growth rate.

Because of the cut-off size of the hollow fiber cartridge (8000-10 000 Da), HSA cannot cross the pores. Thus the observed enhancement of the secretion in experiment 2 versus experiment 3 may be due to fatty acids and other small molecules which are carried by HSA and could diffuse through the pores.

In experiment 3, addition of 0.1 % INTRALIPIDE (9 ml/h) in the intracapillary space on day 25 induced an enhancement of the IgG secretion for 9 days, followed by diminution of the secretion level.

The extracapillary space was washed with SA3S without INTRALIPIDE. The same medium as previously described (SA3S + 0.1 % INTRALIPIDE) was used (9 ml/h). The improvement of IgG production by INTRALIPIDE was confirmed, but, probably due to the toxicity of lipids accumulated in the extracapillary space, the IgG production decreased after 8 days.

Table 1 summarize the data of the 3 experiments :

	Experiment 1	Experiment 2	Experiment 3
Culture time (days)	77	64	53
IgG production (g)	10.21	9.5	6.2
Total medium used (l)	140	316	252
Productivity (μg/ml)	65	29	24
Time necessary to produce the first 2 grams (days)	30	20	30
Total harvest volume (l)	17.0	10.9	8.5
Mean concentration of IgG in harvest (μg/ml)	600	872	729

CONCLUSION

H2D5D2F5 lymphoblastoïd cell line can be cultivated in a hollow fiber cartridge using serum free medium. High medium feed rate allows the system to reach a production phase sooner. The HSA in the intracapillary space has a beneficial effect on IgG secretion which is mainly due to fatty acids. HSA can be replaced by a lipid mixture (INTRALIPIDE) but further experiments are needed to permit long-term production of large amounts of IgG.

REFERENCES

1 - GOOSSENS D., CHAMPOMIER F., ROUGER Ph., & SALMON Ch. Human monoclonal antibodies against blood group antigens. Preparation of a stable immortalised B clones producing high levels of antibody of different isotypes and specificities.
J. Immunol. Methods, 1987, 101, pp 193 -200.

2 - DROUET X., GOOSSENS D., CHAMPOMOER F., LIBERGE G., TSIKAS G., Le BESNERAIS M., ROUGER Ph., & SALMON Ch. Culture de clones de cellules lymphoblastoïdes en milieu défini : application à la production in vitro d'immunoglobulines monoclonales anti-D pour la prévention de la maladie hémolytique du nouveau-né.
Bio-sciences, 1986, 5, pp 75 - 78.

3 - LALEZARI P., A new method for detection of red blood cell antibodies. Transfusion, 1968, 8, pp 372 - 380.

PARAMETERS FOR OPTIMISATION OF FERMENTATION OF AN AT III
PRODUCING CELL LINE

U. Eberhard *, G. Schmid **, R. Johannsen *

 * Behringwerke AG, P.O. Box 11 40, D-3550 Marburg, F.R.G.
** present adress: Hoffmann-La Roche AG, CH-4002 Basel,
   Switzerland

Antithrombin III, a glycosilated human serum protein, was
produced by different CHO cells. Selection of clone and type
of fermenter was done testing different process modes under
aspects of product concentration and productivity. Optimal
results were obtained in long term fermentations using
stirred tank reactors in perfusion mode.

Keywords: AT III, CHO clones, airlift reactor, stirred tank
          reactor, sparging, membrane aeration, cell
          retention, repeated batch, continuous cultivation,
          perfusion

INTRODUCTION

Producing antithrombin III (AT III, MW = 60 kD) as a model
substance for a recombinant glycosilated protein, selection
of cell line and process development and optimisation are
closely connected. An optimal process has to meet the
following attributes of a cell line:

- growth either clearly attached to surfaces or free in
  suspension
- stability of expression system including genomic structure
- constant specific productivity also at high cell densities
  and after prolonged period of time
- product secretion in serum free media
- equipment enabling long term fermentations (up to 100 d)

Different types of fermenters are tested to meet these
demands. Process optimisation was performed regarding
product concentration and productivity as key parameters.

MATERIALS AND METHODS

Cell line: Different CHO-clones expressing AT III:
            - anchorage dependent cells
            - suspension cells

Fermenter: Type: - stirred tank
                                         (B. Braun Melsungen)
                             - fixed bed   (Opticell, CRBS)
                             - airlift   (Chemap)
           Gas supply: - membrane aeration
                             - sparging

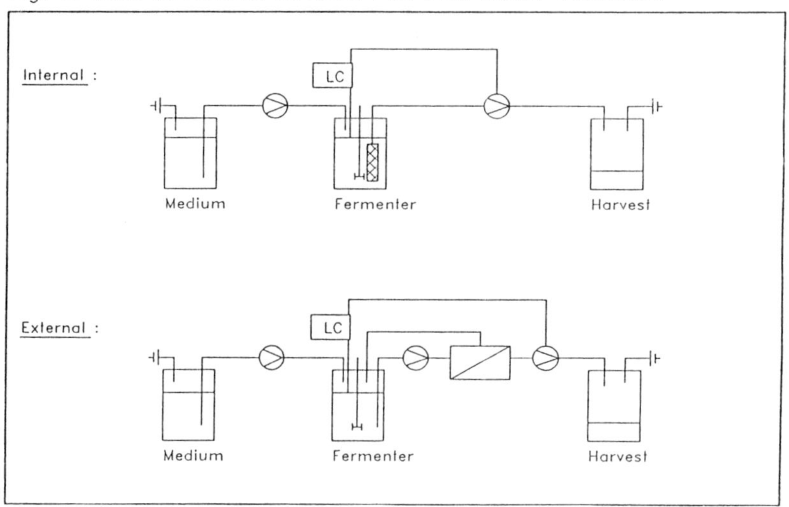

                    Cell retention: - internal (filter/sedimentation)
                                    (Fuji-Filter, Chemap spinfilter)
                                  - external (filter/centrifuge)
                                    (Millipore, Alfa Laval
                                    Centritech)
                    see Fig. 1

Process   : Repeated batch
            Continuous (without cell retention)
            Perfusion

RESULTS

Fermentations using recombinant CHO cells can be run up to
100 days in serum containing and serum free media without
decrease in specific productivity. Sparging or membrane
devices for aeration (oxygen transfer rates:
50 - 100 mg/l x h) are suited to meet the oxygen demand at
cell densities $>10^7$ cells/ml.

Product yields in homogeneous systems (stirred tank or
airlift reactors) were higher compared to those of fixed bed
reactors (see Tab. 1). The lower productivity of fixed bed
systems presumably is due to formation of gradients and
local diffusion limitations of oxygen and nutrients.
Different process modes (repeated batch, continuous harvest
and perfusion mode) in homogeneous systems demonstrated that
cell density and product concentration in perfusion cultures
were optimal (see Fig. 2).

By variation of dilution rates a maximum in product concentration was found under perfusion conditions (see Fig. 3).
Position and level of this maximum were dependent on the
process conditions (cell density, medium composition etc.).

	Stirred tank reactor operation mode:			Fixed bed reactor operation mode:
	batch	continuous	perfusion	perfusion
cell density (10^6 c/ml)	1,3	1,2	13,2	≈ 5*)
AT III concentration (mg/l)	14	18	107	12
specific productivity (mg/10^9 c x d)	7	7	6	≈ 4
productivity (mg/l x d)	6	19	107	18

*) total cell number by total medium volume

Tab. 1: Comparison of process parameters at different operation modes

Fig. 2: FERMENTATION OF CHO SUSPENSION CELL

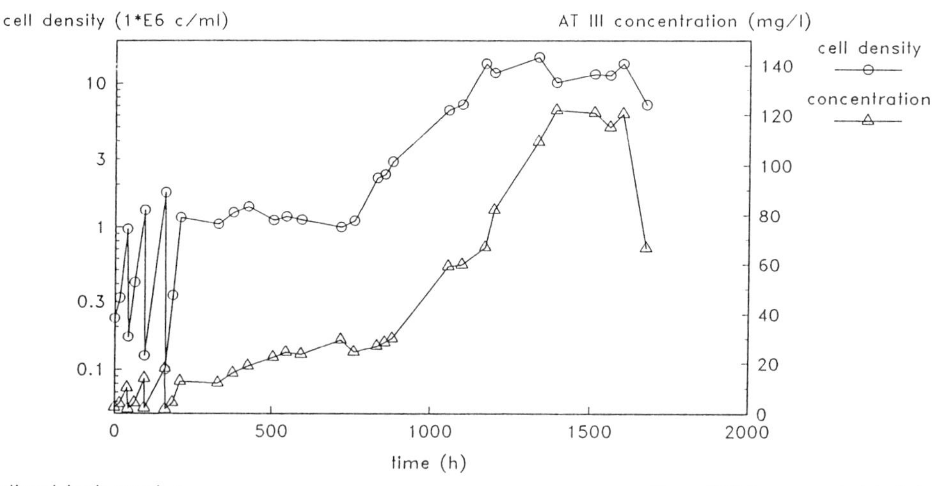

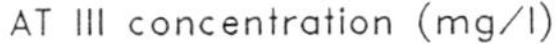

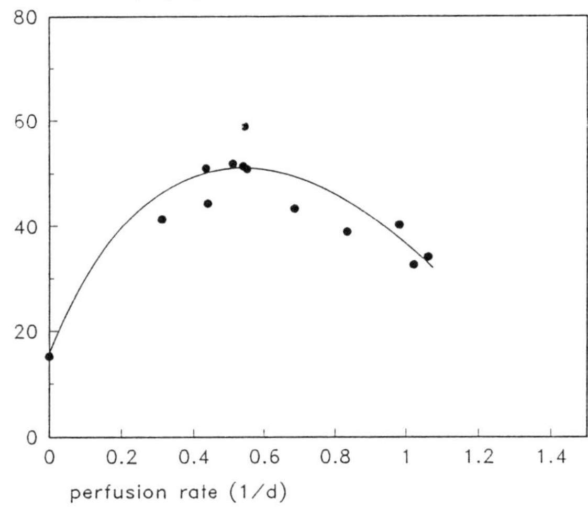

DISCUSSION

Perfusion type cultures show optimal product yields,
resulting from high cell numbers and secretion of product
over prolonged period of time. The expression system
exhibited sufficient biological stability, also process
equipment was suited under aspects of technical stability.

External cell retention devices in perfusion cultures show
the advantage of disposability in case of trouble without
terminating the process, also scaleability of these systems
is feasible. Filter systems for retention of cells like
filters tend to clog within 1 to 2 weeks. Open systems like
continuous centrifuges meet best the demands of long term
process stability.

ENHANCED PRODUCTIVITY OF HYBRIDOMA AND RECOMBINANT CHO CELL
CULTURES BY PLURONIC F-68 AND OTHER MEDIUM COMPONENTS, AND BY
INCREASED PERFUSION RATES, IN FLUIDIZED-BED BIOREACTORS

N.G. Ray, A.S. Tung, P.W. Runstadler, J.N. Vournakis

Verax Corporation
6 Etna Road
Lebanon, New Hampshire 03766 U.S.A.

ABSTRACT

Hybridoma and Chinese Hamster Ovary (CHO) cells are cultured
in continuous fluidized-bed bioreactors. Cells are
immobilized in porous, weighted collagen microspheres which
are suspended in the bioreactor by the recycling of culture
liquid. This paper presents experimental data showing the
response by hybridoma and recombinant CHO cells to changes in
the culture environment brought about by varying process
parameters. The effect of perfusion rate changes, and
limiting nutrient concentration on specific productivity and
metabolic characteristics, was studied. Perfusion rates in
the range of 0.5-2.5 mL/mL fluidized-bed/hr were investigated.
Significant improvements in both population specific
productivity and reactor space-time productivity were observed
at high perfusion rates. Specific metabolic rates, such as
glucose and glutamine consumption rates and lactate and
ammonia production rates, increased with increases in
perfusion rate, whereas by-product yield coefficients, e.g.,
lactate yield on glucose and ammonia yield on glutamine,
remained unchanged. In addition, studies have been carried
out with a number of culture media components that enhance the
productivity of hybridoma cells and recombinant CHO cells.
Results show that pluronic F-68 when added to serum-free
culture medium enhances the productivity of both hybridoma and
recombinant cell cultures in a stable manner. This enhanced
productivity appears to result from an increase in cell number
for hybridomas, whereas enhancement of recombinant CHO cell
productivity is the result of an increase in the cell-specific
productivity.

INTRODUCTION

For commercial production of therapeutic and diagnostic
proteins using mammalian cell culture technology, it is
essential that the product is made at low cost with consistent
product quality and performance predictability. Several
systems have been proposed for culturing mammalian cells in
vitro (1-6) and different modes of operation have been
suggested. The commonly practiced cultivation processes can
be broadly categorized as batch, continuous, and perfusion
systems.

A batch culture is a non-steady-state process where the biochemical environment is continuously changing because of nutrient depletion and accumulation of cell-secreted metabolic by-products. Since the relatively productive culture environment exists only transiently in a batch culture, the overall cell productivity in the culture is expected to be lower compared to that in a continuous or perfusion culture, where the optimized productive environment can be maintained under steady-state conditions.

High density continuous, perfusion systems for mammalian cell cultures have received much attention during the last decade. Different systems have been suggested (7-9). However, none of them have successfully addressed all the critical issues relative to scale-up, productivity, product quality, long-term steady-state operation in low-cost serum-free medium and use of a common system for both anchorage-dependent and anchorage-independent cell lines.

A fluidized-bed, retained cell, perfusion culture system has been developed with an objective to meet all the criteria discussed above (10,11). In this system, cells are cultured in porous collagen microspheres fluidized in a bioreactor. This paper presents the experimental results and analysis of CHO cell and hybridoma cultures in such a system. Also, some data from a batch suspension culture in a stirred tank bioreactor using the same cell line is presented. In the fluidized-bed culture, cell density on the order of 1-3 x 10^8 cells/mL collagen was achieved within 15 days after inoculation. Data on the enhancement of bioreactor productivity by pluronic F-68 for a CHO cell culture are shown. Medium perfusion rate was increased to a maximum 19.2 liter/liter fluidized-bed/day and steady-state data were obtained at four different perfusion rates for the hybridoma cell line. Perfusion rates were increased five-fold in small increments for the CHO cell line. Both productivity and metabolic rates were increased with the increases in perfusion rate. It is suggested that the observed increase was the result of improved cell specific productivity and metabolic rates.

MATERIALS AND METHODS

Cells and Medium

A mouse hybridoma cell line which secretes both IgG1 and IgG2a and a Chinese hamster ovary (CHO) cell which secretes a recombinant thrombolytic protease were used in this study. The base medium consisted of a 3:1 mixture of Dulbecco's Modified Eagle (DME) medium (4.5 gm/L glucose) and Ham's F-12 nutrient mixture (1.8 gm/L glucose). Both the suspension batch and the immobilized perfusion culture experiments were carried out using identical serum-free medium. The glucose and glutamine concentrations in the medium were 3.2 + 0.15 gm/L and 0.46 + 0.05 gm/L, respectively.

Culture Methods

Perfusion Fluidized-Bed: A schematic of the fluidized-bed bioreactor system is shown in Reference 6. The system consists of an external recycle loop through which culture liquid is continuously circulated to fluidize the collagen microspheres in the reactor vessel. The microspheres, approximately 500 microns in diameter, are weighted to achieve a specific gravity approximately 1.6 in order to remain suspended in the recirculating culture liquid flowing upward at about 75 cm/min. superficial velocity. The liquid, separated from the microspheres near the top of the vessel, enters the recycle loop which contains a membrane gas exchanger, the measuring instruments (temperature, pH and dissolved oxygen), a recycle pump, an electric heater, and a recycle flow meter. Independent of the recycle loop, fresh medium is pumped into and harvest is removed continuously. Dissolved oxygen was controlled at 75 + 10 mmHg oxygen partial pressure in the liquid to the gas exchanger inlet, where oxygen tension is the lowest. Culture temperature and pH were controlled at 37 + 0.2oC and 7.2 + 0.05, respectively.

Batch Suspension: Some batch studies were performed in a two-liter stirred-tank bioreactor (Biolafitte). Oxygen was supplied into the culture liquid through a thin-walled silicone tubing coiled around the baffles inside the reactor vessel as well as through the gas-liquid interface at the liquid surface. Culture temperature was maintained at 37 + 0.2oC by circulating warm water from a water bath through the bioreactor jacket. Dissolved oxygen and pH were maintained at 60 + 20 mmHg oxygen partial pressure and 7.2 + 0.1, respectively, by feedback control using a computer.

Analyses: Cell number was determined using a Coulter counter (Model ZM, Coulter Electronics). Matrix cell counts were performed by releasing the cells from the microspheres by collagenase and trypsin at 37oC. Viability was determined with a hemacytometer by erythrosin-B dye exclusion technique. Glucose was assayed by an enzyme electrode analyzer (YSI 27, Yellow Spring Instruments). Lactate levels were determined using an enzymatic kit from Boehringer. Secreted IgG was assayed by an enzyme-linked immunosorbent assay (ELISA) (12).

RESULTS AND DISCUSSION

The perfusion immobilized bioreactor has a maximum fluidized-bed volume of 150 mL (the total system volume, including the recycle loop and a recycle pump, is 750 mL). The starting fluidized-bed (FB) volume in the perfusion bioreactor was 105 mL for the hybridoma culture and 160 mL for the CHO cell culture, having a solids (collagen) content approximately 25%. The systems were inoculated with 1.4×10^8 and 3.7×10^8 viable cells, respectively. The bioreactors were operated in batch mode for 4 and 1 days, and on Days 5 and 2 medium perfusion was initiated. Medium perfusion rate, expressed as liter/liter FB-day, glucose consumption and lactate production rates, expressed as gm/liter FB-day, were obtained. Steady-state data were obtained for the hybridoma culture at four different perfusion rates, ranging from 7.7-19.2 liter/liter FB-day. Perfusion rates were increased more incrementally for the CHO cell culture, from 55-159 L/L-FB-day, thus steady-state levels were not attained. Glucose consumption and lactate production rates increased significantly, with an increase in perfusion rate in the hybridoma culture as presented in Figure 1. These increases

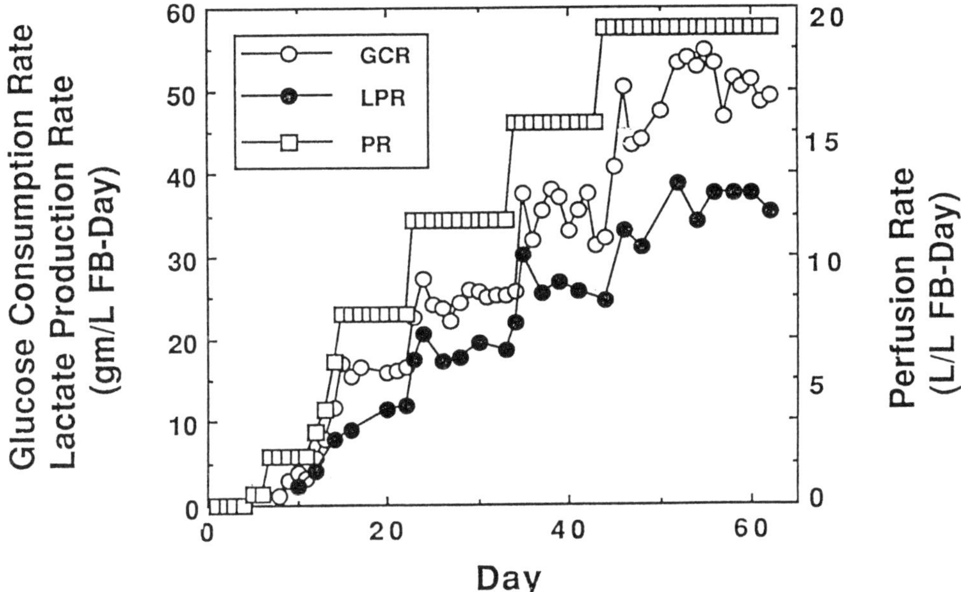

Figure 1 Medium perfusion, glucose consumption and lactate production rates in a fluidized-bed culture of hybridoma cells

seem to have resulted from higher metabolic activities of the immobilized cells at higher perfusion rates. Cell density in the microspheres reached a maximum by Day 22 and Day 80, respectively, for the two cell cultures and no further increase in microsphere cell density was observed, despite increased perfusion rate. The maximum cell densities were 2.3×10^8 and 3.8×10^8 cells/mL collagen for the two cultures. The steady-state lactate yield was unaffected by perfusion rate. Figure 2A presents perfusion rate, antibody concentration and productivity data in the harvest liquid for the hybridoma cell line. The antibody concentration declined transiently each time medium perfusion rate was stepped up; however, the levels rose to steady-state values in a relatively short period of time. The steady-state antibody concentration at all the perfusion rates investigated remained between 85 and 110 mg/L. The normalized bioreactor productivity, in terms of gm-antibody produced/liter FB-day, is shown in Figure 2B indicating that the highest

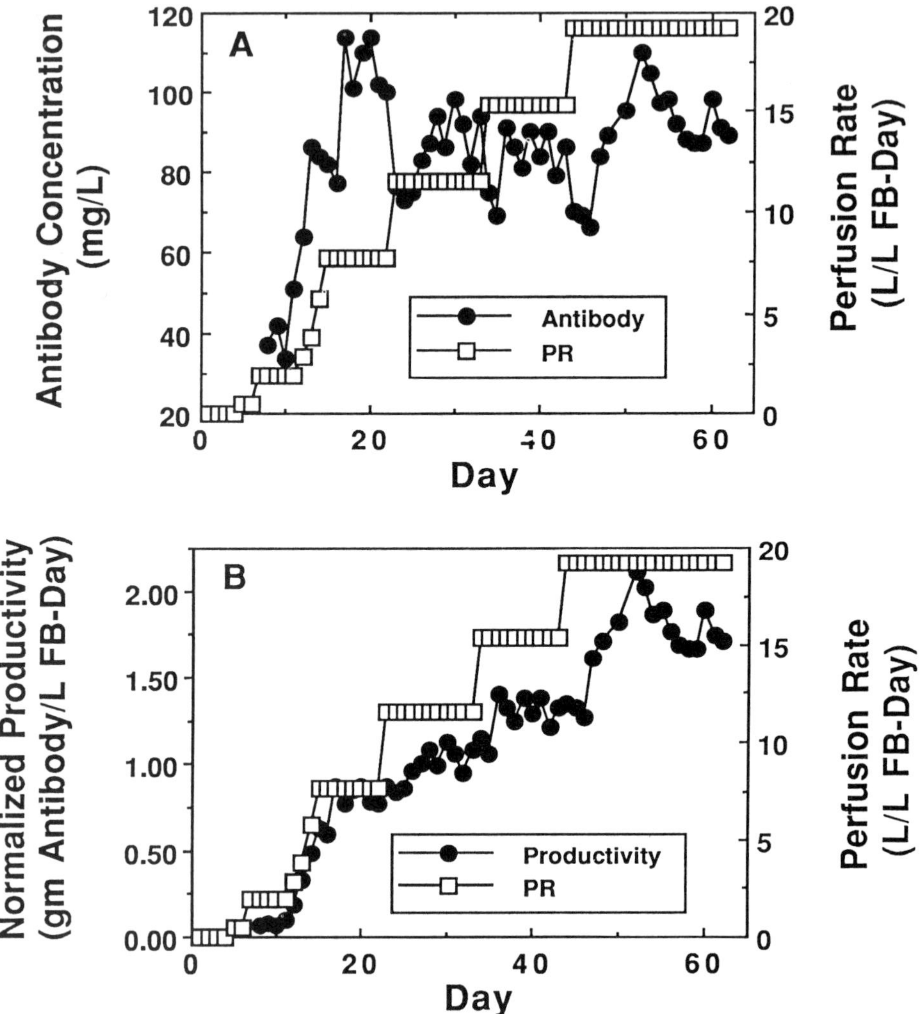

Figure 2   Perfusion culture of hybridoma
cells in fluidized-bed bioreactor:
A   Medium perfusion rate and antibody titer
B   Medium perfusion rate and volumetric productivity

productivity, approximately 2.0 gm/liter FB-day, was achieved
at the maximum perfusion rate investigated in this study.
Similar data are shown for the CHO cell culture in Figure 3.
Concentration of the thrombolytic protein (Figure 3A) reached
and maintained a relatively constant value of 225-250 IU/mL
from Day 30 throughout the remaining 50 days of the run.
Product concentration held essentially constant over a nearly
five-fold increase in perfusion rate. Bioreactor productivity
(Figure 3B) dramatically increased from 7500 to nearly 27,500
units per liter fluidized bed per day in response to increases
in perfusion rate.

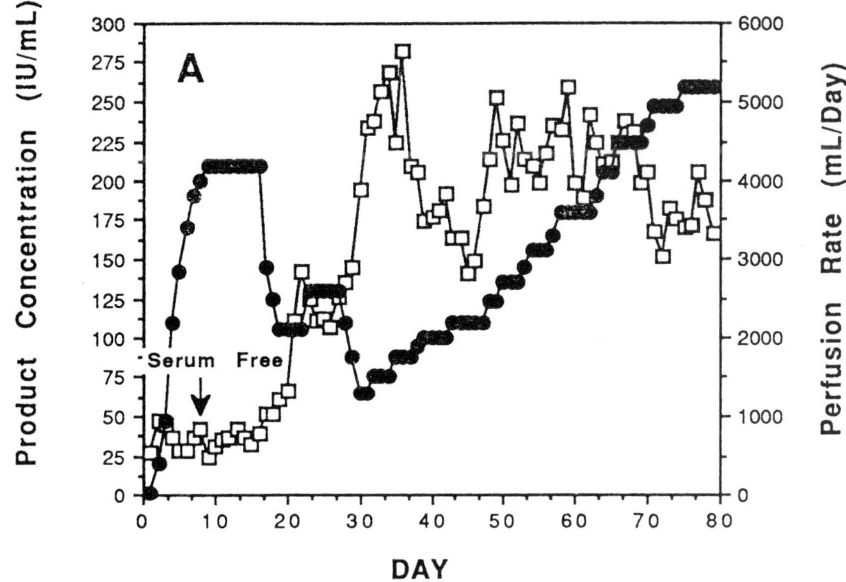
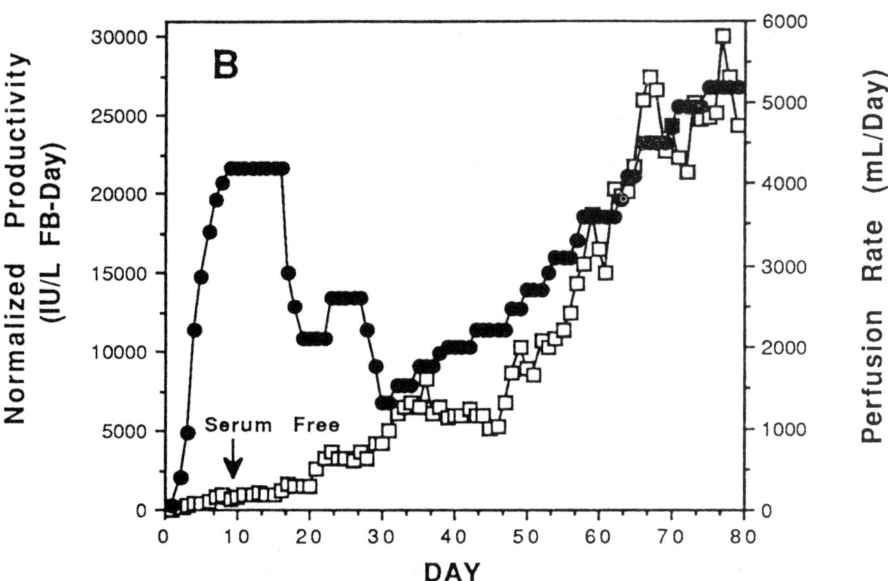

Figure 3 Performance culture of Chinese hanster ovary cells in a fluidized- bed bioreactor:
A Medium perfusion rate (●) and product concentration (□)
B Medium perfusion rate (●) and volumetric productivity (□)

The bioreactor productivities increased from 1.1 to 1.8 gm antibody/liter FB-day and from 7500-27,500 IU/L FB-day, respectively, for the hybridoma and CHO cell cultures with increased perfusion rates Since the cell density during this period is found to be considered to be unchanged for the hybridoma culture, the observed increase in reactor productivity is the result of higher specific productivity. However, the increases observed in the CHO culture are due in part to cell growth as well as an increase in cell-specific productivity.

The highest perfusion rate investigated in this hybridoma study corresponds to a dilution rate, expressed as medium feed rate per unit fluid system volume, of 0.12 hr-1, which is much greater than the maximum cell specific growth rate. Consequently, the primary source of the cells present in the harvest liquid is the dividing, but constant, matrix population. Therefore, a reasonable assessment of cell viability in the microspheres may be made from cell viability in the culture liquid. With this assumption the calculated specific productivity at the perfusion rate of 19.2 liter/liter FB-day is 1.5 μg/v.cell-hr (steady-state cell viability in the culture liquid was 70%). In this specific productivity calculation, it is assumed that the free cells present in the recycle liquid outside the fluidized bed (10%-15% of total cell population is in the recycle liquid) are as productive as the immobilized cells. Table 1 compares productivity of batch suspension culture, carried out as described above, with the steady-state, fluidized-bed culture, for the hybridoma culture.

	Batch Suspension	Perfusion Fluidized-Bed
Specific Productivity (pg/v.cell-hr)	0.9	1.5
Reactor Productivity (mg/liter-day)	10	1740*
Specific medium feed rate (mL/v.cell-day)		4.1 x 10-7

* mg/liter FB-day. 85-90% of the total cells in the bioreactor present in the fluidized-bed.

Table 1 Productivity in batch and perfusion bioreactors

With a different hybridoma cell line, we have observed a four-fold increase in specific productivity in a fluidized-bed bioreactor over T-flask batch culture (6). At the highest specific productivity in that culture, the specific medium

11.5 x 10-7 mL/cell-day and 0.035 hr-1, respectively. In the present fluidized-bed culture study, an increased specific medium feed rate resulted in enhanced specific productivity and growth rate. Also, as mentioned earlier, the specific productivity in the batch suspension culture was observed to be greater in the exponential growth phase. From these observations, it is reasonable to expect that even higher perfusion rates would contribute to further increases in specific productivity in the fluidized-bed culture.

Studies with the addition of pluronic F-68 into the culture medium were performed with the CHO cell in the fluidized-bed system. Pluronic F-68 is often added to stirred-tank and air-lift fermenter cultures of mammalian cells to protect cells from shear damage (13). It was found that the addition of small amounts (50-200 μg/mL) generated an improvement in bioreactor productivity, as illustrated in Table 2.

	Daily Glucose Consumption Rate (g/day)	Perfusion Rate (mL/day)	Product Conc. (U/mL)	Bioreactor Productivity (units/day)
Minus F-68	2.47	800	67	53,600
Plus F-68*	2.77	800	146	116,800

*   F-68 concentration 100 μg/mL.
**   Data is averaged over 40 days of steady-state culture.

Table 2 Pluronic F-68 mediated enhancement of the productivity
of a recombinant thrombolytic producing CHO cell line in a fluidized bed bioreactor

Bioreactor productivity more than doubled with no increase on cell number, indicating that F-68 improved cell-specific productivity.

CONCLUSIONS

Mouse hybridoma and recombinant Chinese hamster ovary cell lines cultured in collagen matrices in a fluidized-bed bioreactor have shown significantly enhanced specific productivity especially when compared to a batch suspension culture in a stirred-tank bioreactor. In the stationary phase of the batch culture, where glucose consumption was negligible, the hybridoma cells continued to secrete antibody although the specific secretion rate was significantly lower compared to that in the exponential growth phase. In the fluidized-bed bioreactor, the specific antibody secretion rates as well as the metabolic rates and cell growth rate were increased significantly with an increase in medium perfusion rate. Similarly, the CHO cell demonstrated dramatic improvement in bioreactor productivity in response to an increase in perfusion rate. In addition, the CHO cell fluidized-bed culture responded to the addition of F-68 by increasing specific productivity and, thus, bioreactor output.

The biochemical environment generated inside the collagen microspheres is a result of a complex set of interactions and regulations brought about by the intimate cell-matrix and cell-cell interactions and intra-matrix concentration of substrates and cell-secreted products, including autocrine factors. Therefore, the cells cultured in the microspheres experience a significantly different culture environment compared to their counterparts in suspension. A similar study in a fluidized-bed bioreactor(s) has suggested that the immobilized cells in collagen microspheres appear to utilize substrates more efficiently toward antibody synthesis than the suspended cells, which allocate more resources toward cell growth. The effect of pluronic F-68 is likely a cell surface phenomenon that facilitates secretion, and has been observed in a wide spectrum of cell types secreting therapeutic proteins.

REFERENCES

1   Feder, J. and Tolbert, W.L., _Scientific American_, __248__, 1983, p.36.

2   Posillico, E.G., _Biotechnology_, __4__, 1986, p. 194.

3   Van Brunt, J., _Biotechnology_, __4__, 1986, p. 505.

4   Arathoon, W.R. and Birch, J.R., _Science_, __232__, 1986, p. 1390.

5   Karkare, S.B., Phillips, P.G., Burke, D.H. and Dean, R.C., Jr., _Large Scale Mammalian Cell Culture_, 1985, J. Feder and W.R. Tolbert, Eds., Academic Press, p. 127.

6   Ray, N.G., Vournakis, J.N., Runstadler, P.W., Tung, A.S. and Venkatasubramanian, K., in _Physiology of Immobilized Cells_ (in press), Elsevier Science Publishers, Amsterdam.

7   Altshuler, G., Dziewulski, D.M., Sowek, J.A. and Belfort, G., _Biotechnol. Bioeng._, 28, 1986, p. 646.

8   Lydersen, B.K., _Large-Scale Cell Culture Technology_, 1987, B.K. Lydersen, Ed., Hanser Publishers, Munich/Vienna/New York, p. 169.

9   Rupp, R., Gilbride, K. and Oka, M., _Large-Scale Culture Technology_, 1987, B.K. Lydersen, Ed., Hanser Publishers, Munich/Vienna/New York, p. 81.

10   Dean, R.C., Jr., Karkare, S.B., Ray, N.G., Runstadler, P.W. and Venkatasubramanian, K., _Ann. N.Y. Acad. Sci._, _506_, 1987, p. 129.

11   Tung, A.S., Sample, J.vG., Brown, T.A., Ray, N.G., Hayman, E.G., and Runstadler, P.W., _Biopharm Manuf._ _1_, 1988, p. 50.

12   Engvall, E., _Methods Enzymol._, _70_, 1980, p. 419.

13   Murhammer, D.W., Scale-up of Insect Cell Cultures: Protective Effects of Pluronic F-68, Goochee, 1988, _Bio/Technology_ _6_, pp. 1411-1418.

<u>**Paper of Vournakis**</u>

Jenkins: In your effect with the glucocorticoids do you see
            it only in myeloma cells, or in the CHO cells as
            well? Also would you like to speculate on what is
            actually happening?

Vournakis: We see this in cells other than myeloma eg CHO.
            It is not a common effect. This is pure
            speculation but it may have something to do with
            the position in which the recombinant genes have
            integrated into the genome of the cell. If the
            integration site is near a glucocorticoid receptor
            binding site then it may be stimulated in the
            presence of glucocorticoid, and an enhanced
            productivity occurs. If this is the reason then
            it could be used as a strategy to make high-
            producers.

Improved Performance of the Fluidized Bed Reactor for the Cultivation of Animal Cells

J. Keller, I.J. Dunn, E. Heinzle

Biological Reaction Engineering Group,
Chemical Engineering Department, ETH Zentrum
CH-8092 Zürich (Switzerland)

Abstract

A fluidized bed reactor system was developed and its performance characterized. Experiments with an anchorage dependent BHK cell line showed the advantages of this reactor system: high cell concentrations (up to $4*10^7$ cells/mL); high cell activity in a small reactor system; on-line oxygen uptake measurements provide an excellent tool for cultivation control and optimization. Porous and nonporous glass carriers were successfully used for cell retention.

Introduction

Fluidized bed reactors have been used in biotechnology for a number of applications for biomass retention. Separation into two compartments for cultivation and aeration allows high mass transfer rates in the conditioning tank and low shear stress for the cells in the reactor.

Materials and Methods

Fluidized bed reactor

The used fluidized bed reactor system (Fig. 1) was explained earlier (Keller *et al.* 1989). The special differential arrangement of the oxygen electrodes allows an accurate measurement of the oxygen uptake rate (OUR) during cultivation. Due to the immobilization of the cells in the reactor continuous operation is easy to perform.

Carriers

The choice of carrier materials for the cell attachment was a critical point during reactor development. Beside the surface characteristics also physical properties (size, density, porosity) are very important. Two different types of glass carriers have been successfully used: nonporous glass beads with a diameter of 105-150 µm or 150 - 210 µm (Polysciences Inc. USA) and porous SIRAN® sintered glass carriers with a diameter of 0.4-1.0 mm and a pore size < 120 µm (Schott Glaswerke, Mainz, West Germany)*.

---

* SIRAN®- samples courtesy of Schott Glaswerke, Mainz, West Germany

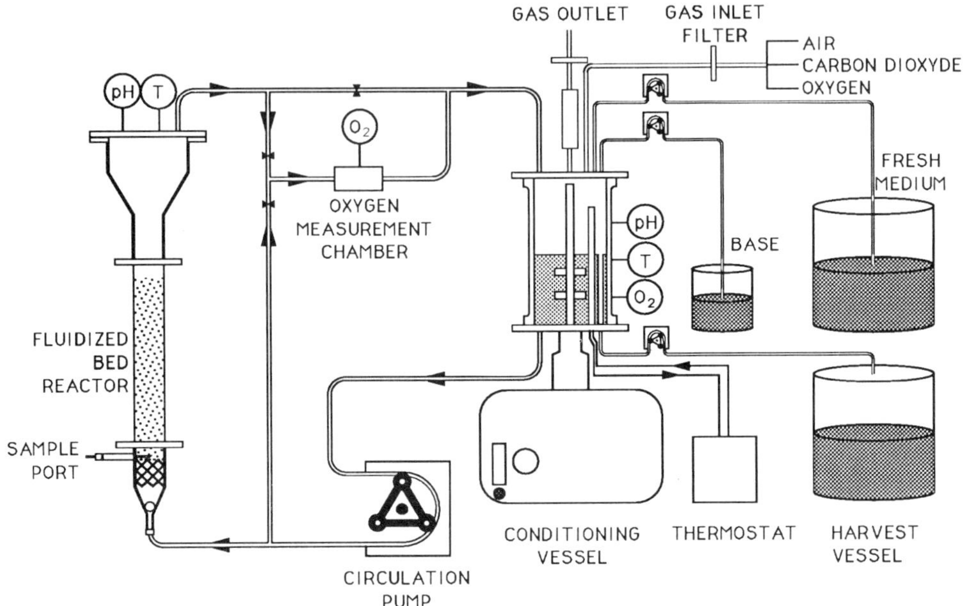

Fig. 1: Fluidized bed reactor: temperature, pH and dissolved oxygen concentration in the conditioning vessel are controlled by a bioreactor control system

Cell line and medium

The experiments were carried out with a BHK 21 (ATCC CCL 10) cell line using Glasgow Modification of MEM containing 10 % tryptose phosphate broth (Gibco-BRL, Basel, Switzerland) and in addition 1-10 % bovine serum (Gibco-BRL, Basel, Switzerland).

Characteristics of the reactor system

The following table shows some typical values used in the experiments and the achieved results:

Maximal volume of the fluidized bed	600 mL
Entire reactor system volume	3.5 L
Medium throughput	up to 5 L/day (210 mL/h)
Glucose consumption	max. 15 g/day (0.6 g/h)
Oxygen uptake rate	3 mmol/h
Max. cell density: nonporous carriers	$2*10^7$ cells/ml expanded bed volume
porous carriers	$4*10^7$ cells/ml expanded bed volume
Ratio of inoculum cell number	approx. 5 % of final cell number

Oxygen uptake rate measurements

The possibility of measuring the oxygen concentration difference between the inlet and outlet of the fluidized bed reactor is an important advantage of this reactor system. An instantaneous measurement of changes in cell metabolism is permitted. Therefore the OUR is useful for optimization of growth and culture conditions. It is also important for process control and validation as shown in Fig. 2.

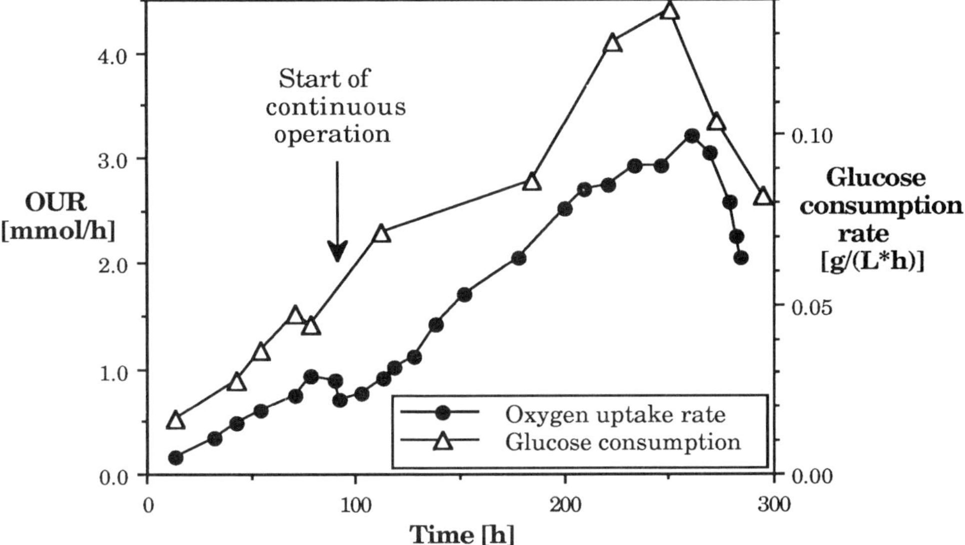

Fig. 2:   OUR correlates with glucose consumption rate during batch and continuous operation of the fluidized bed reactor

Conclusions

Fluidized bed reactors are well suited for the cultivation of anchorage dependent cell lines. High density solid and porous particles have successfully been used. The oxygen uptake rate measurements provide an excellent tool for monitoring cell activity.

Acknowledgement
Research grants from the Swiss Government (KWF) and the Sulzer Company, Winterthur, Switzerland as well as from the ETH Zürich are gratefully acknowledged.

Reference
J. Keller, M. Murkovic, I.J. Dunn, E. Heinzle, J. Prenosil
Development of a Fluidized Bed Loop Reactor for the Cultivation of Animal Cells
DECHEMA Biotechnology Conferences, **3**, 1989, 715

Section 6.6
Bioreactors: comparative studies

BIOREACTORS FOR PRODUCTION OF HIV - A COMPARATIVE EVALUATION
OF FLASK, SUSPENSION, AND FIXED BED CULTURES

J.B. Clarke and J.B. Griffiths

Division of Biologics, PHLS Centre for Applied Microbiology
and Research, Porton Down, Salisbury, Wiltshire, SP4 OJG,
UK.

ABSTRACT

In an attempt to establish a bioreactor system for
generation of HIV that is practicable, efficient,
biologically contained, and capable of scale up, the
production of two strains of this virus was examined in
suspension culture and the 'Porosphere' fixed bed system.
HIV 1 and HIV 2 were grown successfully in both these types
of reactor. The porosphere reactor theoretically appears to
offer a better environment for HIV production, but evidence
for significantly improved yields from this system, compared
to suspension, was equivocal. However, this configuration
facilitated media changes during culture. The data clearly
showed that the culture system and cell environment
significantly affected cell-virus interrelationships.
switches between lytic - and persistent - type infections,
and changes in the virus population were observed.

Keywords: Cell-virus interaction, fixed bed bioreactors,
HIV, suspension bioreactor.

INTRODUCTION

HIV is usually produced in the laboratory in flask cultures
of human T-lymphoblastoid or monocyte cell lines. These
lines are non-adherent, and should be capable of growth and
HIV production in suspension cultures. However,
immobilisation of cells at high density in a fixed bed
bioreactor could provide advantageous conditions for virus
production. Such a system could promote cell-to-cell
contact, which may be important for efficient virus
transfer. It could promote the formation and stability of
syncytia, which for some cell types may be significant sites
of virion assembly and maturation. It could also increase
local concentrations of autocrine factors, which could
affect HIV production. In addition, if cells persistently
infected with HIV could be immobilised, continuous harvests
of virus could be derived over extended periods of time.
Porous glass sphere (Porosphere) bioreactors are fixed-bed
systems which retain non-adherent cells and are readily
capable of both volumetric and cell density scale up (1)
Accordingly, HIV production was compared in porosphere
bioreactors, stirred suspension cultures, and static flasks.
The investigation included examples of HIV/cell systems
exhibiting both persistent and lytic infection, in order to
investigate the effect of different fermenter configurations
on virus productivity with these different types of
behaviour.

METHODS

Bioreactors.

The stirred suspension bioreactors employed were a 2 l fermenter with submerged impeller (Applikon UK.), and a 3 l vessel incorporating a floating impeller (Techne, UK., model BR-06). The fixed bed bioreactor and the experimental procedure were based on those of Looby and Griffiths (1). The carriers were Siran porospheres (Schott Glasswerke).

Cell Growth Monitoring.

Cell concentrations were determined microscopically after staining with trypan blue. Alternatively, for the fixed bed bioreactor, cell nuclei were released by incubating porous glass spheres containing cells with 0.1 M citric acid at 37°C. Cell growth was also monitored indirectly , by measuring glucose utilisation using a Beckmann glucose analyser.

Virus Assays.

HIV was quantified by a $TCID_{50}$ assay utilising syncytium formation in C8166 cells, and by reverse transcriptase (RTase) assay (2).

RESULTS

With U937 cells infected - with HIV 1 ZII, cell concentrations, and virus levels measured by both syncytium formation and RTase activity, increased during the respective culture periods in all three systems (Table 1). Specific virus production (Both SFD_{50}/cell and RTase cpm/ml per cell) was clearly most efficient in the static flask. (Table 2). In addition, the ratios of syncytium forming units to reverse transcriptase levels (SFD_{50}/RTase) was highest in this latter system (Table 2). This suggests that the flask culture may have generated a higher proportion of complete virus particles than did the bioreactors (3).

Table 1. Cell growth and HIV production in flask (F), suspension (S) and Porosphere bioreactor (P) cultures.

Virus	Cell Line	Culture System	Cells			Virus					
			Density ($\times 10^5$/ml)		Time Max Cell Density (h)	$\log_{10}$ SFD_{50}/ml		Time Max SFD_{50} (h)	RTase ($\times 10^3$ cpm/ml)		Time Max RTase (h)
			Start	Max		Start	Max		Start	Max	
HIV 1 ZII	U937	F	0.25	5.4	168	3.5	5.8	120	15	1429	96
		S	0.25	8.0	168	3.5	5.0	144	15	562	144
		P*	0.31	24.0	210	2.0	5.5	210	27	1133	210
	U937	F	1.0	6.4	137	3.5	4.3	89	363	413	137
		S	1.0	6.4	137	3.5	5.3	161	363	5494	113
		P**	0.7	9.8	264	3.8	4.3	168	37	1162	96
		P*	0.9	15.0	360	3.5	7.0	336	57	1023	360
HIV 2 CBL20	JHAN	F	3.0	25.0	168	2.8	4.5	168	190	521	240
		S	3.0	30.0	168	2.8	3.8	120	190	730	240
		P***	1.4	43.0	336	3.3	5.5	192	266	816	312

Media changed at: * : 114, ** : 192h, *** : 168h.

* : cells grown before infection

In contrast U937 cells infected with HIV 2 CBL20 in a static flask showed lytic behaviour, and numbers of viable cells fell during the culture period (Table 1). nevertheless, there was measurable virus production (Table 1). However, in the stirred fermenter cell multiplication occurred as well as virus production (Table 1). It was thus not certain whether U937 cells would show lytic or persistent infection with HIV 1 CBL20 when cultured in a fixed bed, where cells are stationary but medium is circulated. Accordingly, two procedures were compared. In the first, the cells were infected at the outset, as in all previous experiments.

Table 2. Comparison of the HIV specific productivity and SFD_{50}/RTase ratios of different cell lines in flask(F), suspension culture(S), and Porosphere bioreactor(P)

| Virus | Cell Line | Culture System | Specific Productivity | | SFD_{50}/RTase | |
			SFD_{50}/cell	RTase cpm/cell	At Max SFD_{50}	At Max RTase
HIVI	U937	F	37.1	2.7	62.747	1.441
ZII		S	0.13	0.7	0.137	0.178
		P	0.11	0.4	0.275	0.275
HIV2	U937	F	0.11	21.8	0.005	0.002
CBL20		S	0.31	8.6	0.055	0.001
		P	0.05	1.9	0.460	0.0001
		P*	5.9	0.6	40.354	3.092
HIV2	JHAN	F	0.003	0.29	0.026	0.004
CBL20		S	0.007	0.17	0.163	0.006
		P	0.08	0.19	1.237	0.024

*infected after cell growth.

In the second, uninfected cells were introduced into the packed bed and allowed to grow before infection and medium change. When the cells were infected at the outset, virus production measured by syncytium formation was similar to that in static flask, but maximum RTase activity was lower. Glucose levels had fallen by 63% at 192 h, indicating that cells had remained viable and possibly multiplied despite the infection. When the cells were allowed to multiply before infection, particularly high levels of syncytium forming activity were attained, although the maximum RTase level was not as high as with HIV 2 CBL20 in the other systems. Efficiency of virus production measured as SFD_{50}/cell was much higher in this system than in the others, but yields of RTase cpm/ml per cell were lower (Table 2). This system therefore showed the highest SFD_{50}/RTase ration, (Table 2), suggesting that it generated the highest proportion of complete virus particles (3).

For comparison, production of HIV 2 CBL20 in the JHAN cell line was examined in the three culture systems. This virus establishes a persistent infection in JHAN cells in static flasks, which contrasts with its own behaviour in U937 cells but resembles that of HIV 1 ZII in U937. In the present experiments, infected JHAN cells in all three systems multiplied to very high concentrations. However, HIV 2 production was much less efficient than in U937 cells (Tables 1 and 2). The porosphere bioreactor showed the highest SFD_{50} rations (Table 2) and therefore possibly the highest proportion of complete virions (3).

DISCUSSION

These preliminary results have shown that production of HIV
is feasible in suspension and in Porosphere fixed bed
bioreactors. Both systems were readily contained in Class 3
microbiological safety cabinets, and offer a means of
producing large quantities of HIV under controlled
conditions that is less labour intensive than large numbers
of tissue culture flasks. Although the Porosphere
bioreactor offered theoretical advantages for HIV
production, not every HIV-cell combination showed higher
yields in this system than in suspension culture or static
flask. An advantage of the porosphere reactor for
efficiency of virus production is therefore not clearly
established. However, a practical benefit of this system is
that the medium may be readily changed without contained
centrifugation, thus allowing multiple harvests of virus to
be conveniently obtained from persistently infected cell
cultures. U937 cells infected with HIV 2 CBL20 in static
flask showed lytic behaviour. However, in both the stirred
and the fixed bed bioreactors, U937 cells appeared to be in
a physical or physiological state which enabled them to
support HIV 2 CBL20 replication without lysis. The reasons
for this are not clear, but it would allow U937 cells to be
used in the porosphere bioreactor to derive continuous
harvests of HIV 2 CBL20, as well as HIV 1 ZII. In addition,
for each virus-cell combination, the SFD_{50}/RTase ratio was
significantly higher in one system than in the others. With
HIV 1 ZII in U937 cells, this occurred in the static flask;
with HIV 2 CBL20 in U937 and JHAN cells this was in the
porosphere bioreactors infected respectively after cell
growth and at the outset. The SFD_{50}/RTase ratio reflects
the relative proportions of complete and defective virus
particles (2). The states of the cells in flask culture or
the bioreactors could influence virion maturation.
Alternatively, conditions in the different systems could
influence virion stability. The results therefore clearly
show that the cell-virus relationship can be significantly
affected by the culture method.

REFERENCES

1. Looby, D. and Griffiths, J.B. Fixed bed porous glass
    sphere (porosphere) bioreactors for animal cells.
    Cytotechnology 1989, 1, 339-346

2. Hoffman, A.D., Banapour, B and Levy, J.A.
    Characterisation of the AIDs-associated retrovirus
    reverse transcriptase and optimal conditions for its
    detection in virions. Virology 1985, 147, 326-335

3. Harada, A., Yamamoto, N. and Hinumuna, Y. Clonal
    analysis of functional differences among strains of
    human immunodeficieny virus (HIV). J. Virol. Meth.
    1987, 18, 291-304

COMPARISON OF SEMICONTINUOUS CULTURE AND PERFUSION CULTURE IN A 75 L BIOREACTOR

M. Hjertstedt, F. Buzsaky, E. Lindner-Olsson

Summary

Recombinant CHO cells producing a second generation Factor VIII were cultured in a 75 L bioreactor. Cells were cultured in perfusion mode (0,4-0,9 reactor volumes/day) and in a semicontinuous mode with a partial medium change every second or third day.

In perfusion mode cells were grown to approximately $2,5 \times 10^6$ cells /ml and then kept in stationary phase at $1,5 \times 10^6$ cells/ml. In semicontinuous mode cells were grown to slightly lower than 1×10^6 cells/ml. The volumetric productivity was in this experiment shown to be approximately 2-3 times as high in perfusion mode compared to semicontinuous mode.

Glucose consumption was shown to follow the productivity and this is probably a function of nutrient supply/inhibitor removal.

Materials and methods

dhfr negative cells DG44 were cotransfected with the gene for human Factor VIII and the dhfr gene. Cell clones were selected in HGT- deficient medium. Individual clones were subsequently cultured in increasing concentrations of MTX and selected for growth and productivity.

Cells were propagated in 1,5 L spinnerflasks (Techne) and inoculated in a 75 L Chemap perfusion reactor. The cultures were kept at 50% DOT and pH 7,2.

In perfusion mode cells were continuously perfused with 0,4-0,9 reactor volumes/day and cells were recycled to the reactor with a Sulzer dynamic biopressure filter(MBR).

In semicontinuous mode cells were harvested every second or third day with a fresh medium dilution of 40-50%.

Medium was DMEM:F12 (Gibco) 50/50 supplemented with critical amino acids and 5% FCS(Gibco).

In batch/semicontinuous mode cells were freely growing and in perfusion mode cells were kept stationary. The culture period shown was 23 days.The cultures were followed in terms of relative volumetric productivity, glucose, lactic acid and amino acids.

In perfusion mode volumetric glucose consumption was related to volumetric productivity.

Results

In semicontinuous mode cells were shown to have the highest volumetric productivity shortly after medium change. The highest volumetric productivity was found at lower cell densities and normally 24 hours after medium change. During day two and three after change productivity gradually decreased to zero. This was shown in antigen analysis not to be due to degradation.
The relative productivity (related to a perfusion rate of approximately 0,6 reactor volumes/day) was normally between 3 and 8 with peek values of up to 11 when dilution was high. Mean culture period productivity was calculated to 2,3.
In perfusion mode the volumetric productivity was increasing slightly during the culture period and higher productivity was attained at higher dilution rates. When switching mode to stationary culture, the productivity increased even furter.
When lowering the dilution rate productivity decreased.
The relative productivity was roughly 2 during growth phase and almost 7 in stationary phase with a culture mean value of 3,9.
Productivity was 2-3 times higher in a stationary perfusion culture.
The glucose consumtion was found to tightly follow the same pattern as productivity.
The maximum glucose consumption per million cells and day was 0,8 which is several times lower than in a low cell density system. The actual glucose concentration never reached lower values than 1 g/L.

Discussion

The results from this experiment implies that there is a relation between dilution rate/cell and productivity and also between growth rate and productivity.
The glucose consumption is also related to dilution rate which could show a medium depletion or an inhibition.
In this experiment the technical limit for dilution rates was 0,9 reactor volumes/day which was to low for maximum productivity.
In later experiment we have shown that the volumetric productivity is proportional to dilution rate up to several rector volumes per/day.

COMPARISON OF TWO SYSTEMS BASED ON POROUS BEADS FOR THE PRODUCTION
OF RECOMBINANT VON WILLEBRAND FACTOR BY CHO CELLS

*J. JANNIN., *V. GASPARD., *C. ZAOT., °T. FAURE., *F. DHAINAUT and *G. MIGNOT.
* TM Innovation, 3 avenue des Tropiques, F - 91943 Les Ulis FRANCE
° TRANSGENE, 11 rue de Molsheim, F - 67000 STRASBOURG FRANCE

ABSTRACT

The recombinant Von Willebrand factor greatly improves the production of recombinant
factor VIII by CHO cells in serum-free media.
Serum-free productions of von Willebrand factor by CHO cells have been compared on a
laboratory scale using two methods :

1 -   CULTISPHER-G (4g/l), a macroporous microcarrier in a 1 liter fermentor
2 -   SIRAN CARRIERS, a macroporous macrocarrier in a 1 liter fixed bed system.

In the fixed bed of SIRAN CARRIERS the mean volumetric productivity was 1250 Units/l.
day and 720 Units/l. day on CULTISPHER-G beads.
Furthermore, the fixed bed of porous glass beads was found to be the most convenient system
for optimal recombinant Von Willebrand factor production.

INTRODUCTION

New approaches to the high density growth of cells are based on the use of porous macro or
microcarriers in suspension in (1),stirred tanks, (2) fluidized beds or (3) fixed beds .
Increase of the specific area available for the cells, cell protection from shear forces allows
long term maintenance of high density cultures ($1 - 3 \times 10^8$ cells/ml beads) in serum-free media.
Macroporous gelatin microcarriers (CULTISPHER-G) and porous glass beads (SIRAN
CARRIERS) have been compared on a laboratory scale for von Willebrand factor production
by CHO TG 2330 - B32A 1000 6 in serum-free media.

MATERIAL :

Cells :   CHO TG 2330 B 32A 1000 6 (provided by TRANSGENE) are
                                  anchorage-dependent Chinese ovary cells expressing von
                                  Willebrand factor (400-600 mU/10^6 cells/day).

Culture media :   MEM (GIBCO) supplemented with 10 % (FCS) during a
                                  3 day long growth phase. A mixture of 50 % IMDM
                                  (GIBCO) and 50 % HAM F12 (GIBCO) supplemented with
                                  6 mg human recombinant insulin (Eli Lilly) per liter for
                                  production phase. All media have been supplemented with
                                  100 U/ml Penicillin G and 100 µg/ml streptomycin
                                  (GIBCO).

METHODS :

Stirred tank culture :   4 g/l CULTISPHER-G microcarriers (Percell-Biolytica) in
                                  1 liter working volume reactor (SGI). D.O. was maintained
                                  at 50 % air saturation by oxygen diffusion through 3 m of
                                  silicone tubing. Medium was changed every other day.

Fixed bed culture :	1 liter of 3 - 5 mm SIRAN carriers (SCHOTT) in a 1 liter working volume reactor (SGI), connected to a second 1 liter working volume reactor (SGI) which was a media tank. Medium was circulated from bottom to top of the fixed bed at 0,5 - 2 linear cm/mn and increased to 5 linear cm/mn (40 vol.h^{-1}) during production phase. D.O. was maintained at 100 % in the medium tank by circulating fixed bed out flow in an hollow-fiber oxygenator (CD Medical). The two liters of medium contained in the system were changed every day.
von Willebrand factor assay :	vWf concentrations were measured by ELISA (STAGO), using a human pool of plasma as a standard. Results are expressed in international units. (1 IU = 10 µg protein).

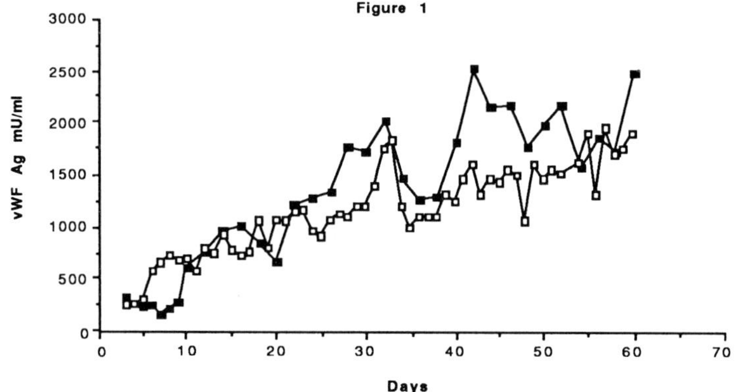

Evolution of von Willebrand factor concentrations in a 1 liter
fixed bed of 3 - 5 mm SIRAN CARRIERS (—□—) and
on CULTISPHER-G in 1liter fermentor (—■—)

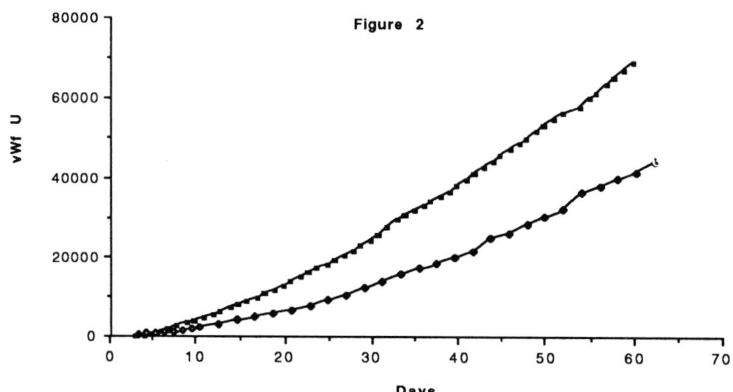

Cumulative von Willebrand factor productions in 1 liter fixed
bed of 3 - 5 mm SIRAN CARRIERS (—■—) and on
CULTISPHER-G in a 1 liter fermentor (—●—)

RESULTS

For 60 days, recombinant Von Willebrand factor production was monitored daily in a fixed bed system and every other day in fermentor system (Figure 1 et 2). Altough vWf concentrations have reached the same level in the 2 systems (1,50 - 2,00 U/ml) mean volumetric vWf productivities have been 1,250 U/l.day and 720 U/l. day in fixed bed and on CULTISPHER-G respectively (ratio 1.73). For SIRAN CARRIERS, total daily production was 2500 units while 720 units were produced daily on CULTISPHER-G (ratio 3.47). On CULTISPHER-G an increase of medium exchange rate did not improve vWf production. Increasing glucose (15 to 3 mM), L-glutamine (4-6mM) or essential amino acid concentration (x2) had no effect on vWf production in both systems. Considering that specific vWf productivities were the same on the 2 types of porous beads and that cell densities of 6.10^6 cells/ml have been maintained from day 20 to day 60 on CULTISPHER-G, we can assume that in a fixed bed of SIRAN CARRIERS, cell density was about 20×10^6 cells/ml of beads during the production phase.
In both cases vWf has been shown to keep its effect when tested on recombinant factor VIII expression in serum-free media.

CONCLUSIONS

In our experimental conditions, the fixed bed of SIRAN CARRIERS system combines the advantages of higher volumetric vWf productivities and cell-free supernatants. Although a scale-up of the fixed-bed system has been previously demonstrated with non porous glass beads (4) specific vessels must be designed for this purpose.

REFERENCES

1 -   NILSSON K., BUSSAKY F. and MOSBACH K. (1986)
      Growth of anchorage dependent cells on macroporous microcarriers.
      Bio/technology, 4, 989 - 990.

2 -   LOOBY D. and GRIFFITHS J.B. (1988)
      Fixed-bed porous glass sphere (porosphere) bioreactors for animal cells.
      Cytotechnology, 1, 339 - 346.

3 -   HAYMAN E.G., RAY N.G. and RUNSTADLER J.P.W. (1988)
      Production of biomolecules by cells cultured in tri-dimensional collagen microspheres.
      In : MOODY D.U. and BAKER P.B (Eds)
      Bioreactors and Biotransformations, (pp 99 - 110)
      Elsevier, London and New York

4 -   GRIFFITHS J.B., THORNTON B. and Mc ENTREE I. (1982)
      The development and use of microcarrier glass sphere culture techniques for the production of Herpès simplex virus.
      Develop. Biol. Stand., 50, 103 - 110.

COMPARISON OF THE PRODUCTION EFFICIENCY OF MAMMALIAN CELLS GROWN IN A FLUIDIZED BED AND IN A STIRRED TANK BIOREACTOR.

R. Kratje, V. Jäger, R. Wagner

Gesellschaft für Biotechnologische Forschung, Arbeitsgruppe Zellkulturtechnik, Mascheroder Weg 1, D-3300 Braunschweig, FRG.

Abstract

A perfused fluidized bed bioreactor packed with porous glass spheres and a stirred tank perfusion bioreactor equipped with a double membrane stirrer for bubble-free aeration and medium perfusion were used for the cultivation of a murine hybridoma cell line which produces a monoclonal murine IgG_{2a} antibody (MAb). The production efficiency of both systems was compared. A productivity per unit reactor volume of 159.7 mg/d/l and 42.8 mg/d/l was obtained with the fluidized bed bioreactor and the stirred tank bioreactor, respectively. The reported results show an approximately 4-fold increase in the MAb production rate attained with the perfused fluidized bed bioreactor based on porous glass spheres.

Keywords: Fluidized bed bioreactor; stirred tank bioreactor;production efficiency; monoclonal antibody.

Introduction

Propagation of mammalian cells for the production of monoclonal antibodies and recombinant products has become of increasing interest during the last few years. Different bioreactor systems have been established in animal cell cultures: basically two concepts are being used. Firstly, suspension of cells within a stirred tank or an airlift bioreactor which can be operated as a batch process or in a continuous or a perfused manner. Secondly, cell immobilization at which we have to distinguish between the immurement and the entrapment approach. All systems are characterized by systematically based advantages and disadvantages (1). Immurement means the retention of cells within a compartment which allows free passage of medium. Finally, entrapment, which provides a substrate with the physical configuration to capture and trap cells.

Entrapment of animal cells in fixed and fluidized bed porous glass sphere reactors have been described by Looby et al. (2,3), but no data about the production efficiency compared with already established systems are available at present. In this report a comparison of the production efficiency of a hybridoma cell line grown in a fluidized bed and in a stirred tank bioreactor is presented.

Materials and Methods

<u>Description and operation of bioreactors.</u>
The fluidized bed bioreactor (Fig.1) consisted of a 1.45 l glass vessel for cell growth which contained a packed bed volume of 0.25 l filled with Siran porous glass spheres (Schott Glaswerke, Mainz, FRG) of a diameter of 0.5-0.7 mm and a pore size of <120 μm. The inoculum was introduced onto the top of the bead bed. Circulation of medium was started immediately by means of a peristaltic pump at an upflow rate of approximately 60 $V_R \cdot h^{-1}$. After 6 h of cultivation the circulation rate was increased to 230 $V_R \cdot h^{-1}$ resulting in a 3-fold bed expansion (0.75 l). Oxygen supply was performed by a hollow fibre gas exchanger inserted into the circulation loop.

The stirred tank bioreactor (Fig.2) consisted of a 2.4 l (working volume) glass vessel equipped with a double membrane stirrer for bubble-free aeration and medium perfusion (4).

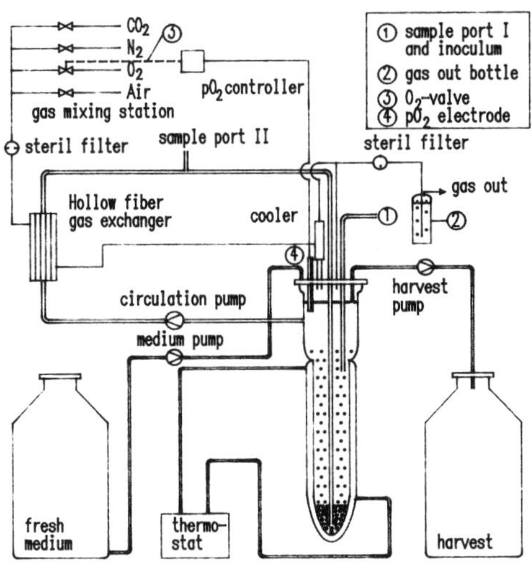

Fig.1: Schematic diagram of the perfused fluidized bed glass sphere bioreactor system.

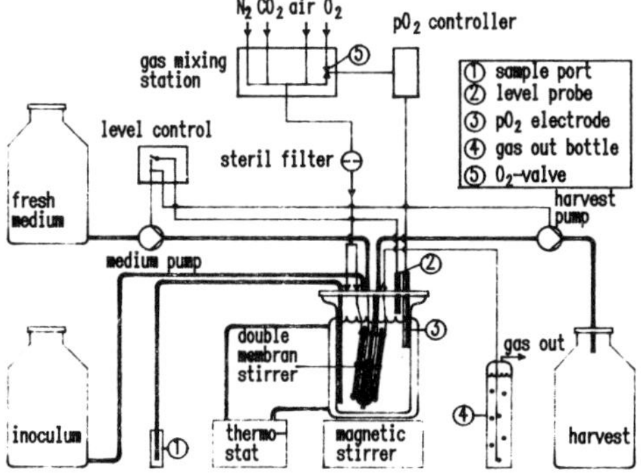

Fig.2: Schematic diagram of the stirred tank perfusion bioreactor system.

Cell line
A murine hybridoma cell line, which produces a monoclonal murine IgG_{2a} antibody was used.

Media and culture conditions
The same serum-free medium (5 mod.) consisting of a mixture of Iscoves and Ham's F12 supplemented with 3.61 g/l $NaHCO_3$, 0.18 g/l sodium pyruvate, 10 mg/l insulin, 10 mg/l transferrin and 1 g/l HSA was used for both fermentations. Oxygen content was maintained at 30 % of air saturation (2.0 mg l^{-1}). pH was maintained between 7.1 and 7.3 and temperature at 37°C.

Analytical methods
Viable and dead cell number were determined by the trypan blue exclusion method. Glucose and lactate contents were assayed with enzymatic analysers (Yellow Springs, YSI, OH). Immunoglobulin concentrations were determined by ELISA.

Terminology
The product and cell yields quoted in this report were expressed per unit reactor volume (unit culture vessel working volume in the stirred tank reactor and unit expanded bed volume in the fluidized bed system). All calculations were based on of viable cell number.

Results

Fig.3 presents a repeated batch process in the stirred tank bioreactor. The reactor was inoculated with $2.3 \cdot 10^5$ cells/ml from roller bottles (90% viability). Maximal cell density of $1.1 \cdot 10^7$ cells/ml was achieved with perfusion ($1.25\ V_R$/d) started at the end of the second batch.

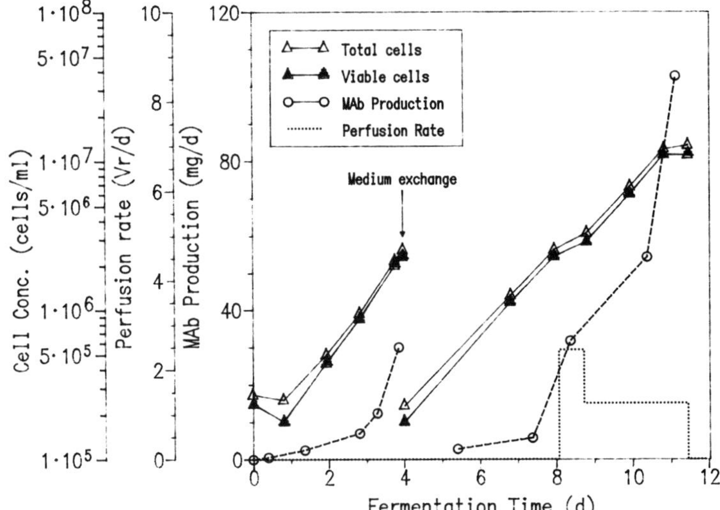

Fig.3: Growth curve and MAb-productivity of a murine hybridoma cell line cultivated in the stirred tank bioreactor system. The perfusion rate is expressed as reactor volumes per day.

MAb production increased during cultivation up to 102.7 mg/d. The specific productivity estimated was $3.9 \cdot 10^{-12}$ g/cell/d. This value is in the same magnitude as reported for other hybridoma cell lines (6).

Fig.4 shows the results obtained during 40 days of continuous fermentation with the fluidized bed bioreactor. The reactor was inoculated with $1.0 \cdot 10^9$ cells growing in the stirred tank bioreactor (second batch). Cell growth was monitored indirectly by glucose/lactate measurements. Glucose consumption, lactate and MAb production rates increased continuously until a steady state was reached. At this state the mean value of glucose consumption rate was 10.5 ± 0.7 g/d. A total cell number of $4.2 \cdot 10^7$ cells/ml was estimated, assuming the same value of the specific glucose consumption rate as determined in the stirred tank reactor ($3.3 \cdot 10^{-10}$ g/cell/d; data not shown).

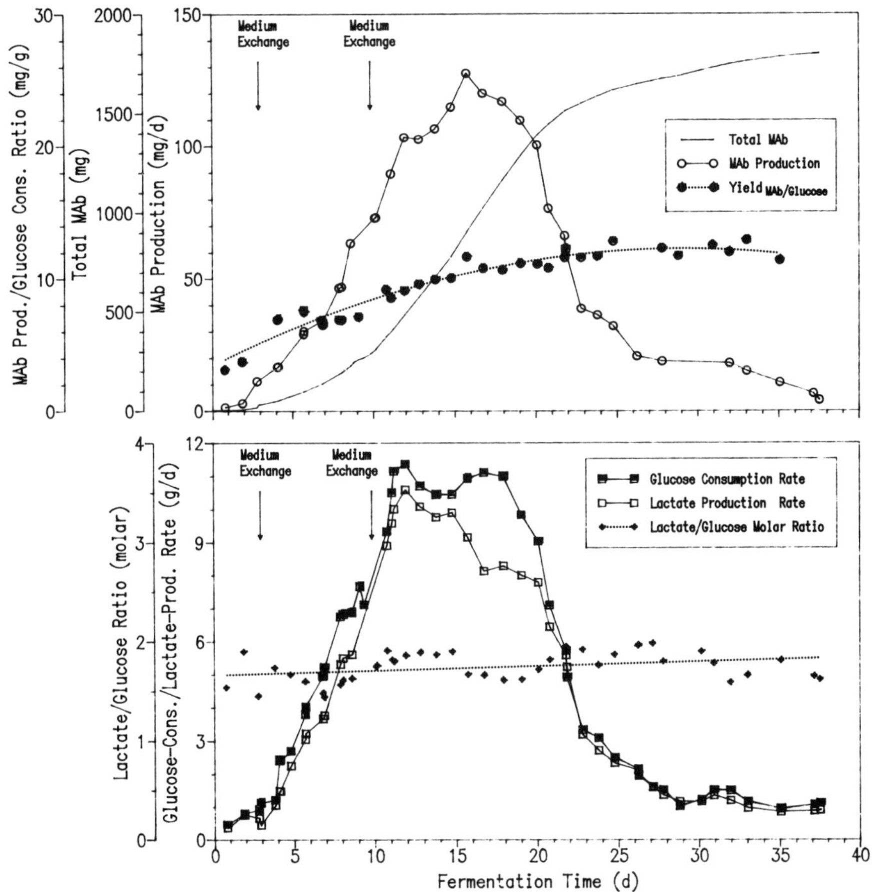

Fig.4: Metabolic Parameters of a murine hybridoma cell line grown in the fluidized bed bioreactor system.

The number of cells not entrapped in the open porous structure of the spheres, which could be measured directly by cell counts was $1.4 \cdot 10^6$ cells/ml, corresponding to a cell release of less than 4%. This is the same value reported by Looby et al. (3) and in accordance with the lack of influence on glucose consumption and lactate production rates when changing the medium (Fig.4).

After 9 days of constant maximum the metabolic rates decreased. In spite of all these variations, the glucose/lactate ratio remained constant and the yield coefficient based on glucose consumption increased constantly up to the end of cultivation.

Table I summarizes the efficiency of both systems. In order to compare both experiments, only the optimum values are given. The results show that the MAb production rate increased approximately 4-fold with the porous spheres perfused fluidized bed bioreactor. This increase in MAb production was well correlated with the increase in cell number estimated upon the glucose consumption rate.

Culture system	Production rate (mg/d/l)	Cell Density (cell/ml)
Fluidized bed	159.7	$4.2 \cdot 10^{7*}$
Stirred tank	42.8	$1.1 \cdot 10^7$

Table I: Comparison of MAb-production rate and cell yield.
* Cell yield estimated as describted in the text.

Conclusion

The results demonstrate quite clearly that the fluidized bed bioreactor filled with porous glass spheres is suitable for the cultivation of hybridoma cells and that the production rate is increased significantly when compared with a stirred tank perfusion bioreactor.

References

1 Griffiths, J.B. (1988) Overview of cell culture systems and their scale-up. In: Animal Cell Biotechnology (Eds. Spier, R.E. and Griffiths, J.B.) Academic Press Ltd., London, p.179-220.

2 Looby, D. and Griffiths, J.B. (1988) Fixed bed porous glass sphere (porosphere) bioreactors for animal cells. Cytotechnology 1: 339-346.

3 Looby, D. and Griffiths, J.B. (1989) Immobilization of animal cells in fixed and fluidized porous glass sphere reactors. In: Advances in Animal Cell Biology and Technology for Bioprocesses (Eds. Spier, R.E.; Griffiths, J.B.; Stephenne, J.; Crooy, P.J.) Butterworths, Guilford, p.336-344.

4 Lehmann, J.; Vorlop, J.; Büntemeyer, H. (1988) Bubble-free reactors and their development for continuous culture with cell recycle. In: Animal Cell Biotechnology (Eds. Spier, R.E. and Griffiths, J.B.) Academic Press Ltd., London, p. 221-237.

5 Jäger V., Lehmann J., Friedl P. (1988) Serum-free growth medium for the cultivation of a wide spectrum of mammalian cells in stirred bioreactors. Cytotechnology 1: 319-329.

6 Seaver, S.S. (1987) Culture Method Affects Antibody Secretion of Hybridoma Cells. In: Commercial Production of Monoclonal Antibodies (Ed. Seaver, S.S.) Marcel Dekker,Inc., New York, p.49-71.

MONOCLONAL ANTIBODY PRODUCTION IN THREE DIFFERENT HOLLOW FIBRE BIOREACTOR CONFIGURATIONS

S. Nikolay, A. Garcia de Castro, M. Chadd and A. Handa-Corrigan

The Wolfson Cytotechnology Laboratory, (c/o The Department of Microbiology), University of Surrey, Guildford, GU2 5XH, U.K.

ABSTRACT

A number of hollow fibre configurations are currently available for the production of monoclonal antibodies. In their simplest form, the cells are held on one side of the fibre and medium is perfused through the other side, nutrient exchange being effected by simple diffusion. In the more sophisticated systems, enhanced mass transfer may be effected by medium flow reversal or by forced ultrafiltrative medium flow. Results will be presented for monoclonal antibody production in three different hollow fibre configurations using the same hybridoma cell line, medium formulation, hollow fibre cartridges (regenerated cellulose; pore size 6-10 Kd; surface area 1.1 square metres), process control set-points and optimisation strategies.
The three configurations are as follows:
(1) Hollow fibre connected to a Stirred tank bioreactor. Simple uni-directional flow of oxygenated medium.
(2) Hollow fibre bioreactor with reversed flow of oxygenated medium.
(3) Hollow fibre bioreactor with forced ultrafiltrative flow of oxygenated medium.
We have demonstrated that monoclonal antibody production may be ranked:
    2 > 3 > 1
The implications of these results will be discussed.

INTRODUCTION

Monoclonal antibody (MCA) production is possible in a wide range of bioreactor systems (1). Several hollow fibre bioreactor (HFB) systems are now commercially available for MCA production. This paper compares the productivity of one hybridoma cell line in three different HFB configurations.

The principle of operation in a HFB involves the cultivation of cells on the exterior of the hollow fibres, the extra-capillary space (EC), and perfusing oxygenated basal medium through the lumen of the fibres, the intra-capillary space (IC). Nutrient, oxygen and low molecular weight metabolic waste transfer occurs across the 6-10 Kd molecular weight cut off membrane. Serum supplemented medium is perfused through the EC, supplying serum to the cells and removing secreted MCA (retained due to its large molecular weight) into a harvest bottle downstream of the EC space.

The three HFB configurations used in this analysis are described below:

(1) Simple, uni-directional (SU) flow of oxygenated, medium in IC: A HFB cartridge was perfused with oxygenated medium circulated in the same direction through the IC throughout the production run. A 2 litre stirred tank bioreactor (SGI) was employed in the IC circuit as a medium reservoir in which pH, D.O.T and Temperature were controlled. (Fig.1).

(2) Reversed flow (RF) of oxygenated medium in IC: The incorporation of a pinch valve assembly in the IC circuit enables the direction flow of oxygenated medium in the IC to be reversed at desired time intervals. pH control and oxygenation was achieved by the addition of Carbon dioxide and air to the IC via a jet pump prior to entry into the medium reservoir. (Fig. 2).

(3) Forced Ultrafiltrative (FU) cycling of oxygenated medium in the IC: Differential pressurisation of the medium expansion chambers connected to the IC and EC resulted in forced ultrafiltrative nutrient, oxygen (rise cycle) and low molecular weight metabolic waste (fall cycle) transfer at desired time intervals throughout the run time course. Oxygenation and pH control was achieved by the addition of Carbon dioxide and air to a gas exchange cartridge in the IC circuit. (Fig.3).

The HFB cartridges used in each system were the same, made from regenerated cellulose and having a surface area of 1.1 square metres.

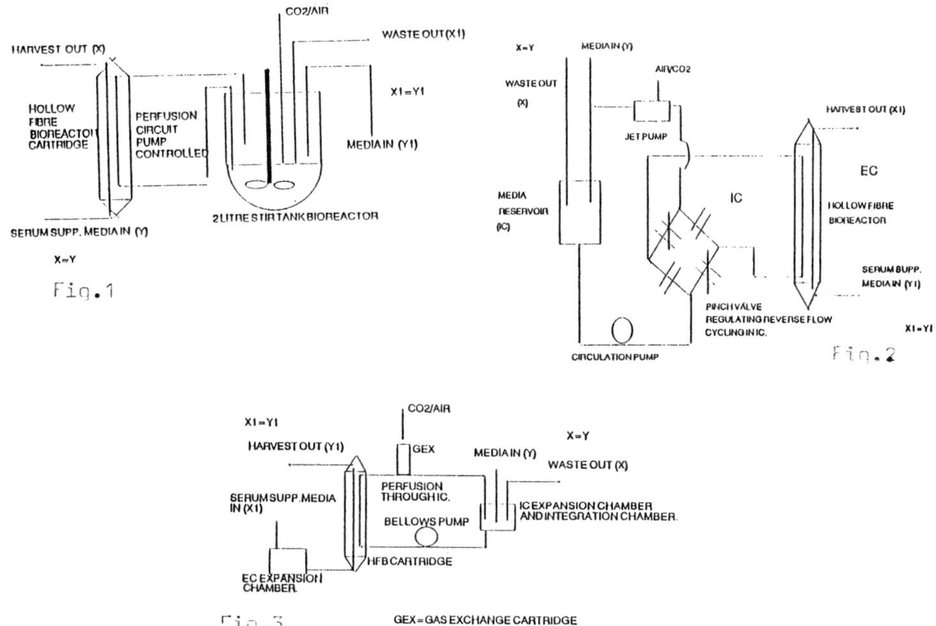

Fig; 1,2 and 3: The three HFB configurations used in this analysis

MATERIALS AND METHODS

Cell line: The three HFB were all inoculated with the same mouse x mouse hybridoma designated R58K secreting IgG_{2a}.

Cell cultivation and medium: Cells for inoculation were expanded in 1 litre surface aerated spinner cultures in 5% New Born Calf Serum (N.B.C.S.) supplemented RPMI 1640, incubated at 37°C in 5% Carbon dioxide atmosphere.

HFB Inoculation: All three HFB were inoculated with 2×10^8 total viable cells (derived from spinner cultures with cell viabilities greater than 95%) in 50 ml of 5% N.B.C.S. supplemented RPMI 1640. Inoculation was achieved by pumping the cells directly into the HFB via the harvest line at 200 mls/hr.

Cell cultivation in HFB: The IC was perfused with RPMI 1640 containing 450 mg/dl D-glucose and 5 mM L-glutamine. The medium perfused through the EC had the same formulation as above, but was supplemented with 5% N.B.C.S.

Metabolic assay and Optimisation strategy: These methods are outlined in a second paper presented at this conference. (2).

MCA production rate calculation: The following equation is used to determine MCA production (3):

$$\frac{(FT)\ (A-AoE)}{1-E}$$

Where:

    FT = total flow rate of medium through EC (ml/hr)
    A = present MCA concentration (mg/ml)
    Ao = previous MCA concentration (mg/ml)
    E = exp (-FtT/V)
    T = time between samples (hr)
    V = volume of EC space (ml)

RESULTS

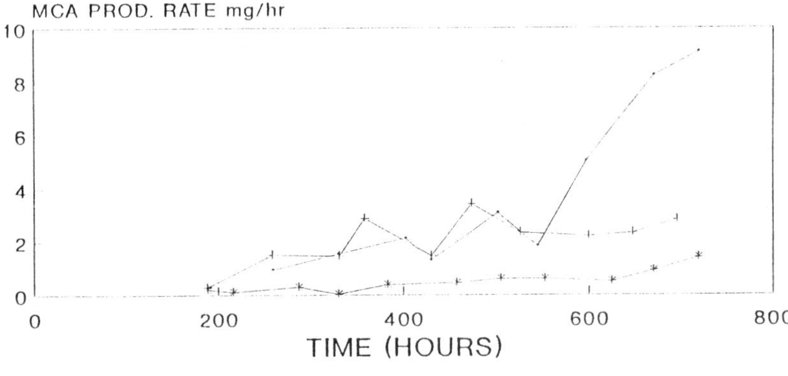

Fig 4. MCA PRODUCTION RATES VS TIME IN THE THREE HFB CONFIGURATIONS

The graph above shows that MCA production rates in the three HFB configurations may be ranked:

RF > FU > SU

DISCUSSION AND CONCLUSION

The reason for low MCA productivity in the simple unidirectional configuration is attributable to concentration polarization effects which result along the length of the hollow fibres, restricting cell growth. Both the Reversed Flow and Forced Ultrafiltrative configuration showed similar productivities up to 550 hours. After this time, the MCA productivity in the Reversed Flow configuration was markedly higher than the Forced Ultrafiltrative configuration. The reason for the poor performance in the latter system is possibly due to a significant (~50%) loss of cells from the HFB cartridge into the EC chamber and product bottle. This loss of cells is believed to be caused by the ultrafiltration process which results in cell dislodgement. In conclusion, the Reverse Medium flow Configuration is the most favourable for MCA production in Hollow Fibre Bioreactors.

REFERENCES

1.   Handa-Corrigan, A.   Large scale _in-vitro_ hybridoma culture: current status. Bio/Technology 1988, <u>6</u>, p. 784.
2.   Handa-Corrigan, A., Nikolay, S. and Spier, R.   Biochemical control of monoclonal antibody secretion in hollow fibre bioreactors. 10th ESACT meeting (to be published).
3.   Anderson, B. and Gruenberg, M.   Optimisation techniques for the production of monoclonal antibodies utilising hollow fibre technology. Proceeding of ECB 1987.

A comparision of two reactors for cell cultivation

H. Rupp-Brunswig, W.-D. Deckwer
Arbeitsgruppe Bioverfahrenstechnik, Gesellschaft für Biotechnologische Forschung, D-3300 Braunschweig

1 Indroduction

A large variety of bioreactors has been designed for the cultivation
of animal cells. In this study two reactor configurations both with
bubble free aeration were compared, namely

- a tank (2 l) equiped with a fixed membrane (silicone) and a
  separate stirrer (BIOSTAT M, B. Braun, Melsungen, FRG) /1/
- a vessel (1,3 l) with a stirring hydrophobic microporous membrane
  (B. Braun Diessel Biotech, Melsungen, FRG) /2/

Tw. cell lines (Hybridoma 187.1 and adherent BHK 21) were cultivated
to test the influence of bioreactor design on cell growth and production rate.

2 Dynamic $k_l a$ Determination

To characterize the physical properities of the two reactors in both
reactors the mass transfer was measured as function of typical aera-
ting conditions. The $k_l a$ values were determined by the dynamic
method. Vessels were first purged with nitrogen to zero dissolved
oxygen and than air was introduced into the tubing and the time
course of dissolved oxygen in the liquid was measured.

3 Fermentation

In the comparative study the same inoculum was used in the two reactors and the pH, pO_2 and $k_l a$ were controlled to the same values. The
length of the membrane and the agitation speed were used as a result
of the measurement of the $k_l a$ values. In the reactor with the fixed
membrane 3 m/l silicone membrane was mounted and the stirrer speed
was adjusted to 100 rpm. In the other fermentor was 2m/l membrane and
the strirrer speed was 30 rpm.

3.1 Hybridoma Fermentation

The hybridoma cells were cultivated in a serum free medium, described
by Jäger /3/. During the cultivation the dissolved oxygen level was
30 % and the pH was 7,0 - 7,2.

3.2 BHK Fermentation

The BHK cells were cultivated in DMEM medium supplemented with 10 %
FCS und 10 % Tryptosephosphatbroth /4/. The dissolved oxygen level
was controlled to 40 % and the pH to 6,9 - 7,1. The microcarrier used
was Cytodex 3 in a concentration of 3 g/l.

3.3 Results

In the figure 1a the results of the comparative batch-fermentation of
hybridoma cells are shown. Identical results were obtained with
regard to growth, production rate and glucose consumption. In an
other experiment the hybridoma cells were cultivated in a continuous
culture. Identical data in both reactors were obtained (data not
shown).

The results of the batch fermentation of the BHK cells is shown in
the figure 1b. The reactor design does not influence the growth and
the glucose consumption rate of the cells. On the fixed membrane
however the cells settle and stick together. Therefore the growth is
less uniform than in the other reactor.

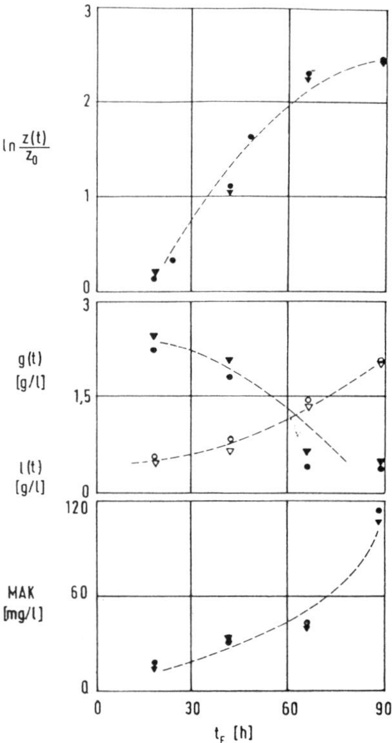

Fig 1a: growth of the Hybridoma
cells, glucose (g), lactate (l),
antibody concentration (MAK) in
the reactor with silicone membrane
(o) and in the reactor with the
hydrophobic membrane (Δ)

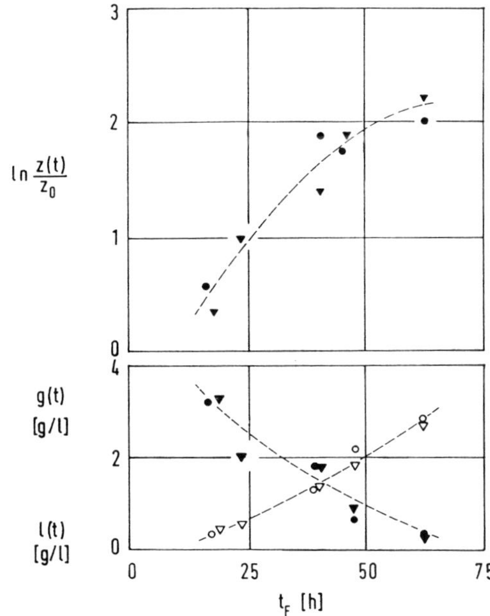

Fig. 1b: growth rate of the BHK cells and the glucose (g) and lactate (l) concentration in the reactor with the silicone membrane (o) and the reactor with the hydrophobic membrane (Δ)

References

1 Kuhlmann, W. Optimization of a membrane oxygenation system for cell culture in stirred tank reactors, <u>Develop. biol. standard.,</u> <u>Vol. 66 (1985)</u>

2 Lehmann, J., et al., Bubble free cell culture aeration with porous moving membranes, <u>Develop. biol. standard., Vol. 66 (1985)</u>

3 Jäger, V. et al., serum-free growth medium for the cultivation of a wide spectrum of mammalian cells in stirred bioreactors <u>Cytotech-</u> <u>nology 1 (1988)</u>

4 Röder, B. personal communication

Section 7
Monitoring and assay of animal cell parameters

STAINING OF CHINESE HAMSTER OVARY CELLS ON MACROPOROUS MATRICES

Bruce Rubin, Luciano Ramos, and Amy A. Murnane

SmithKline Beecham, King of Prussia, PA, USA 19406

ABSTRACT

A great many of the solid supports used for mass culture of adherent cell lines in bioreactors are in the form of beads made of solid materials (ie DEAE-Sephadex, Cytodex, Bioglass, etc). One method of increasing the number of cells produced per unit volume of reactor space is to increase the available surface area for cell attachment by using macroporous beads. Macroporous beads have a "sponge-like" configuration with pores large enough for cells to enter and adhere to the inner walls. This paper describes a rapid method for visualizing the growth of mammalian cells on these supports using hematoxylin.

INTRODUCTION

There are a number of applications using microcarriers for today's biopharmaceutical manufacturing and biological research needs. This paper describes a staining technique developed for Verax Microspheres[TM] (1,2). Visualization of cells grown on these microspheres was previously conducted using scanning electron microscopy, which would prove to be cumbersome and time consuming on a daily basis. Thus, an easy staining procedure was developed using Harris' Hematoxylin. Chinese Hamster ovary cells were grown on Verax microspheres for a period of 24 days. During this time, measurements of cell number and glucose and lactate concentration were recorded, to correlate to the degree of cell staining observed. Using this procedure, a direct relationship between cell staining and cell number, determined by enzymatic digestion, was found.

MATERIALS AND METHODS

Inoculation of Verax microspheres[TM]. Microcarriers were obtained from Verax Corporation (Lebanon, NH). The microspheres (matrices) were hydrated in phosphate buffered saline (PBS) according to the manufacturers specifications. Five mls of microspheres were transferred into a sterile 250ml Erlenmeyer flask (Corning 25600-250), and the residual PBS was removed. The microspheres were pretreated with Alpha(-)MEM/5% FBS by washing the beads with 50 mls of fresh medium twice a day for two days prior to inoculation. An inoculum of 1x10e7 cells in 50 mls of fresh medium was prepared from Chinese Hamster ovary (CHO) suspension cultures. Cells were transferred to the pretreated microspheres and incubated stationary at 37°C overnight. On the first day post seeding, 25 mls of the spent medium was removed, free cells were counted, and 25 mls of fresh medium was added. At this point, the flask was placed on a shaker platform (with a 0.75 inch diacircular orbit), set at 100 rpm, for 2 days. On day three, 50 mls of conditioned medium was removed, 50 mls of fresh medium was added, and the flask was placed on the orbital shaker platform. Beginning on day 5, 50 mls of media was exchanged daily. On day 9, due to increased cell number, the medium feed volume was increased to 100 mls. One hundred mls of fresh medium was exchanged daily for the remainder of the experiment. Due to nutrient and/or oxygen limitation on

day 17, the volume of microspheres in the flask was reduced to 1.0 ml in
order to maintain high cell viability.

<u>Cell Enumeration</u>. Total cells in the microspheres were calculated every
3 to 4 days, starting on day 7. To determine the total cell population
in the macroporous matrices, 0.25 ml of microspheres were removed and
placed in a preweighed tube. The excess medium was aspirated and the
tube was weighed again. One ml of collagenase (1 mg/ml in PBS)(Sigma
type IA) was added to the sample. The sample was placed in a 37°C water
bath, agitating every 30 seconds, until the matrices were completely
degraded. Cell counts and viability (trypan blue dye exclusion) were
performed on the collagenase supernatant using a Coulter Counter and
hemacytometer, respectively. After the collagenase solution was
aspirated from the tube leaving only the weighting elements, the tube was
placed in a oven at 100°C for an hour and weighed again. A mathematical
formula, developed by Verax Corporation, was used to calculate total cell
number per ml of collagen based on the sample weights described above
(Verax VX-100^{TM} product information sheet, 1989). Cell free samples were
taken daily to determine glucose and lactate concentration (YSI
glucose/lactate analyzer).

<u>Cell Staining</u>. Staining was done in conjunction with cell enumeration.
A sample size of 0.1 ml of matrix was removed from the culture on days 3,
7, 10, 14, 17, 21 and 24 and transferred to a 12 mm x 75 mm borosilicate
glass test tube. The microspheres were allowed to settle, and the excess
conditioned medium was removed. One ml of the fixative solution
(Methanol:Acetic Acid, 3:1) was added to the sample for ten minutes, and
then removed. To stain the microspheres for visualization of the CHO
cells, 1.0 ml of Harris' Alum Hematoxylin (Accra Lab, purchase date 1988)
was added to the fixed microspheres for twenty minutes. The stain was
removed and the beads were washed 3 to 5 times with deionized, reverse
osmosis water until the wash water was free of stain. Stained
microspheres were applied to Labtek tissue culture chamber/slides (Miles
Scientific #4804; with the plastic chambers removed), covered with a
glass coverslip, and observed with a Unitron ZST microscope at 60-70X
magnification. Photographs were taken using a Nikon FX-35A camera and a
Nikon HFX automatic light meter with Kodak Ektachrome 160 ASA (tungsten)
film.

RESULTS

The results of the matrix cell counts determined by enzymatic
digestion of the microspheres on days 3, 7, 10, 14, 17, 21, and 24 are
shown in Figure 1. Figure 1 graphs the total cells/ml of matrix and
percent viability versus days in culture. As indicated, the total cell
number/ml of matrix increases from day 3 until day 14. On day 17, the
total cell number/ml of matrix increased to levels where the oxygen
supply and/or nutrients were limiting in the culture, thus the viability
dropped. The cell to medium ratio was changed by removing all but 1.0 ml
of the matrix on day 17 (arrow) which resulted in an increase in both
viability and total cell number per ml of matrix on days 21 and 24.
The daily concentration of glucose and lactate remaining in the
culture medium is shown in Figure 1B. When cell number increased (Figure
1A), a concomitant rise in glucose consumption and lactate production was
observed (Figure 1B). Normally the concentration of glucose in the media
is 4.5 g/L. As indicated in Figure 1B approximately 2 g/L of glucose was
consumed on a daily basis until day 17, when the microspheres per ml of

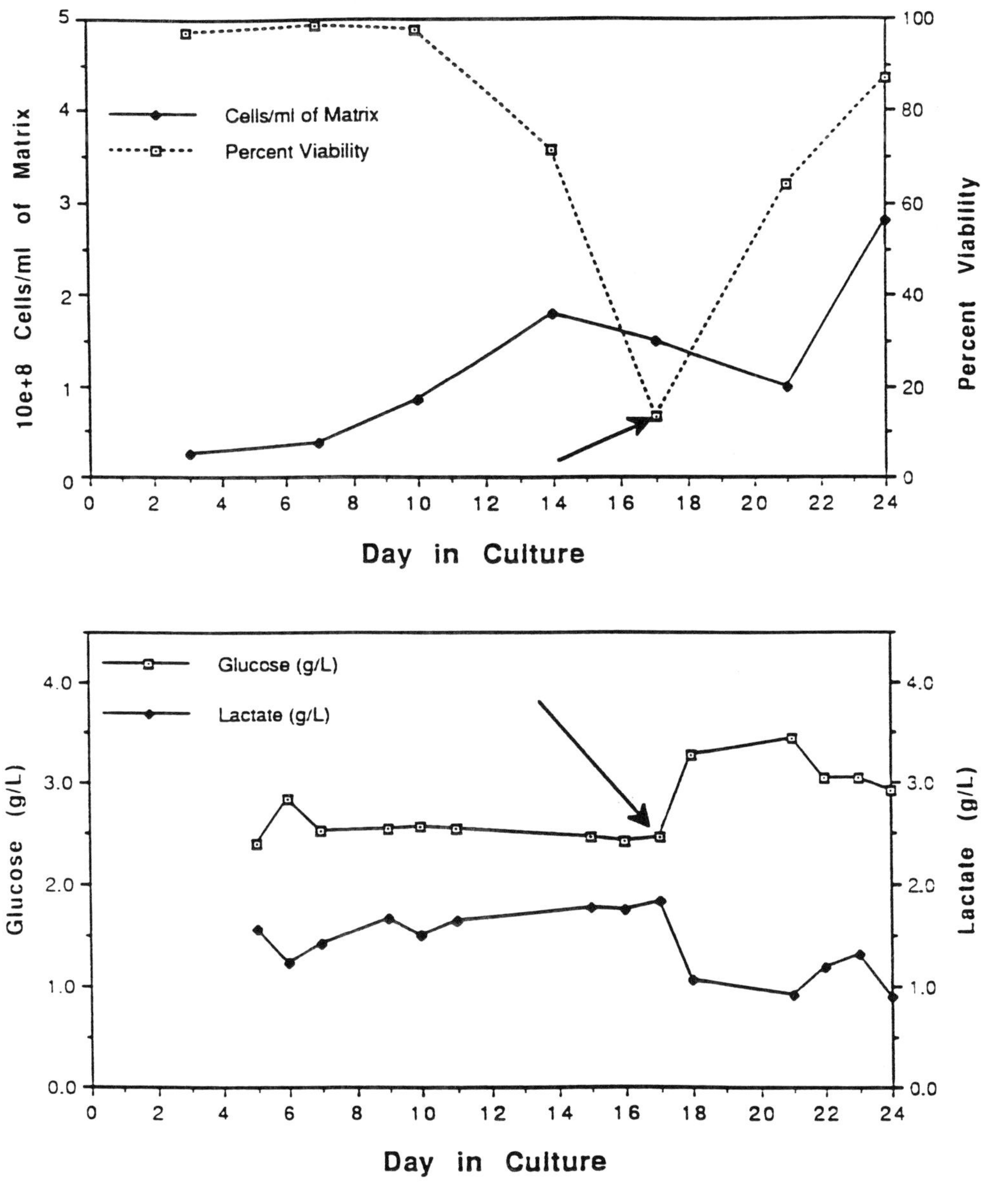

FIGURE 1. (A) Graph of total cells per ml of matrix and percent viability versus day in culture. Arrow indicates the day in which matrix was reduced to 1.0 ml (see material and methods). (B) Daily glucose and lactate concentrations in the culture medium recorded during this period. Arrow indicates the day matrix was removed (see materials and methods). Note on day 9, the volume of media in the flask was increased from 50 mls to 100 mls.

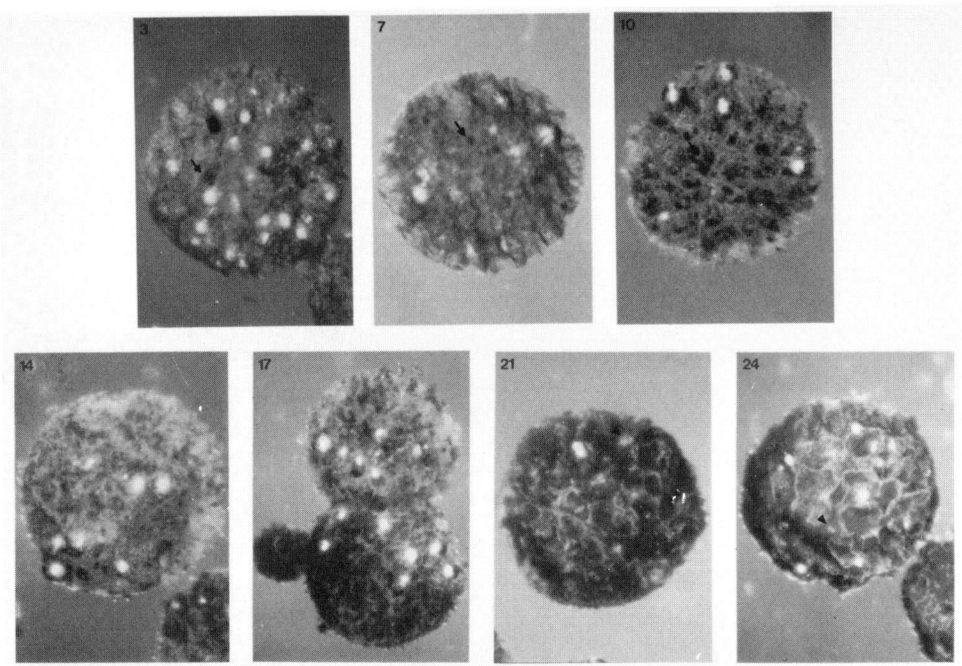

FIGURE 2. Photomicrographs of cells stained on the microspheres. Numbers in upper left corner represent day in culture. Arrows indicate examples of cell population on the matrix. Visualization of cell growth on the weighting elements is shown by arrowheads (day 21 and 24). Day 17: 60X, all other days 70X.

media were reduced (arrow). Daily lactate production prior to day 17 was
approximately 1.8 g/L. On days 17 and 21, a decrease in the amount of
glucose consumed and lactate produced was recorded, due to reduced cell
number and viability. By day 22, the utilization of glucose and
production of lactate increased, but not to the levels seen previously.

To observe cells on and within the matrices, Harris' hematoxylin
stain was used. Microsphere samples taken on the days listed above were
stained and observed using a stereo microscope. Photomicrographs taken of
the stained microspheres indicate a gradual increase in cell density with
time in culture (Figure 2). Samples taken on days 3 and 7 in culture
reveal few stained colonies of cells (arrows). An increased number of
stained cells in the pores and on the surface of the microspheres, was
apparent as the experiment progressed. On day 17 (Figure 2), the smaller
matrix is completely populated with cells, indicating heterogeneity
within the batch of microspheres used. Cell number data and photos
collected on days 21 and 24 indicate significant cell growth.

Note that some stained cells are observed growing on the weighting
elements in addition to layering at the edge of the matrix (Figure 2 days
21 and 24, arrowheads). Significant differences in the size and porosity
of the microspheres were observed during the course of the experiment.
The increase in cell density shown in Figure 1A corresponds to the
observed increase in stained cells on the microspheres (Figure 2) with
time in culture.

DISCUSSION

A means of visualizing cells in macroporous matrices has been
demonstrated above using a hematoxylin-based staining method . A
relationship between culture population numbers, obtained by
enzymatically digesting the collagen microspheres, and the appearance of
hematoxylin stained cells observed on and within the matrices during the
culture period can be made. Advantages of using this staining method over
scanning electron microscopy are the speed and ease of sample processing.
Rapid fixing and staining incubation times allow for a large number of
samples to be processed on a daily basis. Therefore, this method
provides important timely information on the state of the cells in the
macroporous bead culture.

REFERENCES

1. Hayman, E.G., Ray, N.G., and Runstadler, P.W. 1988. Production of
biomolecules by cells cultured in tri-dimensional collagen microspheres.
In: Moody, D.U., and Baker, P.B. (eds). Bioreactors and Biotransformations
(pp. 99-110), Elsevier, London and New York.

2. Runstadler, P.W. and Cernek, S.R. 1988. Large scale fluidized-bed,
immobilized cultivation of animal cells at high densities In: Spier, R.E.
and Griffiths, J.B. (eds) Animal Cell Biotechnology Vol. 3 (pp. 305-320)
Academic Press Ltd., London.

The Role of Oxidation-Reduction Potential in Monitoring Growth of Cultured Mammalian Cells

Christopher Hwang and Anthony J. Sinskey

Biotechnology Process Engineering Center and Department of Biology, Massachusetts Institute of Technology, Cambridge, Massachusetts, U.S.A.

ABSTRACT

We demonstrate that cellular reduction, i.e. the ability of cells to accumulate thiols in the medium is an universial characteristic of cultured cells. Although it is not understood why cells reduce their enviornment, such changes in the extracellular redox state, as indicated by an increase in medium thiol concentration or a decrease in the medium oxidation-reduction potential (ORP), were found to be an excellent indicator for cell growth. Analysis of data from several bioreactor runs shows that the correlation between the medium ORP and viable cell density is reproducible: the average slope of mV vs. ln (viable cells/ml) plots from these reactor runs is -0.0384 ± 0.0028. In addition, we can successfully maintaine the viable cell density of cultures in defined medium as well as serum supplemented medium by on-line measurement and control of medium ORP. Medium ORP is controlled by on-line control of the fresh medium addition rate. Finally, preliminary results with encapsulated mammalian cells indicate that the overall viable cell density in an immobilized culture can be estimated by monitoring the medium redox potential of the culture. Lastly, potential applications of this technology in cell culture is discussed.

Keywords: thiol, oxidation-reduction potential, cellular reduction, process control, encapsulation

INTRODUCTION

1. Problem Statement

Optimization of mammalian cell culture processes is hampered by the inability to monitor cell growth on-line. Such limitation is most evident for immobilized and anchorage-dependent cell culture systems in which viable cell density cannot be readily measured. Several methods for the determination of mammalian cell culture biomass have been reviewed by Merten (1988). These methods are categorized into chemical and physical determinations. Chemical methods, which include measurement of ATP or DNA, have the disadvantage of not being easily automated. Physical methods, which are more readily automated, include nephelometry, infrared nephelometry, turbidimetry, acoustic resonance densitometry (ARD), dielectric (impedimetric) monitoring, and electrical counting. The principles, advantages, disadvantages, and the possibility of detecting the viable or total cell number are summarized by Merten (1988). Additional recent references on on-line cell enumeration analysis includes Kilburn *et al.* (1989) who showed that ARD provides a highly reproducible and stable method for the on-line measurement of human lymphoma culture suspensions at densities above 10^6 total cells/ml; and Blute *et al.* (1988) demonstrate the use of a conductivity technique to perform on-line measurements of hybridoma cell densities within a hollow fiber bioreactor. Many of these physical methods require sophisticated instrumentations, some are limited to suspension cell culture, some cannot distinguish viable from non-viable cells, while others can only measure a limited range of cell densities.

In this paper, we introduce a novel technique for the on-line monitoring of growth of hybridoma cells that can be readily adapted to any cell culture system. It utilizes the measurement of medium oxidation-reduction potential (ORP) as an indicator for viable cell density. The methodology relies on the demonstration that of all cultured mammalian cells evaluated to date reduce their extracellular environment by accumulation of thiols. This increase in the extracellular sulfhydryl/disulfide (SH/SS) ratio results in a decrease in medium ORP, as measured by redox electrode in mV.

2. Cellular Reduction

Cellular reduction, the ability of cultured cells to accumulate reducing compounds, such as thiols, in the environment was first observed by Wiles and Smith (1969). They showed that the medium redox potential level decreases during growth of Earle's L cells and increases during the stationary phase. This observation was later reiterated by Bannai and Ishii (1980) who showed that human diploid fibroblasts IMR-90 reduce a considerable quantity of the medium cystine into cysteine. In addition to cysteine, a very small amount of glutathione (GSH) and GSH/cysteine mixed disulfides also was found to accumulate. Although it is still not known why these cultured cells reduced their environment, thiols such as cysteine, β-mercaptoethanol, monothioglycerol, and ascorbic acid often are used to supplement culture media. Addition of thiols to cell culture mediua has been shown to enhance GSH synthesis, cell activation, and proliferation (Glacken *et al.*, 1988; Zumda and Friedenson, 1983; Noelle and Lawrence, 1981; Lacombe, 1986; Fidelus *et al.*, 1987; Gougerot-Pocidalo *et al.*, 1985&1984; Hallwell and Gutteridge, 1985; Broome and Jeng, 1973). Thiol compounds have also been shown to enhance antibody formation (Click *et al.*, 1972; Chen and Hirsch, 1972; Ohmori and

Yamamoto, 1983a&b; Ohmori *et al.*, 1986). This result may be due to the improved growth characteristics of cells in the presence of thiols.

3. Oxidation-Reduction Potential

The measured oxidation-reduction potential (ORP) relates to all pairs of reducible and oxidizable compounds found in a particular system. In the same manner by which pH provides information about hydrogen ion activity, the redox potential provides information about the electron activity in the medium (Kjaergaard, 1977). The measured potential, which has the unit mV, is the potential generated from the equilibrium established between the electron activity of the sample and the adsorption/desorption process at a electrode's metal surface. For a system in equilibrium, the redox potential is defined by the Nernst equation (Equation 1):

$$E_h = E^0 + RT/nF \cdot \ln[OX]/[RED] \tag{1}$$

where E_h is the redox potential referred to the normal hydrogen electrode, E^0 is the standard potential of the system at 25^0C when the activities of all reactants are unity, R is the gas constant, T is the absolute temperature, F is the Faraday constant. Since biological systems, however, are never in equilibrium, the measured potential is not thermodynamically correct; the measured electrode potential is rather a stationary potential that reflects the redox condition in the medium (Balakireva *et al.*, 1974). Nevertheless, in this paper, the potential is called the redox potential or ORP. Readers are referred to Kjaergaard (1977) and Srinivas *et al.* (1988) for additional discussion on the principle, measurement, and control of redox potential.

In addition to activity ratios of oxidized to reduced compounds in aerobic processes, the redox potential is also a function of the pH, the dissolved oxygen concentration (DO), and the temperature of a given system. Since temperature, pH, and DO concentration, however, are usually controlled in cell culture processes, the redox potential becomes a measure of the activity ratio of the oxidized compounds to the reduced compounds. Furthermore, the redox potential is determined by the redox system present at the highest concentration when the redox buffer capacity of the system is low.

The current application of redox potential in biotechnology is limited, in part, by the difficulties in interpretation of redox measurements. The basic problem lies in the fact that the measurement is highly nonspecific. It is the overall oxidation-reduction capacity of the system that is measured. The multiplicity of redox systems in a biological process does not permit a straight forward interpretation of changes at the molecular level. Despite these problems, several investigators conclude that the redox potential can be a valuable indicator of the metabolic activities inside a fermentor. In microbial systems, for example, many studies show that the carbon flux pathway seems to be dependent on the redox potential. This result was obtained by showing that different metabolic products are formed when the redox potential is controlled at different levels (Kjaergaard, 1977; Radjai *et al.*, 1984; Akashi *et al.*, 1978; Shibai *et al.*, 1974). Levels of TCA enzymes, cytochromes, steady-state ATP pools, growth yields, and levels of hydrogenases all have been shown to be dependent on the redox potential value (Wimpenny and Necklen, 1971).

In mammalian cell culture, the optimum redox potential for growth of Earle's L cells, for maximum cell density and growth rate, was established independently by Wiles and Smith (1969) and Taylor *et al.* (1971). Such a result, however, was not observed for BHK cells (Griffiths, 1984). Instead, Griffiths has shown that changes in redox potential of culture medium during cell growth may have important applications in forecasting the onset of the logarithmic and stationary growth phases for mammalian cell culture systems which cannot be sampled readily.

MATERIALS AND METHODS

1. Cell lines and media

The model cell line that was used was murine hybridoma CRL-1606 (Schoen et al., 1982) and it was obtained from the American Tissue Culture Collection (ATCC, Rockville MD). Other anchorage-independent cell lines examined for thiol accumulation are hybridomas HB-8852 and ID-4; human B lymphomas LB, JY, and Daudi; mouse lymphoma S49 and 653; B lymphoblast HPB.ALL; human cervical carcinoma S3; Pre-B cells BaF3; rat glioma cells, and Preiss cells. The anchorage-dependent cells lines tested include endothelial cell RFP-EC; γ CHO; fibroblasts RAT1 and 3T3; hepatocyte HpG2; and pre-B cell BaF3. These cell lines were obtained from the M.I.T. Cell Culture Center and the Whitehead Institute for Biomedical Research (Cambridge, MA)

Hybridoma CRL-1606 was cultured in standard DMEM medium prepared from a powdered formulation (Sigma D-5500). The defined medium is an improved version originally formulated by Adema (1989). Medium was supplemented with the following additives before medium filter sterilization: 25 mM glucose, 42 μM phenol red, 44 mM sodium bicarbonate, 75 μM monothioglycerol (Sigma M6145), 40 μM aminoethanol (Sigma A5629), 30 nM biotin (Sigma B4639), and 20 nM selenium (Sigma S1382). Prior to use, 6mM glutamine was added to the filtered medium from a 320 mM filtered sterilzed glutamine frozen stock. For serum-containing medium, 5% Donor Bovine Calf Serum (Hazleton Biologics Inc. 12-14378) was supplemented to the prepared medium. For defined medium, 10 mg/l bovine insulin (Sigma I-5500) and 5 mg/l iron saturated human transferrin (Sigma T-2252) were added to the prepared medium. Stock cultures were maintained at 37^0C in a 10% CO_2 environment in the absence of antibotics. During bioreactor runs, gentamycin (50 mg/l) was included. Viable cell density was measured by a combination of Coulter Counter and trypan blue dye exclusion. Viability of cultures in all experiments were greater than 90%.

2. Instrumentation and reactor system

A 1.5 liter bioreactor (B. Braun Instruments model BIOSTAT M) and a 2.5 liter bioreactor (Applikon Dependable Instruments model BTS 06) were used for cultivation of mammalian cells. Each reactor contains a pH (Ingold 465-35-K-9), a DO (ABEC A316), and a redox potential probes (Ingold Pt-4865-35-K). Oxygenation via surface aeration is enhanced by using a custom made impeller which is partially immersed in the medium during cell cultivation. Partially immersed impellers were able to achieve mass transfer coefficient in the order of 5 hr^{-1}. IBM personal computer XT, with two WB-AIO-B8 analog/digital converter cards (Omega Engineering Inc), is used to monitor and control medium pH, DO, and redox potential. The software provided along with these cards is modified to include a PID controller. The controller is able to control pH to $\pm$ 0.1 pH units of the setpoint value via CO_2 addition, DO to $\pm$ 1% air saturation of the setpoint value via nitrogen/air and oxygen addition, and redox potential to $\pm$ 2mV of setpoint value via addition of fresh medium. The addition of fresh medium serves to dilute thiol concentration and increase medium redox potential.

3. Encapsulation of mammalian cells

Encapsulation of hybridoma CRL-1606 is described by Rha *et al* (1988). Essentially, cells suspended in a chitosan/$CaCl_2$ mixture are dropped into an alginate solution resulting in cells enclosed by an inner chitosan/alginate membrane and an outer calcium alginate gel membrane. The permeability of the inner membrane is controlled by varying the pH, ionic strength, and biopolymer concentration of the chitosan solution. An initial cell density of 8 x10^5 cells/ml corresponding to 5 to 10% of the capsule inner core volume was used as the initial inoculum. Encapsulate cells are cultured in either defined or 5% calf serum supplemented medium. For the measurement of overall viable cell density, capsules were ruptured by pushing through a 19G syringe needle. This method of cell sampling has been shown not to affect the viability of cells.

4. Analytical methods

Thiol concentration is measured colorimetrically using Ellman's reagent, 5,5'-dithio-bis(2-nitrobenzoic acid), also known as DTNB (Sigma D8130) with cysteine as the sulfhydryl concentration standards (Bannai and Ishii, 1980). Due to the instability of thiols at neutral and alkaline conditions, cell-free medium samples are stored in dilute HCl at final pH 2. Typically, 0.9 ml of medium is mixed with 0.1 ml of 0.5 N HCl and then frozen at -20°C. Preliminary results demonstrate that under these conditions thiols are stable for at least one month. To measure disulfide concentrations, medium sample is reduced with sodium borohydride and then assayed for thiol concentration (Jocelyn, 1987).

Derivatization with monobromobimane (Calbiochem Thiolyte 596105), a fluorescent compound that react specifically with sulfhydryl group of thiols, followed by reverse phase C-18 HPLC separation was used to identify major thiol(s) produced by hybridomas CRL-1606 and HB-8852 (Fahey and Newton, 1987).

The off-line measurement of medium redox potential is performed in a CO_2 incubator and the procedure is as follows. First a medium sample is used to equilibrate the probe to the medium redox level. Once the probe reaches a pseudo steady state, a second medium sample is taken and immediately measured for approximately 1 to 2 minutes. This sequential methodology for measuring redox potential is necessary because, especially at low thiol concentrations, the response time of redox probe with a given sample can be as long as 5 to 20 minutes, and during this time, the medium conditions can be modified by metabolism of cells and by changes in the environment.

To ensure proper functioning of redox probes, redox probes were cleaned between experiments using the following procedure. 1. Immerse the probe diaphram in Ingold diaphram cleaner (18528) in an inverted position overnight; 2. Immerse the metal ring in concentrated nitric acid for 1 minute to remove proteins and other organic material deposited on the surface; 3. Polish the probe metal ring with a tooth brush and tooth paste; 4. Change the reference electrolyte (Ingold Viscolyte B 18816) and use vaccum to remove air bubbles in the probe; and lastly, 5. Immerse probe in 0.1M $FeSO_4$ for 15 minutes to reduce any platinum oxide to platinum. Ingold redox buffers 9881 and 9883 were used occasionally to check for proper functioning of the probes. We found that different redox probes of the same model and manufacturer can give different redox measurements although the offsets between different probes is consistent for all measurements. As a result, prior to experimentation, all redox probes were calibrated against the redox level of fresh medium (+100 mV), either defined medium or serum supplemented medium, with DO, pH, and temperature at 90% air saturation, 7.25, and 37°C, respectively.

To measure the specific thiol accumulation rate, q_{SH}, the actual medium thiol accumulation rate and the initial thiol autooxidation rate, RX_0, are determined as a function of time. The RX_0 is obtained by monitoring the decrease in thiol concentration employing culturing conditions in the absence of cells within 30 minutes. Once these data are obtained, q_{SH} is calculated according equation 2.

$$q_{SH} = \frac{\Delta[SH]/\Delta t + RX_o}{X_v} \tag{2}$$

where [SH] is medium thiol concentration and X_v is viable cell density.

RESULTS AND DISCUSSION

1. Cellular Reduction

The reduction of medium by hybridoma CRL-1606 cultured in 5% calf serum supplemented medium under DO and pH controlled conditions is shown in Figure 1. The DO was controlled at 90% air saturation and pH was controlled at 7.25. Similar results were obtained for cells cultured in defined medium (results not shown). Typically, the initial redox potential of the medium, prior to cell inoculation and when equilibrated with controlled DO, pH, and temperature conditions is averaged +100 mV with non-detectable medium thiols. Although this value can vary from +90 to +150 mV, depends on the redox probe one uses. In these experiments the probes are calibrated so that the redox value of fresh medium is +100 mV (see Materials and Methods section). The increase medium thiol concentration and the subsequent decrease in medium redox potential demonstrates cellular reduction. Addition of glutamine (4 mM), glucose (25 mM), lactate (25 mM), and ammonium (4 mM) to the culture medium do not affect medium redox potential whereas a mere 10 μM cysteine causes the redox potential to decrease approximately 70 mV (results not shown). Although thiols are readily oxidized in the presence of oxygen, and that this reaction is catalyzed by trace metal ions such as Fe^{3+} and Cu^{2+} (Torchinskii, 1981), thiols are accumulated because as the viable cell density increases, the balance between thiol production rate and thiol autooxidation rate is shifted towards the production side and as such more and more thiols accumulate. The specific cellular thiol accumulation rate for CRL-1606 is approximately 1.5 to 3 x 10^{-5} nmole/cell hr and greater than 90% of this rate is balanced by the thiol autooxidation rate. As cells reach stationary phase, the cellular reduction rate decreases and because thiols are constantly been autooxidized, the medium thiol concentration decreases (Figure 1). These changes in extracellular thiol concentration or SH/SS concentration ratio are reflected by changes in medium redox potential. Essentially, the higher the thiol concentration, or the SH/SS concentration ratio, is in the system the lower the redox potential in that system. These results are in agreement with those of Wiles and Smith (1969). Furthermore, analysis of the thiols(s) accumulated by hybridomas CRL-1606 and HB-8852 indicated that the thiol(s) accumulated is cysteine (Figure 2). Similar results were obtained for human diploid fibroblasts IMR-90 by Bannai and Ishii (1980). Since

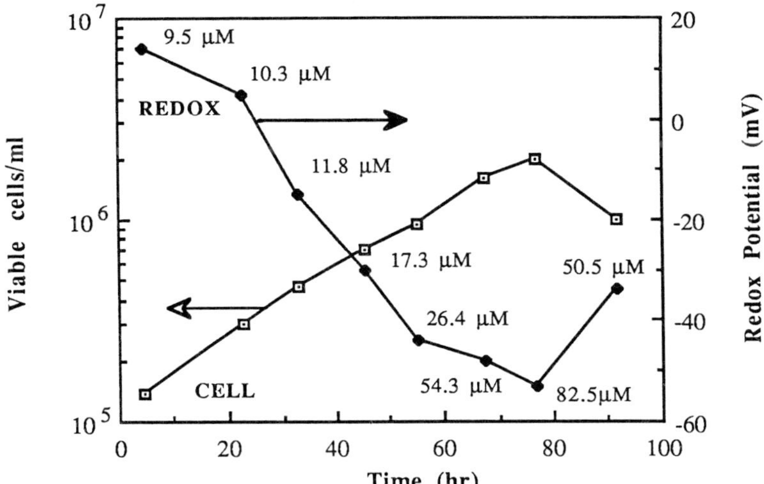

Figure 1. Viable cell density, medium redox potential, and medium thiol concentration profiles of hybridoma CRL-1606 in serum-supplemented medium. DO and pH of the culture is controlled at 90% air saturation and 7.25, respectively.

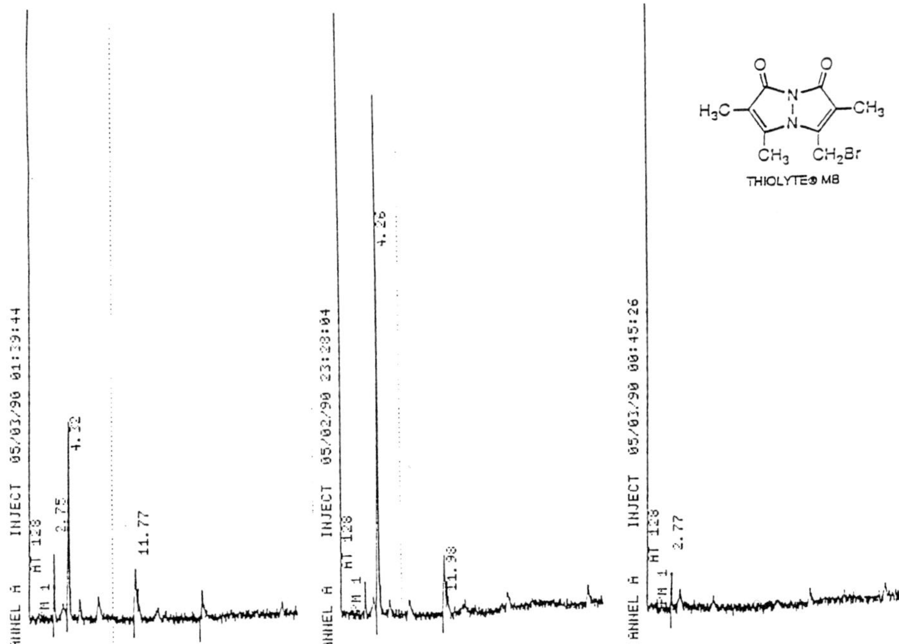

Figure 2. Identification of medium thiols from a culture of CRL-1606 in defined medium (see text). Lane 1. Medium sample only. Lane 2. Medium sample + 50 μM cysteine. Lane 3. Medium sample air oxidized at pH 8 for 5 hr.

the cell culture medium never reaches an equilibrium state, we were not able to mathematically relate the changes in medium [cystine]/[cysteine]^2 concentration ratio to changes in medium redox potential via the Nernst equation.

To determine the universality of cellular reduction, several cell lines were tested for their ability to accumulate thiols in the medium. Clearly, the results show that all cell lines tested were found to accumulate thiols in the medium (Table 1). The specific thiol accumulation rate and the thiol concentration attained for a particular cell density are cell line and medium specific. Although it is not known why and how cultured mammalian cells reduce their environment, review of the limited literature in this area and from our investigations suggests that cellular reduction seems to be a requirement for cells to grow *in vitro*. Many blood and lymphoid cells have very low or no capacity for cystine transport, and since cyst(e)ine is an essential amino acid for cultured cells and that all media is initially thiol-free due to thiol autooxidation, cells require the presence of cysteine or derivatives of cyst(e)ine in order to grow *in vitro* (Ohmori and Yamamoto, 1983a&b; Ishii, *et al.*, 1981; Hankins and Krantz, 1979; Broome and Jeng, 1973). Cysteine and mixed disulfides of cystine and thiols are known to be transported into cells about 5 to 6 times faster than cystine (Ohmori and Yamamoto, 1983a). Studies with mouse lymphoma L1210 cells have shown that the major role of feeder layer used in *in vitro* cultivation is to provide cysteine continuously (Ishii, *et al.*, 1981). In addition, Ishii, *et al.* 1981 show that a thiol-independent variant of L1210, L1210(C), accumulates thiols in the medium and the specific uptake rate of cyst(e)ine was about sixfold higher than that of the parental cell line. Cellular reduction or accumulation of extracellular thiols may also serve to modulate activities of cell surface proteins and regulate intracellular events (Wilden and Pessin, 1987; Noelle and Lawrence, 1981; Inoue *et al.*, 1987; Lash and Jones, 1985; Lorenson and Jacobs, 1982; Robillard and Konings, 1982). Recent studies in our laboratory have shown that the growth enhancement activities of serum is redox-dependent; that the activity of serum was found to degrade with time, and was stablized by addition of thiols (Glacken *et al.*, 1988).

Lastly, cellular reduction may function as a mechanism to maintain the intracellular redox state and/or to prevent buildup of excess intracellular cysteine which is toxic to the cells (Karlsen *et al.*, 1981; Mardashev and Semina, 1960). Cysteine is more reactive, and therefore toxic, than glutathione. This increased reactivity is due to differences of their pKa's. At the physiological pH of 7.4, approximately 6% of cysteine is ionized while glutathione is only 1% ionized; the ionized form or the thiolate anion is the reactive species (Torchinskii, 1981). Therefore, the intracellular cysteine concentration is kept low and is among the lowest concentration observed for any of the amino acids (30-200 μM, Griffith, 1987) while the glutathione concentration can be maintained much higher levels; approximately 4-10 mM in hybridoma CRL-1606 (unpublished results).

Table 1.   Universality of Cellular Reduction in Cultured Mammalian Cells

CELL TYPES	[SH] µM* / (viable cells/ml)
I. Anchorage-independent	
Hybridomas	
CRL-1606	80 µM / 1.2 x 10^6
HB-8852	85 µM / 6.4 x 10^5
ID-4	16 µM / 7.4 x 10^5
Human B-lymphomas	
LB	33 µM / 1.3 x 10^6
JY	38 µM / 5.0 x 10^5
Daudi	38 µM / 1.4 x 10^6
B lymphoblasts (HPB•ALL)	32 µM / 2.5 x 10^6
Mouse lymphoma	
S49	8 µM / 7.2 x 10^5
653	124 µM / 7.5 x 10^5
Human cervical carcinoma (Hela/S3)	105 µM / 1.5x10^6
Rat glioma cells (C6)	32 µM / 2.8 x 10^6
Preiss	28 µM / 8.0 x 10^5
II. Anchorage-dependent (near confluency)	
γ CHO	73 µM
Endothelial cells (RFP-EC)	34 µM
Fibroblasts	
Rat1	32 µM
3T3	30 µM
Hepatocyte (HpG2)	44 µM
pre-B cell (BaF3)	61 µM
mouse smooth aorta muscle cells	30 µM

* Conditioned medium thiol concentration in µM.

2. Medium redox potential as a function of DO, pH, and SH/SS redox state.

As discussed previously, other than temperature, redox potential in cell culture is a function of the DO, pH, and extracellular thiol/disulfide redox state. These functionalities were confirmed experimentally, Figures 3, 4, and 5, and the results are in agreement with previous reports. The linear relationship between the medium redox potential and the logarithm of DO concentration agrees qualitatively with previous reports and the proportionality coefficient of 25 mV/log unit of DO concentration is within the range that has been reported (Srinivas *et al.* 1988). Such linearity generally fails at a DO partial pressures lower than 10^{-2} atm which is also shown in Figure 3 (Srinivas *et al.* 1988). The relationship between medium redox potential and pH agrees qualitatively with results reported by Srinivas *et al.* (1988) in which they found a linear correlation between the redox potential and pH. The proportionality coefficient, however, attained in our system, -48 mV/pH unit (Figure 4), is higher than that reported by Srinivas *et al.* (1988). They report a slope of -60 mV/pH unit. This discrepancy is most likely due to the presence of more than one redox couple in the culture medium in this study that is pH dependent, i.e. the bicarbonate and the cystine/cysteine systems. On the other hand, only one redox couple was used by Srinivas *et al.* (1988). Lastly, the proportionality coefficient of

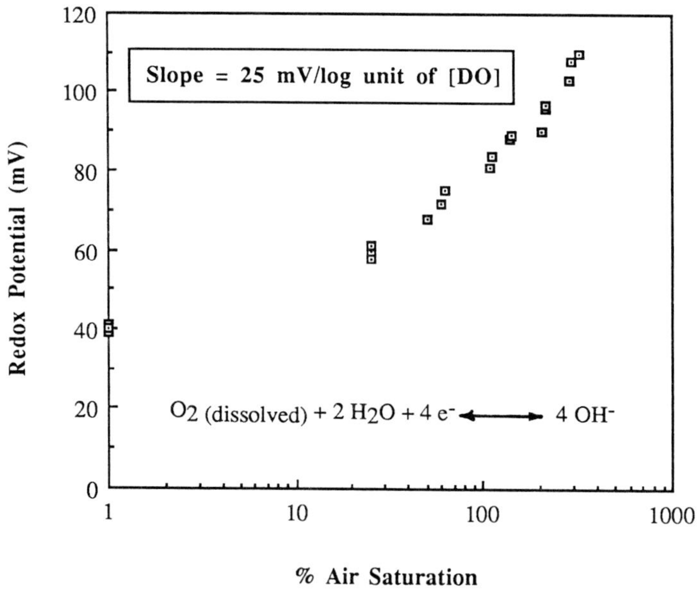

Figure 3. Medium redox potential versus DO relationship in the absence of cells. Temperature, pH, and thiol concentration are 37°C, 7.25 and 0 µM, respectively.

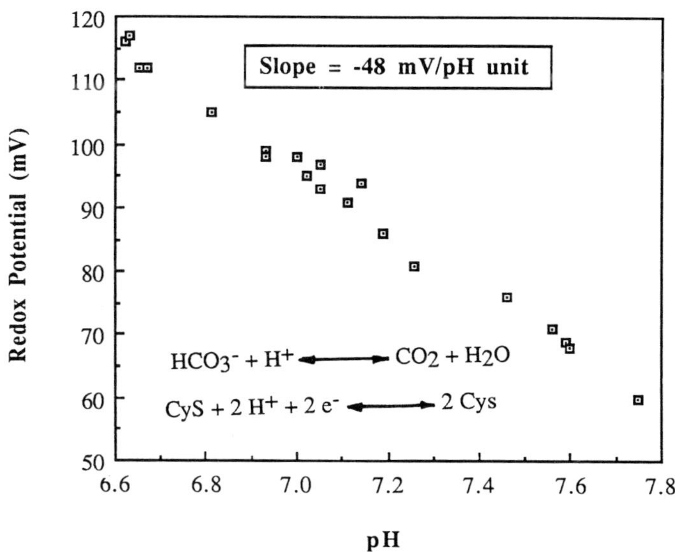

Figure 4. Medium redox potential versus pH relationship in the absence of cells. Temperature, DO, and thiol concentration are 37°C, 90% air saturation, and 0 μM, respectively.

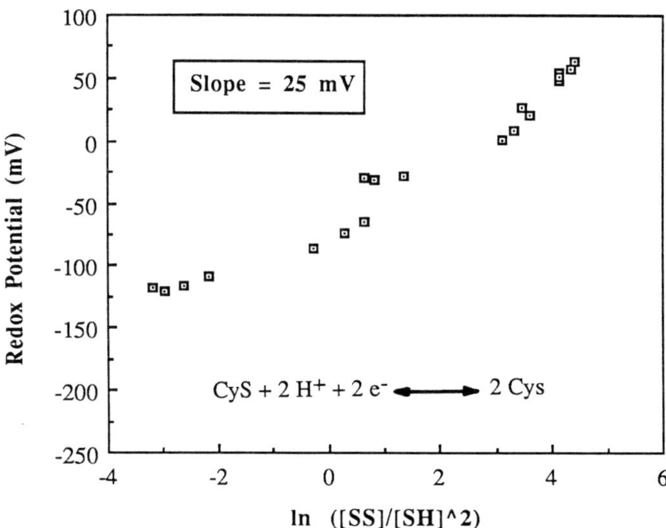

Figure 5. Medium redox potential versus $\ln([SS]/[SH]^2)$ relationship in the absence of cells. Temperature, DO and pH are 37°C, 90% air saturation, and 7.25, respectively.

medium redox potential vs. ln ([SS]/[SH]^2), calculated from Figure 5, was approximately 25 mV; this value is much larger than the 13 mV calculated from the Nernst equation. This discrepancy is expected since cysteine added in culture medium under normal conditions is unstable, due to presence of oxygen, and therefore cannot be assumed to be in an equilibrium state. In other words, the Nernst equation cannot be applied here unless the system is oxygen-free. Nevertheless, this result illustrates how changes in medium thiol/disulfide redox state or thiol concentration can change the medium redox potential.

These experiements clearly show that in cell culture, in addition to changes in medium SH/SS concentration ratio, the medium redox potential is strongly affected by changes in medium DO concentration and pH. Therefore if one were to use changes in medium SH/SS redox state or redox potential to monitor cell growth, medium DO concentration and pH conditions must be taken into consideration. Therefore, for simplicity, and as an aid in result interpretation, the medium DO and pH are controlled in all our bioreactor experiments at 90% air saturation and 7.25, respectively.

3. Medium Redox Potential vs. Viable Cell Density Calibration Curves

To determine whether medium ORP can be used to monitor cell growth, a series of bioreactor runs, in both defined and serum-supplemented media. These studies were conducted over a period of three months to determine whether the cell density vs. medium redox potential profiles were consistent or whether there is a characteristic medium redox state for a particular cell density. Reactors were inoculated with the hybridoma CRL-1606 cell line at approximately 1×10^5 viable cells/ml. Both viable cell density and the medium ORP were monitored during the logarithmic growth phase and the results, expressed as a ln (viable cells/ml) versus mV plot, are summarized in Figure 6. The results indicated that the viable cell density vs. medium redox potential standard curves are reproducible. Although these standard curves were not identical, the average slope and y-intercepts of the lines are -0.0384 $\pm$ 0.0028 and 12.86 $\pm$ 0.26, respectively. Specific cell growth rates of these experiments varied from 0.0319 to 0.0427 hr^{-1}.

These results showed, not surprisingly, that at least for hybridoma cell line CRL-1606, cells will achieve a particular redox state in the medium for a particular viable cell density and that the redox level achieved can be made reproducible upon control of other parameters that affect medium redox potential. This is supported by the fact that this consistency holds under different specific growth rates and also when cells were inoculated at two to three folds lower densities. Together, this suggests that, at least for suspension cultures, that the viable cell density of a actively growing culture can be estimated by monitoring the medium redox potential.

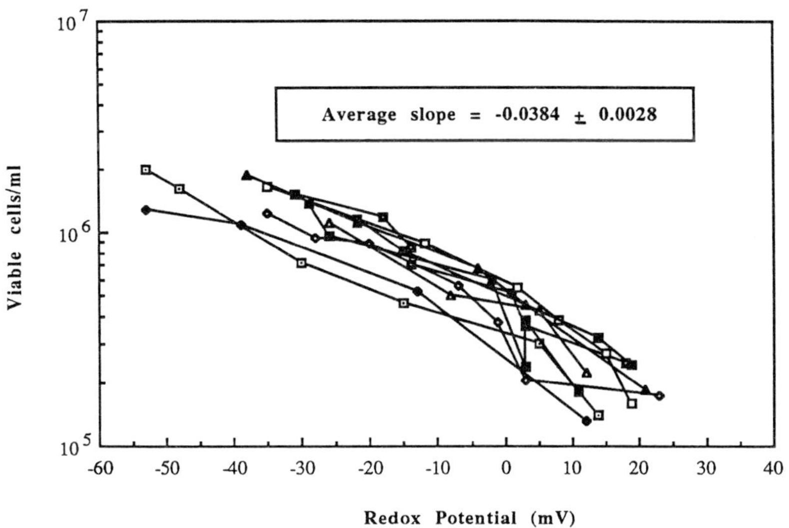

Figure 4. Collection of viable cell density verses medium redox potential profiles from cultures of CRL-1606 in either defined medium or serum-supplemented medium. Medium DO and pH are controlled at 90% air saturation and 7.25, respectively.

4. Maintain Viable Cell Density Experiments.

To further demonstrate that cells achieve a characteristic medium redox state under a controlled culture conditions and that the medium redox potential can be used to monitor cell growth, redox control experiments via addition of fresh medium, either defined medium or serum-supplemented medium, were performed. The predicted result was that the viable cell density of the hybridoma cell line CRL-1606 can be maintained. To prevent decrease in the medium redox potential due to an increase in viable cell density, the computer will activate a fresh medium pump when necessary to decrease culture thiol concentration and thus maintain medium redox potential. The results are summarized in Figures 7 and 8, and Tables 2 and 3.

5. Encapsulation Experiments.

To demonstrate that medium redox potential can be used to monitor viable cell density of immobilized mammalian cell cultures, CRL-1606 hybridoma cells were encapsulated. The viable cell density as predicted from the redox potential calibration curve was compared with what was experimentally measured (Figure 9). When cells reached approximately 1.2×10^6 cells/ml, redox control was initiated to maintain a high viable cell density of the encapsulated culture. The results showed that using empirically determined viable cell density vs. medium redox potential standard curves for suspension cultures, one can estimated the overall viable cell density of an encapsulated culture. Furthermore, upon initiation of medium redox control to maintain viable cell density, culture maintained an overall cell density of 9.8×10^5 viable cells/ml ($\pm$ 10%).

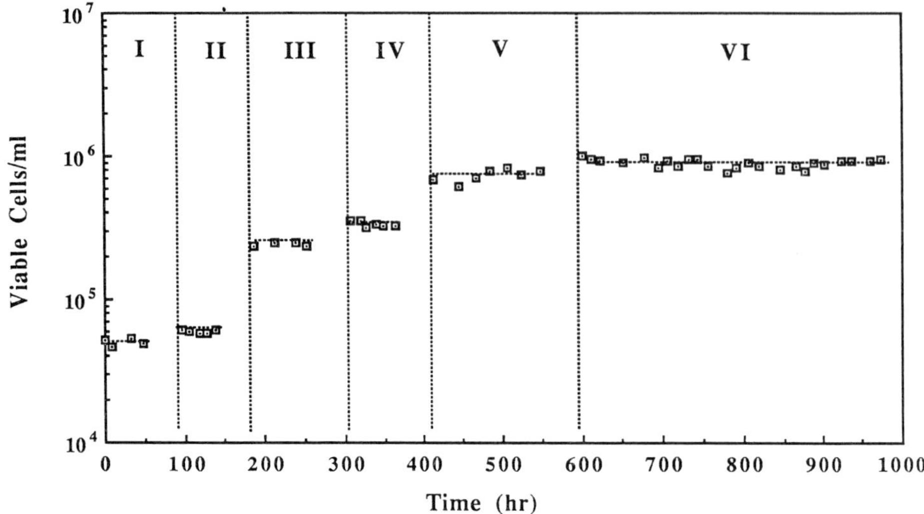

Figure 7. Control of viable hybridoma CRL-1606 cell density in culture via redox control of fresh medium feed rate (Defined medium). Medium DO and pH are controlled at 90% air saturation and 7.25, respectively. See Table 2 for summary of results.

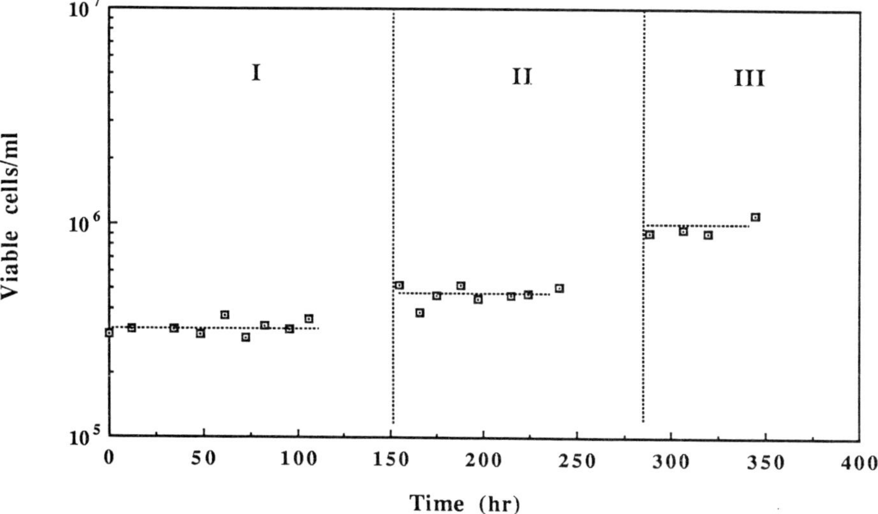

Figure 8. Control of viable hybridoma CRL-1606 cell density in culture via redox control of fresh medium feed rate (Serum supplemented medium). Medium DO and pH are controlled at 90% air saturation and 7.25, respectively. See Table 3 for summary of results.

Table 2 . Control of viable hybridoma CRL-1606 cell density in culture via redox control of fresh medium feed rate (Defined medium).

Run #	mV Controlled	Duration (days)	Viable cell/ml (Std Dev)
I	58 ± 5 mV	2.0	5.00×10^4 ($\pm$ 6%)
II	53 ± 3 mV	1.8	5.94×10^4 ($\pm$ 3%)
III	32 ± 1 mV	2.0	2.41×10^5 ($\pm$ 3%)
IV	17 ± 1 mV	2.3	3.33×10^5 ($\pm$ 5%)
V	-78 ± 1 mV	6.6	7.29×10^5 ($\pm$ 10%)
VI	-85 ± 3 mV	15.6	8.89×10^5 ($\pm$ 7%)

Table 3 . Control of viable hybridoma CRL-1606 cell density in culture via redox control of fresh medium feed rate (Serum supplemented medium). The difference of mV verse viable cell density relationship between Table 2 and this table is due to use of uncalibrated probe for this experiment.

Run #	mV Controlled	Duration (days)	Viable cell/ml (Std Dev)
I	29 ± 3 mV	3.6	3.27×10^5 ($\pm$ 8%)
II	-3 ± 8 mV	2.3	4.73×10^5 ($\pm$ 9%)
III	-38 ± 3 mV	4.4	9.77×10^5 ($\pm$ 10%)

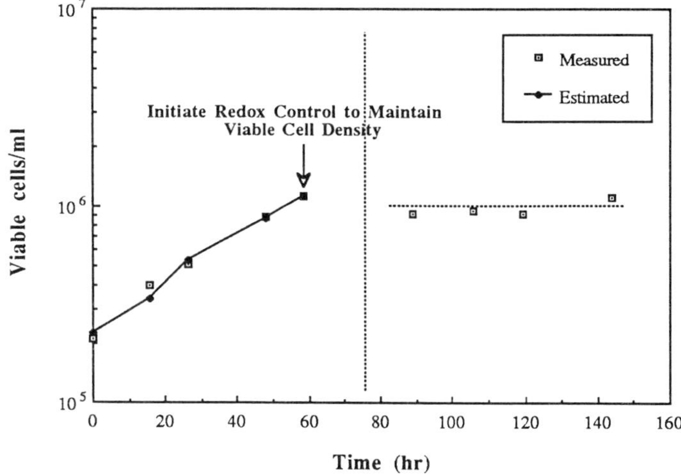

Figure 9. Estimation of viable cell density of encapsulated hybridoma CRL-1606 culture by monitoring the medium redox potential. When cells reached 1.2×10^6 cells/ml, redox control was initiated to maintain overall viable cell density.

SUMMARY

Our investigation shows that cellular reduction, i.e. the ability of cells to accumulate thiols in the medium, is universal for cultured mammalian cells. We have shown that changes in the medium redox potential, under DO and pH controlled conditions, correspond to changes in the medium thiol concentration. Furthermore, based on the effect of accumulated thiols on the medium redox potential and that only viable cells can reduce the medium, at least for murine hybridoma cell line CRL-1606, we have demonstrated that one can monitor the viable cell density of the culture by measuring the medium redox potential. This is demonstrated by the reproducibility of the medium redox potential vs. viable cell density standard curve from several bioreactor experiments, the control of viable cell density of several cultures by control of medium redox potential via computer control of medium feed rate, and the successful estimation of viable cell density of an encapsulation culture. Since cell culture medium has a very low redox buffering capacity, changes in medium redox potential are very sensitive to changes in the medium thiol concentration. As a result, growth of cells at very low densities ($< 10^4$ cells/ml) can still be detected. Together these results suggest that medium redox potential can be used to monitor cell growth of mammalian cells in both suspension as well as immobilized cultures. In addition, redox potential can become an important process control parameter for the optimization of mammalian cell culture. For instance, the principle can be used to maintain a cell culture at its maximum production state, to forecast optimal period for harvest of products, or simply to assess the physiological state of the culture.

ACKNOWLEDGEMENT

This research has been supported by the NSF under the Engineering Research Center Initiative to the MIT Biotechnology Process Engineering Center and Snow Brand Milk Products from Tokyo, Japan.

REFERENCES

Adema, E. 1989. Ammonium toxicity in mammalian cell culture. Ph.D. Thesis. M.I.T. Cambridge, Massachusetts.

Akashi, K., et al.. 1978. Determination redox potential levels critical for cell respiration and suitable for L-leucine production. Biotech. Bioeng. 20:27.

Balakireva, L.M., Kantere, V.M., and Robotnova, I.L. 1974. The redox potential in microbiological media. Biotech. Bioeng. Symp. 4:769-780.

Bannai, S., and Tateishi, N. 1986. Role of membrane transport in metabolism and function of glutathione in mammals. J. Membrane. Biol. 89:1-8.

Blute, T., Gillies, R.J., and Dale, B.E. 1988. Cell density measurements in hollow fiber bioreactors. Biotech. Progress 4:202-209.

Brigelius, R. 1985. Mixed disulfides: Biological functions and increase in oxidative stress. in *Oxidative Stress.* eds.

Broome, J.D., and Jeng, M.W. 1973. Promotion of replication in lymphoid cells by specific thiols and disulfides *in vitro*. J. Exp. Med. 138:574-592.

Fahey, R.C., and Newton, G.L. 1987. Determination of low-molecular-weight thiols using monobromobimane fluorescent labeling and HPLC. Methods Enzymol. 143:85-96.

Gascoyne, P. 1986. The redox-mediated control of enzyme function and cellular structure. Int. J. Quantum Chem.: QBS12:245-255.

Gilbert H.F. 1984. Redox control of enzyme activities by thiol/disulfide exchange. Meth. Enzymol. 107:330-351.

Glacken, M.W., Adema, E., and Sinskey, A.J. 1988. Mathematical descriptions of hybridoma culture kinetics. II. The relationship between thiol chemistry and the degradation of serum activity. Biotech. Bioeng. 33:440-451.

Gougerot-Pocidalo, M-A., Fay, M., and Pocidalo, J.J. 1984. *In vivo* normobaric oxygen exposure depresses spleen cell *in vitro* Con A response. Effects of 2-mercaptoethanol and peritoneal cells. Clin. Exp. Immunol. 58:428:435.

Gougerot-Pocidalo, M-A., Fay, M., Roche, Y. Lacombe, P., and Marquetty, C. 1985. Immune oxidative injury induced in mice exposed to normobaric oxygen: effects of thiol compounds on the splenic cell sulfhydryl content and con A proliferative response. J. Immunol. 135:2045-2051.

Griffiths, B. 1984. The use of oxidation-reduction potential (ORP) to monitor growth during a cell culture. Develop. Biol. Standard. 55:113-116.

Hankins. W.D., and Krantz, S.B. 1979. Effects of sulfhydryl compounds on friend virus-infected spleen cells in vitro. J. Biol. Chem. 254:5701-5707.

Inoue, M., Saito, Y., Hirata, E., Morino, Y., and Nagase, S. ·1987. Regulation of redox states of plasma proteins by metabolism and transport of glutathione and related compounds. J. Protein Chem. 6:207-225.

Ishii, T., Hishinuma, I., Bannai, S., and Sugita, Y. 1981. Mechanism of growth promotion of mouse lymphoma L1210 cells *in vitro* by feeder layer of 2-mercaptoethanol. J. Cell. Physiol. 107:283-293.

Ishii, T., Bannai, S., and Sugita, Y. 1981. Mechanism of growth stimulation of L1210 cells by 2-mercaptoethanol *in vitro*. J. Biol. Chem. 256:12387-12392.

Karlsen, R.L., Grofova, I., Malthe-Sorenssen, D., and Fonnum, F. Morphological changes in rat brain induced by L-cysteine injection in newborn animals. Brain Res. 208:167-180.

Kilburn, D.G., Fitzpatrick, P., Blake-Coleman, B.C., Clarke, D.J., and Griffiths, J.B. 1989. On-line monitoring of cell mass in mammalian cell cultures by acoustic densitometry. Biotech. Bioeng. 33:1379-1384.

Kjaergaard, L. 1977. The redox potential: Its use and control in biotechnology. Adv. Biochem. Eng. 7:131-150.

Lash, L.H., and Jones, D.P. 1985. Distribution of oxidized and reduced forms of glutathione and cysteine in rat plasma. Arch. Biochem. Biophy. 240:583-592.

Lorenson, M.Y., and Jacobs, L.S. Thiol regulation of protein, growth hormone, and prolactin release from isolated adenohypophysial secretory granules. Endocrinology. 110:1164-1172.

Mardashev, S.R., and Semina, L.A. 1960. Inhibition of enzymic decarboxylation of amino acids by DL-penicillamine, L-cysteine, and DL-homocysteine. Biochemistry USSR. 26:27-33.

Merten, O-M. 1988. Sensors for the control of mammalian cell processes. in *Animal Cell Biotechnology Vol.3*, R.E. Spier and J.B. Griffiths. Eds., Academic Press Ltd., London, pp.75-140.

Morrissey, J.J. 1986. Involvement of glutathione oxidation reduction in parathyroid hormone secretion. Am. J. Physiol. 250 (Endocrinol. Metab. 13): E475-E479.

Noelle, R.J., and Lawrence, D.A. 1981. Determination of glutathione in lymphocytes and possible association of redox state and proliferative capacity of lymphocytes. Biochem. J. 198:571-579.

Noelle, R.J., and Lawrence, D.A. 1981. Modulation of T-cell function. II. Chemical basis for the involvement of cell surface thiol-reactive sites in control of T-cell proliferation. Cell. Immun. 60:453-469.

Ohmori, H., and Yamamoto, I. 1983a. Mechanism of augmentation of the antibody response in vitro by 2-mercaptoethanol in murine lymphocytes. II. A major role of the mixed disulfide between 2-mercaptothanol and cysteine. Cell. Immunol. 79:173-185.

Ohmori, H., and Yamamoto, I. 1983b. Mechanism of augmentation of the antibody response in vitro by 2-mercaptoethanol in murine lymphocytes. III. Serum-bound and oxidized 2-mercaptoethanol are available for the augmentation. Cell. Immunol. 79:186-196.

Radjai, M., Hatch, R., and Cadman, T. 1984. Optimization of amino acid production by automatic self-tuning digital control of redox potential. Biotech. Bioeng. Symp. 14:657.

Kim, S-K., and Rha, C-K. 1989. Chitosan for encapsulation of mammalian cell culture. in *4th International Conference on Chitin and Chitosan.* in press.

Robillard, G.T., and Konings, W.N. 1982. A hypothesis for the role of dithiol-disulfide interchange in solute transport and energy-transducing processes. Eur. J. Biochem. 127:597-604.

Shibai, H., et al.. 1974. Simultaneous measurement of dissolved oxygen and oxidation-reduction potentials in the aerobic culture. Arg. Biol. Chem. 38:2407.

Srinivas, S.P., Rao, G., and Mutharasan, R. 1988. Redox potential in anaerobic and microaerobic fermentation. in *Handbook on Anaerobic Fermentations.* Erickson, L.E. and Fung, D.Y-C. Marcel Dekker Inc. pp.147-186.

Taylor, G.W., *et al.* 1971. Growth and metabolism of L cells in a chemically defined medium in a controlled environment culture system. I. Effects of oxygen tension on L-cell cultures. Applied Microbiol. 21:928-933.

Tietz, F. 1969. Enzymic method for quantitative determination of nanogram amounts of total and oxidized glutathione. Analytical Biochem. 27:502-522.

Torchinskii, I.M. 1981. *Sulphur in Protein.* pp.3-8;48-65;199-217, New York:Oxford.

Wilden, P.A., and Pessin, J.E. Differential sensitivity of the insulin-receptor kinase to thiol and oxidizing agents in the absence and presence of insulin. Biochem. J. 245:325-331.

Wiles, C.C., and Smith, V. 1969. Oxidation-reduction potential controlled submerged tissue culture fermentation in pilot-scale fermentors. Amer. Inst. Chem. Eng. Symp. Bioeng. Technol. November, 85-93.

Williamson, J.M., Boettcher, B., and Meister, A. 1982. Intracellular cysteine delivery system that protects against toxicity by promoting glutathione synthesis. Proc. Natl. Acad. Sci. USA 79:6246-6249.

Wimpenny, J.W.T., and Necklen, D.K. 1971. The redox environment and microbial physiology. I. The transition anaerobiosis to aerobiosis in continuous cultures of facultative anaerobes. Biochim. Biophys. Acta. 253:352-359.

Ziegler, D.M. 1985. Role of reversible oxidation-reduction of enzyme thiols-disulfides in metabolic regulation. Ann. Rev. Biochem. 54:305-329.

Zumda, J., and Friedenson, B. 1983. Changes in intracellular glutathione levels in stimulated and unstimulated lymphocytes in the presence of 2-mercaptoethanol of cysteine. J. Immunol. 130:362-364.

<u>**Paper of Hwang:**</u>

Finter:

If you operate a fermenter for periods in excess of several months it become impossible to measure dissolved oxygen because of probe fouling. So for the last 25 years the Wellcome group has used Redox measurements in place of dissolved oxygen. So Dr. Sinsky's paper is not a new observation as it is already a well established technique for controlling fermenters.

Hofmann:

Your redox potential decreased when your cells are increasing in number, is this an effect of conditioning the medium. Would it help to add cysteine as opposed to cystine or add ascorbic acid.

Hwang:

If you make the medium too reduced by addition of cysteine the cells will die. If you poise the medium to the level where the cell metabolises normally we did not see any effect.

Spier:

Did you control dissolved oxygen and pH levels because if not your redox reading becomes a reflection of variations in these other two parameters.

Hwang:

Every experiment we did was DO and pH controlled with the DO maintained at 90% saturation.

The results of Wildsmith indicate an optimum redox level for cell growth. If we control redox by manipulating DO we see increase growth rates and obtain a 50% increase in the maximum cell density.

Estefanell:

How do you calibrate your redox potential probes; We find that if you have two probes in one fermenter they might give two different readings.

Hwang:

We calibrate our probes to the conditions in the medium at the commencement of the culture which is about 100mV.

Estefanell:

With the use of charged membranes as used in media filtration we have found a switch in the redox values of the fresh medium; have you experienced this in your work?

Hwang:

I have not worked with charged membrane sterilizing filters.

POTENTIAL AND PITFALLS OF USING LDH RELEASE FOR THE EVALUATION OF ANIMAL CELL DEATH KINETICS

A. MARC[1], A. WAGNER[1], A. MARTIAL[1], J.L. GOERGEN[1], J.M. ENGASSER[1], V. GEAUGEY[2], H. PINTON[3]

1 Institut National Polytechnique de Lorraine, Laboratoire des Sciences du Génie Chimique, CNRS, BP 451, F - 54001 NANCY Cedex
2 Bertin et Cie, BP 3, F - 78373 PLAISIR Cedex
3 SGI, 15 allées de Bellefontaine, F- 31100 TOULOUSE

ABSTRACT

The release of lactate dehydrogenase (LDH) in the culture medium can represent a good qualitative and quantitative indicator of cellular death. An overview of the kinetics of LDH release in batch and continous cultures, with both suspension and adherent cell lines is presented. Under controlled conditions the intracellular LDH activity of living cells is relatively constant during the culture. It varies however with the pH, the dissolved oxygen level, the nature of the carbon source and the type of cells. Monitoring the release kinetics of LDH in the culture medium allows the evaluation of the actual growth and death rate of cells inside bioreactors.

KEY WORDS

Lactate dehydrogenase, animal cells, cell death, enzyme release, intracellular activity, kinetics, monitoring.

INTRODUCTION

Cellular death is an important event in mammalian cell cultures. Its influence can become quite appreciable, if not predominant, at the end of batch and fed-batch cultures or during the stationary phase of continuous cultures. Thus for the kinetic analysis or for the optimal control of animal cell processes a convenient and accurate procedure to evaluate the rate of cell death must be available.

The classical way for dead cells measurement is the Trypan Blue staining method. Dead cells having a permeabilized membrane can no longer exclude the Trypan molecules and become blue when exposed to the dye. This staining technique, however, requires the sampling of cells and is difficult to automate. Moreover it does not account for cells which have been lysed.

An alternative method which is increasingly used for cell death detection is the release of lactate dehydrogenase (LDH) in the culture medium [1,2]. The level of measured enzyme activity has often been reported to be simply proportionnal to the amount of dead cells [3,4]. A main advantage of the procedure is to account for both dead and lysed cells.

Yet when using LDH measurements for a quantitative determination of cell death several questions must be adressed concerning the amount of LDH inside living cells and the rate of LDH release during cell death (Figure 1). Is the calibration curve between released enzyme activity and dead cells dependent on the type of cells, the medium composition and the culture conditions ? Is LDH totally or partially released when a cell is considered as dead by the Trypan Blue staining ?

This paper presents an overview of recent kinetic data on the release of LDH in batch and continuous cultures with both suspension and adherent cell lines and under a wide range of operating conditions and medium composition. It also illustrates how LDH measurements can be used to achieve a more precise understanding of cell kinetics.

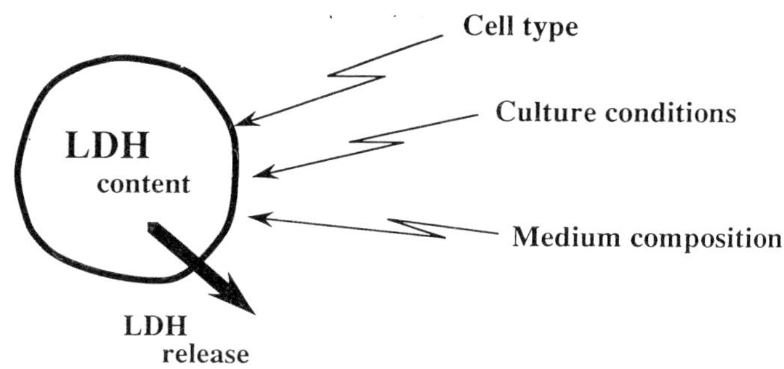

Figure 1: *Schematic representation of the factors which may influence the intracellular LDH content and the kinetics of LDH release of mammalian cells.*

RESULTS AND DISCUSSION

Influence of culture conditions on the intracellular LDH content

A first point to consider is how culture conditions may affect the level of LDH inside living cells. Under standard conditions (controlled pH, negligible nutrients and oxygen limitations) the intracellular LDH content of viable cells seems relatively constant (+/- 50 units per 10^9 cells) both during batch and continuous cultures (Figure 2). It can, however, considerably vary from one cell type to the other. For instance, whereas for different hybridoma internal LDH has been found to range between 150 and 400 units per 10^9 cells, larger quantities, up to 4000 units LDH per 10^9 cells, have been measured in kidney cells.

For a given cell line the intracellular LDH level can be modified by several parameters related to the medium composition, and particularly by the pH and the dissolved oxygen concentration. With hybridoma cells, LDH content has been found to increase with pH. When cultured under oxygen limitations mammalian cells also contain larger amounts of the enzyme [5].

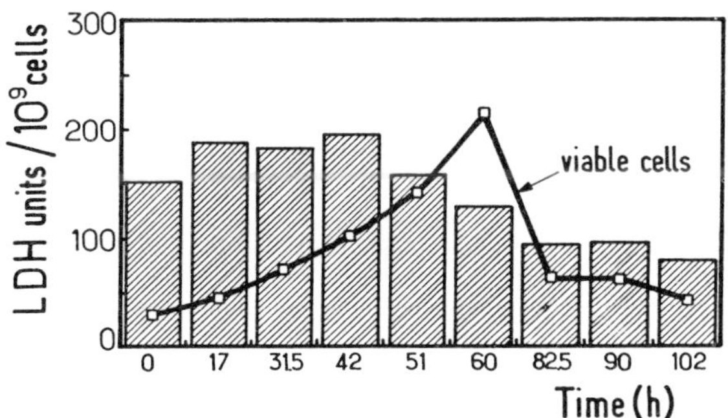

Figure 2: Time variation of the LDH content of living cells during a batch culture of hybridoma.

An additional modulating factor is the nature of the carbon source. Indeed kidney cells growing on glucose contain 4000 LDH units per 10^9 cells, whereas on a mixture of glucose and galactose they only contain 900 LDH units per 10^9 cells. On the other hand prolonged nutrient limitations in continuous cultures can also interfere with the LDH level. Thus exposure of hybridoma to amino acids limitations has been found to increase intracellular LDH from 400 to 700 LDH units per 10^9 cells.

Kinetics of LDH release

An accurate evaluation of cell death from LDH activity measurements also requires sufficient knowledge on the kinetics of LDH release during the death process. Especially if one tries to correlate the LDH level in the culture medium to the dead cells counted by the Trypan Blue staining, it is necessary to know how LDH release is kinetically related to the membrane permeabilisation to the Trypan Blue molecules.

The few data presently available seem to indicate different schemes of LDH release depending on the considered cell line (Figure 3). The simplest case is found with hybridoma which have released most of their intracellular LDH when taking up Trypan Blue. The situation can be quite different with other types of cells, for instance CHO and kidney cells, which can still contain large amounts of LDH though they are counted as dead by Trypan Blue. For these cells loss of LDH appears as a more lenghty process which is only complete when cells are lysed. Under these conditions a more precise distinction has to be made between dead and lysed cells when analysing data on enzyme release.

Use of LDH measurements for kinetic analysis

In addition to its interest for the detection of cell death in bioreactors, a major application of LDH activity measurements is for the more advanced kinetic analysis of cell cultures.

Either in batch or in continuous cultures the cellular growth rate is usually evaluated from the time variation of the measured concentration of living cells.

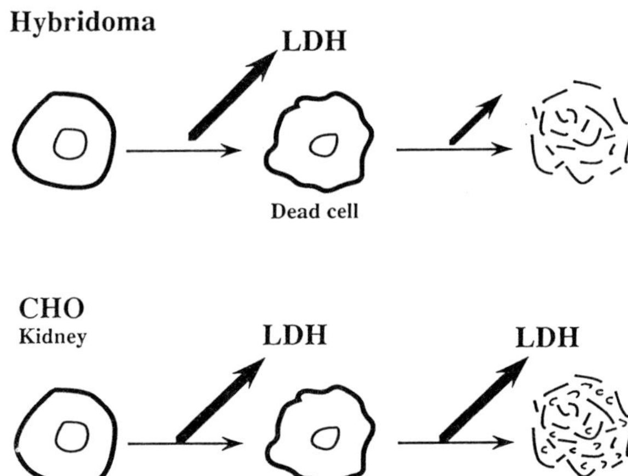

Figure 3: Schematic representation of the LDH release during the death process for different types of cells.

Yet at a given time the level of living cells is the result of two simultaneous processes: the production of new cells and the death of cells. Thus from the level of living cells only the apparent growth rate can be calculated. More interesting for the kinetic interpretation is the actual growth rate of cells, which can be evaluated by adding to the apparent growth rate the death rate evaluated from the rate of LDH release into the medium.

Death rate and actual growth rate determinations are particularly relevant when considering perfusion cultures (Figure 4). After an initial growth phase, they often yield a stationary phase at a high cell density. A simultaneous detection of LDH in the medium shows the presence of a significant cellular death which can be evaluated using a previously established calibration curve for the intracellular LDH of activity of living cells. Under these conditions protein production occuring during the stationary phase should not be related to an absence of cell growth, but, instead, should be correlated to the actual cell growth which compensates the cellular death [6].

CONCLUSIONS

Measuring the release of LDH in the culture medium can represent a good qualitative and quantitative indicator of cellular death. When using the kinetics of LDH appearance for the evaluation of cellular death rate, care should be taken with respect to the influence of the medium composition, especially pH, dissolved oxygen and nutrients limitations, on the intracellular LDH content of living cells. One should also consider the possibility for LDH excretion to proceed during a length of time which may extend to the total lysis of cells.

Under standard culture conditions simple proportionalities between released LDH and dead cells can be directly used to determine the rate of cell death. Under the more complex conditions of varying LDH content or of delayed LDH excretion, the evaluation of the actual cell death and growth rate can still be performed by

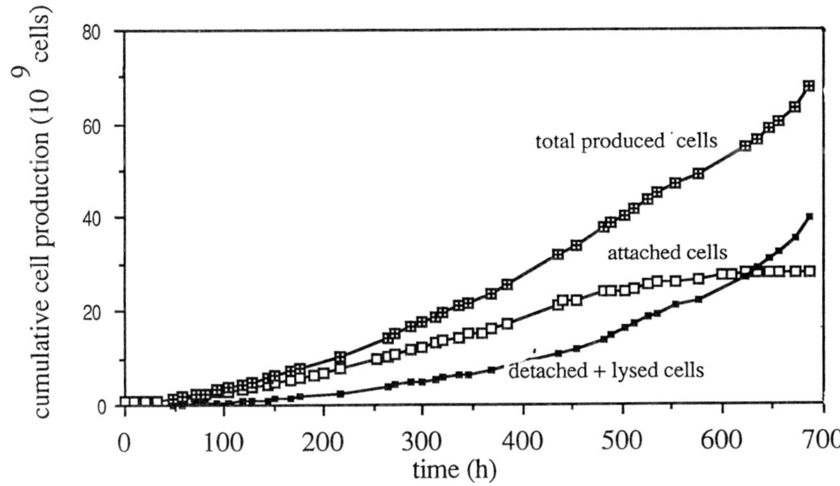

Figure 4: Use of LDH excretion data for the evaluation of the cell death and actual growth during a perfusion culture of human kidney cells on microcarriers

using a more elaborate estimator strategy [7]. LDH production and release are integrated in a kinetic model of the cellular process, together with other variables representing the medium composition in nutrients and metabolites. The model can then be used to estimate on-line the amount of living and dead cells from a limited number of measurements on the culture medium. Moreover, if the enzyme assay can be coupled to an automatic medium sampler it is possible to achieve an on-line LDH analysis which can be further integrated in a computer control strategy.

In the future the interpretation of released LDH data should also be considered in the framework of a more precise definition of cellular death. Clearly the presently used evaluation of cell death by the Trypan Blue method represents an oversimplification of cellular death, which only discriminates between a living cell and a permeabilized cell. It seems preferable to regard cell death as a progressive process where cells are successively loosing their different properties. And measurements of the release of intracellular enzymes such as LDH may represent one of the indicator of the progressive loss of cell viability.

ACKNOWLEDGEMENTS

This study was partly supported by grants of the CEC (Biotechnology Action Program), of the French Research Ministery, and of the Biotechnology Institute of Nancy (IBN). The scientific guidance and analytical assistance of Professors P. NABET and G. SIEST (IBN) are acknowledged.

REFERENCES

1   Petersen J.F., McIntire L.V. and Papoutsakis E.T. Shear sensitivity of cultured hybridoma cells (CRL-8108) depends on mode of growth, culture age and metabolite concentration, J. of Biotechnol 1988, 7, 229

2   Abu-Reesh I. and Kargi F. Biological responses of hybridoma cells to defined hydrodynamic shear stress, J. of Biotechnology 1989, 9, 167

3   Bour J.M., Maugras M., Capiaumont J., Dousset B., Straczek J., Gelot M.A., Nabet P. Marqueurs biochimiques de la prolifération et de la mort des hybridomes en culture, Bio-Sciences 1988, 7, 2, 35

4   Gervaise C. Cultures de cellules d'hybridomes et de cellules productrices d'hGH, PhD Thesis, INPL Nancy France, 1989

5   Geaugey V., Pascal F., Engasser J.M. and Marc A. Influence of the culture oxygenation on the release of LDH by hybridoma cells, Biotechnol. Techn. in press

6   Wagner A. Etude de la production de pro-urokinase par des cellules humaines tumorales cultivées en réacteurs discontinus et perfusés, PhD Thesis, INPL Nancy France, 1990

7   Mailly E., Fonteix C., Engasser J.M., Marc A. Mathematical estimator for the evaluation of cell density and medium composition in hybridoma cultures. Proceedings of the 10th ESACT Meeting, Avignon (1990)

<u>**Paper of Engasser**</u>

Kilburn: You need a kinetic model when you use LDH and you don't
             appear to have included the stability of the enzyme in
             the culture supernatant.   LDH has a relatively short
             half life under some conditions and therefore one can
             be misled.

Engasser: We checked the stability of LDH in our cultures and we
             found it to be stable - we loose 1% of the activity per
             day.

Kilburn: We experience LDH half lives as short as 12 hours with
             5% calf serum in DMEM.

Engasser: We still observe a stable enzyme.

Steiner: You have shown that the LDH content of the cells
             depends on the type of carbon source, have you seen an
             effect dependent on the concentration of the carbon
             source which as it varies during the course of the
             culture might cause a change in the LDH concentration.

Engasser: We did not do this study.   We only examined the
             difference between glucose and galactose in a constant
             concentration perfusion culture.

Steiner: There could be a glucose concentration effect.

Engasser: Possibly.

Arathoon: The stability of LDH is cell type dependent.   The
             material found in the supernatant of certain cells can
             be very unstable.

FLOW CYTOMETRIC (FCM) ANALYSIS ON THE GENETIC STABILITY OF CONTINUOUS CELL LINES

G. Fertig, M. Klöppinger and H.G. Miltenburger

Institute of Zoology, Cell Biology Laboratory, Technical University, D-6100 Darmstadt

INTRODUCTION

The characterization and identification of cell lines used in production processes of biologicals is a fundamental requirement. Growth kinetics, microscopic karyotyping and iso-enzyme-analysis are the usually applied criteria. As alternative methods, flow cytometric karyotyping by measurement of single chromosomes as well as cell cycle kinetics and DNA-index-determination by the application of an internal DNA-reference-standard can be performed routinely.
The genetic stability of continuous cell lines (V79-Chinese hamster cells and mouse-mouse hybridoma cells) was evaluated by flow cytometric karyotyping and DNA-index determination. Additionally, G-banding and iso-enzyme-analysis was carried out, to support the results obtained by flow cytometric DNA-analysis.

MATERIALS AND METHODS

Cells. V79 cells were cultured in Hank's minimum essential medium (MEM) with 10% fetal calf serum (FCS). Cells were adapted to suspension growth during a six months cultivation in spinner flasks. Hybridoma cells (HBD1) were grown in RPMI-medium with 10% FCS and supplemented with additional amino acids and 1mM sodium pyruvat. Cultivation was performed in spinner flasks as well as in a fermenter (Biostat MC, B.Braun Melungen). Trout erythrocytes (TE), obtained by vein puncture and stored in 1ml aliquots at -70°C in a citrate buffer (5%DMSO, 250 mM sucrose, 40 mM sodium citrate, pH7.6) were used as DNA controls.
Flow cytometry. An arclamp-based flow cytometer (PAS II, Partec GmbH, 4400 Münster, F.R.G.) was used to analyze the DNA-content of single chromosomes or cells. For DNA-index-determination TE were mixed with the monodispersed cells, before staining. The DNA of the cells was stained by a DAPI-solution (2µg/ml 4'6-Diamidino-2-phenylindole, 2mM MgCl$_2$, 0.1% Triton-X-100, 0.9% NaCl and 0.1 M Tris-HCl, pH 7.2). For flow cytometric karyotyping, a suspension of

metaphase chromosomes was prepared by the method of VAN DEN ENGH (1985) and stained with 2µg/ml DAPI.
G-banding was performed as described by SEABRIGHT (1972) and iso-enzyme-analysis according to the protocol of MASKOS & MILTENBURGER (1983).

RESULTS

DNA-index-determination

Fig.1a+b show the DNA-histograms of two different cell lines measured in combination with TE for DNA-index-determination (DI). The ratio of G_0 (erythrocytes) and G_1 (cell line) determines the DNA-index ($DI_{V79}=1.229\pm0.013$, $DI_{HBD1}=2.75\pm0.037$). The validation-data of the DNA-index for V79 cells exhibit a dispersion of 1.14%. Thus, it is possible to detect a subpopulation that has lost one single chromosome.
An example for the establishment of a subpopulation with differing DNA-content during a hybridoma batch-fermentation is shown in figure 1c. The DNA-index of the new subpopulation is 3.280, which is significantly different from the original population (DI=2.750).

Chromosome-histograms

During a six months cultivation period, V79 cells were examined for genetical constancy by flow cytometric karyotyping. Figure 2 shows chromosome histograms of the cells at the beginning and at the end of the culture period. The arrows point out the appearance of new chromosome classes, which are further characterized by G-banding (figure 3). Additionally, iso-enzyme-analysis was performed, which also shows differences in the lactate-dehydrogenase (LDH) pattern.

CONCLUSIONS

Flow cytometry provides a reliable and rapid method for the characterization and identification of cell lines. The DNA-index and chromosome-histograms are suited to detect genetic differences, developing during cultivation processes. Thus, flow cytometry can be routinely used to screen cell lines for their genetical constancy.

REFERENCES

1 Van den Engh, G.J., Trask, B.J., Gray, J.W., Langlois, R.G. and Yu, L.-C. Preparation and Bivariate Analysis of Suspensions of Human Chromosomes. <u>Cytometry</u> 1985, <u>6</u>, 92

2 Seabright, M. The use of proteolytic enzymes for the mapping of structural rearrangements in the chromosomes of man. <u>Chromosoma</u>, 1972, <u>36</u>, 204

3 Maskos, C.B. and Miltenburger, H.G. Isoenzym-Analyse von Insektenzellinien durch isoelektrische Fokussierung in Dünnschicht-Polyacrylamid-Gelen. <u>Z. Mitt. Dtsch. Ges. allg. angew. Ent.</u>, 1983, <u>4</u>, 44

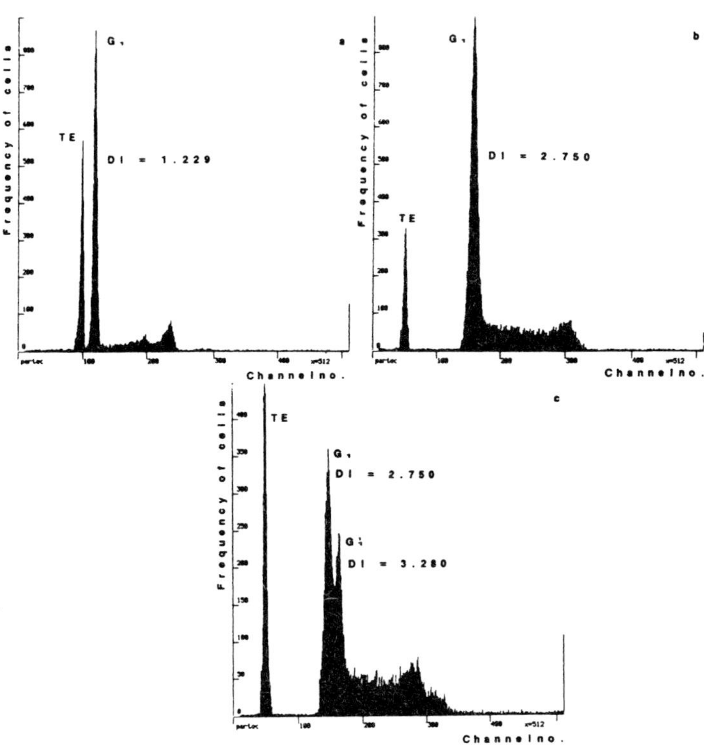

figure 1: Histograms of the DNA-content from different cell lines for DNA-index-determination (DI).
a) V79-cells, grown for 72h b) Hybridoma-cells (HBD1) at the beginning of a batch fermentation c) HBD1-cells, grown for 96h in a batch fermentation, showing a subpopulation with higher DNA-content.
TE = Trout erythrocytes, DI = DNA-index.

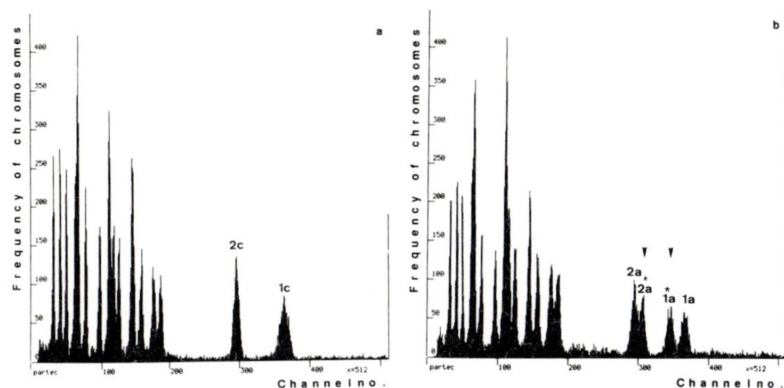

figure 2: Chromosome-histograms of V79-cells.
a) control-cells stored in liquid nitrogen,
b) cells, continuously cultured for 6 months in
   spinnerflasks
The arrows indicate new chromosome classes.
c = control, a = 6 months in culture, * = new
type of chromosome, 1 = chromosome number 1,
2 = chromosome number 2.

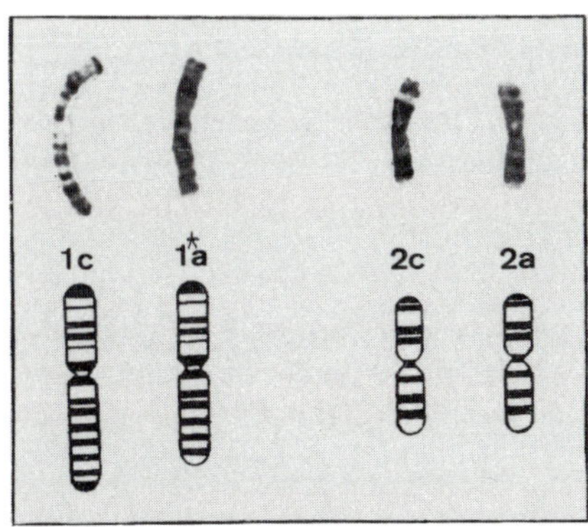

figure 3: G-banding of V79-chromosomes. 1c = chromosome 1
of the control population, 1*a = chromosome 1 of
the cells grown in suspension, which shows a
deviating banding pattern, 2c = chromosome 2 of
the control cells, 2a = chromosome 2 of the 6
months spinner culture, which shows no
alterations.

BIOMASS ESTIMATION IN ANCHORAGE-DEPENDENT ANIMAL CELL CULTURES.

Véronique CHOTTEAU[1]*, Luc FABRY[2], Serge LOWAGIE[1] and John WERENNE[1].

[1] Animal Cell Biotechnology Group, Faculty of Sciences, Université Libre de Bruxelles, Brussels, Belgium.

[2] Molecular and Cellular Biology Departement, Smith-Kline/Biologicals, Rixensart, Belgium.

ABSTRACT

In order to develop a reliable method to follow the growth of anchorage-dependent animal cell in bioreactor, we have measured a number of biological parameters (lactate, ammonia, glucose, amino acids, lactate dehydrogenase, ...) available in the culture medium and we have evaluated the possibility of using them for an on-line estimation of the cell biomass.

An approach which is derived from methods already established for microorganisms - the adaptive estimation - was compared to linear estimation to estimate on-line the cell biomass. This method was applied succesfully to VERO cells culture on microcarrier. These first results are therefore promising they are discussed.

key words : biomass estimation, anchorage-dependent animal cell culture, adaptive estimation, VERO cell culture / ammonia, lactate, glucose, amino acids, lactate dehydrogenase, aspartate aminotransferase.

INTRODUCTION

Biopharmaceutical productions rely more and more often on the use of anchorage-dependent animal cell cultures. The development of optimized process production would require control of several biological parameters, involved in cell metabolism, cell growth and biomass evaluation.

Although progresses have been made for a better monitoring of the physical and biochemical environment in bioreactors, no reliable and general method is yet available for on-line estimation of cell density and cell physiology (1). A good knowledge of the biomass concentration and of the cell physiology by on-line method is critical for an optimised production of a protein or vaccines by the cells.

The aim of the present study is to evaluate the variation of those parameters and to provide an automatisable method to estimate the cell biomass in culture.

As they are used for industrial production of vaccines, we selected VERO cell culture as a model for this approach. Metabolites and nutrients were measured (i.e. glucose, ammonia, lactic acid and amino acids) as well as some marker enzymes for cell physiology (i.e. lactate dehydrogenase, aspartate aminotransferase).

Given the physiological changes observed during cell growth, we have also analysed the activity of an intracellular enzyme (the 25Asynthetase) which could be involved in control of cell proliferation and virus replication (2,3).

MATERIAL AND METHODS

VERO cells (passage 138-150) were cultured in spinner flasks (250 ml) on Cytodex 1 (3 g/l) using M199 medium supplemented with foetal calf serum (10 % at the inoculation and 5 % for medium renewals) and antibiotics. Cell counting was performed with haematocytometer using crystal violet staining and biomass is expressed in cells per ml. Lactic acid and glucose were measured with a Yellow-Spring analyser (YSI 2000). Ammonia, lactate dehydrogenase and aspartate aminotransferase were determined with Sigma kits (n°170, 228 and 505 respectively). The amino acids analysis were performed by an ion exchange HPLC method.

The 25Asynthetase activity was measured according to Lowagie et al. (4). For this experiment VERO cells were cultivated in 600 ml spinner flask, each measure needing 100 ml culture sample.

RESULTS

Our first approach was to correlate the cell biomass to the ammonia, lactate or glucose concentration (A).

Furthermore, we attempted to establish the relationship between the concentration of lactate dehydrogenase and the cells released from the microcarriers in the supernatant during growth (B).

In a second, step we refined our results by applying algorithms of adaptive estimation as developed for microorganisms by Dochain and Bastin (C).

Finally, we studied the evolution of 25Asynthetase activity during the growth of VERO cells (D).

A) <u>Correlation between the biomass and the ammonia, lactate or glucose concentration</u>

A.1) A linear correlation was established in exponential growth phase using the ratio of the biomass concentration and the quantity of ammonia [1], lactate [2] or consumed glucose [3].

The results are summarized in table 1.

In these experiments, the glucose concentration was not limiting and cells grew exponentially (see also figure 1). Indeed, we observed that the production of lactate is similar for the different conditions reported above. However ammonia production depended on the culture conditions, i.e. medium change resulted in lower cumulative ammonia production. On the other hand, the specific consumption of glucose was increased when glucose was more abundant (i.e. in case of daily changes -a- and initial glucose concentration of 3 g/l -d-).

A.2) When glucose became limiting (i.e. after day four with an initial glucose concentration of 1 g/l, see figure 1), a reduction of the growth occured. The rate of production of ammonia remained unchanged while glucose concentration fell to near zero. On the contrary, lactic acid concentration fell off slowly, suggesting that lactic acid was further metabolised. At the end of the culture, cell lysis resulted in further accumulation of ammonia.

conditions	ammonia [1]	lactate [2]	consumed glucose [3]
	(million cell /ml) / mg ammonia	(million cell /ml) /g lactate	(million cell /ml) /g glucose
-a-	0.22 0.19	2.2 2.0	1.8 2.0
-b-	0.13 0.14	2.0 2.2	2.4 2.6
-c-	0.14	2.1	2.6
-d-	0.14	2.2	2.0

Table 1 : the mean of the ratio between the biomass concentration and the ammonia [1], lactate [2] or consumed glucose [3].
Following conditions were tested :
 -a- culture medium was renewed daily (with medium containing 1 g/l of glucose),
 -b- culture medium contained initially 1 g/l glucose,
 -c- culture medium contained initially 2 g/l glucose,
 -d- culture medium contained initially 3 g/l glucose.
(For -a- and -b- : data from duplicate experiment)
(In case of medium change, the cumulative concentrations were used.)

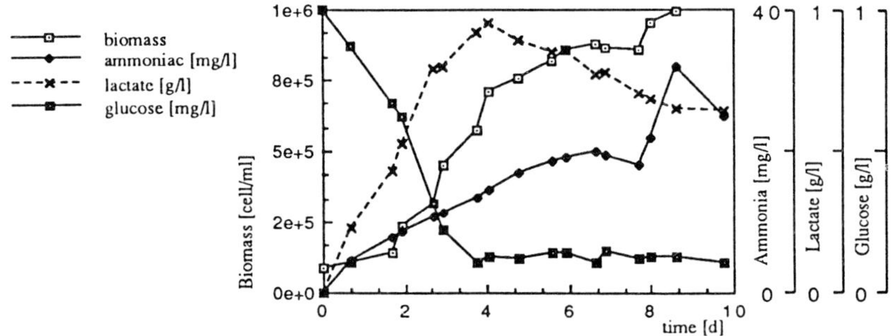

figure 1 : VERO cell culture, growth in experimental conditions -b- of table 1.

B) Correlation between some marker enzymes and the cells in the supernatant

A correlation between lactate dehydrogenase accumulation in the medium and detachment of cells from the microcarriers was observed. We found a good linear relationship between those parameters as mentionned earlier by Kim and Hu (5), suggesting that the cells released from the microcarriers are dying.

An other marker enzyme, the aspartate amino tranferase, was also tested in the supernatant; first results indicate that aspartate aminotransferase concentration increases as cells are released from microcarriers.

C) Application of an algorithm of adaptive estimation

The methods of adaptive estimation successfully developed by Dochain and Bastin successfully for bacteria or yeast (6,7) were applied to our data. These methods are based on mass balance (*)[1], i.e. the principle is to use an on-line measured parameter in an algorithm (*)[2] to estimate the biomass concentration. We compared this adaptive estimation to an other approach based on a simple linear fitting of a measured parameter to the biomass concentration.

Figures 2 and 3 present data obtained with serine and ammonia as measured parameters.

In this comparison, we found that the adaptive estimation gave a better fitting with the biomass measured than the linear estimation.

A same approach was also applied with lactate with similar results.

However, it was noticed that the choice of the design parameters is critical in the adaptive method for the convergence of the estimate to the measured biopmass. On the other hand, the behaviour of serine is highly dependent of culture conditions, so the choice of this parameter is not the most appropriate for the biomass estimation.

(*)1   Mass balance

$$\frac{dX}{dt} = \mu X; \qquad\qquad \frac{dS}{dt} = -\frac{1}{Y_s} \mu X + D (S_{in} - S);$$

$$\frac{dL}{dt} = \frac{1}{Y_l} \mu X - D L; \qquad\qquad \frac{dA}{dt} = \frac{1}{Y_a} \mu X - D A.$$

where X : biomass concentration; μ : specific growth rate, t : time, S : glucose concentration, S_{in} : influent glucose concentration, L : lactate concentration, A : ammonia concentration, Y_s, Y_l, Y_a : yield coefficient of the biomass to glucose, lactate or ammonia respectively, D = 'dilution rate' = influent flow rate / volume of the culture.

(*)2   The algorithm of adaptive biomass estimation of Dochain and Bastin (6) :

$$\frac{d\underline{P}}{dt} = \frac{1}{Y_p} R - D P + C_1 (P - \underline{P}); \qquad\qquad \frac{d\underline{X}}{dt} = R + C_3 (P - \underline{P});$$

$$\frac{d\underline{R}}{dt} = C_2 (P - \underline{P}).$$

where P : metabolite concentration (metabolite is ammonia, lactate, alanine or serine), $\underline{P}$: estimated metabolite concentration, $\underline{R}$: estimated auxiliar variable, $\underline{X}$: estimated biomass, C_1, C_2, C_3 : design parameters.

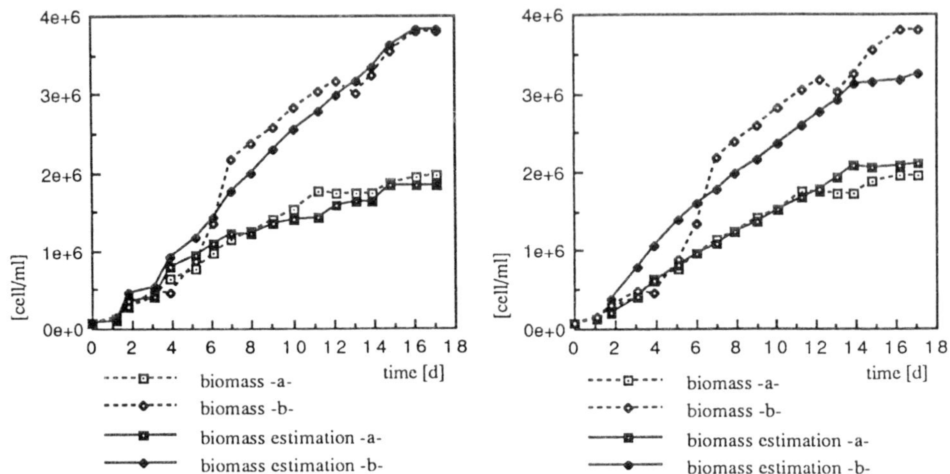

figure 2 : comparison of adaptive estimation (left) and linear estimation (right) of the biomass based on ammonia measurement (culture medium was 3 times renewed for -a- and daily renewed for -b-)

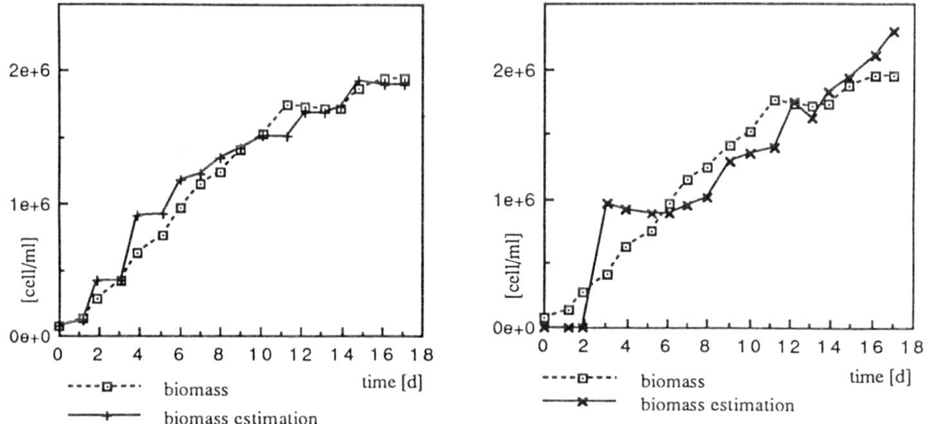

figure 3 : comparison of adaptive estimation (left) and linear estimation (right) of the biomass based on serine measurement (culture medium was 3 times renewed).

D) 25Asynthetase activity

We measured the activity of an intracellular enzyme involved in the antiviral and antiproliferative activity of interferon (3,2). The figure 4 represents the basal (non induced) activity of this enzyme in VERO cell culture. It was shown that this specific activity increased as the growth rate decreased.

The relationship between cells and viruses related to the interferon system could be different depending on the growth phase of the cells. This will be further investigated.

CONCLUSION

Using the linear fitting, we have shown that the ratio of the biomass to the lactate production is the same for different conditions during the exponential growth phase of VERO cell culture. This indicates that lactate could be used as a marker of biomass estimation in the exponential growth phase. On the other hand, the relationship between cell

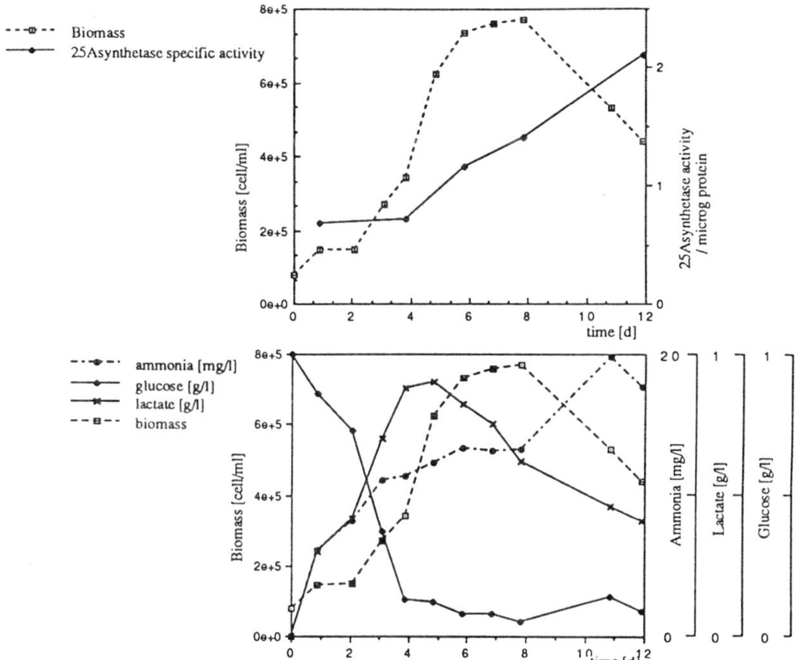

figure 4 : 25Asynthetase specific activity (non induced) of a VERO cell growth in experimental conditions -b- of table 1.

biomass and ammonia production does not depend on initial glucose concentration but varies according to the conditions of medium renewal.

The utilisation of a second approach - the adaptive estimation - showed that this method developed for microorganisms by Dochain and Bastin is, according to our first results, also valid for biomass estimation in animal cell culture. With this method, lactate and ammonia seem to be usefull parameters for biomass estimation of VERO cell culture on microcarriers.

ACKNOWLEDGMENTS

*Véronique CHOTTEAU and Serge LOWAGIE hold a Fellowship from the IRSIA (Institut pour l'Encouragement de la Recherche Scientifique dans l'Industrie et l'Agriculture).

REFERENCES

1. Merten, O.W., Animal Cell Biotechnology, 1988, 3, pp 76-140.
2. Rysiecki, G., Gewert, D.R. and Williams, B.R.G. J. Ifn. Res., 1989, 9, 649.
3. Van den Broecke, C., Plasman, O., Hauzeur, K., Goossens, A., Ligongo, G., Piscitelli, S. and Wérenne, J. in "The 25A system : Molecular and Clinical Aspects of the Interferon-regulated Pathway" Eds B.R.G. Williams and Silverman (A.R. Liss, Inc. N.Y.), 1985, pp 339-344.
4. Lowagie, S., Herrera, A., Sexsmith, E., Chotteau, V., Ledent, E., Williams, B. and Wérenne, J. in "Production of Biologicals from Animal Cells in Culture : Research, Development and Achievements" in press.
5 . Kim, K.-H. and Hu W.-S. Cytotechnology, 1989, 2, 135-140.
6. Dochain D. in "On-line Parameter Estimation, Adaptive State Estimation and Adaptive Control of Fermentation Processes" Ph. D. Thesis, 1986, University of Louvain, Louvain-la-Neuve, Belgium.
7. Bastin, G. and Dochain, D. Automatica, 1986, 22, pp 705-709.

<u>**Paper of Chotteau**</u>

Bushell: We would like to measure ammonia on-line because of its non-linear response; can you recommend a good method?

Chotteau: There are some new probes but the best method is to sample and make off-line determinations.

Bushell: How can you use such a method with an adaptive algorithm for control?

Chotteau: Our experiments were designed to select the best methods but we have not yet achieved the on-line determinations.

DYNAMIC ASSAY OF SYNTHETIC ACTIVITIES IN SINGLE HYBRIDOMA CELLS

Mohamed Al-Rubeai, S. Chalder, A.N. Emery

Centre for Biochemical Engineering, School of Chemical Engineering
University of Birmingham, Birmingham B15 2TT. U.K.

ABSTRACT :

Laser flow cytometry has been used to study hybridoma cell cultures. DNA
analysis provided relevant information on the influence of serum on
growth/death kinetics. Mitochondrial staining provided an indication of
cell viability which reflected metabolic and membrane integrity. Changes
in propidium iodide fluorescence and cell size distributions in cultures
subjected either to high speed mechanical agitation or to bubble sparging
conditions were found to be essentially different. Increasing
hydrodynamic forces enhanced the rate of efflux of fluorescein out of
hybridoma cells. No clear evidence was found of differential sensitivity
of cell cycle phases to hydrodynamic forces.

KEYWORDS :
Hybridoma; cell culture; flow cytometry; cell cycle; hydrodynamic stress.

INTRODUCTION :

Flow cytometry (FC) is a rapid and sensitive analytical technique with an
increasing number of applications.   The technique has the facility for
detection and quantitation of specific biochemical and morphological
changes in each cell within a population.   This may provide powerful
evidence in the assessment of effects of chemical and physical agents on
cellular activity and enable the identification and characterisation of
heterogeneous cell populations.   In large scale mammalian cell culture
there is growing interest in the use of FC for near on-line process
monitoring and control as it allows rapid rates of cell analysis with high
precision and sensitivity (1-5).   In hybridoma culture the technique can
be applied to the provision of additional and more accurate information
about the proliferative capacity of cultured cells (3) and on changes in
cell-specific productivity (5).

The quantification of cell viability is important in hybridoma culture but
there are several problems with the routine procedures used to assess
viability (e.g. counting following trypan blue staining) that limit their
usefulness. A major problem is that although cells which let in trypan
blue are considered and counted as dead, cells which do not let in trypan,
blue are not necessarily viable in the sense that they are metabolically
or reproductively inactive. Moreover the stain is only reliable when
applied to situations in which cells are killed by loss of integrity in
their plasma membranes. This situation is not necessarily applicable
where hydrodynamic and other stresses may affect cellular metabolism and
proliferation without disrupting the plasma membranes. The first purposes
of the present work are therefore to extend the applications of FC in

biotechnological processing using mammalian cells by: 1.   The use of mitochondrial staining with Rhodamine (R) 123 to provide an indication of cell viability which is based upon metabolic integrity as well as membrane integrity.   2.   Analysis of cell growth/death in an intense hydrodynamic environment by staining cells with fluorescein diacetate (FDA) and propidium iodide (PI).   Another area of interest which can be investigated by FC methods is the possible variation in the response of cells to hydrodynamic forces during different stages of the cell cycle. It might for example be postulated that cell death which is related to the action of intense hydrodynamic forces occurs when the newly dividing cell is prematurely separated during cytokinesis thereby.   Larger cells which correlate with G2 and M might then be expected to be more sensitive to hydrodynamic stress than others.   Other possibilities for using FC as a tool are in the assessment of the actions of induction agents and nutrients which affect cellular growth and viability and in monitoring the heterogeneity of immobilised cell populations.

MATERIALS AND METHODS :

Cells and Cell Culture Conditions : The following murine hybridomas were used in this work : TB/C3, producing antibodies to the C2 region of human IgG. PQXB 1/2 and PQXB 2/2 producing antibodies against paraquat, and EBNA, a non-producing cell line. All cell lines were grown in RPMI 1640 supplemented with either 5% or 10% newborn calf serum.

Hydrodynamic Effects : Cells were incubated at 3-5 x 10^5/ml in 50ml cultures agitated with magnetic followers (8mm x 35mm) in 100 ml Duran bottles (60mm in diameter).   Stirring was maintained at 200 rpm (low agitation condition) and 600 rpm (high agitation condition).   A bubble sparging condition was achieved by introducing air/CO_2 continuously at 100ml/min through a tube directly above a magnetic follower stirred at 200 rpm.   60 ppm of antifoam was added.

Flow Cytometric Analysis : FC analysis was made with a Becton-Dickinson FACS 440 using an argon laser with excitation at 488nm and filtering the emitted light with a 530nm filter for FITC, 620nm for PI, 514-540nm for FDA and R123 and 620nm for dual staining with PI and R123.

Staining Procedures :

Rhodamine 123 : At required times 3-5 x 10^5 cells/ml were incubated at 37 C in RPMI 1640 medium containing R123 (0.5 mg/ml) for 30 minutes. After incubation cells were collected by centrifugation and resuspended in PBS for FC analysis.   For dual staining PI was added to cells for 2 minutes prior to analysis of cells in order to stain dead cells only.
DNA Staining with Propidium Iodide : Cell samples were centrifuged, resuspended in cold 70% ethanol and fixed for > 1 hour.   The fixed cells were washed in PBS and DNA was specifically stained with 50 mg/ml PI for 15 minutes.
IgG Staining with FITC : Cells were fixed with cold 70% ethanol, centrifuged, washed with PBS, resuspended in 0.1 ml PBS and stained with FITC-conjugated goat anti-mouse (H+L) IgG (50 μl of 1:10 dilution) for 30 minutes at room temperature.   Cells were washed twice with 0.5% Tween 20 in PBS, resuspended in 0.5 ml PBS and placed on ice for subsequent FC.

RESULTS AND DISCUSSION :

Fig.1. shows the growth and viability of PQXB1/1 cell line in 1, 5 and 10% serum-supplemented (SS) medium. The viable cell number in 1% SS culture remained unchanged for 110 hr, but the viability was significantly decreased. It could be suggested that even, when the cells are deprived of sufficient serum to support an observed increase in cell number, the cells remain in active division, though at a slow rate. This interpretation is supported by the results from FC presented in Fig.2. Each spectrum of Fig.2. is a DNA histogram whose dominant feature is the G_1 peak. Cells with the DNA content intermediate between that of G_1 and G_2 are representative of the S phase while the smaller peak to the left represents cells with the DNA content of the late S, G_2 and M part of the cell cycle. Although an apparent similarity is noted between the histograms for 10, 5 and 1% SS cultures, a significant decrease during late exponential and decline phases in S and G_2 cells is observed in 10% SS culture and a slightly similar decrease but not as distinct occurred in 5% SS culture. In contrast to this, in 1% SS culture the relative cell numbers in S and G_2 are essentially unchanged, indicating that cells remain in active division but, due to an equal rate of cell death, the net apparent growth rate remains zero.

In Fig.3., the results of staining fixed cells of TB/C3 with goat anti-mouse IgG are shown. The modal fluorescence intensity decreases with the duration of culture, whereas the overall heterogeneity remains unchanged. Therefore, the reduction in fluorescence staining intensity does not reflect the appearance of population bimodalism (5) but may be associated with the gradual loss of cell synthetic or/and IgG storage capability.

The batch cell growth of the 4 cell lines shown in Fig.4a illustrates widely varying growth curves. PQXB 1/2 and PQXB 2/2 proliferated faster than TB/C3 and EBNA (inoculated at lower cell density) reaching at day 2 of cultivation 1.4 and 1 x 10^6/ml respectively compared to 6.4 and 3.8 x 10^5/ml for TB/C3 and EBNA respectively. Nonetheless the measurements of R123 fluorescence intensity (Fig.4b) showed a consistant and general decrease with time for the 4 cell lines. Assuming that R123 fluorescence intensity reflects changes in mitochondrial transmembrane potential which are linked to the processes of energy metabolism (6), the results indicate that such decrease in the dye uptake reflect the deteriorating metabolic and membrane integrity as the cultures grow old, independantly of the final cell number.

The data in Table 1 shows that trypan blue staining typically gives an exaggerated estimate of viability. Dead cells may undergo lysis and thus are not included in the count when trypan blue is used. However in R123-P1 staining the nuclei of the lysed cells are stained with PI and can still be counted. It could be argued that PI can stain fragmented nuclei or chromosomal fragments. These fragments, can be removed from analysis by setting window boundaries to provide a count of "real" cells only.

In Fig.5. data on viability and cell size distributions are presented for TB/C3 cells subjected to two hours of either high speed agitation (vortexing was observed) or bubble sparging. Viable cell numbers were reduced to 14% and 28% of the control value (at low speed agitation) respectively. In contrast to the effect of high speed agitation, bubble sparging had no effect on viability as measured by the trypan blue method. However, the light scattering histograms indicated that the mean relative "cell" size was more reduced by sparging than agitation and was characterised by the presence of a larger peak of small-sized cellular debris. The scattergram of PI fluorescence and "cell" size clearly showed that sparging had not only led to lysis of the cells but also their total destruction. As PI specifically stains DNA, the scattergram also showed the complete absence of intact or moderately damaged nuclei which may reflect a different mechanism of damage from that of high speed agitation. In the latter case cells death was associated with loss of plasma membrane integrity. Once membrane damage existed, it appeared that secondary injury was inflicted on the cytoplasmic matrix and organelles, thus leading to metabolic death. On the other hand in sparging condition cells were destroyed by catastrophic rupturing of their plasma membranes and internal structures and even shearing of DNA. It appeared that the nuclei may be ruptured at the same time as the plasma membranes. Fig.6 shows the efflux of fluorescein out of TB/C3 cells. The rate of efflux was increased by high agitation. The nature of membrane damage by hydrodynamic forces cannot be elucidated from measurements of efflux only; however, it is very likely that the measured increase in efflux is due to an increase in leakage and passive transport caused by the changes of the overall state of the plasma membrane. The relative rates of efflux of fluorescein as a function of the stress level are still needed to understand the type of damage caused by hydrodynamic forces.

The response of cells to hydrodynamic forces during different stages of the cell cycle was studied with the aid of FC and no clear evidence found of differential sensitivity . First, we observed normal cell cycle distribution in a population of cells that had died as a result of high agitation. Next, we exposed cells to a constant rate of sparging and analysed them at various time intervals. The proportion of cells in G2,M, S and G1, as well as cell sizes remained constant during the 105 minutes of sparging, although the cell number was reduced during this time by 28%. Finally, we subjected the cells to various rates of sparging for a constant time. Again we failed to see any changes in the proportion of the surviving cells in each cycle phase, in-spite of a 51% reduction in cell number under the most extreme condition tested.

ACKNOWLEDGEMENTS

We gratefully acknowledge the help of R. Bird and A. Milner for the FACS analysis. We thank ICI plc for the supply of PQXB hybridomas.

REFERENCES

1 Altshuler, G.L., Dilwith, R., Sowek, J. and Belfort, G. Biotechnol. Bioeng. Symp. 1986, 17, 725
2 Schliermann, M., Beckers, C. and Miltenburger, H.G. Develop. Biol. Standard. 1987, 66, 101
3 Kloppinger, M., Fertig, G., Fraune, E. and Miltenburger, H.G. In : Advances in Animal Cell Biology and Technology for Bioprocesses, Eds. Spier, R. et al., 1989. Butterworth, pp 125-128
4 Al-Rubeai, M., Rookes, S. and Emery A.N. Ibid, pp 241-245
5 Rupp, R.G., Tahe, E. and Peterson, L. Ibid, pp 129-131
6 Martinez, A., Vigil, A. and Vila, J.C. Exp. Cell Res. 1986, 164, 551

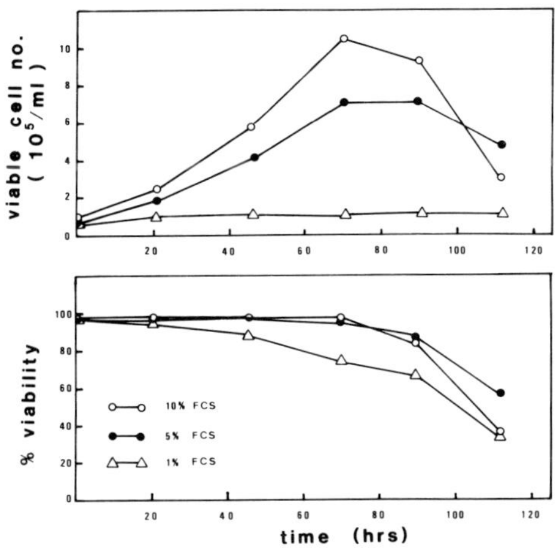

Fig.1. Growth of PQXB1/2 hybridoma cells

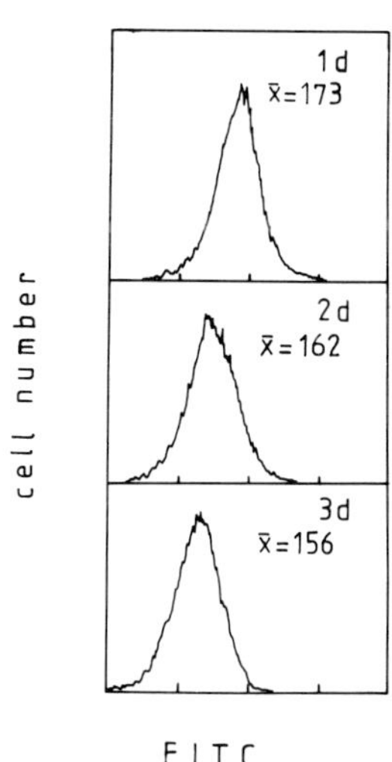

Fig.3. IgG distribution of hybridoma cells at different time of batch cultivation

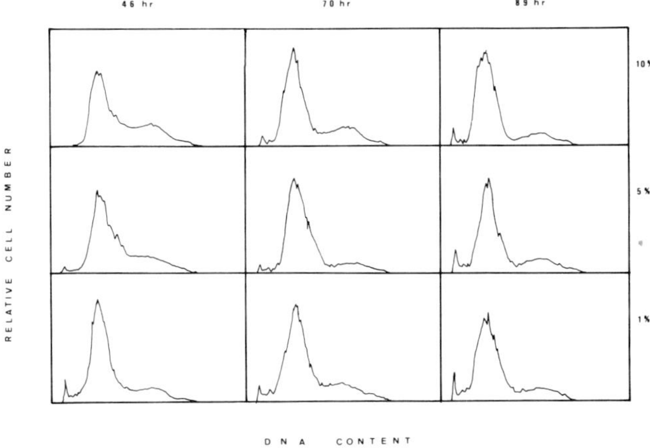

Fig.2. DNA distributions of cells grown in different serum concentrations

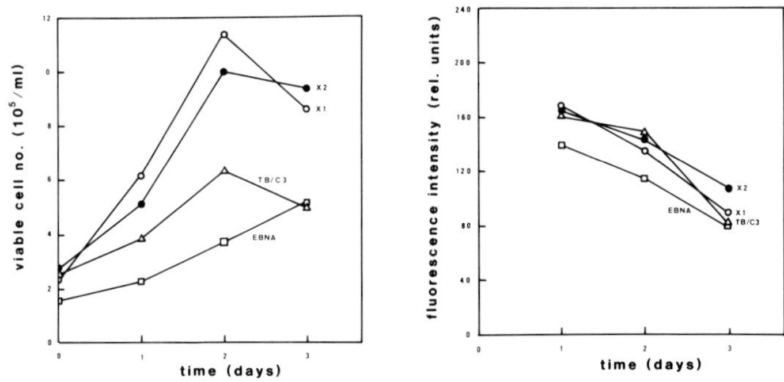

Fig.4.a. Growth of 4 hybridoma cell lines b.R123 fluorescence intensity of 4 cell lines during batch cultivation

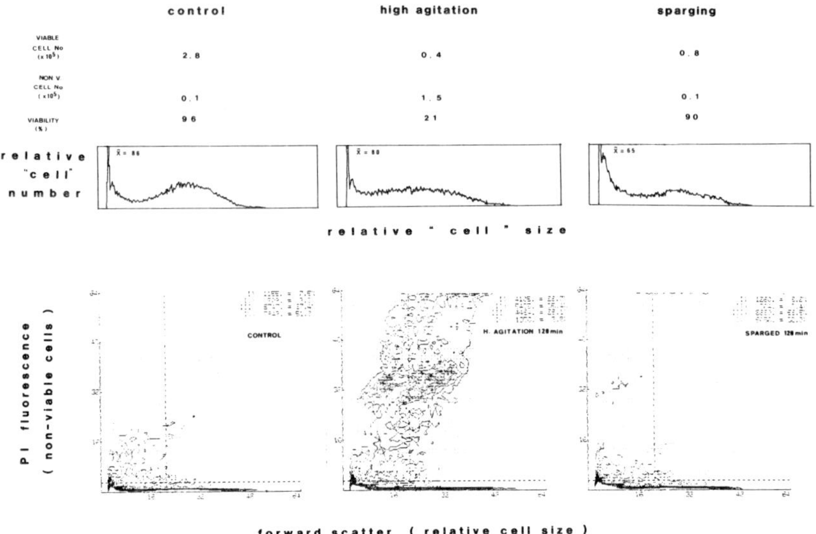

Fig. 5. Effect of high agitation and sparging on growth/death and cell size distributions

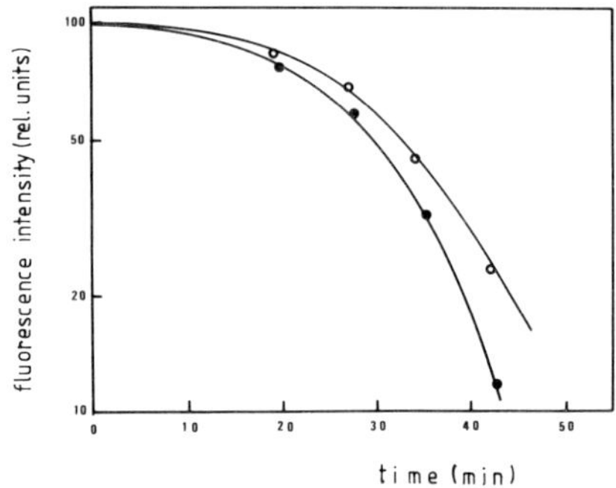

Fig. 6. Efflux of fluorescein out of hybridoma cells, open circles: low agitation, closed circles: high agitation

Table 1.
Comparison of cell viability (%) determined by trypan blue or rhodamine 123 – propidium iodide

Cell line & incubation time (d)	trypan blue	Rhod(+) PI(−)
TBC3		
2	97	77
3	76	44.5
PQX1		
2	91	77
3	73	49
PQX2		
2	96	86
3	83	58
EBNA		
2	91	59.9
3	79	42.6

<u>Paper of Al-Rubeai</u>

Litwin: I always thought living cells were more interesting
                than dead cells but Dr. Al-Rubeai has raised the
                interesting question of how do we define a viable cell.
                We need better methods to define the living cell than
                we need to define an uninteresting dead cell.

Al-Rubeai: To understand living cells we need to understand the
                process of death. We need better definition of living
                cells in terms of proliferation and productive
                capacity. A metabolically inactive cell is dead as far
                as a process technologist is concerned so we need to
                define viability in terms of biosynthetic capability.

RAPID MONITORING OF MONOCLONAL ANTIBODIES IN CELL CULTURE MEDIA BY HIGH PERFORMANCE LIQUID AFFINITY CHROMATOGRAPHY (HPLAC)

Ann Holmberg[1], Sten Ohlson[2], Torgny Lundgren[3]

[1] HyClone AB, S-223 70 Lund, Sweden
[2] HyClone Laboratories Inc, 1725 South State Highway, Logan, Utah 84321, USA
[3] Monocarb AB, S-223 70 Lund, Sweden

ABSTRACT

The ProAnaMabs^{TM} system is an efficient chromatographic monitoring device to follow the production of a monoclonal antibody all the way from fermentation medium through downstream processing to finished product. This new technology is based on an affinity HPLC column which contains a bacterial immunoglobulin receptor capable of recognizing most monoclonal antibodies in a rapid accurate and cost effective manner. In addition the ProAnaMabs^{TM} will give valuable information about the purity status of the processed product.

INTRODUCTION

The quantitative detection and characterization of monoclonal antibodies has become an area of considerable interest to many biotechnology companies. The antibodies are often present in complex mixtures such as cell culture media which, up till now, has made rapid detection difficult.

BASIC FEATURES OF THE PROANAMABS

ProAnaMabs is a complete set-up for monitoring of monoclonal antibodies. The core of the system is an HPLAC column containing a proprietory bacterial Fc-receptor covalently attached to the SelectiSpher^{TM} silica support. Together with special buffers and standards it can be used for quantitative analysis of most IgG from various species and subclasses. The basic features of this technique are illustrated in Fig. 1, where mouse monoclonal IgG1 in a cell culture broth was bound specifically by the ProAnaMabs column and, after the washing of contaminants (i.e. cell culture components) the

IgG1 was eluted in a pure form and monitored by UV
absorption.

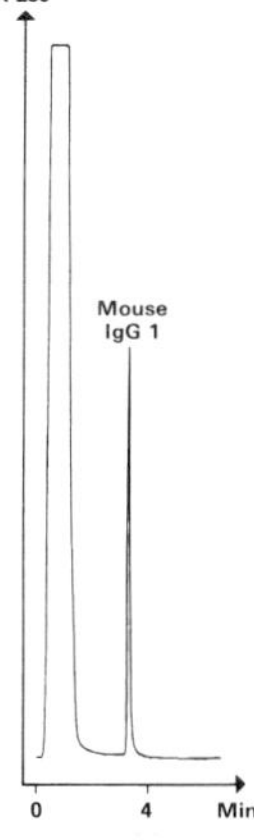

Figure 1. Analysis of monoclonal antibodies
(murine IgG1) in cell culture supernatant
using the ProAnaMabs.

Conditions:	Binding Buffer	0-2 min
	Elution Buffer	2-4 min
Flow rate:	2 ml/min	0-2 min
	3 ml/min	2-4 min
Injection:	1 ml cell culture supernatant	
Detection:	280 nm	
Temperature:	23°C	

The recovery of various IgG from different species was
quantitative (95-100%). The ProAnaMabs system featured high
precision when intra and interassay variations were estimated
by repeated measurements of mouse monoclonal IgG1 in cell
culture fluid. The within day variations were CV = 1-3 % and
the day-to-day variations were CV = 3-7 %. The detection
limit for the system (1-5 ug with UV detection at 280 nm) is
adequate for most purposes.
A number of different monoclonal antibodies of different
species and subclasses were evaluated as to their response
and retention in the ProAnaMabs system (4). They gave only
minor variations (CV=1-5%) in peak area, probably reflecting
the minor variation in absorbtion coefficient of the
antibodies.
When a new analysis method is on trial, it has to be
validated against established technologies such as in this
case ELISA, As a critical test of ProAnaMabs, a variety of
samples from a production run including various stages of
purification were analyzed in a comparative study with ELISA
(4). An excellent correlation with a correlation coefficient
of 0.997 was obtained.

MONITORING DURING PRODUCTION AND DOWNSTREAM PROCESSING

The ProAnaMabs was used to monitor the level of monoclonal
antibodies during a production. The antibodies were produced
in roller bottles. Samples were extracted from one bottle
twice a day and analyzed with regards to IgG concentration
(ProAnaMabs), cell density and viability.
The production was terminated after 10 days as the cell
viability level reached 10 %. In Fig.2 it can be seen that
the IgG concentration reached its maximum after 6 days and

subsequently the production could have been terminated at
that time.

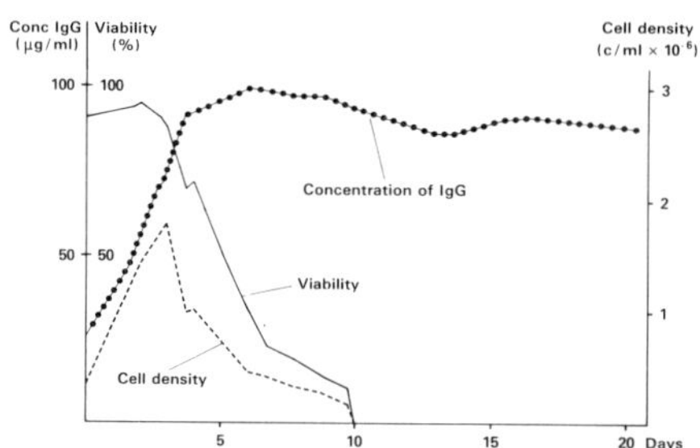

Figure 2. Monitoring of monoclonal antibody (murine IgG1) concentration, cell density and viability during production. The Igg concentration was monitored with ProAnaMabs.

As shown in Fig. 1, ProAnaMabs gives to peaks; one front peak
illustrating the non-retarded substances which do not have
any affinity for the the Fc-binding receptor and an elution
peak containing the pure antibody. This means that it is
possible to get two pieces of information from one
chromatogram, concentration and purity of the antibody.
ProAnaMabs was used during downstream processing, both for
following the antibody concentration and determining the
purity of the preparation (5).

CONCLUSIONS

The ProAnaMabs system has the ability to rapidly quantify
most IgG species in various intermediate production stages,
ranging from cell culture fluid to finished product. It
offers rapid analysis, adequate response, high
reproducibility and excellent recovery in both buffers and
media. The ProAnaMabs system is well adapted for process
control of monoclonal IgG production. It is a useful tool in
downstream processing since it gives information not only of
antibody concentration but also on purity.

REFERENCES

1. Ohlson, S., Hansson, L., Larsson, P.O. and Mosbach, K.,
FEBS Lett., 1978, 93, 5

2. Larsson, P.O., Glad, M., Hansson, L., Månsson, M.O.,
Ohlson, S. and Mosbach, K., Adv. Chrom., 1983, 21, 41

3. Ohlson, S., Hansson, L., Glad, M., Mosbach, K., and
Larsson, P.O., TIBTECH, 1989, 7, 179

4. Tedesco, J.L., Ohlson, S., Holmberg, A., and Rupp, R.,
BioChrom., 1989, 4, 216

5. Ohlson, S., Holmberg A., Lundgren, T., Int. Lab, In
press

APPLICATION OF THE PCFIA TO RAPID OFF-LINE PROCESS MONITORING

E. JERVIS, D.W. LEE, and D.G.KILBURN, Biotechnology Laboratory, University of British Columbia, Vancouver, B.C., Canada. V6T 1W5

ABSTRACT

The Particle Concentration Fluorescence Immunoassay (PCFIA) technique provides a sensitive and rapid method for the quantification of specific proteins in mammalian cell culture systems. We have used this technique to measure cell-associated and supernatant concentrations of product: either monoclonal antibody from hybridoma cells or recombinant human transferrin from stably transfected BHK cells. The cell associated concentration of these proteins correlates with their cell-specific production rate. Total assay times in the order of 5-10 min can be achieved making it feasible to use this technique for process monitoring and control. This offers a powerful new technique for feedback control to optimize cell productivity.

INTRODUCTION

Most methods, such as ELISA, presently used for quantifying protein concentration require relatively long assay times. Analysis turnaround time therefore, makes these techniques inappropriate for investigating dynamic systems when feedback interaction is desired. Furthermore, the formulation of control models or laws for bioprocesses is restricted because of this long measurement time. The Particle Concentration Fluorescence Immunoassay (PCFIA) uses submicron spheres as the capture solid phase, greatly increasing the available surface area to volume ratio hence reducing the required incubation time[1]. A rapid off-line method using the PCFIA system is presented in which repeated assays were used to monitor supernate and cell-associated protein products during batch cell cultures.

METHODS AND MATERIALS

Cell Line

The transformed BHK cell line produces human transferrin half-molecules[2]. The BHK cells express transferrin under the control of the metallothionein (MT-1) promoter. Cells were maintained in DMEM medium with 5% FCS in 80 cm^2 Nunclon T-flasks at 37°C. Cell concentrations were determined using a hemocytometer. Trypan blue exclusion was used for determining cell viability. Cells in late exponential phase (i.e. 7-9 x10^5 cell/ml) were used to seed individual 250 mL Bellco spinner flasks.

PCFIA

Analyte concentrations in the supernate and cell extract samples prepared from detergent lysed cells (0.1% Triton X-100, Boehringer Mannheim) were determined using the Pandex FCA. Briefly, 20 μL of samples, standards or controls at appropriate dilutions, were added to wells in the special FCA 96-well plate. Ten wells were used per process measurement (4 standards, 2 controls and two each of supernate and intracellular samples), permitting a single plate to be used for 9 process measurements. Standards at .25, .15, .1, and .05 μg/mL were used for calibration curve preparation. 20 μL of the appropriate capture Ab coated on polystyrene spheres (0.7 μM @ 0.25% v/v, Baxter/Pandex Healthcare Corp.) was added to each well containing a sample. The samples were gently mixed and incubated at room temperature (21°C). Following the first incubation, 20 μL of appropriate secondary Ab-FITC conjugate (ICN, Costa Mesa, CA) was added to each sample and incubated, at room temperature in the dark, after gentle mixing. The plate was then evacuated using the Pandex FCA. Samples in wells were washed three times with PBS and read using the 485/535 filter pair at 25X gain.

RESULTS AND DISCUSSION

The efficiency of this assay with respect to calibration and sample throughput was examined. A power transformed, linear calibration model is used to minimize standard curve sample requirements (see y-axis of figure 1, Fluorescence$^{1.5}$). The power transform model is developed using maximum likelyhood analysis by pooling results obtained over several assays. This approach has two main advantages. Firstly, the calibration models developed become relatively insensitive to chance peculiarities in any single analysis. Secondly, assay quality control becomes an integral part of the calibration process. For example, when results are pooled to determine the appropriate transform value, trends or drifts in calibration become quite evident through analysis of residuals.

The Effect of Incubation time

The linear range and sample throughput of the assay using various incubation time schedules was investigated. Figure 1 shows the effect of incubation time on calibration linearity and assay sensitivity (i.e. slope). Generally it was found that the assay sensitivity increased with increased incubation time. However, the minimum required incubation times varies depending upon analyte and antibody used. Results demonstrate that acceptable assay performance could be obtained with a total incubation time of six minutes.

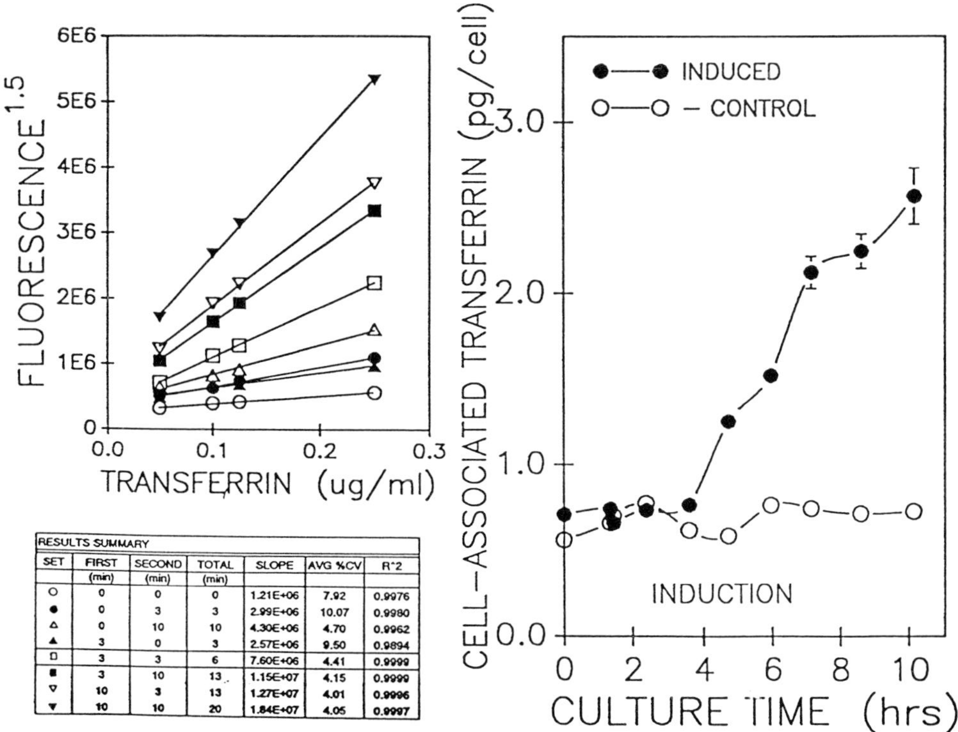

RESULTS SUMMARY						
SET	FIRST (min)	SECOND (min)	TOTAL (min)	SLOPE	AVG %CV	R^2
O	0	0	0	1.21E+06	7.92	0.9976
●	0	3	3	2.99E+06	10.07	0.9980
△	0	10	10	4.30E+06	4.70	0.9962
▲	3	0	3	2.57E+06	9.50	0.9894
□	3	3	6	7.60E+06	4.41	0.9999
■	3	10	13	1.15E+07	4.15	0.9999
▽	10	3	13	1.27E+07	4.01	0.9996
▼	10	10	20	1.84E+07	4.05	0.9997

Figure 1- The effect of incubation time on the assay sensitivity

Figure 2- The effect of zinc addition on cell-associated transferrin concentration

Induction of MT-1 promoter with $ZnSO_4$

The mouse metallothionein (MT-1) promoter is known to be activated by the presence of heavy metals[3]. Sterile $ZnSO_4$ solution was added to the suspended BHK cells in one spinner flask to induce expression of the human transferrin gene. The zinc concentration was then maintained at 60 μM throughout the experiment. The short analysis turnaround time (less than 25 min including cell lysis and sample preparation) permits the assay system used to effectively track the increase of the transferrin product in the intracellular protein pool. Figure 2 shows the induction time course for the recombinant BHK cells in suspension.

CONCLUSION

The successful engineering of bioreactor systems requires the application of improved and rapid sensing techniques for the monitoring of specific biomolecules. With the rapid assay presented, a measure of the cell culture's productivity was available within 25 minutes. The rapid sample throughput of the PCFIA offers a unique opportunity for dynamic optimization and feedback control of culture conditions for maximum fermenter productivity.

ACKNOWLEDGEMENTS

This work was supported by grants from the British Columbia Science and Technology Development Fund and the British Columbia Foundation for Non-animal Research.

REFERENCES

(1) Jolley, M.E, Wang, C.J., Ekenberg, S.J., Zuelke, M.S., and Kelso, D.M., Particle Concentration Fluorescence Immunoassay (PCFIA): a New, Rapid, Immunoassay Technique with High Sensitivity, J. Immunological Methods, 1984, 67, 21.

(2) Funk, W.D., MacGillivray, T.A., Mason, A.B., Brown, S.A., and Woodworth, R.C., Expression of the Amino-Terminal Half-Molecule of Human Serum Transferrin in Culture Cells and Characterization of the Recombinant Protein, Biochemistry, 1990, 29, 1654.

(3) Kelder, B., Chen, H., and Kopchick, J., Activation of the Mouse Metallothionein-I Promoter in Transiently Transfected Avian Cells, Gene, 1989, 76, 75.

Section 8
Kinetics and modelling

MATHEMATICAL ESTIMATOR FOR THE EVALUATION OF CELL DENSITY AND MEDIUM COMPOSITION IN HYBRIDOMA CULTURES.

E. Mailly, C. Fonteix, J.M. Engasser, A. Marc

Laboratoire des Sciences du Génie Chimique, CNRS, ENSIC-INPL, BP451, 54001 Nancy Cedex, France

ABSTRACT

An estimation technique has been developped for the evaluation of the medium composition (concentrations of cells, nutrients, products) using a kinetic model for mammalian cells coupled to a data filtering procedure. A single experimental measurement, for instance the ammonia concentration, was found sufficient to obtain good evaluations of the other main medium components both in batch and continuous cultures of hybridoma cells.

INTRODUCTION

Only very few sensors are presently available for the on-line monitoring of bioreactors for mammalian or microbial cell cultures. This represents the main limitations for computer control of biological processes.

Recently, new computational techniques have been developped for the control of bioreactors (1). Based on the use of kinetic models and filtering techniques, they are able to estimate the concentrations of cells, substrates and metabolites from only a limited number of experimental measurements. With the general objective of the optimization of monoclonal antibodies production, this study aims at selecting a convenient mathematical tool for this purpose.

MATERIAL AND METHODS

CELL CULTURE :
Cell line : Murine hybridoma producing IgG1 monoclonal antibodies.
Culture medium : RPMI 1640 (Intermed, France) with 5% FCS (Biosys, France) and 1-2 mM Glutamine (Intermed).
Bioreactor : Hybridomas are cultivated in a 2 l reactor (Biolafitte, France)
Analytical methods : NH_4^+ is measured with a NH_3 electrode (Orion). Monoclonal antibodies are determined by an ELISA method. Glucose is measured by an enzymatic method (Boehringer). Cell count and viability are determined using the Trypan blue dye exclusion procedure.

MATHEMATICAL ESTIMATOR :
The estimator procedure is adapted from techniques previously developped for microbial fermentations (2,3). It entails a kinetic model for hybridoma cultures capable of simulating cell growth and death, glucose and glutamine consumptions, and lactate, ammonia and antibodies productions (4). For a given initial medium composition and inoculum, the model predicts the time variation of the different concentrations in the medium. Because of approximations in the model and uncertainties in the initial medium composition and cell physiological state, these predictions are corrected by a numerical filtering technique : for one or several species, the actual concentration has to be measured, and the estimation of the concentrations of all the species is then

corrected by a term proportional to the difference between the estimated and the actually measured values. The filtering technique used is the Extended Kalman Filter (EKF) suited for non linear kinetic models.

RESULTS AND DISCUSSION

The estimator technique has been validated on batch and continuous hybridoma cultures using the measurement of a single species, ammonia, to correct the model estimation. The procedure is performed off-line by using previously obtained experimental results.

Figure 1 shows the experimentally determined and the estimated values of the cellular density and the antibody concentration during a batch hybridoma culture, with estimation corrections based on the measurement of the ammonia concentration every two hours. Two situations are illustrated with respect to the initial evaluation of the cell density : one with a correct initialization, another with a 40% initial error. In both cases good estimations of medium composition are provided by the estimator.

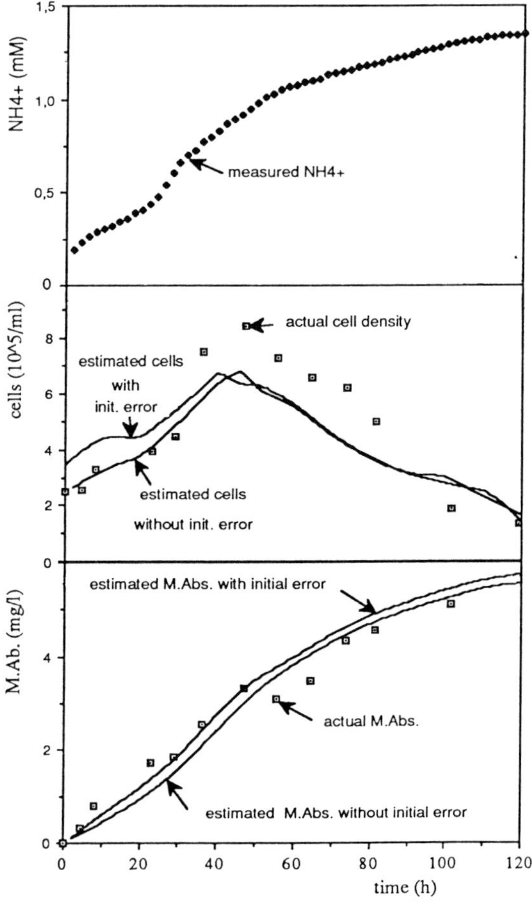

Figure 1 : *Cell density and M.Ab. estimation by Extended Kalman Filtering with and without initial error on cell count.*

Figure 2 presents the prediction capacity of the estimator for a continuous hybridoma culture operated at three consecutive dilution rates. Again using only the measurement of ammonia concentration every two hours, the time variation of the cell density and the residual glucose concentration is satisfactory evaluated.

REFERENCES

1- Bellgardt, K.H. ; Meyer,H.D. ; Kuhlmann,W ; Schügerl,K. ; Thoma, M. ; On line estimation of biomass and fermentation parameters by a Kalman-filter during a cultivation of *Saccharomyces cerevisiae*; in : 3^d E.C.B., München, Verlag Chemie 1984, 2,607-615

2- Ghoul,M. ; PhD thesis; Cinétique, modélisation, contrôle et conduite automatique de la fermentation de *Candida utilis* ; 1983, INPL, France.

3- Dantigny,P ; PhD thesis; Cinétique, modélisation de la croissance de *Saccharomyces cerevisiae* ,commandes non-linéaires de type L/A ; 1989, INPL, France.

4- Goergen, J.L. ; Martial,A. ; Marc,A. ; Engasser,J.M. ; A kinetic model for the influence of serum in batch and continuous hybridoma cultures. in: Proceedings of the ESACT 10th meeting, Avignon 1990.

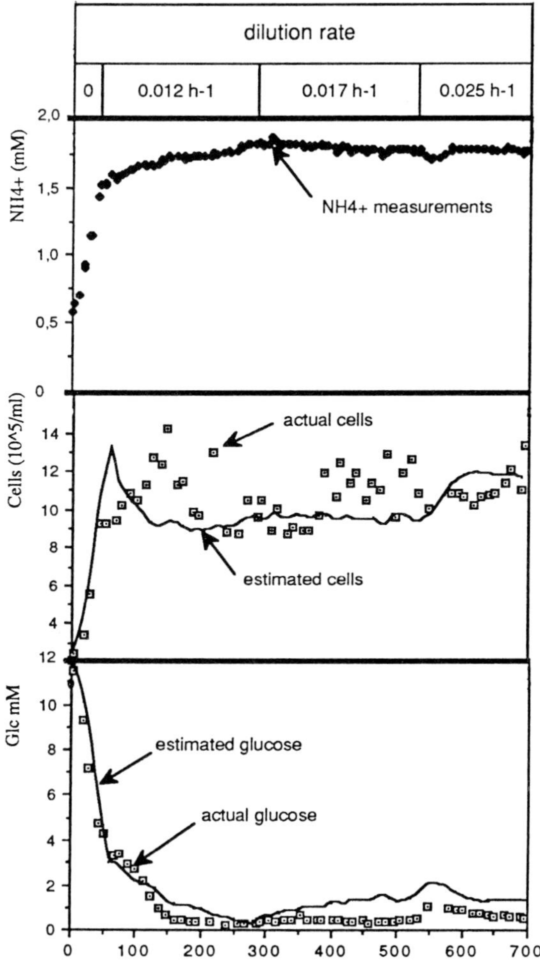

Figure 2 : *Cell density and Glucose estimation by Extended Kalman Filtering in continuous hybridoma culture.*

KINETIC EFFECTS OF GROWTH FACTORS ON BATCH AND CONTINUOUS HYBRIDOMA CULTURES

A.MARTIAL[1], P.NABET[2], J.M.ENGASSER[1] and A.MARC[1]

1 Laboratoire des Sciences du Génie Chimique, CNRS-ENSIC-INPL, BP 451, F-54001 NANCY
2 Laboratoire de Chimie Biologique, Université Nancy 1, BP 184, F-54505 VANDOEUVRE

ABSTRACT

In batch and continuous hybridoma cultures fed with a serum-free medium, insulin is consumed, ascorbic acid produced, whereas the level of transferrin remains constant. Insulin is inhibitory to cell growth above 5 mg/L. Continuous cultures can be maintained at a relatively high density (2 $\times 10^6$ cells/mL) in the absence of added insulin.

INTRODUCTION

Serum-free media are increasingly used for the culture of mammalian cells in bioreactors[1-2]. In addition to the basal components - sugars, amino acids, vitamins, minerals - they may contain different amounts of growth factors, hormones, lipids and other functional proteins[3-4]. For the optimization of serum-free media very few data are presently available concerning the rate of utilization of these components by the cells and their kinetic influence on cell growth and protein production. This study presents kinetic results for the time variation of insulin, transferrin, ascorbic acid during batch and continuous cultures of hybridoma. It also investigates the influence of insulin concentration on the production of cells and antibodies.

MATERIAL AND METHODS

Inoculation conditions

Cell line: A mouse hybridoma cell secreting IgG1 monoclonal antibody.
Culture conditions: Batch: 250mL spinner flasks (Techne); Continuous: 2L stirred reactor (Biolafitte) at pH 7, D.O. 40% of air saturation.
Medium: Basal medium: 50% IMDM +50% Ham F12 with 15-20mM glucose , 4mM glutamine (Intermed S.A.); Supplements: 20-25mg/L insulin, 30mg/L transferrin, 0.2% w/v polyethylene glycol, 20μM aminoethanol, 50μM ß mercapthoethanol, 12nM sodium selenite, 20mg/L ascorbic acid, 20ml/L of liposomes containing cholesterol, oleic acid, L α phosphatidylcholine dipalmitoyl and BSA 200mg/L (Sigma).

Analytical methods: Cell count and viability are determined by the Trypan Blue dye exclusion method using an haemocytometer. MAb concentration is evaluated by an ELISA test. Insulin concentration is determined with a radioimmunoassay kit (CIS Bioindustries) (standard deviation less than 15-20%; linearity from 1-20μg/L; insulin stability in cell-free medium at 37°C during 7 days). Ascorbic acid assay is based on its oxydation with copper in the presence of 2-4DNPH (linearity from 2 to 25mg/L; standard deviation less than 10%). Transferrin concentration is determined by a nephelemetric method (linearity from 2 to 38mg/L; standard deviation less than 10%).

RESULTS AND DISCUSSION

When the hybridoma are cultivated batchwise on the defined serum-free medium the time variations of the concentrations of cells, antibodies, insulin transferrin and ascorbic acid are shown in Fig1. Cells inoculated at 2.10^5 cells/mL grow during the 80 first hours until reaching a maximal density of about 10^6 cells/mL. The antibody concentration increases during cells growth and reach a plateau in the cellular decline phase. Very different kinetics are observed from the three investigated medium components. The concentration of insulin decreases steadily during the whole culture from an initial 25 mg/L to a final level of 5 mg/L, which corresponds to an average insulin consumption rate around 0.15 mg/10^9 cells.hour. The level of transferrin, on the contrary, remains constant until the end of the culture. Whereas the concentration of ascorbic acid increases both during the cellular growth and decline phase from about 10 to 15 mg/L.

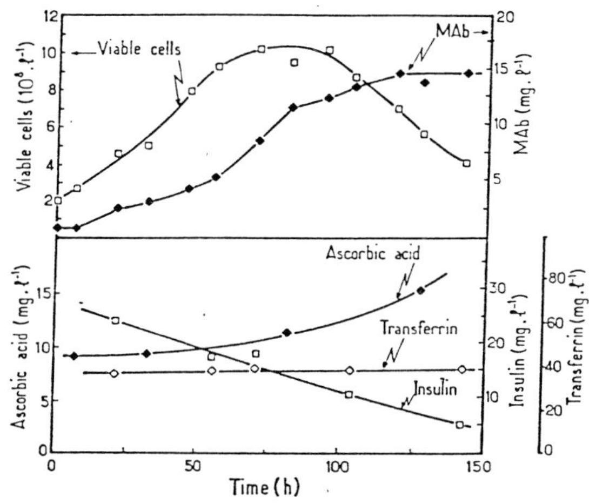

Fig1: Evolution with time of cells, MAb, ascorbic acid, transferrin and insulin concentrations during a batch hybridoma culture.

The kinetics of cell growth and metabolism were also investigated during a continuous culture maintained at a dilution rate of $0.017h^{-1}$ for 90 days (Fig 2). After an initial batch culture lasting 180 hours, the reactor is continuously fed with the serum-free medium containing constant concentrations of transferrin and ascorbic acid but varying ,concentrations of insulin. When insulin is initially maintained at 30 mg/L a steady-state is reached with 1.10^6 cells/mL, 11 mg antibodies /L and 22 mg insulin /L. As previously observed in the batch culture, insulin is consumed, ascorbic acid is produced (15 mg/L in the feed, 20 mg/L in the outlet), whereas the level of transferrin remains constant. The specific consumption rate of insulin amounts to 0.15 mg/10^9 cells.h, which is comparable to the value determined in the batch culture.

In order to determine the influence of insulin on the cellular kinetics, after 530 hours the insulin concentration in the feed is stepwise decreased to 5 mg/L. This results in a concomitant decrease in the insulin level inside the reactor, which becomes practically negligible after 1400 hours of culture. Interestingly, after a transitory decrease, both the cell and antibody concentrations strongly increase until reaching 3.10^6 cells/mL and 30 mg antibodies/L, respectively.

607

This indicates an inhibitory effect of insulin in the investigated range of concentrations. Inhibition of growth by excess insulin is confirmed when the insulin feed concentration is again increased to 20mg/L. During the whole continuous culture the concentration of produced antibodies closely follows the level of viable cells. Thus the specific rate of antibody production is essentially unaffected by the level of insulin in the medium.

During a last phase the culture vessel was fed with the serum-free medium containing no insulin. We found that the continuous culture can be maintained at least during 200 hours at a high level of cells (2 x 10^6 cells/ml). This result suggests that for the considered cell line the addition of insulin in the serum-free medium is not essential for cell growth and antibodies production. At the relatively high cell density reached in the continous culture the production of autocrine growth factors may be sufficient to sustain cell growth.

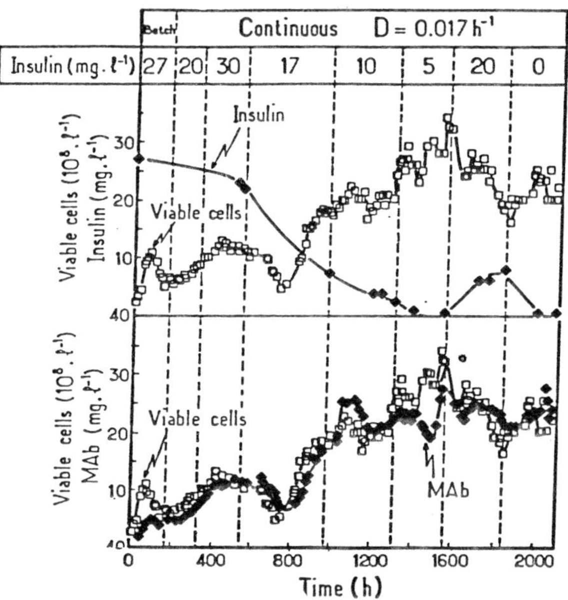

Fig 2: Continuous culture with step feed insulin variation. Evolution with time of insulin , cells and MAb concentrations.

ACKNOWLEDGEMENTS

The authors would like to thank Professor Nabet-Belleville, Professor Didierjean and Mrs.Dousset for technical assistance in insulin, transferrin and ascorbic acid assays.

REFERENCES

1.Louis Cleveland ,W.Wood,I.Erlanger,B.F.(1983).J.Immunol.Meth.56,221-234.
2.Jäger,V.Lehmann,J.and Friedl,P.(1988).Cytotechnology.1,319-329.
3.Shintani,Y.Iwamoto,K.Kintano,K.(1988).Appl.Microbiol.Biotechnol.27,533-537.
4.Glassy,M.C.Tharakan,J.P.Chau,P.C.(1988).Biotechnol.Bioeng.32,1015-1028.

BATCH PRODUCTION KINETICS OF HYBRIDOMAS: PULSE-EXPERIMENTS.

Merten, O.-W., Keller, H., Siami, K., Cabanié, L., Leno, M.

Institut Pasteur, Laboratoire de Technologie Cellulaire,
25, rue du Docteur Roux, F-75015 Paris, France

<u>Abstract:</u>

Pulse-experiments, avoiding changes in the cellular physiology, have been
conducted, in order to establish, (a) wether the secretion of monoclonal
antibodies (mAbs) by mouse hybridomas occurs mainly by a de novo synthesis
or by a release of intracellularly stored IgG/M, and (b) to verify if the
calculated specific productivity (pg produced IgG/cellxh) gives a real
indication about the cellular mAb-production-activity or not.
The results, obtained from two hybridoma cell lines (10/8/20, I.13.17),
indicate that during the growth phase (lag and/or exponential phase) the
calculated specific productivity correlated well with the incorporation of
S-35-methionine or H-3-leucine into cytoplasmic IgG. However, hybridoma
cultures, showing a second peak of calculated specific productivity during
the death phase (so called dead production), did not show any incorporation of S-35-methionine or H-3-leucine into cytoplasmic IgG. This may be
interpreted as mAbs secreted during the death phase were not synthesised
de novo, but were released from an intracellular pool.
By conducting a second set of pulse-experiments using cell line I.13.17,
we were able to show, that this non-correlation between the effective
production during the death phase (Merten et al. Cytotechnology (1990) in
press) and the incorporation of radiolabeled amino acid (H-3-leucine) into
IgG was due to (a) the development of the intracellular leucine-concentra-
tion (strong reduction); and (b) the profound reduction of the incorporation and utilisation of leucine during the stationary and death phase. The
results indicate, that both pulse-methods, ours, which avoids most of the
physiological changes during the pulse-periode, and the classical one,
which follows the incorporation/synthesis kinetics of a new batch culture
after a complete medium change, are not applicable for this type of study,
because both are influenced by, or influence the actual state, of cellular
physiology. The results will be discussed with those obtained from pulse-
chase experiments.

<u>Introduction:</u>

A lot of work has been done in the last few years to elucidate the parameters which influence growth and monoclonal antibody (mAb)-production of
hybridomas. Nevertheless, little is known about these influences, and the
regulation of growth with respect to mAb-synthesis and -secretion, or vice
versa, is still not understood. One of the uncertainties is the question
of the mAb-synthesis during the death phase of hybridoma batch cultures;
if mAbs are synthesized and secreted at once, or if they are liberated
from a cytoplasmic Ig-stock, in particular during the death phase. Some
groups have favored the hypothesis of de novo synthesis (Birch et al.
1987, Walker et al. 1987), others demonstrated that a part of IgG released
during the death phase is of storage origin (Al-Rubeai et al. 1989, Merten
et al. 1990). To get a more detailed insight of the mAb-production during
the death phase we have conducted pulse-experiments, modified, in order to

reduce the physiological changes due to the medium change. The results of
these experiments (no incorporation of radiolabeled amino acid (AA) into
the IgG during the death phase) lead us to investigate the incorporation
and utilisation of some amino acids during different growth phases. Also
these tests give an explanation why pulse-experiments are not always
suitable for elucidating production/incorporation kinetics during different phases of batch cultures.

Materials and Methods:

Cells: I.13.17 and 10/8/20 are mouse hybridomas, based on X63.653 and
SP2/0-myelomas, respectively. They have been obtained from Dr. Mazié and
Dr. Michelson, both Institut Pasteur. The cells have been cultivated as

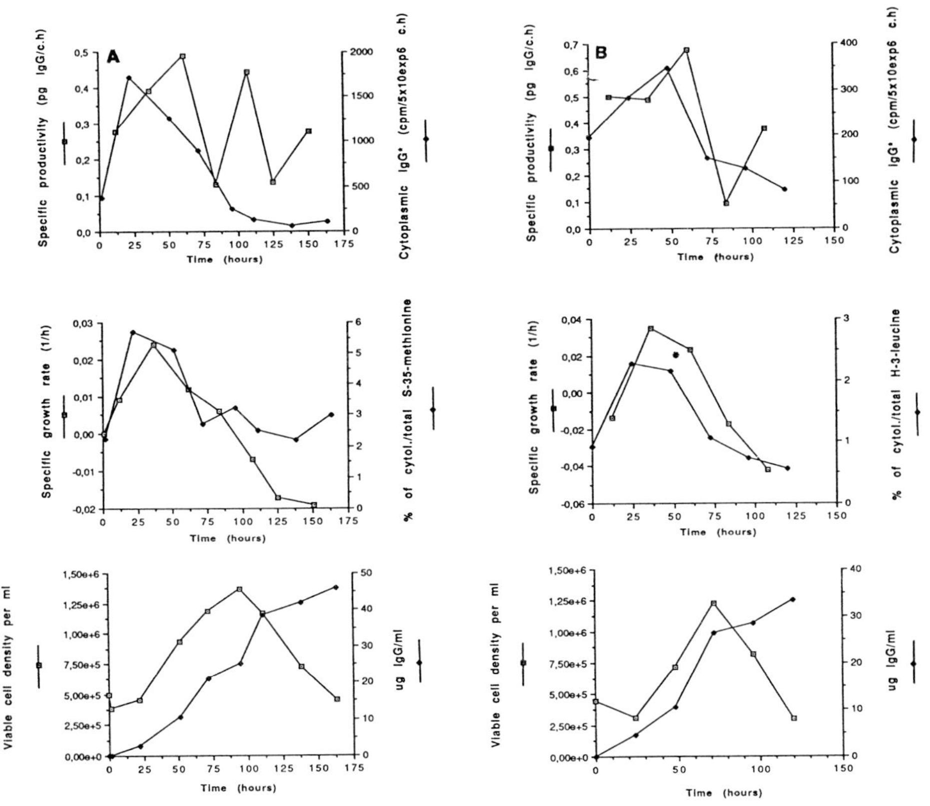

Fig. 1.A. Batch culture of I.13.17, B. Batch culture of 10/8/20. Notes:
bottom diagrams: viable cell density/ml; µg IgG/ml. Central diagrams:
ratio of cytoplasmic to total S-35-methionine for I.13.17 and H-3-leucine
for 10/8/20, respectively; specific growth rate (1/h). Top diagrams: cell
specific productivity (pg IgG/c.h); incorporation of S-35-methionine (A)
or H-3-leucine (B) into cytoplasmic IgG, after pulsing 5x10exp6 cells for
1h using 50µCi.

610

published elsewhere (Merten et al. 1990).

Medium: All cultures were conducted in 75cm2 or 150cm2 Roux-bottles (Corning); using Dulbecco's modified Eagle's Medium (DMEM, mixed in the laboratory), containing 3g/l glucose and 5% newborn calf serum (Medical & Veterinary Supplies Ltd. Botolph, Buckingham, U.K.). The cultures (always two in parallel) were inoculated at about 4-5x10exp5 cells/ml. The starting volume was 60ml (Fig. 1) and 150ml (Fig. 2, 3).

Dayly pulses have been conducted as described elsewhere (Merten et al. 1990), whereby for each day 2.5 (Fig. 2, 3) or 5 (Fig. 1) x10exp6 cells/ml were separated by centrifugation (5min., 800rpm, 25°C) and incubated for 1h (Fig. 1) or 1.5h and 3hrs. (Fig. 2, 3) in the old supernatant, to which 40-50 μCi of labeled AA (L-(4,5-H-3)-leucine (Amersham TRK.636, 126 Ci/mmol) or L-S-35-methionine (Amersham SJ-1015, >1000 Ci/mmol)) have been added. The pulsed cultures have been stopped and treated as described elsewhere (Merten et al. 1990).

Analysis, calculations, and corrections for the ratio of cytoplasmic labeled AA to total labeled AA: Merten et al. (1990).

Amino acid analysis: Cytoplasm. Preparation of cells: Every day 2x10exp7 cells were separated (1000rpm, 5min., 4°C) and washed twice in PBS. The cell pellet (about 150μl) was lysed in 500μl H2O dest. and frozen at - 30°C. Three cycles of freezing and thawing were added in order to complete the cell lysis. The cytoplasm was separated (3000rpm, 10min., 4°C), the cellular proteins (200μl sample) were precipitated by using 20μl of 50% sulfosalicylic acid in water. After mixing and precipitation, the solution was centrifuged at 13000rpm for 10min. After mixing 1:1 with sample dilution buffer (pH 2.2) and adding the interne standard (norleucine), 100μl of this supernate was analysed using the method of Spackmann et al. (1958)(HPLC: Biotronik LC 5001, ninhydrin post column derivatation) by Mme. Gilles (Institut Pasteur, Laboratoire de Regulations cellulaires).

Supernatant: The supernate was centrifuged (1500rpm, 10min., 4°C) and deproteinized by ultrafiltration (cut-off 10Kd) using Millipore UFC3 LGC filters. The derivatation and determination of the amino acid concentration has been performed with the help of Mlle. Mauyart (Univ. de l'Etat, Unité de Biotechnologie Appliquée, Mons/B) by using Water's Pico-Tag-method.

Using the results of the AA-analysis, utilisation rates and concentrations have been calculated for leucine with respect to cell density and time.

Results and Discussion:

Classical pulse experiments are carried out as following: the cells to be pulsed are separated from the previous culture supernate and a new culture is started at a fixed cell density (e.g. 10exp6 cells/ml) in a **new** medium containing one or several radiolabeled compounds (e.g. AA). However, this procedure implies that pulse experiments always give a response about the incorporation, synthesis and/or secretion kinetics at the **onset** of a culture, because each medium change is inherently a new start of a batch culture (e.g. shown by Al-Rubeai and Emery (1989a) for the incorporation of labelled AA into cytoplasmic and secreted IgG during batch cultures). This may be a reason why no real pulse-kinetic studies of complete batch cultures have been published up to now.

In order to obtain more knowledge about the production (synthesis, storage and/or secretion) of mAb by hybridomas during the different phases of batch cultures, we have conducted pulse-experiments of 1h duration during

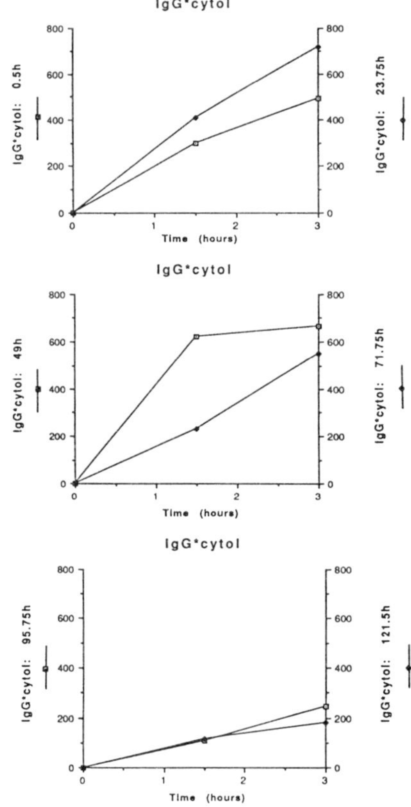

Fig. 2. Incorporation-kinetics of H-3-leucine into cytoplasmic IgG for 1.5 and 3 hrs., during the I.13.17-batch culture, shown in Fig. 3 (at: 0.5h, 23.75h, 49h, 71.75h, 95.75h, 121.5h). 2.5x10exp6 cells have been pulsed with 40μCi of H-3-leucine.

different phases of hybridoma batch cultures, where in all cases, the supernatant of the batch culture has been used as pulse medium. This duration was convenient to get a response of the incorporation of radiolabeled AA into the intracellular IgG (synthetic activity), but too short for following this incorporation into secreted IgGs. The speed of synthesis and secretion of mAbs generally ranges from 1 1/4 and 2 1/2 hrs. (Parkhouse 1973, Walker et al 1987, Merten et al. 1990).

The cultures of cell lines I.13.17 and 10/8/20 are shown in Fig. 1A and 1B, and lasted for 7 and 5 days respectively. Both cell lines showed two production phases, one during the beginning of growth and a second one during the decline phase, which showed a lot of variability in case I.13.17. The incorporation of labeled AA (S-35-methionine for I.13.17 and 10/8/20 (not shown) and H-3-leucine for 10/8/20) followed, to some extent, the specific IgG-production during the growth phase. However, no correlation was seen during the death phase. Only negligible quantities of labeled AA were incorporated into cytoplasmic IgG, but a considerable amount of IgG was produced and secreted during this phase. We could show for the same cells (Merten et al. 1990) that most of the IgG secreted during the decline phase of a batch culture (50-86%) was newly synthesized, which signifies that a certain incorporation of labeled AA into cytoplasmic IgG should have been found during the dying phase. This non-correlation is certainly due to profound changes of the cellular physiology during batch cultures. One indication for this hypothesis is shown in Fig. 1. It is evident, that the incorporation of labeled AA into the cytoplasm (ratio of labeled cytoplasmic AA to total labeled AA) followed the specific growth rate. The highest incorporation rate of labeled AA into the cytoplasm was found during the maximal growth (= highest metabolic activity). During the decline phase this incorporation rate was considerably reduced. The incorporation of labeled AA into cytoplasmic IgG followed, therefore, the specific growth rate and not the cell specific IgG productivity. Although we have tried to correct the values of the AA-incorporation into the cytoplasmic IgG for the differences of the AA-incorporation into the cytoplasma, it was not possible to obtain the real and expected values.
To solve this problem and to determine the influence of cellular physi-

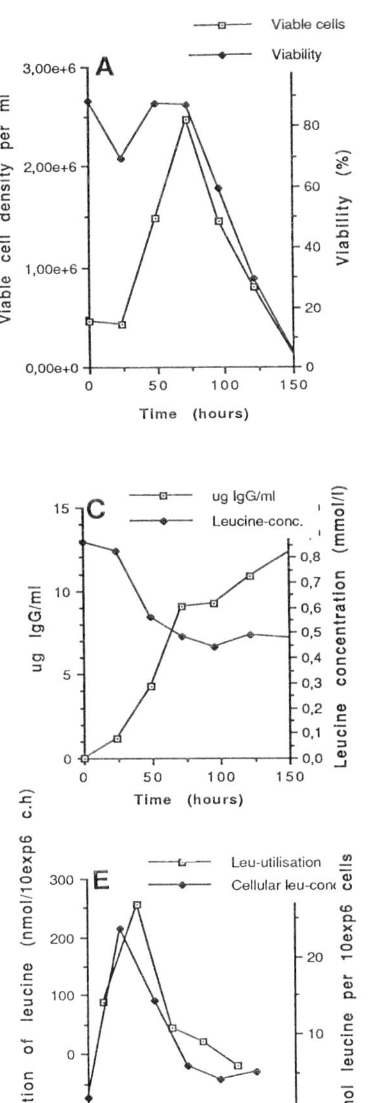

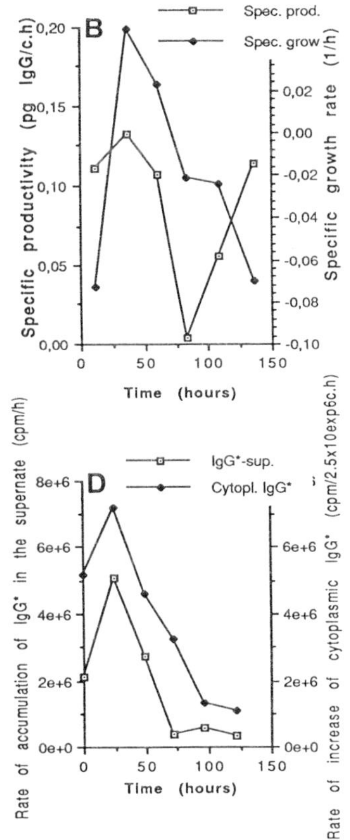

Fig. 3. Batch culture of I.13.17 (pulse-kinetics inb Fig. 2): A. viable cell density/ml; viability (%). B. Cell specific productivity (pg IgG/c.h); specific growth rate (1/h). C. IgG-accumulation (µg IgG/ml); leucine concentration of the supernate (mmol/l). D. Accumulation rate of labeled IgG (IgG*) in the supernate and increase of cytoplasmic IgG*; both (cpm/2.5x10exp6 c.h), both have been corrected for the molar ratio of labeled to cold leucine in the medium of the different sampling points. E. Leucine utilisation (nmol/10exp6 c.h); intracellular leucine concentration (nmol/10exp6 cells).

ology on the incorporation kinetics of labeled leucine or methionine into cytoplasmic IgG, we conducted a second set of pulse experiments with H-3-leucine by using cell line I.13.17. In addition we analysed the intracellular AA-concentration and utilisation during the batch culture (Fig. 2, 3). As already shown, the incorporation of labeled leucine into the cytoplasmic IgG depended largely on the state of the batch culture (Fig. 2), the maximum rate was found between 23.75 and 49 hrs. Afterwards (95.75 and 121.5 hrs.) a strong reduction could be seen. Fig. 3 shows the most

important kinetics of the culture: diagrams A, B, and C present the development of the batch culture (viable cells/ml, viability, specific IgG-
productivity, specific growth rate, µg IgG/ml, and leucine concentrati-
on/ml). The diagrams in Fig. 3 D and E show, that, on the one hand, the
maximal incorporation of labeled leucine into cytoplasmic IgG and secreted
IgG (theoretically IgG-synthesis-rate) took place during the growth phase,
as already shown for the cytoplasmic IgG in Fig. 2; and that, on the other
hand, the specific utilisation of leucine and the cytoplasmic leucine
concentration showed maxima during the same phase, the growth phase.
During stationary and decline phases a strong reduction of the incorporation of labeled leucine into cytoplasmic and secreted IgG (during the
pulse periods) could be seen, which followed directly the intracellular
leucine concentration and the specific leucine utilisation and of course
the specific growth rate. However, no correlation exists between the
specific IgG-productivity during this phase and the incorporation of
labeled leucine into cytoplasmic and secreted IgG during the pulses.
Similar kinetics were found for methionine (not shown). These amino acid
kinetics are in full accord with recent communications about the utilisation of amino acids by hybridoma cells (e.g. Geaugey et al. 1989, Reid et
al. 1988, own unpublished results). However, these results signify that
the kinetics of mAb synthesis during batch cultures cannot be followed by
this type of pulse-experiment, because the incorporation of the labeled AA
into the cell and the IgG depends too much on the physiological state of
the cells (culture phase).
The facts, that neither classical nor modified pulse-experiments were
usable for elucidating the kinetics of mAb-synthesis during batch
cultures, has lead us to design pulse-chase experiments, which avoid
physiological changes during the chases to a large extent (Merten et al.
1990).
In conclusion: -Classical pulse experiments are not suitable to follow the
kinetics of mAb-synthesis during batch cultures, because the pulsed
cultures are always started by using fresh medium. Therefore, one can only
investigate the beginning of a new batch culture.
-Modified pulse experiments, using the culture supernate of the same
culture to which the labeled compound has been added, in order to prevent
a perturbation of the physiological state of the culture, are not suitable
to follow the kinetics of mAb-synthesis during batch cultures, because the
AA-utilisation and incorporation into the cells is strongly influenced by
the culture conditions. In this case rates were reduced during the stationary and death phases of the batch culture, and only insignificant amounts
of labeled AA was incorporated into newly synthetized IgG.
-The only possibility is the use of pulse-chase experiments, whereby the
batch culture is pulsed at the onset of the culture, and each day one or
several aliquots of the culture are chased by the use of the supernate of
a non-labeled parallel culture. Using this method and material balances it
could be shown that a certain amount of IgG (50-86%), which was secreted
during the stationary and death phase, was newly synthesized (Merten et
al. 1990).

References:

- Al-Rubeai M, Emery AN (1989a) Cytotechnology 89.
- Al-Rubeai M, Rookes S, Emery AN (1989) In "Advances in Animal Cell
  Biology and Technology for Bioprocesses", eds. Spier RE, Griffiths JB,

Stephenne J, Crooy PJ, pp. 241-245, Butterworths, Borough Green, Sevenoaks/U.K.
- Birch JR, Thompson PW, Boraston R, Oliver S, Lambert K (1987) In "Plant and Animal Cells: Process Possibilities", eds. Webb C, Mavituna F, pp. 162-171, Ellis Horwood Ltd. Publishers, Chichester/U.K.
- Geaugey V, Duval D, Geahel I, Marc A, Engasser JM (1989) Cytotechnology 2, 119-129.
- Merten O-W, Keller H, Cabanié L, Leno M, Hardefelt M (1990) Cytotechnology, in press.
- Parkhouse RME (1973) Transplant Rev 14, 131-144.
- Reid S, Forbes L, Abeydeera P, Greenfield PF, Randerson DH (1988) Presented at the 8th Int. Biotechnol. Symp., 17th-22nd July 1988, Paris/F.
- Spackmann DH, Stein WH, Moore S (1958) Anal Chem 30, 1190-1206.
- Walker AG, Davison W, Lambe CA (1987) Proc 4th European Congress on Biotechnology, Vol. 3, eds. Neijssel OM, van der Meer RR, Luyben KChAM, p. 587, Elsevier Science Publishers B.V., Amsterdam/NL.

ANALYSIS OF HYBRIDOMA GROWTH, METABOLISM, AND PRODUCT FORMATION IN CONTINUOUS SUSPENSION CULTURE

G. Schmid[#], C. R. Wilke, and H. W. Blanch

Department of Chemical Engineering, University of California,
Berkeley, CA 94720, USA
[#]Present address: Central Research Laboratories, ZFE/MB, Bld.
66/302, F. Hoffmann-La Roche AG, CH-4002 Basle, Switzerland

ABSTRACT

Hybridoma growth, metabolism, and product formation was evaluated in continuous suspension culture experiments under controlled environmental conditions using HEPES-buffered medium. Steady-state values for viable and total cell counts as well as metabolite and product concentrations were determined for five different dilution rates. Specific growth and death rates were recorded as a function of dilution rate. The following parameters were estimated as function of specific growth rate μ: specific substrate consumption and byproduct production rates (metabolic quotients) and apparent molar yield coefficients. Results are briefly discussed with respect to changes in mammalian cell metabolism.

INTRODUCTION

A limited number of publications on animal cell (hybridoma) growth, metabolism and product formation in continuous culture experiments under well controlled environmental conditions have been published to date (1-14). Most of the studies – except those by Miller et al. (9-13) – did cover a narrow range of dilution rates and/or provided only very sparse data on nutrient, byproduct, and product concentrations, metabolic quotients, and yield coefficients, etc. With the same hybridoma cell line that Miller (10) used in his experiments we here report on preliminary results for continuous suspension culture in HEPES-buffered medium.

MATERIALS AND METHODS

Cell line and medium

A mouse hybridoma line AB2-143.2 (15) was grown in Dulbecco's Modified Eagle's medium supplemented with 10% fetal bovine serum, nonessential amino acids, and Na-pyruvate. Buffering capacity was provided by 25 mM HEPES (N-2-Hydroxyethyl-piperazine-N'-2-ethanesulfonic acid) sodium salt (16). For continuous suspension cultures initial (and feed) concentrations of glucose and glutamine were 13.5 mM and 4.9 mM, respectively. All experiments were performed without the use of antibiotics and periodic mycoplasma samples were negative.

Cell culture reactor

A 1-L glass reactor (Pegasus) was used with 600 mL working volume. Agitation was provided by a 5-cm diameter axial flow turbine operating at 180 ± 10 rpm. Oxygen transport was via surface aeration and the partial pressure in the liquid was

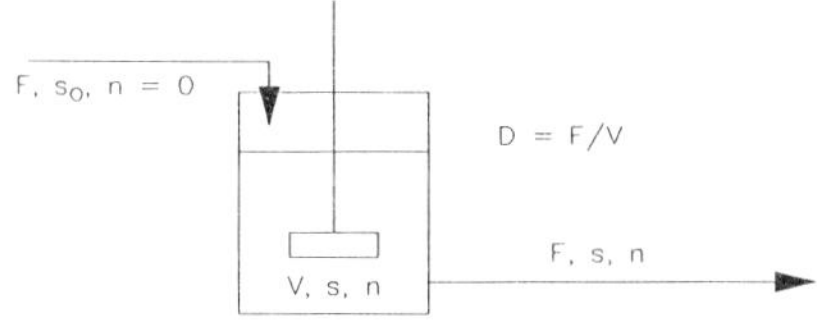

EQUATIONS FOR CONTINUOUS CULTURE

CELL GROWTH

$$dn_V/dt = \mu\, n_V - k_d n_V - Dn_V$$
$$dn_d/dt = k_d n_V - Dn_d$$
$$dn/dt = \mu\, n_V - Dn$$

$$\boxed{\mu = D(n/n_V) = D + k_d}$$ at steady state

SUBSTRATE CONSUMPTION

$$q_S = (D(s_F - s) - ds/dt)/n_V$$

PRODUCT FORMATION

$$q_p = (D(p - p_F) + dp/dt)/n_V$$

Figure 1

Determination of specific growth rates μ and metabolic quotients

controlled at 110 ± 10 mm Hg (i.e., 70% air saturation) by varying the oxygen concentration in the headspace. Temperature was maintained at 37.0°C with a circulating water bath. The pH was controlled at 7.2 ± 0.1 by the addition of 0.5 N sodium hydroxide. Samples were taken twice daily. A multi-channel peristaltic pump (Gilson) was used for medium addition and product removal.

Sample analyses

Viable and nonviable cells were estimated by hemacytometer counting (trypan blue staining). Glucose and lactate were determined by enzymatic assays; ammonia was measured with an ion-selective electrode. Fluorescent amino acid derivatives were separated by reversed phase HPLC and antibody concentrations quantitated by high pressure Protein A affinity chromatography.

Some mathematical equations for the determination of specific growth rates μ and metabolic quotients are derived in Figure 1. Details on the hybridoma cell line, medium composition, and growth conditions as well as the assay procedures for metabolite and product concentrations are given elsewhere (17,18).

RESULTS AND DISCUSSION

Experimental data for the continuous suspension culture of a murine hybridoma cell line in HEPES-buffered medium were obtained. A laboratory scale bioreactor was operated at pH 7.2 and 70% air saturation using DME medium supplemented with 10% serum as sterile feed. Steady-state values for viable and total cell counts

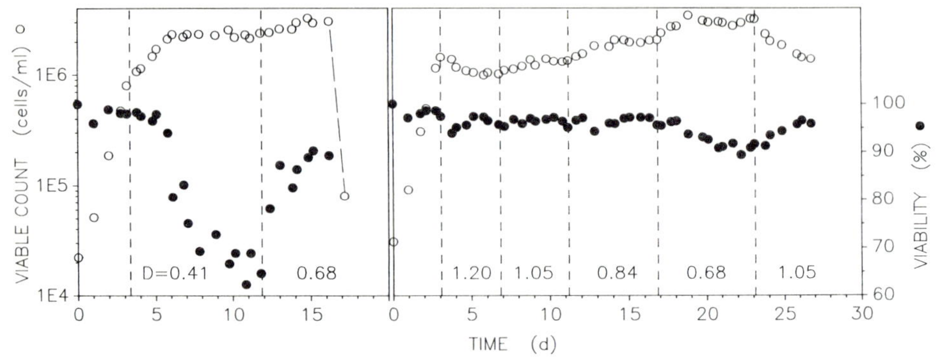

Figure 2

**Continuous hybridoma suspension culture:
Viable cell growth curves and percent viability**

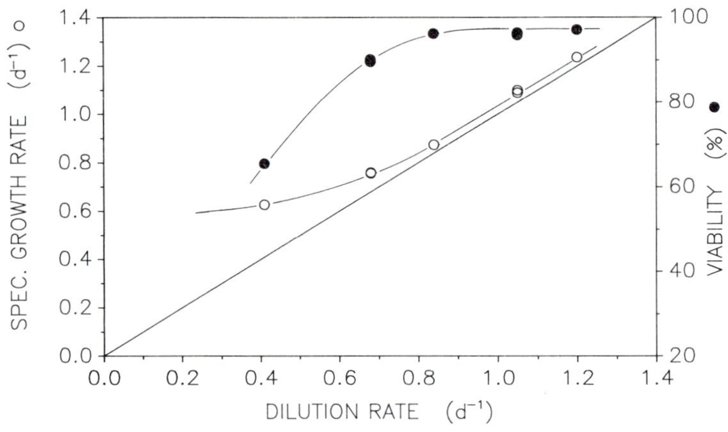

Figure 3

**Effect of dilution rate on steady-state growth rate μ
and percent viability**

(Figure 2) as well as metabolite (glucose, lactate, ammonia, glutamine, amino acids) and product (antibody) concentrations were determined for five different dilution rates (Figure 4a and b). Besides glutamine and glucose being exhausted at dilution rates < 0.6 d^{-1}, methionine, arginine and asparagine were limiting substrates under those conditions (data not shown). Specific growth and death rates were recorded as a function of dilution rate (Figure 3). The decrease in viable cell concentrations at lower dilution rates and the dramatic decrease in viability at these dilution rates may be a result of high toxin concentrations and/or increased hydrodynamic stress due to the longer residence times of cells within the bioreactor.

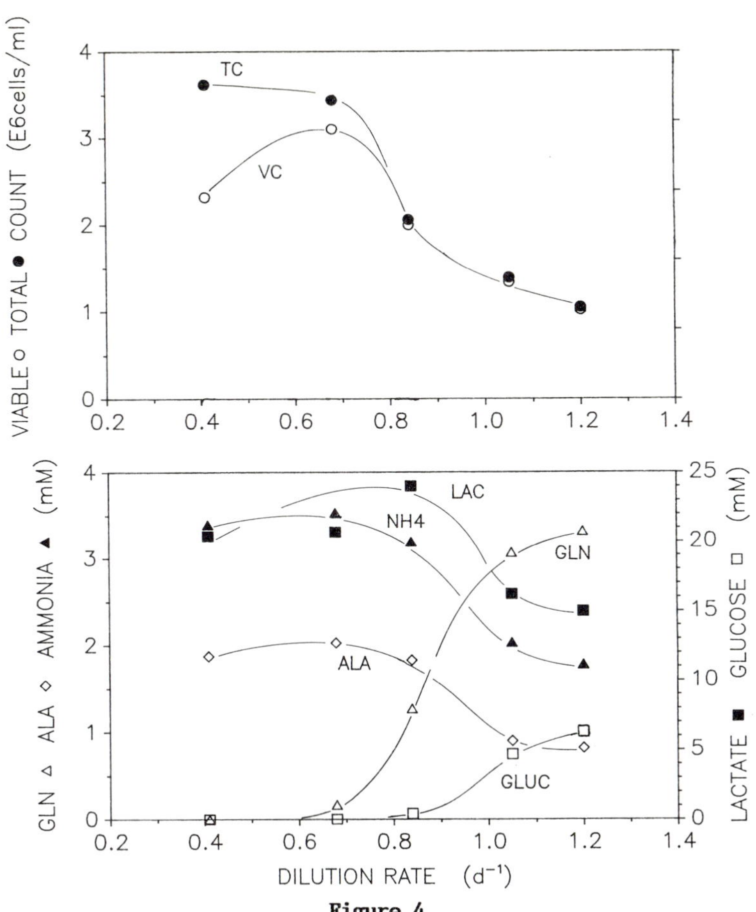

Figure 4

**Effect of dilution rate on steady–state cell
and (selected) metabolite concentrations**

μ (d^{-1})	$Y'_{lac,gluc}$ (mol/mol)	$Y'_{NH4,GLN}$ (mol/mol)
0.63	1.49	0.69
0.75	1.56	0.76
0.87	1.84	0.88
1.09	1.79	1.02
1.24	2.01	1.00

Table 1

**Effect of specific growth rate μ on (selected) steady–state
apparent byproduct yield coefficients**

Figure 5 shows the effect of specific growth rate μ on selected nutrient and by-
product metabolic quotients. As was observed by Miller (9,10) the experimental
data for glutamine seem to fit the maintenance energy model whereas the specific
glucose consumption rate is not linear with μ. Possible explanations for this
deviation include changes in the apparent yield coefficients Y'[lac/gluc] and
Y'[ALA/gluc] with specific growth rate (Table 1). Lower values for Y'[lac/gluc]
indicate a more efficient glucose utilization at lower dilution rates and glucose concentrations. Furthermore, different amounts of glucose will be channeled
via pyruvate into acetyl CoA or serve as building blocks for biosynthetic needs
of cells. The decreased ammonia production from glutamine at low specific growth
rates (Table 1) may in part reflect differing metabolic pathways being taken in
the conversion of glutamate to α-ketoglutarate (i.e., dehydrogenase vs transaminase activity).

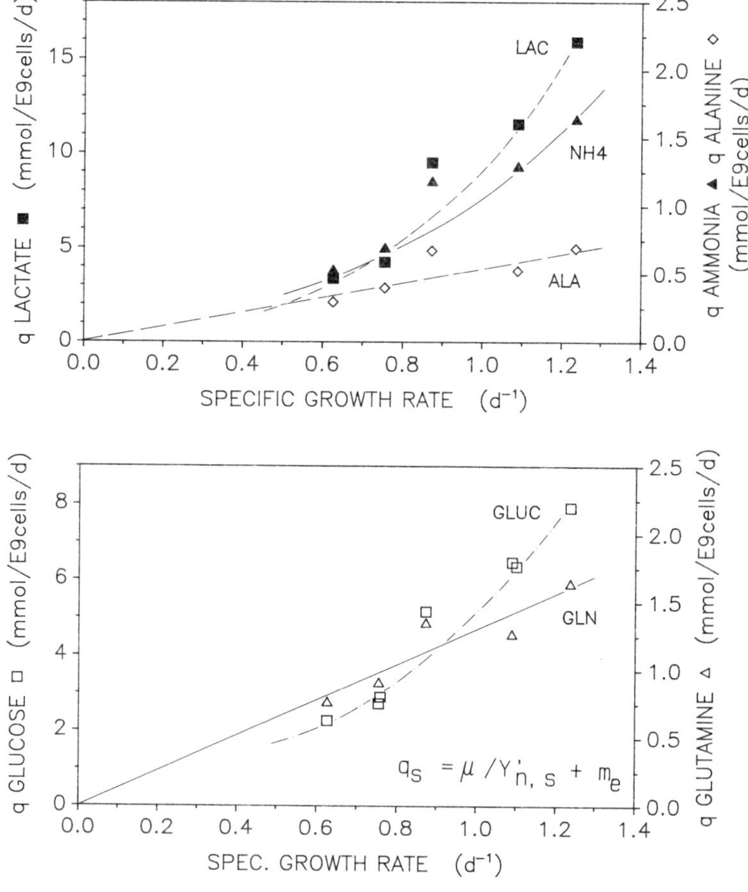

$$q_S = \mu / Y'_{n,s} + m_e$$

Figure 5

**Effect of specific growth rate μ on (selected) nutrient and
byproduct metabolic quotients**

A complete analysis of hybridoma growth, metabolism, and product formation as a function of the specific growth rate μ in HEPES-buffered medium including data on amino acid metabolic quotients, the various yield coefficients Y′, ATP production rates from oxidative phosphorylation and glycolysis, and specific antibody production rates and space-time yields will be published elsewhere (18).

ACKNOWLEDGEMENTS

G. S. was supported by a postdoctoral fellowship from the Deutscher Akademischer Austauschdienst (DAAD).

REFERENCES

1 Griffiths, J. B., and Pirt, S. J. Proc. Roy. Soc. B. 1967, 168, 421
2 Tovey, M., and Bouty-Boye, D. Exp. Cell Res. 1976, 101, 346
3 Sinclair, R. In vitro 1974, 10, 295
4 Moser, H., and Vecchio, G. Experientia 1967, 23, 120
5 Boraston, R., Thompson, P. W., Garland, S., and Birch, J. R. Dev. Biol. Standard. 1984, 55, 103
6 Fazekas de St.Groth, S. J. Immunol. Methods 1983, 57, 121
7 Ray, N. G., Karkare, S. B., and Runstadtler, Jr., P. W. Biotechnol. Bioeng. 1989, 33, 724
8 Low, K. S., Harbour, C., and Barford, J. P. Biotechnol. Tech. 1987, 1, 239
9 Miller, W. M., Blanch, and H. W., Wilke, C. R. Biotechnol. Bioeng. 1988, 32, 947
10 Miller, W. M. Ph.D. Thesis 1987, University of California, Berkeley, CA
11 Miller, W. M., Wilke, C. R., and Blanch, H. W. Biotechnol. Bioeng. 1989, 33, 477
12 Miller, W. M., Wilke, C. R., and Blanch, H. W. Biotechnol. Bioeng. 1989, 33, 487
13 Miller, W. M., Wilke, C. R., and Blanch, H. W. J. Cell Physiol. 1987, 132, 524
14 Schmid, G., Wilke, C. R., and Blanch, H. W. 1987, 194th ACS National Meeting, New Orleans, LA, paper no. 74
15 Hornbeck, P. V., and Lewis, G. K. J. Exp. Med. 1985, 161, 53
16 Shipman, Jr., C. PSEBM 1969, 130, 305
17 Schmid, G., Blanch, H. W., and Wilke, C. R. Biotechnol. Lett. 1990, in press
18 Schmid, G., Wilke, C. R., and Blanch, H. W., in preparation

KINETICS OF NUTRIENT UTILIZATION IN A HYBRIDOMA BATCH CULTURE

Frieberg, H.+, Persson L.+, Grönvik KO.+, Häggström L.#

+National Veterinary Institute, BMC Box 585, S-75123 Uppsala, Sweden.
#Royal Institute of Technology, S-10044 Stockholm, Sweden.

INTRODUCTION

The aim of this investigation is to gain some knowledge about the environmental factors affecting cell growth and monoclonal antibody production by studying the kinetics of nutrient consumption and metabolite formation in batch culture.

MATERIALS AND METHODS

Cells, a hybridoma producing rat anti mouse CD 4 antibodies, were grown grown in fDMEM supplemented with 2 % FCS in 2 liter stirred tank reactors with temperature (37 degrees), pH (7.0) and DOT (30 % air sat.) control.
Samples were analyzed with respect to cell density and viability by trypan blue exclusion. To determine monoclonal antibody concentration a sandwich elisa employing polyclonal anti rat IgG antibodies was used. Glucose and lactate concentrations were determined enzymatically using commercial kits. For amino acid analysis the samples were deproteinized with 4 volumes of buffered sulfosalicylic acid (containing an appropriate amount of norleucine as internal standard) according to Mondino et al (J. Chromatog. 74, 255-263, 1972). Following centrifugation, 0.05 ml aliquots were analyzed with a Biotronik LC-5001 amino acid analyzer using the extended Li-citrate physiological system and ninhydrin as detection reagent.
The specific consumption or production rate $q(t) = (dC/dt)/n$ were calculated by fitting the concentration data by the least squares method to an appropriate function, taking the derivative with respect to time of this function and then dividing by the total

amount of cells per liter as calculated from a curve fit of the cell concentration during the exponential growth phase.

RESULTS AND DISCUSSION

Figure 1 illustrates the identification of an exponential growth phase from t = 18 h to t = 87 h (growth rate=0.043 per h, R=0.99). The mAb concentration reaches almost 30 mg/L while the specific production rate falls from 0.00028 mg/million cells/h to 0.00020 mg/million cells/h (Figure 2). During culture, the glucose concentration falls from 22 mmole/L to 2 mmole/L while the lactate concentration rises from 1 mmole/L to 37 mmole/L. This is slightly less than the theorethical amount of lactate that could be produced from the consumed glucose (Figure 3). From Figure 4 it can be seen that the decline in specific consumption rate of glucose (0.0008 mmole/million cells/h to 0) and specific production rate of lactate (0.0013 mmole/million cells/h to 0) are essentially parallel to each other. Thus it would seem that the fall in glucose concentration decreases its consumption rate which also leads to a decrease in lactate production rate. However the quotient of qlac to qgluc (Figure 4) shows that the fraction of glucose converted to lactate is rather low during the first part of the culture, while towards the end of the culture more than the theoretical 2 moles of lactate per mole glucose are produced.

Figures 5 and 6 shows the concentrations and specific metabolic rates of glutamine and some of its metabolically related compounds. The qs falls asymptotically towards 0 in all cases. Of the 2 mmole/L ammonium formed, 1.3 mmole/L can be stoichiometrically coupled to the biochemical pathway leading from glutamine to alanine. Not shown are the concentrations and specific consumption rates of the essential and nonessential amino acids. The qs falls to 0 for these nutrients also, with the exception of glycine and proline that are produced during the second half of culture.

We have seen that in the course of batch culture of this hybridoma cell specific consumption rates decreases during exponential growth. We suggest that specific consumption rates are concentration dependent. The question of how cells can maintain a constant growth rate while specific consumption rates decreases remains. A decrease in qs means lower energy and substrate availability. This can be explained by, for instance, compensation by other metabolic routes, storage and use of intracellular energy sources, change in cell composition, decline in macromolecular synthesis or reduction in cell size.

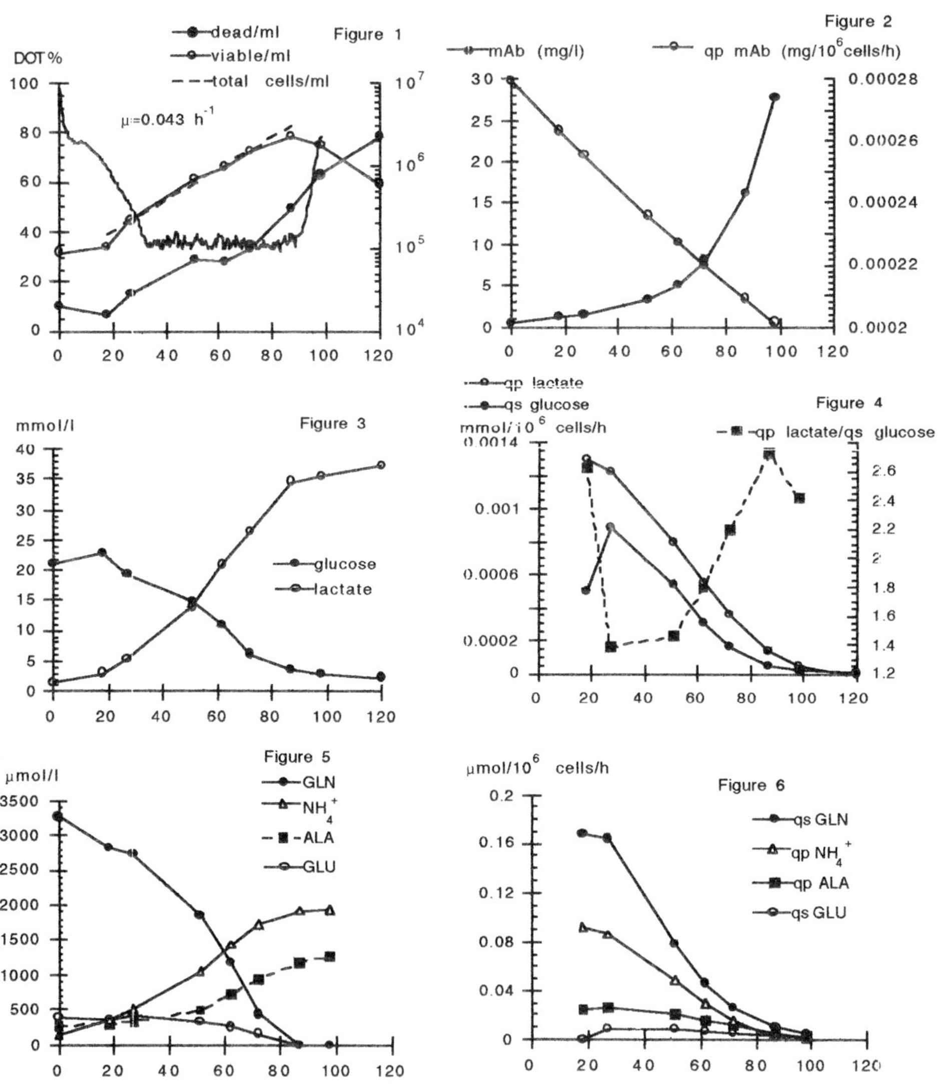

MODELLING GROWTH OF AND ANTIBODY PRODUCTION BY HYBRIDOMAS IN GLUTAMINE
LIMITED SUSPENSION CULTURES

Lars Keld Nielsen, Wardono Niloperbowo, Steven Reid, and
Paul F. Greenfield

Department of Chemical Engineering, The University of Queensland,
St.Lucia, Queensland, Australia 4067

ABSTRACT

Growth and antibody production in glutamine limited hybridoma cultures
were modelled using an unstructured model based on novel concepts for
medium requirements, energy metabolism, and inhibition. Batch
propagation in a protein free medium was fully described by the model
with parameters estimated in serum containing batch cultures. The model
suggests that high antibody titres can be obtained by linearising the
increase in total cell density through controlled feeding. This limiting
fed batch strategy extended the growth phase 50% and the antibody titre
400% as compared to batch propagation.

Keywords: hybridoma, antibody, model, protein free medium, fed batch,
          growth inhibition

INTRODUCTION

Mathematical models are important not only for process control but also
as tools facilitating our understanding of complex biological systems.
We have developed a general unstructured model describing growth and
antibody production for hybridomas in suspension culture (to be
published). The model was formulated on basis of a thorough analysis of
papers concerning hybridomas and other mammalian cells. We here present
some of the novels concept introduced llustrate the model for glutamine
limited batch cultures. Finally, fed batch propagation is discussed in
light of the model.

THEORY

An unstructured model was selected as we believe the present limited
understanding does not justify the use of complex structured models.
Critics point out unstructured models inability of describing changes in
biomass over time[1]. In batch, fed batch, and continuous culture,
however, we have not observed changes in cell yield on essential amino
acids, indicating that changes in biomass - at least for proteins - are
minor[2].

Parameters

Recent years work on formulating protein free media has added
substantially to our understanding of the qualitative requirements for
growth of hybridomas (table 1).

Glucose (sugar)
Glutamine (nitrogen)
Oxygen
Essential amino acids
Lipid-alcohols, B-vitamins, metals

Ammonia and lactate
pH, osmolarity, shear, etc.
Reactive oxides, endotoxins, etc.

Table 1 Growth Parameters.
Growth parameters are divided into
nutrients essential for growth and
factors which can inhibit growth

For some cell lines – including ours – serum, lipids and hormones are
obsolete when cells are carefully weaned[3-5], and it appears that many of
the positive serum effects reported in the literature are related to
serum's toxin buffering capacity (especially against reactive oxides)
rather than nutritional or hormonal requirements[2].

Energy metabolism

In our view (to be submitted) hybridomas are not limited by energy
except under extreme conditions (figure 1).

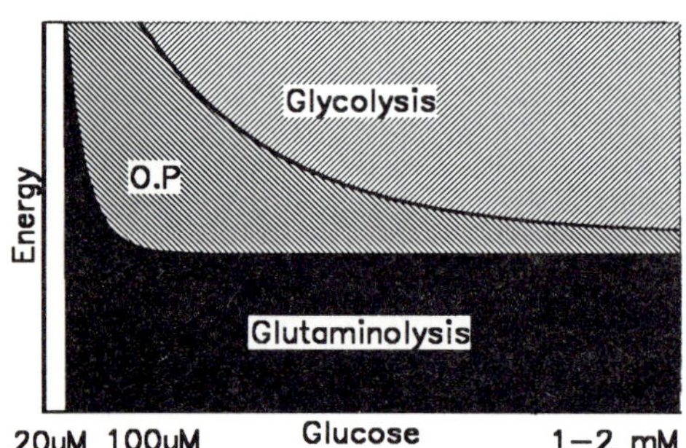

Figure 1 Energy Metabolism.
Hybridomas balance glycolysis and
oxidative phosphorylation to meet
without exceeding energy requirements at a growth rate given by
other factors. An energy deficit
at low glucose levels is met by
increased glutamine metabolism and
glucose limitation of growth is
only observed when anabolic
requirements can not be met.
The values are only indications of
the level.

Hybridoma's large glutamine consumption partly reflects the essential
requirement for glutamine as precursor for non-essential amino acids
(60% of the glutamine amino group enters biomass) and as nitrogen donor
in the synthesis of nucleotides, asparagine, NAD, and amino sugars (40%
of the glutamine amido group enters biomass).

Transient inhibition

The traditional static view of inhibition does not describe the
inhibitory effects of ammonia, lactate, pH, and osmolarity. Over normal
ranges inhibition by these factors is mainly transient, i.e. depends on
the rate of change rather than the actual level (figure 2). The
mechanism behind the transient inhibition of ammonia and pH could be

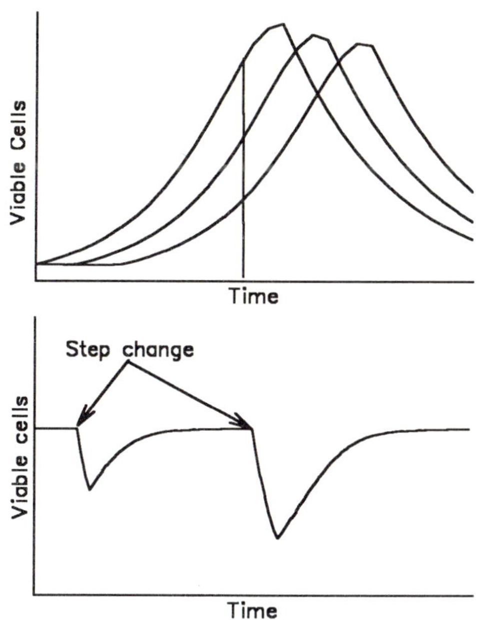

Figure 2: Transient inhibition.
In a standard one-point experiment
(illustrated with a vertical line
in A) the transient nature (here
modelled as a lag-phase) is not
appreciated. Consequently, large
inhibition has been reported for
low ammonia levels and small
increases in osmolarity[6-8].
The transient nature is most
obvious in continuous cultures (B)
for which adaptation to 8.2 mM
ammonia and pH 7.7 has been
reported[9-10].
One can speculate that the lag-
phase often observed in flasks and
sometimes in fermentors is a
transient inhibition from the pH
change at inoculation.

transient decoupling of ATP-production. For osmolarity, it appears that
hybridomas overcome hyperosmotic stress by accumulating the non-
essential amino acids proline and glycine[2,11].

Mathematical formulation

For a typical batch culture limited by glutamine our model is very
simple. Firstly, depletion is likely to occur before any transient
inhibition is observed[12-14] (no inhibition term in growth rate eqs. 6
and 7). Secondly, we have observed constant yields for cells, ammonia,
and alanine on glutamine in batch, fed batch, and continuous culture[2]
(Y and Y_A are constant). Thirdly, the change from the exponential to the
decline phase occurs over a very short period and can be modelled by
assuming some threshold requirement below which growth and antibody
production cease and the death rate increases (eq. 7).

$$\frac{dn_V}{dt} = (u - k_D)n_V \qquad \frac{dn_D}{dt} = k_D n_V \qquad (1-2)$$

$$\frac{dG}{dt} = -(u/Y)n_V - d_G G \qquad \frac{dA}{dt} = d_G G + Y_A(u/Y)n_V \qquad (3-4)$$

$$\frac{dI}{dt} = q_I n_V \qquad f = \frac{G}{k+G} \qquad (5-6)$$

For G>L: $u=u_{max}f$, $k_D=a_D$, $q_I=a_I$ $\qquad (7)$

For G<L: $u=0$, $k_D=a_{DD}$, $q_I=0$

MATERIALS AND METHODS

A SP/2 derived murine hybridoma was propagated in serum containing (RPMI1640/2.5% FCS) or protein free medium (DMEM:HAM F12 with 0.1% Pluronic F68 and SSR A+C). The serum substitute SSR was kindly provided by HI Nielsen, MediCult A/S, Kanalholmen 12, DK-2650 Hvidovre, Denmark. Two different reactor systems were used: LH Fermentation (experiments in serum containing medium) and Setric Genie Industrial both equipped with Ingold pH and oxygen probes. Setpoints for pH and oxygen were 7.1 and 30% DOT, respectively. Feeding was controlled with a peristaltic pump (Pharmacia).

In batch experiments 2 mmol/L glutamine (Sigma) was added. The non-limiting fed batch was fed at 4-8 hour interval with a mixture of amino acids (Sigma) and glucose (Ajax) to maintain glutamine concentration above 1 mM and other nutrients in excess. The feed medium for the limiting fed batch contained 100X BME vitamins (Cytosystem) and SSR A+C in addition to amino acids and glucose and was dissolved in medium instead of water. The feed rate in the limiting fed batch was maintained constant at 0.05 mmol glutamine/hour.

Cells were stained with Trypan blue (Filtron) and enumerated using a haemocytometer. Glutamine was measured using an enzymatic kit (Boehringer Mannheim), ammonia using an ammonia probe (Orion), and antibody using ELISA.

RESULTS AND DISCUSSION

Glutamine limited batch

The model was implemented in Pascal using a fourth-order Runga-Kutta to solve the differential equations. With parameters estimated in serum containing medium (table 2) the model fully described growth in protein free medium (figure 3), supporting our claim that serum, lipids and hormones are obsolete, if the toxin level is kept under control.

Y	0.43 Gcells/mmol G	Table 2 Estimated parameters.
d_G	0.0027 1/h	d_G was estimated in a separate
Y_A	0.70 mmol A/mmol G	batch experiment without cells.
k	0.60 mM	L was given a small, arbitrary
u_{max}	0.059 1/h	value. Other parameters were
a_D	0.002 1/h	estimated to give best visual fit
a_{DD}	0.035 1/h	to four RPMI/2.5% FCS batch
a_I	0.54 mg/Gcells/h	experiments (see figure 3)
L	0.05 mM	

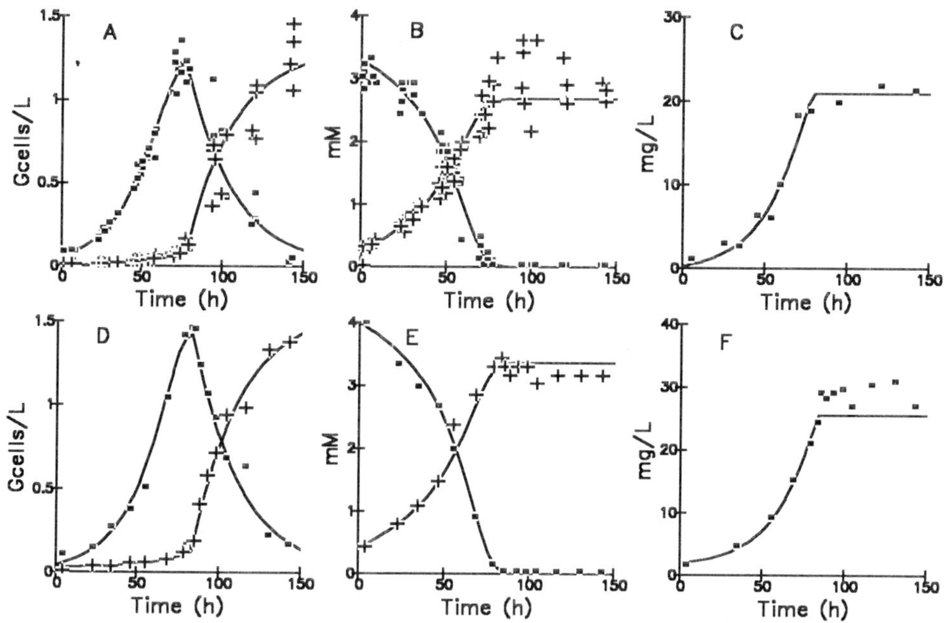

Figure 3 Modelling glutamine limited batch cultures.
Observed (marks) and predicted (solid line) in serum containing (A-C)
and protein free (D-F) batch cultures. A+D: viable (square) and dead (+)
cell density, B+E: glutamine (square) and ammonia (+) concentration,
C+F: antibody concentration

Limiting fed batch

Depletion can not be allowed in a production situation. Feeding
nutrients in excess, however, only extended the growth period 20 hours
with a 60% increase in the antibody titre (figure 4A). We believe the
cells entered the decline phase in response to transient inhibition
(during a 6 hours period around peak density the ammonia level increased
1 mM and the osmolarity 20 mOsmol/kg) and/or due to excessive sparging
required to maintain the oxygen concentration.
These problems do not occur in a limiting fed batch with constant –
rather than exponential – growth in total cell density (and hereby
constant production and consumption rates). The model indicate that a
limiting fed batch can be implemented by feeding glutamine at a constant
rate. This approach gave a 50 hour increase in growth period and a 400%
increase in antibody titre as compared to batch (figure 4B). The
prediction, however, failed as the cell yield on glutamine increased
markedly at low growth rates. The increased efficiency in glutamine
utilisation was obtained by the cells lowering the alanine yield from
40% to 7% (not illustrated).
Presently, we investigates the irreversible nature of the entrance to
the decline phase observed in both fed batch experiments. Possibly, the
medium's toxin buffer capacity deteriorates over time as the death rate
– despite exponential growth – increased markedly after 80 hours in both
cultures (not illustrated).

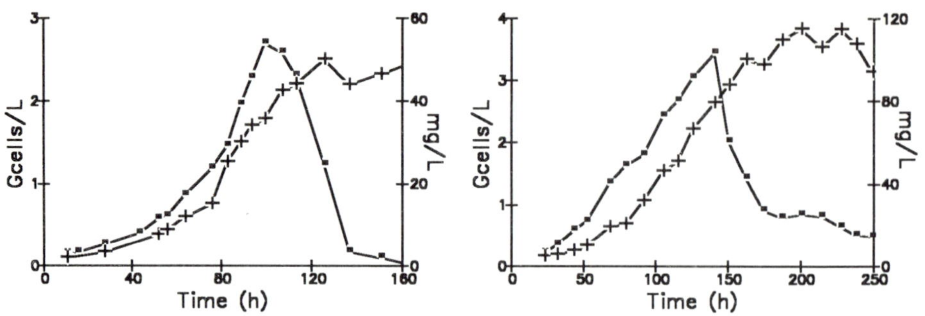

Figure 4 Fed batch and limiting fed batch.
Cells were fed either to maintain the glutamine concentration above 1 mM
(A) or to maintain a constant increase in total cell density (B). The
figures show viable cells (square) and antibody titre (+). The solid
line in (B) is the predicted viable cell density

NOMENCLATURE

Gcells	10^9 cells
n_V, n_D	viable and dead cell density (Gcells/L)
u, k_D	specific growth and death rate (1/h)
G,A	glutamine and ammonia concentration (mM)
Y, Y_A	cell and ammonia yield on glutamine
d_G	glutamine decomposition constant (1/h)
I	antibody concentration (mg/L)
q_I	specific antibody production rate (mg/Gcells/h)
k	Monod constant for glutamine (mM)
u_{max}	maximum growth rate (1/h)
a_D, a_{DD}	specific death rate, G above and below threshold (1/h)
a_I	growth independent antibody production (mg/Gcells/h)
L	glutamine threshold value (mM)

REFERENCES

1. Fredrickson, A.G. _Biotechnol.Bioeng._ 1978, _18_, 1481
2. Nielsen, L.K. M.Sc. thesis, 1989
3. Kovar, J. and Franek, F. _Methods in Enzymology_ , 1986, _121_, 277
4. Schneider, Y-J. _J. Immunol. Methods_ 1989, _116_, 65
5. Radford, K. et. al. submitted to Cytotechnology
6. Reuveny, S. et. al. _J. Immunol. Methods_ 1986, _86_, 53
7. Dodge, T.C. et. al. _Enzyme and Microbial Technology_ 1987, _9_, 607
8. Harbour, C. et. al. _Biotechnology Techniques_ 1989, _3_, 73
9. Miller, W.M. et. al. _Bioprocess Engineering_ 1988, _3_, 113
10. Miller, W.M. et. al. _Biotechnol.Bioeng._ 1988, _32_, 947
11. Oeyaas, K. et. al. In: _Advances in Animal Cell Biology and
    Technology for Bioprocesses_ (Eds. Spier, R.E. et. al.) Butterworth,
    London, 1989, p.212-220
12. Luan, Y.T. et. al. _Biotech.Lett._ 1987, _9_,691
13. Geaugey, V. et. al. _Cytotechnology_ 1989, _2_, 119-129
14. Nielsen, L.K. et. al. presented at Engineering Foundation
    Conference on Cell Culture Engineering II, 1989, Santa Barbara, CA

A COMPUTER SIMULATION OF THE KINETICS AND ENERGETICS OF
HYBRIDOMA CELL GROWTH AND ANTIBODY PRODUCTION

John Barford*, Colin Harbour**

*Department of Chemical Engineering
**Department of Infectious Diseases
University of Sydney, 2006, NSW, Australia

ABSTRACT

A computer simulation of hybridoma cell growth and antibody
production has been developed for batch, fed-batch and
continuous culture. It is capable of simulating all major
metabolic variables of interest, e.g. specific growth rate, cell
yield (viable and total), sugar and amino acid uptakes, and
antibody yield. It also includes such effects as membrane
composition, media composition, substrate and product
inhibition, and osmolarity. As a result, the simulation allows a
rational assessment of different cell lines, media compositions
and modes of cultivation (particularly fed-batch) for optimising
antibody yields.It may also be used to assist in the selection
of fusion partners for optimal antibody production and the
identification and evaluation of the role of various physical
and biochemical factors which affect cell growth and antibody
production. These may assist in rationally based genetic
engineering approaches.

MODEL AIMS

The simulation has the following aims:
(1) Understand the role of kinetics and energetics of hybridoma
cell growth in the observed variations in cell yield, antibody
yield and growth rate (and indirectly put into perspective their
role in such variations compared to random mutation to
non-secreting cells).
(2) Understand the internal metabolism of animal cells with
respect to the relative extent of various biochemical pathways
(e.g. glycolysis, respiration, pentose phosphate pathway).
(3) Understand the effect of defined variations in media
composition and variations from cell line to cell line with
respect to energies and nutrients uptake, cell composition,
antibody composition, antibody excretion mechanisms, and
substrate and product inhibition effects.
(4) Understand the role of cultivation methodology (batch versus
fed-batch versus continuous cultivation).
(5) Effect "What if?" scenarios.

MODEL DEVELOPMENT

The major steps in model development may be identified as:
(1) Identify major energy producing pathways and biosynthetic
pathways for hybridoma cells.
(2) Simplify pathways to limit their detail to major energy and
nutrients uptake and major metabolic intermediates which focus
on pathway interactions.
(3) Simplify by grouping metabolisms together (e.g. families of
amino acids not individual amino acids).
(4) Obtain stoichiometric and energetic details from biochemical
sources.
(5) Write detailed equations for each pathway:

$$A + a\ ATP + b\ NADH + B \qquad = \qquad C$$

(6) Solve differential equations:
For batch and fed-batch: Runge-Kutta numerical methods
For continuous (steady-state and dynamic): SPEEDUP - an
interactive simulation designed to solve both steady-state and
dynamic problems.
(7) Calculate derived quantities (e.g. specific growth rate,
yield(s), specific uptake and excretion rates etc.).

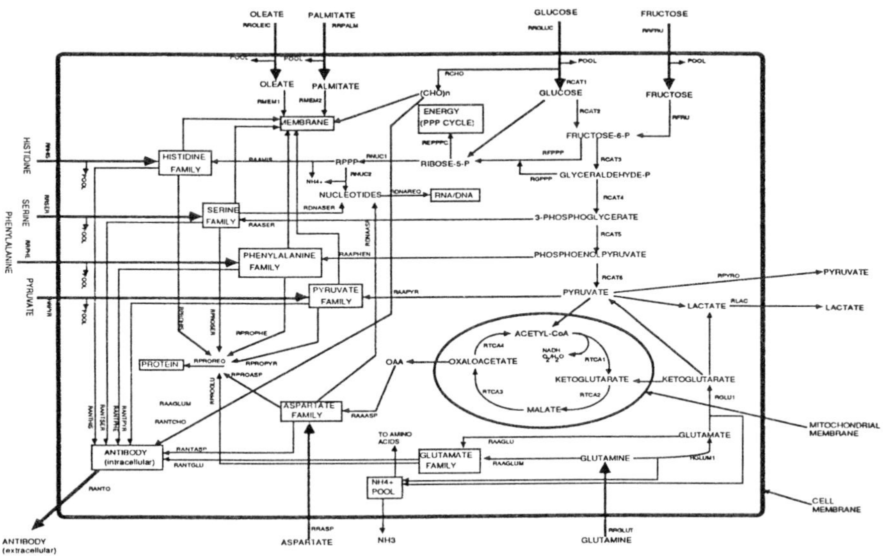

Figure 1 Hybridoma growth model structure

RESULTS

Figure 2 illustrates typical model simulations for batch
cultures (1). Figure 3 illustrates typical model simulation for
continuous cultures. The utilisation of this simulation is the
subject of other publications (2,3) and a computer simulation
package.

DISCUSSION

The examples chosen illustrate that the simulation that has been
developed is able to fit batch and continuous experimental data.
It is now being used to rationally assess a range of
commercially important aspects of hybridoma growth and antibody
production including the assessment of the metabolic fusion
features of the partners and the resultant hybridoma, and the
effect of media composition and cell cultivation methods.

REFERENCES

1   Low, K.S., Harbour, C., Barford, J.P., de Zwart, R. and
    Marquis, C.P. Hybridoma cell growth and antibody production
    kinetics. _Aust. J. Biotechnol._ 1987, _1_ (2), 59

2   Barford, J.P., Harbour, C. A mathematical model of hybridoma
    growth and antibody production - batch culture. _Biotechnol.
    Bioeng._   (submitted)

3   Barford, J.P., Harbour, C. A mathematical model of hybridoma
    growth and antibody production - continuous culture.
    Biotechnol. Bioeng.   (submitted)

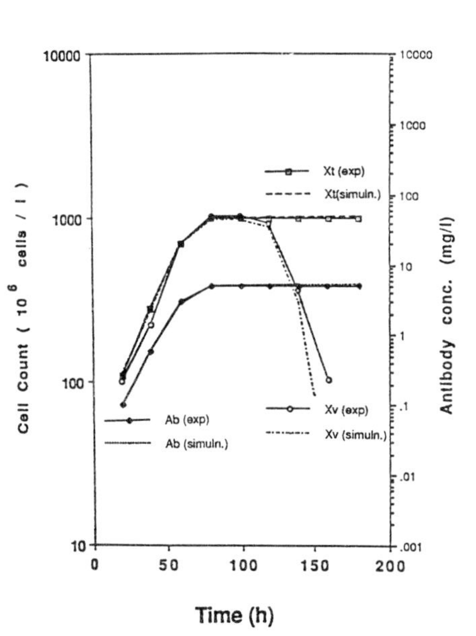

Figure 2 Typical batch simulation
of total and viable cells and
antibody concentration.

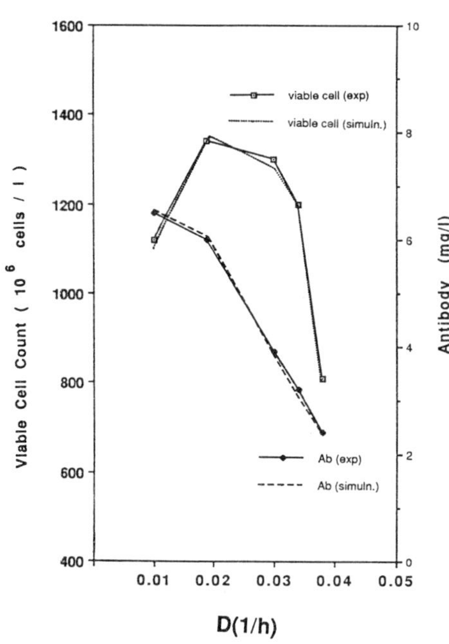

Figure 3 Typical continuous
simulation of viable cells
and antibody concentration.

A KINETIC MODEL FOR THE INFLUENCE OF SERUM IN BATCH AND CONTINUOUS HYBRIDOMA CULTURES

J.L. GOERGEN, A. MARTIAL, A. MARC and J.M. ENGASSER

Laboratoire des Sciences du Génie Chimique, CNRS-ENSIC, Institut National Polytechnique de Lorraine, BP 451, 54001 Nancy Cedex-FRANCE

ABSTRACT

The kinetics of batch and continuous cultures of hybridoma has been investigated at levels of foetal calf serum varying from 10 to 0.5 % v/v. A model taking into account the limiting effect of serum on cell growth and the increased glucose uptake at reduced serum levels correctly describes the kinetics of cell growth and metabolism in the two culture modes.

KEY WORDS

Hybridoma, foetal calf serum, kinetics, modelling, batch cultures, continuous cultures

INTRODUCTION

Serum has been traditionaly added to culture media to grow mammalian cells, but only few quantitative data are available on the influence of serum level on the kinetics of cellular growth, metabolism and proteins production[1-3]. This study examines the kinetics of batch and continuous cultures of hybridoma with different levels of foetal calf serum and proposes a model able to simulate the serum effect.

MATERIAL AND METHODS

Cells: Murine hybridoma, resulting from the fusion of mouse BALB/C spleen cells with mouse myeloma cells, secreting an IgG1 monoclonal antibody.

Culture medium: RPMI 1640 (Intermed) with 0.5 - 10 % FCS (Biosys), 2-4 mM Gln (Intermed).

Cultures : Cultures were performed in spinner flasks (Techne) in batch mode (250ml working volume, 30 rpm, 37°C, 5% CO2) or in a bioreactor (B.Braun) in continuous mode (2 liters; pH=7; T°= 37°C; pO2= 50% of air saturation; 40 rpm).

Analyses : The cell viability was determined with the Trypan-Blue method. Glutamine, glucose and lactate were measured by enzymatic methods (Boehringer) while $NH4^+$ ions are measured with a selective electrode (Orion). Monoclonal Antibodies were determined according to the ELISA method.

RESULTS AND DISCUSSION

The kinetic model

A model previously developped, simulates the growth and death of cells, the uptake of glucose and glutamine, the production of ammonia, lactate and proteins [4]. It takes into account the limiting effects of nutrients, the inhibitory and toxic influence of metabolites in the different rate expressions. Based on the new experimental results obtained in this study, the model has been completed

to include the kinetic effect of the serum concentration. Two important modifications are
reported. A first influence of serum is the growth limitation at reduced level, which can be
represented by a Monod type contribution to the specific growth rate expression:

$$\mu = \mu_{max} \cdot \left[\frac{[Glc]}{K_{Glc} + [Glc]}\right] \cdot \left[\frac{[Gln]}{K_{Gln} + [Gln]}\right] \cdot \left[\frac{[Serum]}{K_{Serum} + [Serum]}\right] \cdot \left[\frac{K_{Lac}}{K_{Lac} + [Lac]}\right] \cdot \left[\frac{K_{NH4}}{K_{NH4} + [NH4]}\right]$$

where [Glc], [Gln], [Serum], [Lac], [NH4] are the concentration of glucose, glutamine,
serum, lactate and ammonia in the medium, μ_{max}, K_{Glc}, K_{Gln}, K_{Serum}, K_{Lac}, K_{NH4} are
kinetic constants.

A second introduced modification is an increase of the specific rates of glucose consumption
and of lactate production at a reduced serum level:

$$V_{Glc} = -\left[Y\frac{Glc}{x} \cdot \mu + m_{Glc}\right] \cdot \left[\frac{K1}{K2 + [Serum]}\right]$$

$$\pi_{Lac} = \left[Y\frac{Lac}{x} \cdot \mu + m_{Lac}\right] \cdot \left[\frac{K1}{K2 + [Serum]}\right]$$

where $Y_{Glc/x}$ and $Y_{Lac/x}$ are respectively the glucose and lactate to cell yields; m_{Glc}, m_{Lac}, K1,
K2 are kinetic parameters and x is the cell density.

The influence of serum level in batch cultures

Figure 1 shows the experimentally measured and modelled time variation of the hybridoma
concentration during batch cultures carried out at four different initial serum levels ranging
from 0.5 to 10 %. A decrease in serum concentration below 5 % yields a reduction in the
specific rate of cellular growth, thus a lower maximal cell density. The model that considers
the limiting effect of serum is capable of simulating the cell density evolution at the different
initial serum concentrations.

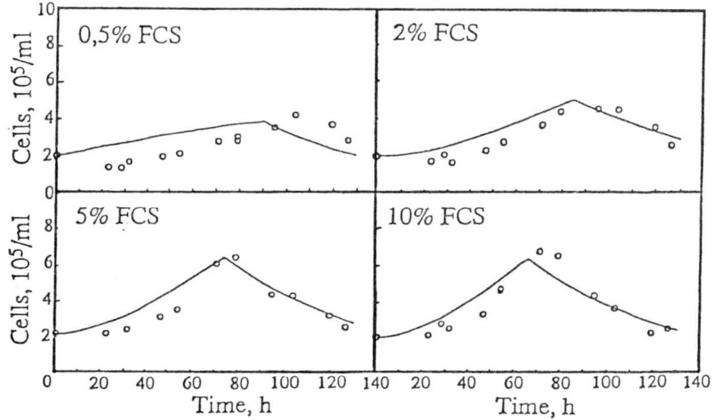

*Fig.1: Variation of the cell density with time for different serum supplements (0.5 % FCS, 2% FCS, 5%
FCS, 10% FCS). empty circles = experimental points; solid line = model .*

The influence of serum level in continuous cultures

Figure 2 shows the experimentally measured and modelled kinetics of a hybridoma continuous culture with successive variations of the serum level in the feed from 4% to 1%, 2% and back to 4%. The continuous culture has been maintained for more than 1300 hours. A decrease in serum level results in a decrease in the production of cells and antibodies, a higher glucose uptake and lactate production rate, but has no significant effect on glutamine consumption. An adaptation of cells to low FCS level is observed: cells which have been maintained at a low serum level show a higher growth rate but a lower antibody production and glucose consumption rate when reexposed to a 4% FCS level. The model with the kinetic effect of serum concentration on glucose uptake and lactate production correctly simulates the dynamic and steady-state kinetics of hybridoma growth and metabolism at least before cell adaptation.

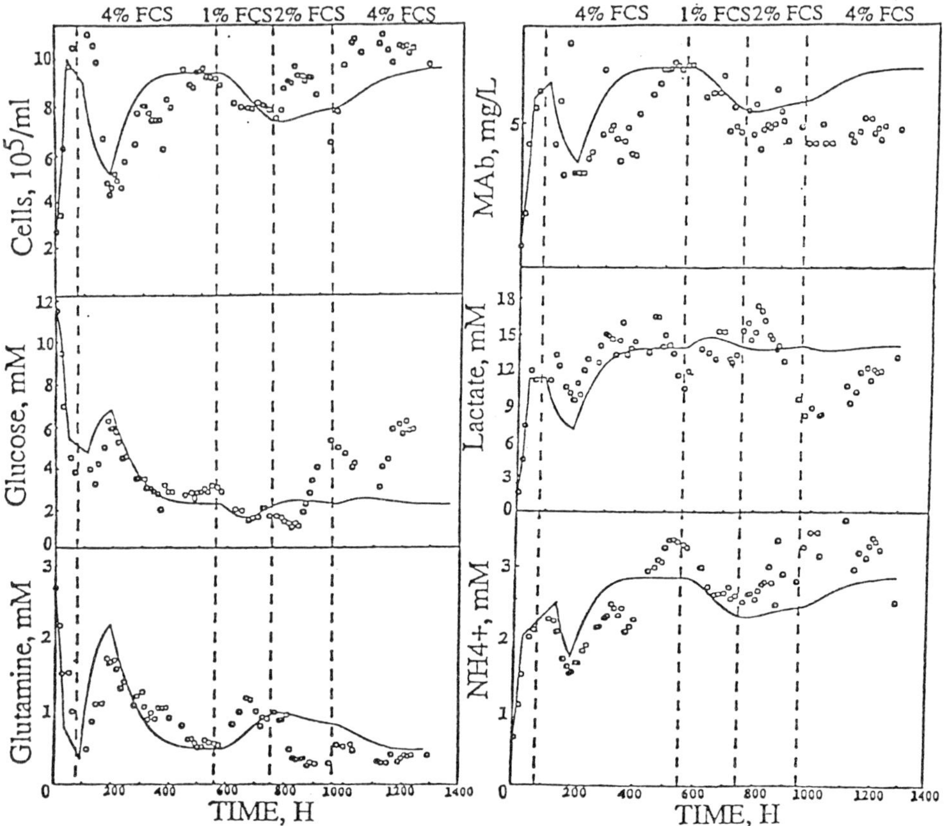

Fig. 2: Evolution of cell density, and glucose, lactate, glutamine, ammonium ions and antibodies concentrations for differents FCS levels vs time; empty circles = experimental points; solid line = model.

REFERENCES

1   M. Dalili and D. Ollis (1988). Biotechnol. & Bioeng., **33**, 984-990
2   S.Ismet Gürhan and N. Özdural (1990). Cytotechnology, **3**, 89-93
3   J. P. Tharakan, A. Lucas and P. C. Chau (1986). J. of Immunol. Methods, **94**, 225-235
4   A. Wagner, PhD thesis, I.N.P.L.-Nancy-France (1990).

Section 9
Downstream processing

ISOLATION OF BIOLOGICALS

LEACHABLES AND CLEANING IN PLACE BECOME A CRUCIAL ISSUE IN LIQUID CHROMATOGRAPHY

E. BOSCHETTI

I B F Biotechnics, Villeneuve-la-Garenne 92390 France

ABSTRACT

It is now clearly admitted that the diversity of separation methods and their applicability mainly depend upon the sample and its properties. There are many examples demonstrating that the crude material origin must be associated with specific pretreatment and chromatographic cycle. Moreover, the choice of separation "tools" sequence is related to the nature and pretreatment of the sample.

Although the available separation techniques lead satisfactorily to pure biologicals, they have to be utilized with care. Actually, these manipulations could introduce unacceptable contaminations either biological (microbial or pyrogen) or chemical (leachables from separation tools).

Cleaning in place should be defined according to the process adopted and to the nature of sorbents and membranes. Precise examples will be given on chromatographic sorbent cleaning making use of acidic and alkaline solutions.

Leachables should be detected, identified and tested for their toxicological properties. If present, they must be eliminated using a final polishing step. Examples on this matter will also be discussed.

INTRODUCTION

The objective of downstream processing is to reach a highly pure protein starting from a crude material, by assembling different available separation technologies in a best configuration ; that means overcoming the problems connected with the nature of the starting raw material, the characteristics of the protein to be isolated, the suited degree of purification and the cost of entire process.

A purification process can be divided into three main steps : extraction, fractionation and purification.

The common feature to different purification steps is playing upon the intrinsic properties of proteins. This leads, on the one hand, to the recognition and separation between proteins and salts, and on the other hand, to the separation between proteins themselves.

Among the primary factors affecting the fractionation of a mixture, there are in fact the molecule size and shape, different solubility in aqueous buffers, diffusivity, ionic charge and biological activity.

The extraction if of course restricted to the insoluble starting material such as cells, cell debris, animal or vegetal tissues. Extraction involves the use of crushing machines homogenizers, stirrers and then filters or centrifuges in order to separate clear water-soluble material from the solid pellet. As it is a very classical operation, this step needs not really sophisticated material, the most important imperatives being temperature control, choice of machines compatible with the stability of investigated protein and the right choice of aqueous solution (composition, ionic strength, pH, additives) so as to reach a high extraction yield. Sometimes, the destruction of cell wall or tissues is optimized by alternating steps of freezing and thawing or ultrasonic treatments.

The characteristic of an aqueous crude extract is to be diluted in term of protein content, to be rich in salts, small organic molecules and often in pigments.

The fractionation can be summarized as an enrichment step where proteins are separated from other small undesirable molecules and yielded in a concentrated clear aqueous solution. This step can also remove a group of contaminant proteins.

The most know and performant technologies used in fractionation are precipitation and ultrafiltration. The former is based on the insolubility of proteins when the aqueous solution contains some specific salts (e.g. ammonium sulfate), organic compounds (e.g. polyethylene glycol, ethanol, acetone) and when the pH is modified by acidic or alkaline solutions. Since precipitation is an easy way to recover proteins in the insoluble phase, all other molecules are in the supernatant. The collected proteins can then be solubilized in a minimum volume of buffer.

Fractionated precipitation can also be carried out when separating two groups of proteins. This is particularly done for instance, by increasing progressively the quantities of ammonium sulphate.

In downstream processing, ultrafiltration involves the use of microporous flat membranes or microporous hollow fibers that separate in the aqueous phase, the large molecules (proteins) from the small ones (e.g. salts). This method is advantageous as it acts like a real molecular sieving and at the same time, excess water is eliminated from the diluted protein solutions. Ultrafiltration can be used not only as an alternative precipitation (separation) method, but also as a complement to precipitation (elimination of remaining salts or solvents).

Ultrafiltration, diafiltration and microfiltration are three different aspects of this technology and are applied at different levels of downstream processing.

The purification step is an isolation operation where all or most of the contaminants are removed. The most suitable techniques for protein purification are the chromatographic methods.

Except gel filtration, liquid chromatography is based on the interaction between proteins solubilized in the buffer and the column solid phase. When the protein solution runs through the column, the proteins interact differently with the solid phase according to their composition and can thus be separated.

TAB I - GENERAL OUTLINE OF BIOSYNTHESIS AND PURIFICATION OF DNA DERIVED PRODUCTS

PROCESS STEP	GOAL AND PROCESS INVOLVEMENTS
Choice of the cell host	Characterization
Choice of culture media	Growth, secretion level, contaminations
Bioreactor	Productivity, agitation mode, sampling possibilities
Cell separation	Concentration without cell lysis, microfiltration
Sample treatment	Clarification, ultrafiltration, precipitation
Ion exchange chromatography	Removal of largest part of contaminating proteins
Bioaffinity adsorption	Selective recovery of active proteins and concentrations
Gel filtration	Polishing step to remove final traces of contaminants
Concentration of pure products	Ultrafiltration, sterile filtration
Acidic/alkaline treatments	Virus inactivation
Formulation of final product	Concentration or dilution, adjustment of active ingredient, biological activity calibration

Among different types of chromatography, the most important ones are ion exchange chromatography, adsorption chromatography, affinity chromatography and hydrophobic chromatography.

Ion exchange chromatography is based on the ionic interaction between a support electrically charged and the net charge of a protein which may be modified by the pH and ionic strength of the aqueous solution. The isoelectric point and the charge density command the type of ion exchanger to be used.

Affinity chromatography is based on the highly specific interaction between the molecule to be purified and a ligand chemically immobilized on the solid support.

Hydrophobic chromatography exploits its ability of creating hydrophobic complexes between the proteins possessing long-chain aliphatic amino acids and the hydrophobic ligands immobilized on the solid phase. This association occurs in particular when the proteins medium has high ionic strength.

When designing a whole purification process for biological, different techniques must be associated. They include in fact pretreatment of the samples, membrane technology (filtration or ultrafiltration) and chromatography steps.

These different methods are associated in a most suitable way to save time, labour and to fulfill the economic requirements. There is there a real strategic approach permitting to create very integrated and effective industrial systems as described earlier.

A purification process must furthermore meet the necessary purity requirements in accordance with the final application of the biological and the regulatory agencies recommendations.

In most of the cases, the purity of a biological means :

- absence of any other contaminating proteins,
- absence of microorganisms (cells, bacteria, yeasts, viruses)
- absence of pyrogenic substance
- absence of leached material from fractionating tools (membranes, filtration aids, chromatographic sorbents, ...)
- absence of DNA.

All these imperatives imply the application of a number of more or less defined operations which are :

- application of CIP methodologies
- utilization of "clean" samples and any aqueous solutions.
- Elimination of small impurities by final polishing steps.

A general outline of the purification of DNA derived products is illustrated on table I.

CLEANING IN PLACE OF SEPARATION TOOLS (chromatographic sorbents)

Cleaning in place includes three different notions which are the regeneration, the pyrogen removal and the sterilization.

Regeneration is clearly effected to remove any mineral and organic compound non specifically adsorbed on the chromatographic sorbent (this is also true for any other separating tool like ultrafiltration membranes). The most frequent chemicals bonded on the solid sorbents after repeated operations are the lipidic substances (including pyrogens), protein aggregates and pigments, polyphenols and metal complexes. All these products contribute to decrease the level of separation efficiency, the sorption capacity while introducing non specific adsorptions sites. These phenomena diminish also the operation yields and decrease the level of purity of the final products . To overcome these problems several solutions have been proposed (see table II), which are applicable according to the nature of the contaminating material.

Sterilization implies the destruction of any living cell (bacteria, yeast) by particular chemical treatments of the separating tools.

Sodium hydroxide is well known as an aqueous solution for the sterilization of chromatographic packings. Ethanolic mixtures containing acetic acid or sodium hydroxide are less know but not necessarily less efficient.

In an internal experimental study, we tried to quantify the sterilization power of sodium hydroxide at different concentrations, of a 60 % ethanol 0.5 M acetic acid mixture and of a 0.2 M - 0.5 M sodium hydroxide-ethanol (at different concentrations) mixtures.

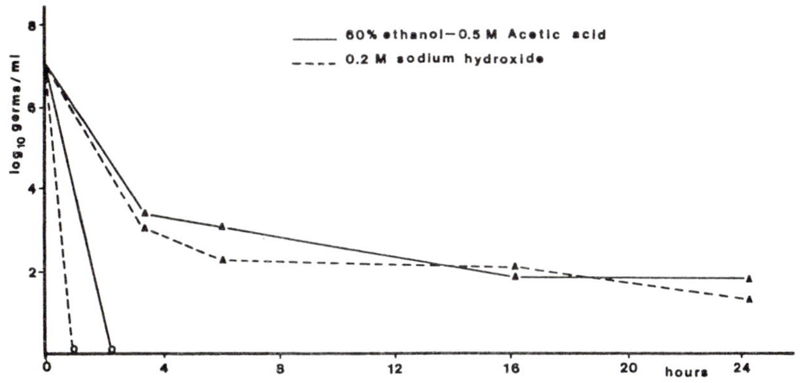

Fig 1 .   Inactivation kinetic of germs (Bacillus subtilis   (△), and Escherichia coli, Staphylococcus aureus, Candida albicans (o)) using two CIP solutions at room temperature

Chromatographic sorbents were first contaminated with a large amount of defined microorganisms (*Escherichia coli, Staphylococcus aureus, Candida albicans* and sporulated form of *Bacillus subtilis*) and then decontaminated by washing with appropriate solutions.

After contamination, the sorbents were treated with three volumes of the appropriate sanitizing solution (up to 24 hours at 25°C). The remaining germs were then detected by a standard culture after neutralization of the sorbent-cleaning solution mixtures (or column effluents).

It was found that the inactivation of germs by sodium hydroxide washing was dependent on the nature of the strains used. (*Escherichia coli* was the most sensitive to alkaline media ; it was in fact totally inactivated by sodium hydroxide at concentration as low as 0.05 M. *Candida albicans* and *Staphilococcus aureus* were also sensitive to NaOH treatment but their total inactivation was observed when the NaOH concentration was 0.1 M or higher. However, sodium hydroxide at any concentration (and at a temperature of 20-25° C for 3 hours) was not found to be very effective in the inactivation of the sporulated form of *Bacillus subtilis*, even when the sodium hydroxide treatment was extended up to 24 hours (fig. 1). In the best cases, the decrease of the amount of *Bacillus subtilis* was about 5 logs, which means that, from an initial concentration of about ten millions germs/ml, about 100 germs per ml were still present at the end of the treatment.

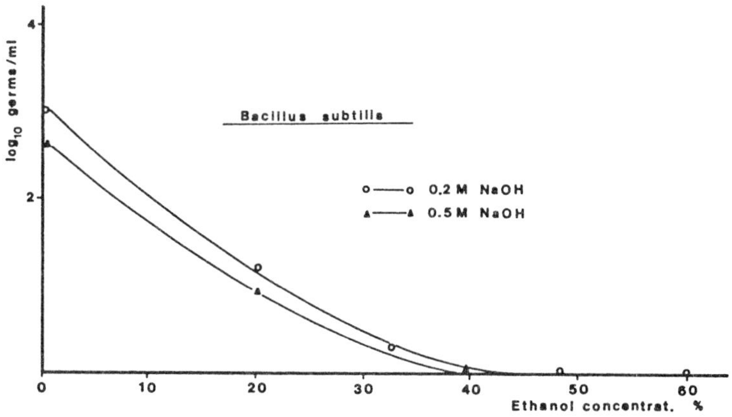

Fig 2 . Influence of ethanol concentration on Bacillus subtilis (sporulated form) inactivation with ethanol sodium hydroxide mixtures at room temperature for three hours. initial germ content : 10 millions/ml

The treatment of contaminated supports by an aqueous mixture of 60 %
ethanol and 0.5 M acetic acid evidenced an extreme sensitivity of all the
strains studied, except *Bacillus subtilis*. While in an ethanol-acetic acid
treatment of less than 1 hour, *E. coli, C. albicans and S. aureus* germs
were quantitatively inactivated, the number of *B. subtilis* decreased
greatly during the first hours of treatment (4 logs) and then very slowly
in the subsequent hours. After 24 hours of treatment, a significant level
of contamination (180 germs/ml) still persisted (fig. 1).

It was found however than an alternated treatment of a contaminated
sorbent for 1.5 hour each with 0.2 M sodium hydroxide and acetic acid-
containing ethanol inactivated totally *B. subtilis*. The results obtained
with these experiments led us to imagine a treatment with a solution
composed of 0.2 M or 0.5 M sodium hydroxide and ethanol at a concentration
between 20 and 60 % for three hours. When the ethanol concentration was
superior to 40 %, he inactivation of sporulated *B. subtilis* was total.
While decreasing this concentration to 20 %, the efficiency of this
mixture in sterilizing contaminated solutions was very good for *E. coli,
C. albicans* and *S. aureus*, but *B. subtilis* was not totally destroyed (fig.
2). From these results, it can be ascertained that, if total elimination
of germs in a chromatographic support is to be achieved, it is necessary
to proceed either to an alternated treatment using 0.2 M sodium hydroxide
and ethanol-acetic acid mixture or to an alkaline treatment of low
concentration in the presence of ethanol.

Besides of the differences found in the sterilizing efficiency all of the
investigated solutions were able to remove pyrogens (determination with
limulus lysate test).

LEACHABLES : DETECTION AND ELIMINATION

Chemicals of different nature can come from separating tools (membranes or
chromatographic packings) and in a certain extent could contaminate the
final pure biological. These chemical products can be generated by two
different phenomena :

- some chemical could be present in the separating tools from this
  manufacturing steps,

- leached material (or extractables) can be generated by strong
  CIP operations.

In any cases, any leached material of whatever origin should be detected
and then eliminated by appropriate validated steps. If a certain level of
chemicals is detected it could be necessary to determine the level of the
potential toxicity.

TAB II – OPERATIONS OF CLEANING IN PLACE ACCORDING TO THE NATURE OF THE ADSORBED PRODUCT

TREATMENT	REGENERATION (elution of greatly adsorbed molecules)	STERILIZATION	DEPYROGENATION
1 - 2 M sodium chloride	Molecules greatly charged	Inefficient	Inefficient
Buffer pH 3-5	Molecules greatly charged	"	"
Pronase, neutral pH, ions calcium	Hydrolysis of adsorbed proteins	"	"
Pepsine pH 1,5-2	Hydrolysis of adsorbed proteins	"	"
Non ionic detergents (Triton X-100, Tween 80)	Elimination of hydrophobic proteins and lipidic substances	"	"
Cationic detergents pH 9-11	" " " " "	"	"
Non ionic detergents in acid solution pH ≃ 3 (acetic acid)	" " " " "	"	"
Urea 6 M - 8 M	Elimination of aggregates of proteins	"	Not determined
1 mM - 100 mM EDTA (in a neutral or slightly acidic solution)	Elimination of metal complexes	"	Inefficient
0.1-1 M sodium hydroxide	Elimination of hydrophobic proteines, lipopolysaccharides and other unknown contaminants	efficient	efficient
Ethanol 60 % - 0.5-1 M acetic acid	Elimination of lipids, pigments, lipopolysaccharides and other lipophilic substances	very efficient	efficient
Acetic acid 50 - 80 %	Solubilization and elimination of precipitated proteins	not determined	not determined
Ethanol 40 - 60 %	Elimination of some proteins and of subtances of a family close to the one of lipids	"	"
Isopropanol gradient till 100 %	Elimination of non polar lipids	inefficient	"
Mineral or organic acids 0.1 - 1 M	Elimination of various adsorbed molecules and hydrolysis of ligands	not determined	"

It is obvious that on the level of industrial exploitation leading to the purification of a therapeutic product, the chromatographic support must be sufficiently stable and not leach polymer or oligomer traces which could be toxic or have a parasite action. In this view, many research works tried to determine the level of leachables or undesirable products which may be present in the chromatographic supports. In vivo and in vitro toxicity studies were also made. Two examples are detailed in this paper : DEAE-TRISACRYL   and BLUE-TRISACRYL

In the case of DEAE-TRISACRYL,   the trials to evidence free acrylic monomers (N -acryloyl-2-amino-2-hydroxymethyl-1, 3-propane diol and diethylaminoethyl acrylamide) were carried out in the effluents of a column washed with a 1 M NaCl solution. HPLC analyses done on Nucleosil 5 C18 in perchloric acid medium (70 %), acetonitrile and distilled water in the proportions of 3 : 10 : 987 evidenced that the monomer content was extremely low and in any cases below the sensitivity of the method (< 0.1 mg/l). Moreover, washings with a sodium chloride solution would remove these traces and permit to work in the most appropriate conditions (figure 3).

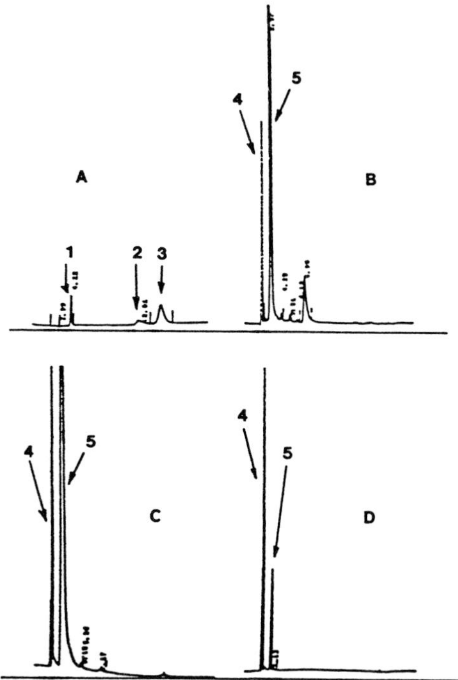

Fig 3. *Analytical HPLC of DEAE-Trisacryl original supernatant (B) compared to standard monomers (A) (N-acryloyl-2-amino-2-hydroxymethyl-1,3-propano-diol "1", N,N'-methylene-bis-acrylamide "2" and DEAE-acrylamide "3"). C and D represent the column effluents after one and five column volumes washings with classical buffer 4:sodium chloride ; 5:sodium azide*

The toxicity studies carried out with those free monomers demonstrated they were well tolerated in classical standard assays (DL-50 and in vivo irritation studies).

Another example in the field of leachable and toxicity is given by special immobilized dyes. Blue Cibacron F3 GA immobilized on a solid matrix provides adsorbents whose efficiency and specificity are so high that they are very attractive for application at the preparative level. However, the dye may leak under certain physico-chimical conditions (acidic hydrolysis on agarose-based supports or desorption of molecules chemically unfixed) and it is then necessary not only to assay the ligand amount in the column effluents but also to know the eventual toxic effects.

The results of specific studies carried out in vitro (effect on human cell culture, chromosome study, genotoxicity study) clearly show that even in the presence of a large quantity of dye, there is practically no effect. MRC-5 human cells cultured in the presence of dye during six passages (between the 29th and the 35th passage, according to World Health Organization (WHO)'s recommendations) showed neither modification in their growth curve nor morphological anomalies. The lethal dose was around 250 ug dye/ml of medium.

However, when cells were cultured in the presence of the leached dye coming from an agarose based sorbent then the growth ratio was significantly lower (see fig. 4).

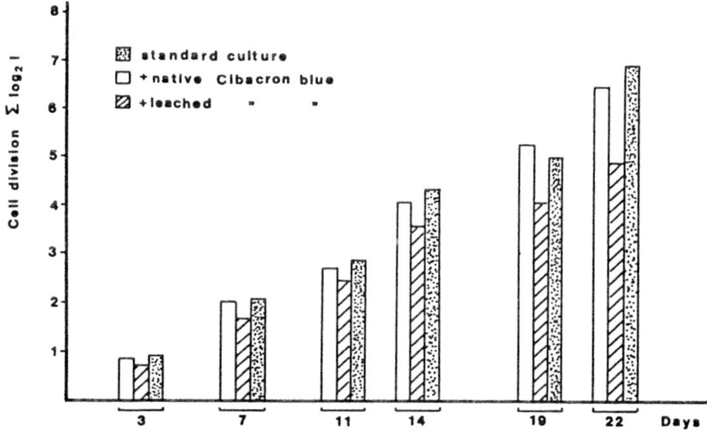

Fig 4 . Growth rate of MRC-5 human cells in vitro over six passages in classical conditions (from the 29th and the 35th passage). The cultures were performed in DMEM medium containing 10 % fetal bovine serum in the presence of 25 ug/ml of native free cibacron blue or leached cibacron blue compared to a standard cell culture.

Additionally, a chromosome analysis effected on more than 500 metaphases of these cells evidenced that the level of polyploidia in the presence of 25 ug/ml of free dye was of the same magnitude than that of the reference. The obtained values of 6/514 or 9/520 for the polyploidia level are significantly inferior to WHO's requirements (17/500). When the cells were cultured in the presence of 25 ug/ml of leached dye the level of polyploidia was significantly higher (from 18/500 to 23/500). This last result can be explained by the difference between the chemical structure of native and leached Cibacron Blue Dye. Investigations demonstrated that the leached dye contained a certain amount of polysaccharide resulting from the matrix hydrolysis and so explaining the leakage phenomenon.

CONCLUSION

When using polymeric separation material (membranes and chromatographic packings) for the production of pure biologicals special precautions must be taken.

The necessity of working in clean, sterile and apyrogenic conditions supposes the application of very drastic washings (strong acidic or alkaline solutions, hydroorganic mixtures) which could generate by-products. These by-products must be identified, quantified and tested for their possible toxicity. Specific washing procedures should in this case be defined to remove any polymeric by-product. To be sure that any traces of this kind of leached material are completely eliminated, a final gel filtration polishing step must be used. This last approach becomes more and more popular since it assures not only the elimination of small molecules or fragments and possibles aggregates but also permits the final formulation of the pure product.

<u>Paper of Boschetti</u>

Estefanell: Would you recommend your clinician process for the affinity gels or at least the ethanol acetic acid.

Boschetti: We did a lot of experimentation of ways of cleaning affinity chromatography columns with protein ligands like Conconavalin A and bacterial proteins like Protein A and antibodies. We found the anti human IgG supported this washing with 60% Ethanol/0.5M acetic acid for 45 minutes for 5 cycles. After this we found a decrease of adsorption capacity of between 12-18%. If the desanitizing solution was a mixture of NaOH with 60% Ethanol then the decrease in adsorption capacity was about 40% after 5 cycles of sanitization.

Estetanell: Did you try to wash the column with detergent?

Boschetti: We tried detergents. A way to clean the column is to mix a non-ionic detergent like Tween 80 or Triton X 100 mixed with 1M acetic acid. This can wash out a lot of impurities but it does not guarantee sterilization so you have to do 2 steps one to regenerate the gel and then to resterilise the gel.

Handa-Corrigan: There is a school of thought which holds that if you use stainless steel implants in the human body material leached from the metal can cause cancer. Could you tell me if there is leaching of metallic ions from fermenter walls into the bioproducts.

Boschetti: We recommend that after using acetic acid solutions we pass through the system buffer containing citric acid or EDTA to complex as much as possible any leached metal ions.

COMPOSITE HIGH FLOW RATE ION EXCHANGERS FOR ECONOMICAL
SCALE-UP

Magnus Glad and Stefan Schornack

Perstorp Biolytica AB, S-223 70 Lund, Sweden

ABSTRACT

A novel type of high flow rate ion exchanger - ProCell - has
been developed. The base material is a composite which
combines the biocompatibility of cellulose with the high
mechanical strength of polystyrene. ProCell DEAE and CM were
used in a process to to purify immunoglobulin and albumin in
gram quantities from bovine plasma. The rigidity of the
composite sorbent allowed for the use of high flow rates
which kept the total cycle time short. Efficient
sanitization of the ion exchangers was easily achieved using
sodium hydroxide and urea.

INTRODUCTION

Protein purification is one of the most demanding steps in
modern biotechnology. From a usually extremely complex
mixture present in microorganisms or cell cultures one
single component must be isolated and highly purified to be
suited for human injection. Several separation steps
including chromatography must often be employed and the
purification cost usually stands for a major part of the
total production cost. Many different chromatographic
methods are today available but ion exchange chromatography
still seems to the most commonly used method (1). Especially
cellulose ion exchangers have been widely used for a long
time (2) because of the hydrophilic nature of cellulose
resulting in low tendency to denature proteins and in high
recoveries. Some of the features of ion exchange
chromatography are stable adsorbents, reproducable results,
high recovery of active proteins, predictable scale-up and a
relatively low cost.

A NEW COMPOSITE ION EXCHANGER

A new type of composite high flow rate ion exchanger,
ProCell, and its applications have been jointly developed by
Cultor (formerly Finnish Sugar) and Perstorp Biolytica in
order to supply an attractive alternative to traditional ion
exchangers for process applications. The base material is
manufactured by an extrusion process which gives a composite
of cellulose and polystyrene combining the well known
biocompatibility of cellulose with a highly rigid core of

polystyrene. After crushing and sieving to 150-350 um the
material is derivatized with DEAE or CM groups (Fig.1).

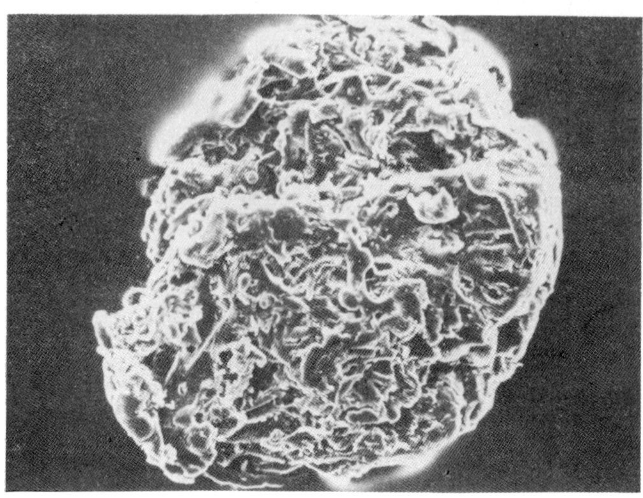

Figure 1   SEM picture of ProCell
cellulose/polystyrene composite particle

Some relevant chemical and physical properties of the
ProCell ion exchangers are found in Table 1. The most
characteristic feature of the new sorbent is its high
mechanical stability in a packed bed which allows for the
use of simple and long columns if needed and the use of high
flow rates (up to 2500 cm/h) and pressures up to 3 bar which
is unusual for sorbents of carbohydrate origin. The binding
capacity for the DEAE-derivative (30 mg BSA/ml) and for the
CM-derivative (20 mg haemoglobin/ml) is in the same range as
most other common medium or high pressure ion exchangers but
lower than the fully porous carbohydrate-based gels. This
can be explained by the observation (SEC) that only 30-40%
of the particle volume is accessible to protein solutes. The
rest of the particle volume is occupied by the rigid
polystyrene core which only contributes to the mechanical
stability of the ion exchanger.

	ProCell DEAE	ProCell CM
Titrated capacity	50 uekv/ml	70 uekv/ml
Protein capacity	30 mg BSA/ml	20 mg bov.Hb/ml
Particle size	150-350 um	
Flow rate	up to 2500 cm/h	
Pressure	up to 3 bar	
pH stability	2 - 14	

Table 1   Technical characteristics of ProCell ion exchangers

A similar ion exchanger has already proven very reliable for column immobilization of enzymes, e.g. glucose isomerase, in process scale food applications. Furthermore, some large scale applications of enzyme purification in kilogram quantities per cycle are also in progress.

FRACTIONATION OF BOVINE PLASMA

A procedure to purify IgG and albumin from bovine plasma was developed (3). The new high flow rate ion exchangers ProCell DEAE and ProCell CM were both employed to speed up the total procedure (Fig.2).

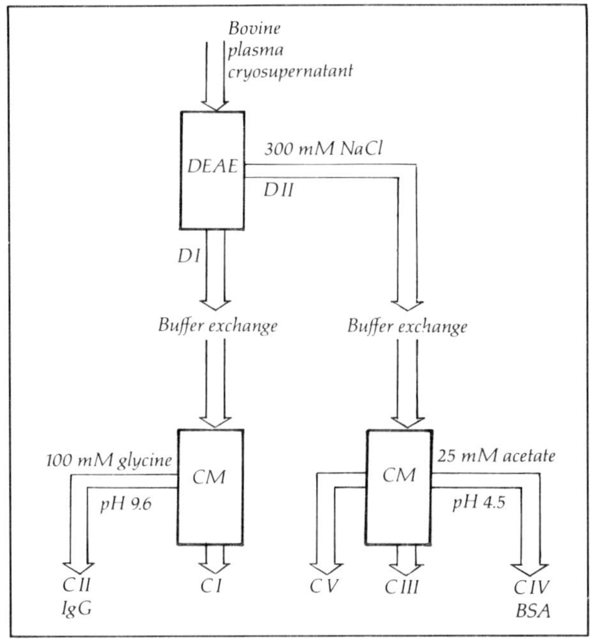

Figure 2   Scheeme for the fractionation of bovine plasma with high flow rate ion exchange chromatography

Columns of approximately 5 L bed volume were utilized with a linear flow rate of up to 900 cm/h. A centrifuged and diluted (1.5L to 4.0L with 25 mM Tris-HCl, 80 mM NaCl, pH8.3) cryosupernatant from bovine plasma was applied to a column packed with 5.0 L of ProCell DEAE (32 x 14 cm I.D.) at a linear flow rate of 460 cm/h which corresponds to 20 bed volumes/h (Fig.3). The flow through fraction (DI) contained IgG with a purity of approximately 60%.

The BSA-rich fraction (DII) which was bound to the DEAE-adsorbent could be eluted with a high ion strength buffer (300 mM NaCl). The peak shape was acceptable despite the

high flow rate used and the separation could be completed
within less than 20 minutes.

After diafiltration the IgG fraction (DI) was applied to a
column with 5.0 L of CM ion exchanger at a flow rate of 260
cm/hour.The IgG was eluted with 0.1 M glycine, pH 9.6, with
a purity of 80-85 %, the main impurity being transferrin.
The BSA fraction (DII) was also diafiltrated and then
applied to a 5 L column with CM-ion exchanger. The albumin
was eluted in 25 mM acetate, pH 4.5 with a purity of 95 %.

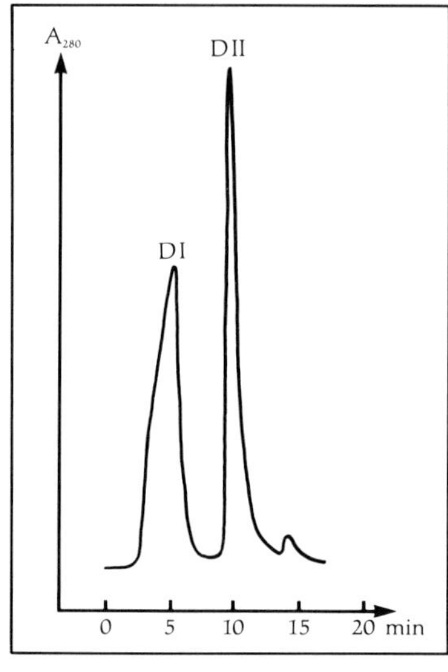

Figure 3   Bovine plasma
on DEAE ion exchanger

The protein recovery was in each chromatographic step 70-
80%. The regeneration of the columns with high salt and
binding buffer was performed at a flow rate of 900 cm/h. The
gels were stored in 0.1 M NaOH when not in use.

The fractions were analyzed for protein with BCA (Pierce
Chemical Company), for IgG with ProAnaMabs HPLAC (Perstorp
Biolytica), for BSA with anti-BSA antibodies coupled to
agarose, and for purity with IEF and SDS-PAGE.

In order to investigate the durability of the ion exchanger
bovine serum was chromatographed on a smaller ProCell DEAE
column (80 mm x 10 mm I.D.) in 40 concequtive runs. Bovine
serum samples (0.5 ml diluted 1:10) were applied in 5 mM
potassium phosphate, pH 7.6 and subsequently step-eluted
with 0.1, 0.2 and finally 1.0 M sodium chloride. Negligible
variation in performance were found between runs since
elution times, peak areas and resolution remained essential
constant during the series of experiments. This long time
stability makes the ion exchanger suited for automated
processes.

COST ANALYSIS

A cost analysis for a one step fractionation of bovine serum
albumin with DEAE ion exchange chromatography is shown in
Table 2. The comparision is made between a traditional
carbohydrate-based gel and the new high flow rate ion
exchanger. The main object was to investigate how the flow
rate and the binding capacity influence the production cost
for the final product. It should be noted that not all the
costs involved in the production have been taken into
consideration. Thus is neighter the price of ion
exchanger nor the hardware costs included in the
calculation. It can be seen that despite a lower protein
binding capacity it is possible to more than enough
compensate for that with a higher flow rate.

	DEAE ion exchanger (5 liter column)	
	Conventional gel	ProCell
Flow rate (l/min)	1.2	7.5
Albumin loading (g)	368	160
Cycle time (min)	199	30
Albumin yield (g/cycle)	331	144
Cycles per day	3	17
Buffer use (l/day)	660	3740
Buffer cost (SEK/day)	54	305
Labour cost (SEK/day)	275	275
Total cost (SEK/day)	329	580
Albumin yield (kg/day)	1.0	2.45
Albumin cost (SEK/kg)	329	237

Table 2   Cost analysis for purification of bovine serum
albumin with ion exchange chromatography

CLEANING

Proteins which are to be suited for human injection must not
only be highly purified but also free of process-derived
contaminants such as bacteria and endotoxin. Endotoxins are
lipopolysaccharides (LPS) from gram negative bacteria which
induce fever and shock. ProCell cellulose/polystyrene
composite ion exchangers can withstand sodium hydroxide
which is effective in removing endotoxins from
chromatographic systems and behave much like classical
cellulosic ion exchangers except they can handle very high
flow rates without compacting.

A convenient procedure to achieve low endotoxin ion exchange
chromatography with ProCell has been developed by A.R.
Torres (4). In short the procedure is as follows:

1) After use of the column wash with 1-2 column volumes
   of 10 mM NaOH in 3 M urea.

2) Wash out the urea with 3 column volumes of 10 mM NaOH
   and store the column in this.

3) When the ion exchanger is to be used wash with 2
   column volumes of water followed by 1-2 column
   volumes of a ten-fold concentrated buffer.

4) Equilibrate with 6-10 column volumes of buffer before
   application of sample.

Ion-exchange columns often take 10-20 column volumes of
buffer for equilibration and there is always a risk for
rapidly growing bacteria to contaminate buffers and sorbents
during prolonged equilibration. The high flow rates on the
ProCell ion exchangers allows for rapid buffer and pH
equilibration. Complete protein separations with very low
endotoxin levels (below 0.1 ng/ml concentrated protein
solution) can be accomplished in a normal working day as the
columns can be rapidly equilibrated in about 2 hours (4).

REFERENCES

1   Bonnerjea, J., Oh, S., Hoare, M. and Dunhill, P. Protein
    purification: The right step at the right time.
    Biotechnology 1986, _4_, 954

2   Peterson, E.A. _Cellulosic Ion Exchangers_ Elsevier/North
    Holland, 1980

3   Glad, M., Schornack, S., Myöhänen, T. and Lommi, H.
    ProCell DEAE And CM - Novel Composite Ion Exchangers For
    Rapid Separations In Biotechnology. _BioMedia_ Vol.2
    Perstorp Biolytica, Lund, Sweden, 1989   pp 14-15

4   Torres, A.R. Low Endotoxin Ion Exchange Chromatography.
    BioMedia Vol.3 Perstorp Biolytica, Lund, Sweden, 1990
    pp 3-4

<u>**Paper of Glad**</u>

Hofmann: It appears to me that you have a conventional gel
             geometry and you are still in a diffusion driven
             process and the superficial residence time is the same
             as that needed in a conventional gel, so if you changed
             your geometry would you not have a high capacity and a
             high flow rate.

Glad: The geometry is not different but we have a gel with
             macropores which gives a lower superficial residence
             time.

SERUM FREE MEDIA (SFM) AND SERUM SUBSTITUTES (SS) IN ANIMAL CELL CULTURE: DOWNSTREAM CONSIDERATIONS.

H. Graf[1], J.N. Rabaud[1], J.M. Egly[2] .

1. S.G.I. 15, Allées de Bellefontaine 31100 Toulouse.
2. INSERM U184 11, rue Human 67085 Strasbourg.

ABSTRACT

We have analysed 14 of the 35-40 SFM or SS available on the market today, in order to determine their protein content and their behaviour on three chromatographic supports (Gel filtration, ion exchange, hydrophobic interaction). Those media mainly developped for hybridoma cell culture, generally contain serum albumin (95 % of total protein), insulin, transferrin and poorly defined low MW compounds. All of these compounds will interfere with monoclonal antibody (MAb) purification especially in ion exchange chromatography. Several examples of behaviour of "serum free " cell supernatants containing MAbs on DEAE resin are presented.

INTRODUCTION

Recovering biological reagent, recombinant protein or monoclonal antibody from cell culture supernatant is a critical part of biotechnology manufacturing. To developp a downstream strategy, it is of first importance to characterize the starting material in detail but this is a very difficult task when one use commercial SFM (so-called chemically defined media) or SS (often undefined media) in animal cell culture, because of fabrication secrets. For these reasons, we will review and characterize some SFM or SS available on the market.

MATERIALS AND METHODS

Determination of protein content was assayed according to Bradford (ref.1) using B.S.A. as standart. SDS-PAGE and silver staining were performed according to Laemmli (ref.2) and Wray (ref.3), respectively. HPLC experiments were performed at room temperature using an LKB apparatus. HPLC columns, e.g. TSK G3000 SW (600x7.5), DEAE 5PW (75x7.5) and Phenyl 5PW (75x7.5) were supplied by Toyo Soda (Japan).

RESULTS

Determination of protein content

Good reproductibility was observed between commercial data (when given) and experimental results (Bradford assay and HPLC quantitation). As deduced from table 1, there are two groups of SFM according to the protein content (reflecting the BSA content): Low protein content SFM (<0,03 g/l), and high protein content SFM (>0.8 g/l) where serum albumin (S.A.) is the main component (90 to 95% of total protein).

Media	Protein content (g/l) c.d.	e.r.	Albumin (g/l) c.d.	e.r.	Polymer%	Transferrin (g/l) c.d.	e.r.	Other protein c.d.	e.r.
BMS ** 10% (Biochrom)	1,50	1,46	+	+	2,8	n.a.	+ (n.d.)	pept., GF[3]	Ins.[1]
Feb 100 * (Biochrom)	1,50	1,45	+	1,40	8,7	+	0,02	Ins.	Ins.
ADCM ** 2% (Caryoser-IBF)	n.a.	0,60	+	0,60	1,0	+	0,07	Ins. Fib.	/
NU Serum ** 10% (Coll. Res.)	1,36 [4]	1,44	+[5]	1,10	11,3	+	0,12	EGF,Ins,Ig[6]	/
H.M. high protein * (Gibco)	0,73	0,80	+	0,80	7,4	+	0,02	Ins, Gluc.	Ins.
H.M. low protein * (Gibco)	0,03	0,03	-	0	0	+	0,03	Ins.,Gluc.	Ins.
Opti MEM I * (Gibco)	n.a.	0,01	-	0	0	n.a.	<0,01	G.F.	Ins.
Ultroser HY ** 4% (IBF)	0,80	0,88	+	0,83	9,5	+	0,02	Ins.	Ins.
Ultroser G ** 2% (IBF)	1,50	1,44	+[2]	1,30	22,5	n.a.	0,07	G.F., A.F.	Ins.
Imocell * (IBF)	1,00	1,00	+	1,00	5,0	+	0,01	Ins	Ins.
Hyb. Sf-p* (ICN Bioch.)	n.a.	2,50	+[7]	1,90	26,7	+	0,11	Ins.	Ins.
DCCM * (PBS Orgen.)	n.a.	2,00	+[8]	1,95	6,7	n.a.	0,02	n.a.	Ins.
SFRI4 * (Sfri Labs)	n.a.	2,00	+[8]	1,90	10,0	n.a.	0,01	n.a.	Ins.
HL-1 * (Ventrex)	0,03	0,02	-	0	0	+	0,02	Ins. S.P.[7]	Ins.

* = SFM, ** = Serum Substitute
1. not quantifiable, 2. Binding protein , 3. Peptides 500mg/l, Growth factor 2,5 mg/l, 4. Assumes that one OD280 = 1mg/ml, 5. Bovine serum albumin 6. Bovine Ig 7. Stabilizing protein, 8. BSA Cohn fraction V; Polymer % represent % of protein of M.W. higher than 80 Kd, n.a. = not available, n.d. = not determinated, G.F. = Growth factor, A.D. = Adhesion factor, Ins. = Insulin, Gluc. = Glucagon, Fib. = Fibronectine.

Table 1: Protein content of various SFM and SS: Commercial data (c.d.) and experimental results (e.r.)

Chromatographic behaviour of SFM and SS

In a second step of our investigations, 3 HPLC columns have been used in order to study the size (TSK G3000 SW), the charge (DEAE 5PW) and the relative hydrophobicity (Phenyl 5PW) of the various components of SFM. As seen on panel a (fig.1), several size family can be defined. Known size will be more than helpfull to design UF or dialysis steps. Chromatography according to the charge indicated that usually the main part of low MW compounds are not bound to the anionic resin. Nevertheless in some cases (fig.2), removal of these compounds (by dialysis) is necessary in order to limit interferences and competition for protein adsorbtion. In addition, BSA and transferrin behaviour on DEAE can be of great interest for Mabs purification (fig.2). Hydrophobicity of components is particulary important in view of membrane based systems, downstream the bioreactor (such membrane are often hydrophobic such as PTFE, polysulfone...).As seen on panel b (fig.1), small compounds are usually not adsorbed on phenyl support in our conditions, unlike to proteins. S.A. and transferrin (low hydrophobicity) can be separated from Immunoglobulin (high hydrophobicity).

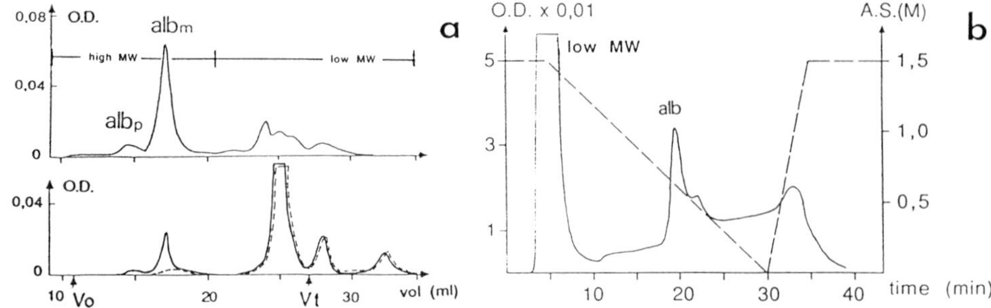

Figure 1: a.Gel filtration analysis of Ultroser HY 10% (top), HM high (—) and low (--) protein (bottom). 200 µl were loaded in 0,1 M ammonium acetat pH 7.0 at 0.25 ml/min. b.HIC analysis of HM high protein.1000 µl were loaded in 1,5 M ammonium sulfate (A.S.) 0,5 M ammonium acetat pH 6.0 at 1 ml/min.

Isolation of MAb from "serum free" derived cell supernatant

As a practical approach of this study, we have attempted to purified several MAbs on DEAE 5PW using different "serum free" supernatants. Good separation between MAb (IgG) and S.A. can be achieved (peak 1 and 2, fig.2). On the other hand, transferrin often contaminates MAb fraction, this depends on mouse IgG pHi (known to be of great variability) and on initial ratio [MAb] / [Transf.]. In serum free conditions, this ratio is low comparing to a 10% FCS supernatant (high content of bovine transferrin) and thus good purity can be achieved (fig.2).

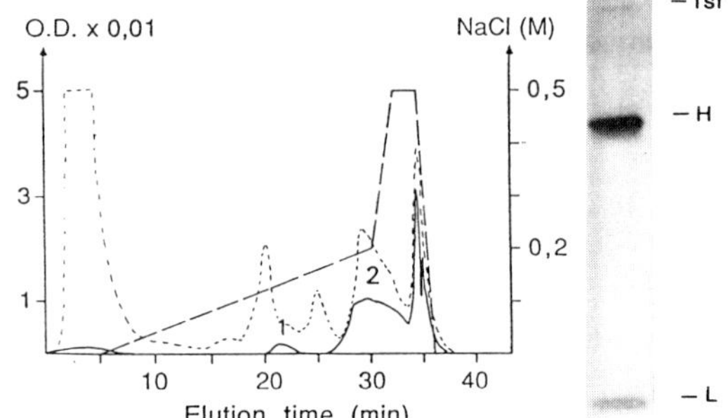

Figure 2: DEAE 5PW analysis of serum free supernatant (Imocell) containing MAb (30 mg/l). 2 ml were loaded onto the column, before (--) and after (—) dialysis, in 20mM Tris HCl pH 7,6. Flow rate is adjusted to 1 ml/min. MAb purity is checked on a 10% SDS PAGE as shown.

CONCLUSIONS

This systematic analysis allowed us to establish a sort of "identity map" for each medium in order to predict it's behaviour in downstream processes. Although SFM have to be dialysed before a chromatographic step because of the large amount (comparing to RPMI1640) of low MW compounds, the great advantage of using these media for hybridoma growth and MAbs production is their low content of transferrin and the lack of host Ig, the major contaminating proteins on DEAE. Moreever, several SFM are now free of albumin, this allows high throughputs of cell supernatant on DEAE resin until saturation unlike to other SFM (high S.A. content) or 10% FCS media.

REFERENCES

1   Bradford, M.M. A Rapid and Sensitive Method for the
        Quantitation of Microgram Quantities of Protein utilizing
        the Principle of Protein Dye Binding. <u>Analytical</u>
        <u>Biochemistry</u> 1976, 72, 248.

2   Laemmli, U.K. Cleavage of Structural Proteins during the
    .   assembly of the Head of Bacteriophage T4. <u>Nature</u> 1970,
        <u>227</u>,280.

3   Wray, W. et al. Silver Stain of Proteins in Polyacrylamide
        Gels. <u>Analytical Biochemistry</u> 1981, <u>118</u>, 197.

THE USE OF AFFINITY CHROMATOGRAPHY FOR THE PURIFICATION OF MONOCLONAL ANTIBODIES

H. Büntemeyer, D. Lütkemeyer, B. Bernat and J. Lehmann

Institute for Cell Culture Technology, Faculty of Technical Science
University of Bielefeld, D-4800 Bielefeld, FRG

INTRODUCTION

Monoclonal antibodies are widely used for diagnostical and therapeutical purposes. Depending on their use the antibodies have to be purified to a defined quality. In most of the purification strategies several chromatographic techniques are used. Affinity chromatography becomes a suitable method to purify antibodies from cell culture fluids [1]. Commercially available chromatographic media are Protein A and Protein G coupled to several matrixes.

In this study another affinity medium is presented. A rat-mouse hybridoma secreting a monoclonal antibody against æ light chain of mouse antibodies was cultivated in serum free medium. This antibody was purified from the cell culture supernatant by Protein G affinity and ion exchange chromatography. Then, the antibody was coupled to CNBr activated Sepharose^R (Pharmacia) and filled into FPLC columns. These columns were tested for the purification of a mouse monoclonal antibody type IgG_1. The antibody was also coupled to an epoxy activated silica HPLC column for analytical quantification of mouse antibodies.

The results are compared to the results obtained from Protein G purification. Purification success was monitored using kinetic ELISA techniques and PhastGel electrophoresis.

MATERIALS AND METHODS

The antibody specific for mouse æ light chain was produced by serum-free cultivation with rat-mouse hybridoma cell line 187.1 (ATCC: HB 58) in a 2 l perfusion bioreactor (Biostat BF/MD, Braun, FRG, equipped with a hydrophilized polypropylene membrane for perfusion) [2]. First, the cells were adapted to a serum-free medium consisting of a 1:1 mixture of IMDM and F12 supplemented with 2-4 mM glutamine, 20 μM ethanol-amine, 10 mg insulin/l, 10 mg transferrin/l and 1 g bovine serum albumine/l [3]. High viable cell density during perfusion led to an antibody concentration of more than 500 mg/l. A total amount of several grams were produced. From this supernatant the antibody was purified by Protein G affinity chromatography followed by cation exchange chromatography (same conditions as described below) and coupled to CNBr activated Sepharose 4B (Pharmacia).

Coupling conditions: coupling procedure according Pharmacia data file; blocking: PBS
Chromatography conditions: Temperature 4°C; Biopilot system
Buffer system for Protein G Sepharose FF column (Pharmacia) and anti mouse affinity column (Sepharose 4B):
Buffer A: 20 mM sodium phosphate pH7.0; Buffer B: 20 mM sodium phosphate pH2.5
IEX-column (S-Sepharose FF): Buffer A: 50 mM MES pH 5.8; Buffer B: Buffer A + 0.5 M NaCl

The antibody was also coupled to a HPLC column for rapid analytical detection of mouse hybridoma from fermentation supernatant. The HPLC column was an ULTRAFFINITY EP, 50 x 4.6 mm, (Beckman) filled with epoxy activated silica. Coupling was followed by the procedure given by Beckman using etanolamine as blocking agent. HPLC runs were performed on a Kontron D450 HPLC system. The buffer system was the same as used for the Sepharose affinity column.

The columns were tested with supernatant from serum-free perfusion cultivation of a mouse hybridoma producing a monoclonal antibody IgG_1 æ light chain [4]. The supernatant was concentrated 10 fold by ultrafiltration (Amicon SP20) before application to the columns.

Antibody concentrations were determined by kinetic ELISA methods (for rat and mouse) using peroxidase and OPD. Gel electrophoresis was done on a Phast System (Pharmacia) using SDS-PAGE under unreducing conditions with 4-15% gradient gels.

RESULTS AND DISCUSSION

The binding capacity for the used mouse antibody were 20 mg for the Protein G column and 17 mg for the anti mouse æ light chain column, respectively. That means a column effectivety of only 26%, because 65 mg anti mouse æ light chain antibody were coupled to the matrix. The testing solution (UF concentrate from mouse hybridoma cultivation) contains also many free light and heavy chain fragments (lane 1) which lower the binding effectivity for complete antibody. Therefore, the elution fraction of anti mouse æ light chain column contains also heavy and light chain fragments of the antibody (lane 3) which are not present in the elution fraction of the Protein G column (lane 2).

From gel electrophoresis it can also be seen that in both cases most of the albumine is removed (lane 2 and 3, respectively). But there is still a lot of pollution. These proteins in the range between 70 and 100 kD (secreted by the cells during cultivation) can be removed by cation exchange chromatography (lane 5).

This 2 step purification for mouse antibody with æ light chains is a rapid and satisfactory method also scalable to bigger columns with higher binding capacity. The preparation of the rat-mouse antibody coupled to the matrix can easily be done by cultivation of hybridoma 187.1.

We achieved very similiar results as the results described in [1] with our rat-mouse antibody. The use of 187.1 antibody in HPLC affinity chromatography is useful for rapid detection of æ light chain antibody, although coupling effectivity is very low. Quantification can be done when no free æ light chains are present.

FPLC - Columns

Column 1	:	5 ml Protein G Sepharose FF
Flow rate	:	0.5 ml/min
Sample	:	60 ml UF concentrate of serum-free hybridoma supernatant (90 mg/l)
Column 2	:	65 mg anti mouse æ light chain (187.1) coupled to 3g (14 ml) CNBr act. Sepharose
Flow rate	:	0.5 ml/min
Sample	:	60 ml UF concentrate of serum-free hybridoma supernatant (90 mg/l)

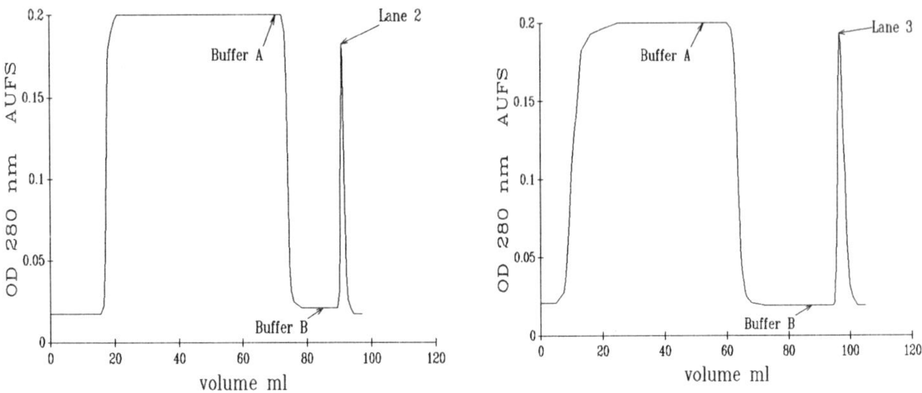

Figure 1: Protein G Chromatography   **Figure 2:** Affinity Chromatography with anti mouse æ light chain antibody

HPLC - Column

38 mg of anti mouse æ light chain antibody (187.1) were coupled to the Beckman Ultraffinity EP column according to the Beckman procedure. The column was also tested with the UF concentrate from mouse hybridoma cultivation.
The maximum column capacity for this antibody was 34 µg. Therefore, only 0.1% of the coupled anti mouse antibody was active, but this was enough for analytical quantification.

Gradient:

6 min Buffer A

in 7 min from Buffer A to Buffer B

3 min Buffer B

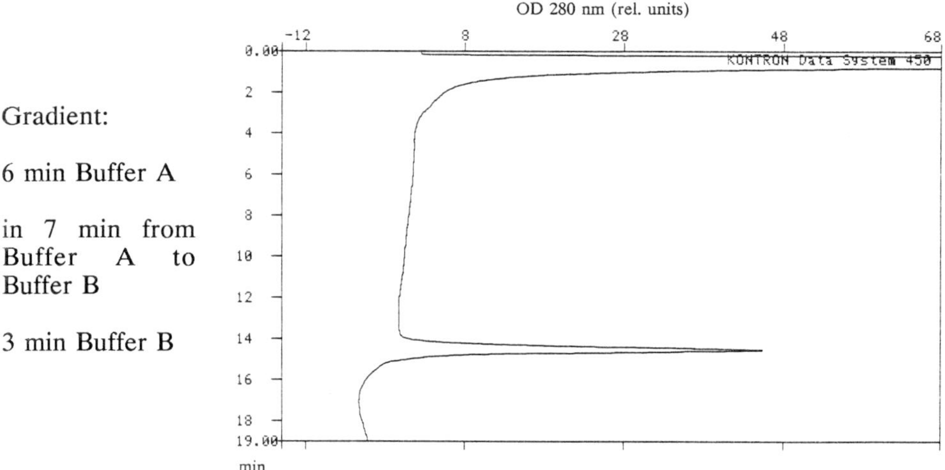

Figure 3: HPLC - Chromatography of 250 µl mouse supernatant UF concentrate.

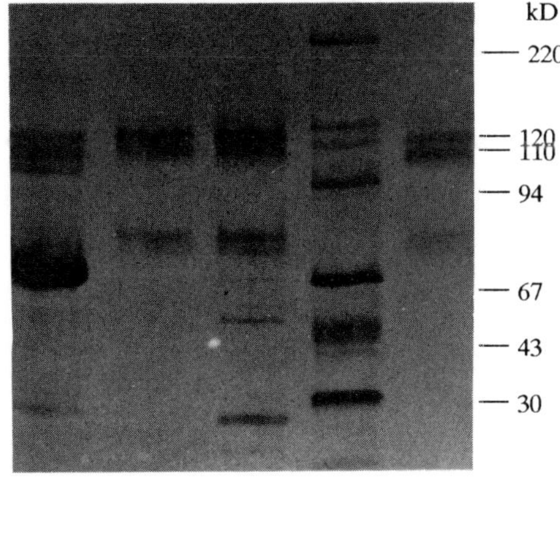

Figure 4:   Phast Gel Electrophoresis

4 - 15 % gradient SDS-PAGE Gel
unreducing conditions

Lane 1:   UF concentrate
Lane 2:   Protein G column elution
           fraction
Lane 3:   anti mouse æ column
           elution fraction
Lane 4:   Molecular weight marker
Lane 5:   IEX column elution
           fraction

LITERATURE

1   Bazin, H.; Malache, J.M.; Nisol F. and Cormont F. In: <u>Advances in Animal Cell Biology and Technology for Bioprocesses</u> (Eds. Spier R.E.; Griffiths J.B.; Stephenne J.and Crooy P.J.) Butterworths, Kent, UK, 1989, p.421-427

2   Büntemeyer H.; Bödeker B.G.D. and Lehmann J. In: <u>Modern Approaches to Animal Cell Technology</u> (Eds. Spier R.E.and Griffiths J.B.) Butterworths, Kent, UK, 1987, p. 411-419

3   Jäger V.; Lehmann J. and Friedl P. Serum-free growth medium for the cultivation of a wide spectrum of mammalian cells in stirred bioreactors <u>Cytotechnology</u> 1988, 1, 319

4   Lütkemeyer D.; Büntemeyer H. and Lehmann J. Production of a monoclonal antibody against gesolin Presentation at the 10th ESACT Meeting, Avignon, 1990

Section 10
Products

Production of a pharmaceutical enzyme : Animal Cells or E.coli ?

Terence Cartwright
and
André Crespo

RHONE-POULENC SANTE
Institut des Biotechnologies
13, quai Jules Guesde
B.P. 14
94403 Vitry Sur Seine
FRANCE

Introduction

Recombinant DNA technology has permitted production of biologically and therapeutically active proteins in effectively unlimited quantities. The structural genes encoding such proteins may be expressed in a range of different systems including bacteria, yeast, mammalian cells and insect cells. Each of these systems has special characteristics that may influence the nature of the product produced and the process required to obtain it. Here, we compare our experiences with tissue plasminogen activator (tPA) produced in E.coli and in Chinese Hamster Ovary (CHO) cells.

tPA belongs to the group of serine proteases that convert plasminogen to plasmin by cleavage between arginine 560 and valine 561. Plasmin can degrade several protein substrates including fibrin, and plasminogen activators are thus used clinically as thrombolytic agents.

tPA is considered to be particularly promising for clinical use since it requires fibrin as a cofactor for effective plasminogen activation and its action is therefore mainly limited to sites of fibrin deposition. This is important for avoiding generalized depletion of circulating fibrinogen and other clotting factors which could create a risk of haemorrhagic side effects (1). tPA is currently used in treatment of acute myocardial infarction and is under evaluation for use in deep vein thrombosis, pulmonary embolism and other indications.

The human tPA cDNA (2) and gene (3) have been cloned, and the primary structure of the protein confirmed by sequence analysis (4). The tPA molecule is large (527 amino acids) and complex, involving a large number of disulphide bonds and several glycosylation sites. The molecule can also be divided into several discrete domain structures. The overall structure of tPA is summarized in Fig 1.

<u>tPA MOLECULE</u>

* **527 AMINO ACIDS : A SINGLE POLY-PEPTIDE CHAIN.**

* **35 CYSTEINES; 17 DISULPHIDE BONDS**

* **3 POTENTIAL GLYCOSYLATION SITES**
  (ONE APPEARS NEVER TO BE GLYCOSYLATED)

* **5 SEMI-INDEPENDANT DOMAINES**
  (FINGER, EGF, TWO 'KRINGLES', SERINE PROTEASE)

Fig. 1   Overall characteristics of the tPA molecule

<u>Choice of production system</u>

Several key factors have to be considered when choosing a production system for a protein intended for clinical use. These include the likely scale of production and the acceptable cost, the need for accurate post-translational modification of the product and whether the system under consideration can

produce a product of adequate quality and safety. This last point obviously
implies that purification can be satisfactorily achieved, potential biological
risk factors eliminated and that an adequately characterized product of
appropriate potency can be reproducibly achieved.

Given the complexity of the tPA molecule, most production of tPA
undertaken so far has used recombinant animal cells as a production vehicle (5).
Several groups have shown, however, that glycosylation of tPA is not essential
for its biological activity (4). After evaluation of the quantities of tPA
required for clinical studies and for commercial production of tPA (summarized
in Fig. 2) we decided to evaluate in parallel production of tPA in E. coli, and
in CHO cells.

tPA Production: Objectives

For clinical trials .... **about 100g**

Probable production level........ tens of kgs

Therefore evaluation of two systems:

Animal cells and E. coli

Fig. 2   tPA production objectives

Table I illustrates our initial appreciation of the relative
advantages and disadvantages of the two tPA production systems under
consideration.

Table I   Initial evaluation of the factors for and against production of tPA
in animal cells or in E.coli.

tPA Production: starting positions

CHO	E. coli
+	
Fidelity of expression	Ease of scale up of fermentation
Secretion of product	Cheap and simple medium
	Expression vectors well understood
–	
Expression vectors less well developed	No glycosylation
Scale up of culture relatively less simple	Correct processing and secretion not guaranteed
Medium potentially more expensive	

tPA production by E. coli

Human tPA cDNA was cloned from the Bowes melanoma cell line (2) and used in two types of expression construct based either on the E. coli tryptophan promoter Ptrp or on the phage lambda left lytic promoter P_L (6). The types of vector used are shown in Fig. 3. The tPA coding sequence was fused to a ribosome binding site derived from the lambda CII gene and placed under the control of the Ptrp or P_L promoter. Vector stability could be improved by addition of the T7 transcriptional terminator (6). When tPA expression was de-repressed by

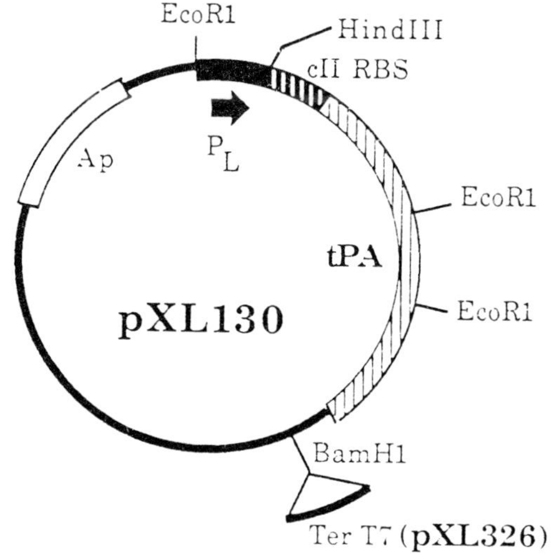

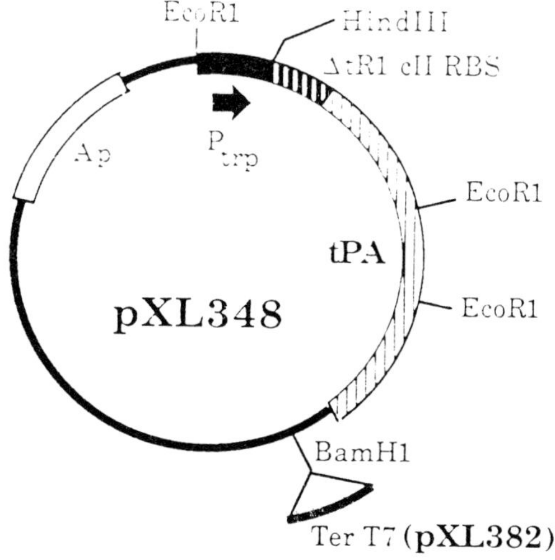

Fig. 3   Schematic drawing of the tPA expression plasmids used in _E.coli_
Derivatives with the T7 terminator inserted into the unique
Bam H1 site were also constructed.

warming to 42°C in the case of plasmid pXL130 containing the P_L promoter or by tryptophan deprivation in the case of plasmid pXL348 containing the P<u>trp</u> promoter, (Fig. 3) tPA was produced as 5-10 % of total cell protein (6). In both cases tPA was produced in an insoluble denatured form which migrated in SDS PAGE with an apparent molecular weight of 59 kDa, the expected value for non-glycosylated, single chain tPA (Fig.4). A maximum yield of 700 mg/litre of tPA was obtained after optimization of induction and fermentation conditions.

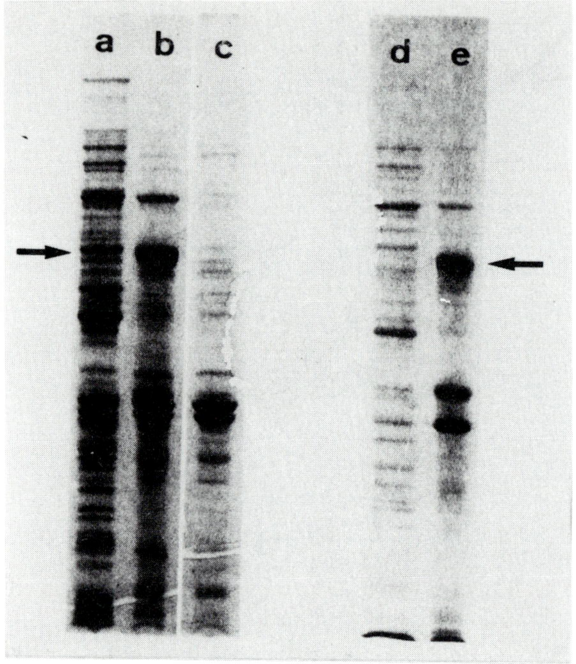

Fig. 4   Expression of tPA in <u>E.coli</u>. Arrowheads indicate the position of the unglycosylated tPA band at 59 kDa.

(a) Soluble protein fraction from <u>E.coli</u> transfected with pXL348

(b) Insoluble fraction from (a) above

(c) As in (b) but with tryptophan added during the expression phase.

(d) Soluble protein fraction from pXL130 transfected cells.

(e) Insoluble fraction from (d) above under de-repression conditions

In an attempt to obtain secretion of tPA from E.coli, the mature tPA gene was inserted behind either the natural tPA leader sequence, or behind the Omp A leader sequence which is known to promote efficient secretion of E. coli proteins. In both cases, only insoluble, unprocessed tPA was produced. Also no secretion was obtained when the tPA leader sequence was placed upstream of the pho A gene is whose product is normally secreted by E.coli. These data show that the tPA leader sequence is not effective as a secretion signal in E.coli and that furthermore, the tPA gene product itself is not effectively processed by E. coli even when fused to a normally efficient E.coli leader peptide. In consequence it appears that secretion from E. coli is unlikely to be a viable approach to tPA production (6). Our experience with production of tPA in E.coli is summarized in Table II.

Table II   Summary of experience with tPA production in E.coli

tPA: E. coli production

* **Easy fermentation with cheap medium**

* **High levels of tPA (ca 700 mg/l)**

* **tPA insoluble and inactive**

tPA production in CHO cells

Several groups have shown that tPA that is essentially identical to natural circulating tPA can be produced in recombinant animal cells. Amplified CHO cells have been most widely used and we used CHO contructions very similar to those described by Collen et al (5) in which the SV40 early promoter and

enhancer sequences flank an inserted dihydrofolate reductase (DHFR) gene and the
structural gene for tPA. DHFR⁻ CHO cells were transfected with a plasmid
containing the above elements (Plasmid pXL261, Fig. 5), then grown in presence
of increasing quantities of the antimitotic agent methotrexate (MTX) which
functions by inhibition of DHFR. One mechanism by which cells may become
resistant to the cytotoxic effects of methotrexate is by increasing production
of the DHFR enzyme by amplification of the DHFR structural gene (7). This
amplification involves co-amplification of large segments of DNA adjacent to
the DHFR gene, and this results in over-production of all proteins whose genes
an located in these amplified regions. (8) MTX resistant clones were thus
selected and tested for their capacity to produce increased amounts of tPA.

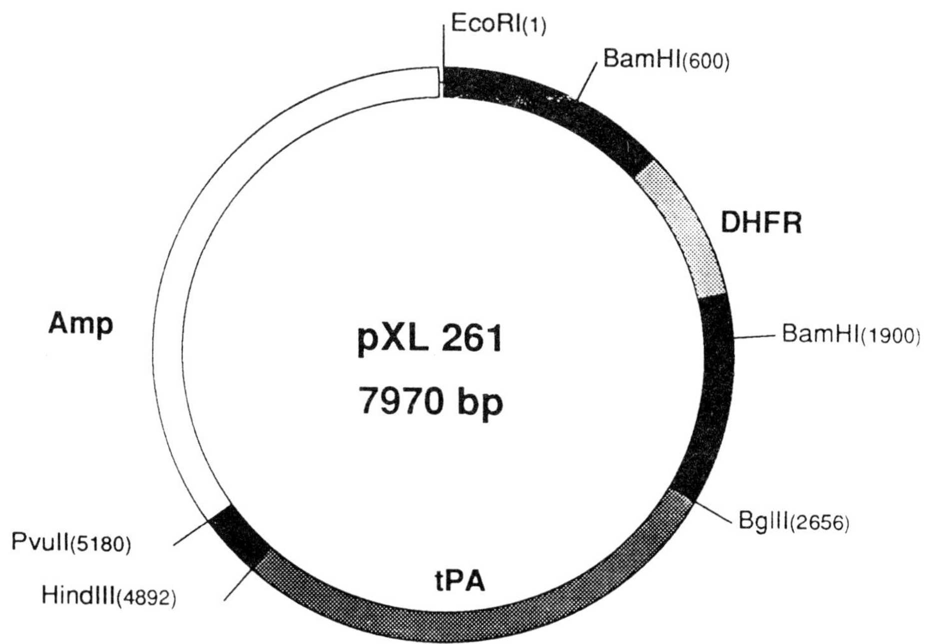

Fig. 5   Schematic drawing of the tPA expression plasmid used in CHO-cells.

Table III summarizes results obtained with amplification of
recombinant CHO clones carrying the tPA gene compared with results obtained with
the Bowes melanoma cell line which naturally produces low levels of tPA and from
which the tPA structural gene was cloned (2). Although higher tPA levels were

Table III   Influence of MTX levels on tPA production in recombinant CHO cells.
Doubling time and tPA yield from nine transfected CHO lines are
compared with the Bowes melanoma cell line.

CLONES	DOUBLING TIME (h)	MTX LEVELS (μM)	mg of tPA/10^9 ¢ /24 H
Bowes	24	0	0.93
48501	34	0.25	6.10
4840012	30	2	5.50
134003	48	2	9.80
AR 25	34	25	3.95
AR 23	33	25	4.30
AR 11	35	25	4.70
AR 9	26	25	9.40
AR 17	30	25	4.50
AR 14	35	25	5.25

obtained in the presence of MTX, there was no clear relationship between the tPA
production level and the MTX concentration to which the cells were exposed. The
highest tPA levels produced were about 10 times greater than the level obtained
with Bowes melanoma cells. In addition to the increase in tPA production
observed, MTX also had other, less desirable consequences including increased
doubling time of the selected cells and also, in some cases, increased cell
fragility which prevented efficient cell growth in stirred fermenters (Table
III). For these reasons, AR9 was selected for further study as being the line
which showed the best compromise between good tPA production and acceptable
culture characteristics.

tPA production by hybridomes

Determination of the number of copies of the tPA gene in different
amplified clones, and the level of tPA mRNA produced (data not shown) showed
that cells resistant to the highest MTX concentrations produced less tPA then

would be predicted from the degree of amplification and transcription of the gene obtained. This suggests that some other, post-transcriptional, factor may be limiting for production of the mature protein such as the capacity for glycosylation or for secretion of the protein.

This possibility led us to examine the possibility a creating a hybrid cell by fusion between an amplified CHO clone and another cell of known high performance in the secretion of glycosylated proteins. It was also proposed to use as a fusion partner, a cell with good growth characteristics capable of being grown on a large scale in a stirred tank fermenter. The parental cells chosen for production of the hybridoma were thus the tPA producing CHO clone AR9 and the murine myeloma Sp 2/0 Ag14. Cells were fused as described by Duchesne et al (9) and hybrids were selected that were capable of growth in Dulbeccos MEM supplemented with 20 % foetal calf serum which had been dialysed to eliminate proline and containing 25 μM MTX. Since AR9 cells are autotrophic for proline (Fig. 6) and Sp 2/0 Ag 14 cells are MTX sensitive, only hybrid cells are capable of growth in the selective medium ased. Cells capable of multiplication in this medium were cloned by the limiting dilution technique and clones were selected according to their tPA production capacity. The procedure used is summarized in Fig. 7. Several hybrids were obtained that produced more tPA than the parent AR9 clone, the best being HYB F2 with an initial tPA production of 32.6 mg of tPA per 10^9 cells per 24 hours when adapted to grow in serum free medium in stirred fermenters (Table IV). When grown in batch culture, HYB F2 reached a plateau of tPA production of 100 mg per litre per 10^9 cells after 6 days in culture. In these conditions, tPA in the culture supernatant was about 40 % of total secreted protein and could be visualized directly by HPLC of the crude culture supernatant (Fig. 8).

At this level of production, a substantial development programme would be needed to increase the scale of cell culture to that needed to produce commercially viable quantities of tPA in animal cells. A summary of our

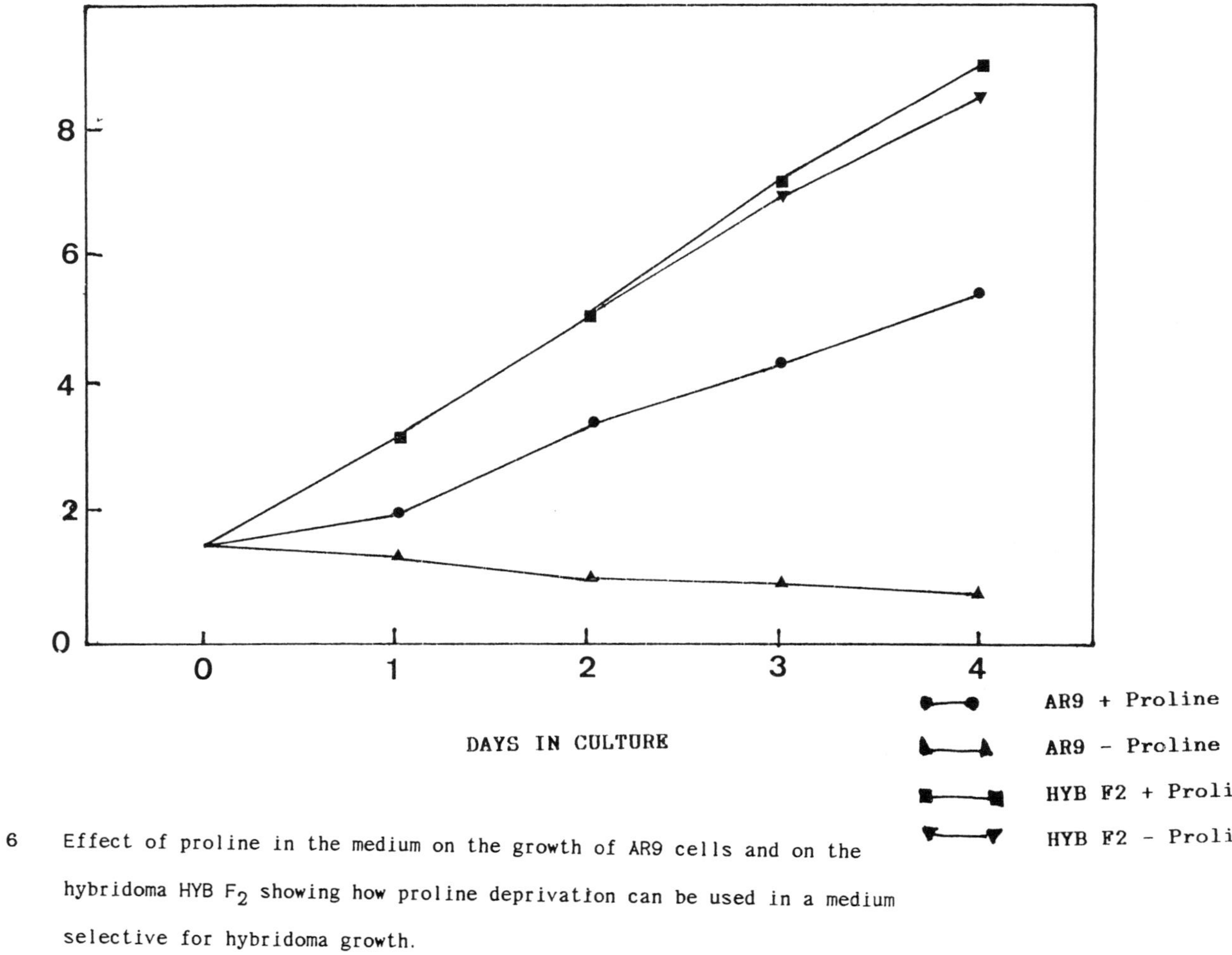

Fig. 6   Effect of proline in the medium on the growth of AR9 cells and on the hybridoma HYB F_2 showing how proline deprivation can be used in a medium selective for hybridoma growth.

CELL FUSION and SELECTION OF HYBRIDES

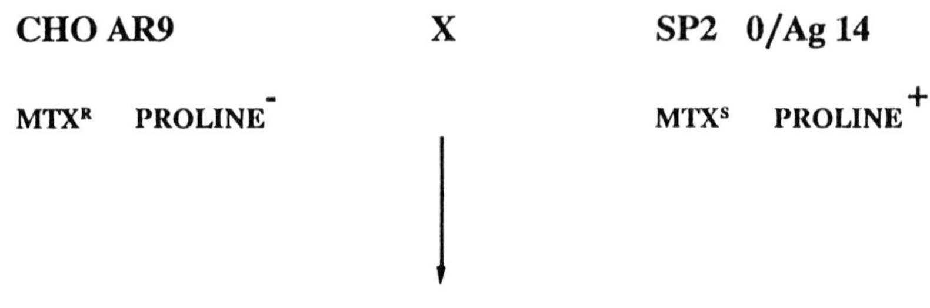

Fig. 7   Summary of the protocol used for selection of tPA secreting hybrids following fusion of AR9 cells and the mouse myeloma SP$_2$ 0/Ag4.

experience with tPA production in animal cells in given in Table V.

Down stream processing

In terms simply of product yield, the E.coli system appears attractive since up to 700 mg of tPA per litre has been obtained in a few hours of fermentation in a system which could easily be extrapolated to an industrial scale. With animal cells, only 100 mg/litre at best was obtained after 6 days of culture in a system that would require major development and investment for industrialization. However, this evaluation changes radically when product

Table IV   tPA production from five CHO-SP$_2$ O/Ag4 hybridomas compared with yield from AR9, the best amplified CHO line.

CLONES	mU I / cell / 24 H	mg / 10^9 ℓ /24H
AR 9	4.70	9.40
HYB A8	5.45	10.9
HYB D6	8.30	16.6
HYB G12	11	22
HYB B9	11.60	23.2
HYB F2	16.30	32.6

t.PA in the culture serum free medium was assayed by the chromogenic substrate method using S 2251.

Table V   Summary of experience with tPA production in recombinant animal cells.

<u>**tPA : Production in animal cells**</u>

* **Product secreted in native, active form**

* **Yield of tPA: plateau at 6 days (100 mg/l)**

* **Medium complex but simplified substantially during development**

* **Scale up of CHO culture needed with its attendant problems and investments**

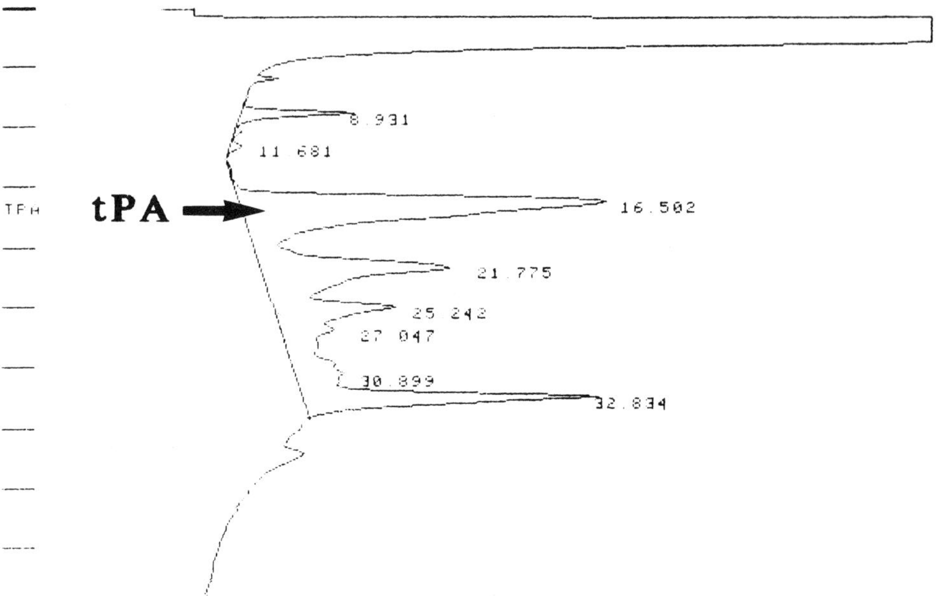

Fig. 8   Reverse phase HPLC applied directly to the culture supernatant obtained from HYB F_2 cells. tPA is directly visible in the HPLC profile and represents about 40 % of total protein.

recovery is considered. In animal cells, tPA is produced as the soluble, mature protein, and, if the medium used has been selected appropriately, purification presents no particular problems.

In <u>E.coli</u> however, tPA is produced as insoluble 'inclusion bodies" that contain denatured, inactive enzyme (2,10). Recovery of the active enzyme from such inclusion bodies involves the solubilization of the protein in 7M guanidine, reduction of incorrectly arranged disulphide bonds, removal of the denaturants used and controlled re-oxidation of disulphide bonds to produce the correctly folded protein. We developed procedures that permitted recovery of tPA from <u>E.coli</u> of about 3 mg per litre of culture and per OD unit of fully active tPA (6). The tPA obtained was purified to better than 95 % pure, was essentially (>95 %) in the single chain form and showed the same specific activity in several plasminogen activator assays as the International tPA Reference Preparation isolated from the Bowes melanoma cell line.

The need to renature the tPA adds very considerably to the complexity of the product recovery flow sheet as indicated in Fig. 9. Although the technical problem of renaturation of tPA is soluble, production scale renaturation of tPA is not practical due to the very low concentration of tPA at which it is necessary to work to obtain reasonably efficient (20 %) renaturation. In our hands, it was not possible to exceed 2 mg/litre of tPA in the final renaturation mixture without unacceptable product losses. In addition, tPA refolding apparently occurs very slowly and 48 hours is required in the final renaturation mixture to obtain efficient refolding (6).

It should be noted that these conditions are by no means general for all proteins and examples exist of efficient refolding at concentration exceeding 1g/litre (11) and sufficiently rapidly to permit renaturation on a flow through basis rather than by prolonged incubation (12).

In practice, the limitation on tPA concentration mentioned above has serious process implications in terms of the volumes which would need to be treated and the large scale process plant that would be immobilized by this operation. This is illustrated in Fig. 10 for the production of 1000 doses (ie about 100g of tPA). In the diagram, the encircled figures represent the volume in cubic metres at each stage of the treatment. The concentration of tPA is shown in brackets for each stage. The figures in square brackets represent the number of tonnes of urea [2.3 t] and guanidine [12 t] used respectively. These reagents represent major cost factors (and subsequently major waste disposal problems) in the possible industrial scale production of tPA by renaturation.

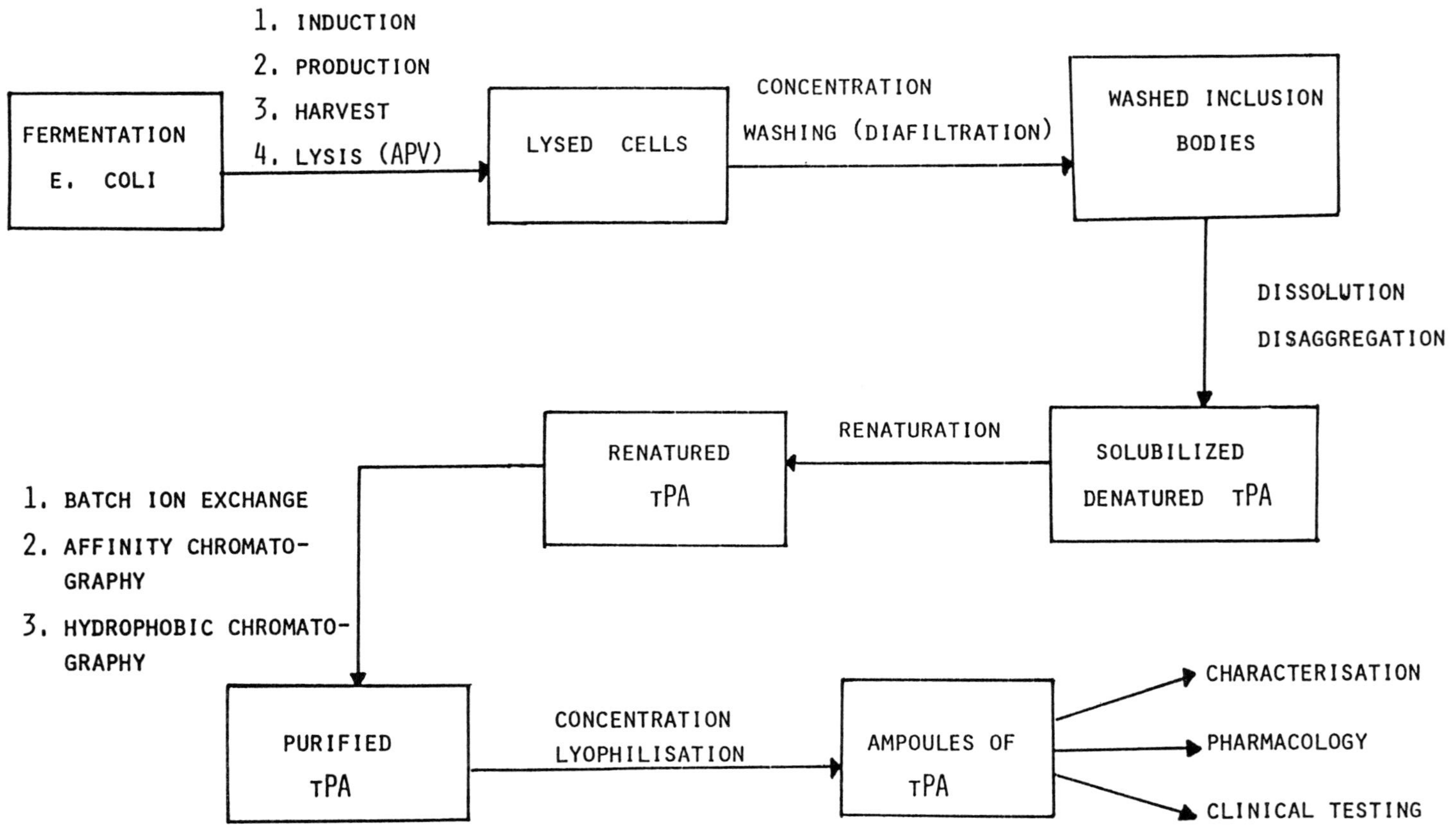

Fig. 9   Summary flow shect of the different steps for production of injectable tPA from E.coli.

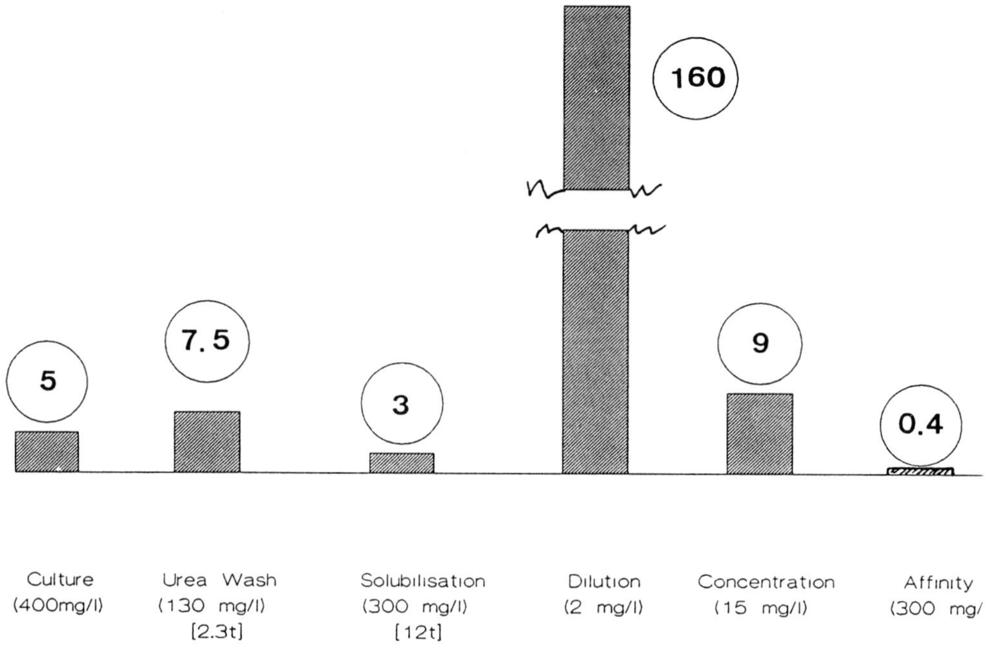

Fig. 10   Scale up problems associated with renaturation of tPA. Figures represent volumes in cubic metres for 1000 doses of tPA at different points in the renaturation process.

Relative production costs of tPA in animal cells and in E.coli

As predicted, fermentation costs for production of tPA in _E.coli_ represented a small fraction of the total cost of production and were much lower than the cost of production of tPA by animal cell culture. However this cost advantage for _E.coli_ production was completely negated by the high cost of the tPA renaturation procedure which was a direct consequence of the low tPA concentration imposed by the renaturation characteristics of the protein. A similar purification procedure was used for tPA derived from the two production systems. Overall materials and labour cost per gram of tPA were of the same

order for tPA produced in animal cells and in <u>E.coli</u>. The breakdown of costs for
the two systems in given in Fig. 11.

Purity and quality of the tPA produced

tPA from both production systems was purified by variations of the
same purification protocol involving batch purification on SP Trisacryl followed
by affinity chromatography on Lysine Sepharose. (6) A 'polishing step' on phenyl
Sepharose was also employed. Purity for both products was greater than 95 % by
reverse phase and gel filtration HPLC and by SDS PAGE in reducing and in
non-reducing conditions. In both cases the tPA was produced in the single chain
form. About 2-3 % of lower molecular weight contaminants were detected and shown
by immunoblot procedures to represent fragments of tPA. Specific plasminogen
activator activity and stimulation by fibrin were close to the values obtained
with the international reference standard tPA preparation (83/157). For <u>E.coli</u>
produced tPA, particular regulatory concerns include the possible persistance of
pyrogens in the final preparation and the presence of imperfectly renatured
forms of the protein potentially able to behave as immunogens.

Analysis of the pyrogen load at different stage of purification
showed that a greater that 99.999 % clearance of endotoxin was achieved during
purification and that the final preparation was within the acceptable limits of
endotoxin concentration for an injectable product.

In addition to the tests of biological activity and the
physicochemical tests which showed no evidence of persistance of incorrectly
folded forms of tPA, the <u>E.coli</u> tPA was also analysed with a panel of monoclonal
antibodies raised against natural tPA. No differences in antigenicity were
observed.

tPA E. coli

Percentage costs for production of 1kg

tPA Animal Cells

Percentage costs for production of 1kg

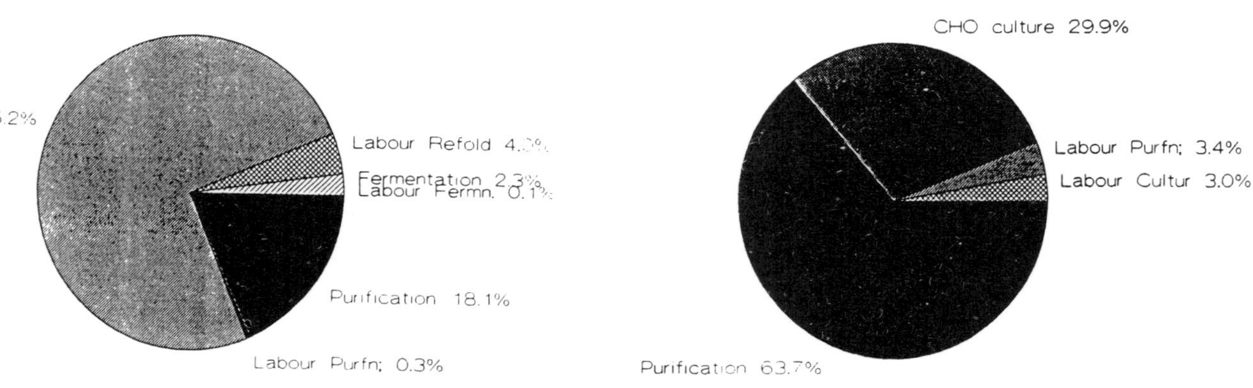

Fig. 11   "Pie Chart" indicating the relative costs of the different stages of tPA production in E.coli (left) on amplified CHO cells (right).

Production of tPA in the HYB F_2 hybridoma was not considered to pose any unusual regulatory problems, and the cells and product were analysed basically as suggested in the "points to consider" documents relevant to the production of products from animal cells (13) with particular attention being paid to possible persistance of host cell DNA and proteins in the final product.

Biological activity of animal cell and E.coli derived tPA

The biological activity of tPA purified from HYB F_2 and from _E.coli_ was tested and compared to that of a commercially available recombinant tPA producet in CHO cells (Actilyse[R], Boehringer).

HYB F_2 derived tPA showed identical biological properties to Actilyse[R] in all systems tested. _E.coli_ derived tPA however showed similar properties _in vitro_ but important differences were seen _in vivo_.

Thus, _E.coli_ derived tPA had comparable specific activity to the control tPA when tested in clot lysis, synthetic substrate or fibrin plate assays. The affinity of _E.coli_ tPA for fibrin was determined and was not significantly different from that of the control tPA used. The same was true for the degree of stimulation of plasminogen activator activity by fibrin. _E.coli_ tPA showed no fibrinogenolytic activity or fibrinolytic activity in the absence of plasminogen, and thus behaves as a specific plasminogen activator (14).

When _E.coli_ tPA was perfused into rabbits or into dogs, activation of plasminogen was achieved (as determined by the measurement of-englobulin lysis on fibrin plates, 15). No signifiant diminution of circulating plasminogen or fibrinogen was observed suggesting that the plasminogen activation was specific. Importantly, the plasma half-life of _E.coli_ tPA was about 4 times longer than that of the control tPA and the measured cleareance rate was similarly lengthened.(14). These observations are compatible with the notion that the carbohydrate moiety of natural tPA is not involved in its enzymic activity, but contributes to the rapid clearance of the glycosylated molecule. Non-glycosylated tPA could thus present certain advantages in therapy where it would be very desirable to reduce the dose of tPA and the duration of the perfusion (16).

Conclusions

As has already been shown by other groups, these studies confirm that transformed animal cells are capable of producing and secreting significant quantities of tPA in a correctly processed and fully active form. However, in our hands, continued amplification of the tPA gene did not result in concomitant increases in tPA production. This suggested that other factors may be limiting , and that cells better adapted than CHO cells, to the secretion of glycoprotein should be developed for future production of large quantities of therapeutic proteins. In addition, we found that highly amplified cells grew poorly in fermenters, and we consider that the development of more "fermenter friendly" cell types should also be a target for future research.

As a first step in this direction, we evaluated the tPA producing capacity of CHO/mouse myeloma hybridomas, and obtained cell lines that were well adapted to growth in suspension and that produced reasonable amounts of tPA. However the system was not fully optimized, and other approches should also be undertaken to develop more efficient cell lines for the production of recombinant proteins of similar complexity to tPA.

It should be noted that glycosylation patterns of such proteins may alter as translation levels are increased and thus that a complete analysis of the product at different levels of production is required, and not simply measurement of biological activity (our unpublished data).

We have also shown that complex eukaryotic proteins can be efficiently expressed in E.coli and that procédures can be designed that permit recovery of acceptable yield of fully active product. However, with our present knowledge, secretion of tPA from E.coli or from other microbial systems cannot be achieved (6). A consequence of the absence of effective secretion mechanisms for tPA is the deposition of the protein as inclusion bodies in the bacteria. This necessitates the development of renaturation procedures for product recovery. In the case of tPA, but not of several other proteins, the low protein concentration permissible for efficient renaturation ($\simeq$ 2 mg/litre) limits the practicability of a production process based on renaturation.

In terms of biological activity, unglycosylated tPA derived from E.coli shows a longer in vivo half life than does animal cell derived, glycosylated tPA. This is because, in the case of tPA, the carbohydrate does not apparently contribute to the biological activity of the enzyme but does contribute significantly to its rapid clearance from the blood (16). E. coli tPA may thus show advantages in the clinic by reduction of the dose needed to maintain a thrombolytic state. It is not yet known whether the absence of glycosylation could give rise to undesirable secondary effects such as, for example, the development of antibodies after prolongéd treatment due to the exposure of epitopes on the unglycosylated molecule that are not present on endogenous tPA.

Thus for tPA, the ideal production process has not get been developed. Animal cells can produce an apparently faithful copy of the endogenous protein but very large scale cultures are necessary to produce the kilograms of tPA that the market requires. E.coli production, while yielding large quantities of a product that may be more effective in vivo, suffers from the need to operate an extraction and refolding process that is scarcely practical on an industrial scale.

With tPA as with all other therapeutic proteins it is necessaray to evaluate the process as a whole   to obtain the best integrated production system. Each protein has its own requirements in terms of folding, glycosylation, maturation cleavage or other post-translational modification, as well as other conditions imposed by the likely production scale and the added value of the product. As with many other aspects of biotechnology, it is a question of "horses for courses" which underlines once again the necessity for a laboratory which intends to produce recombinant therapeutic proteins to have several expression and production systems operational to permit their rigorous comparative evaluation when the production of a new protein is contemplated.

References

(1)   Rijken D.C., Hoylaerts, M. and Collen D. (1982)

        Fibrinolytic properties of one or two chain human

        Extrinsic (tissue type) plasminogen activator

        J. Biol. Chem. 257 : 2920-2925

(2)   Pennica, D., Holmes, W.E., Kohr, W.J., Harkins, R.N., Vehar, G.A.,

        Ward, C.A., Bennet, W.F., Yelverton E., Seeburg, P.H., Heyneker H.L.,

        Eodal, D.R. and Collen, D. (1983).

        Cloning and expression of tissue type plasminogen activator in E.coli

        Nature 301 : 214-221

(3)   Ny, T., Elgh, F. and Lund, B., (1984)

        The structure of the human tissue-type plasminogen activator gene ;

        correlation of intron and exon structures to functional and structural

        domains.

        Proc. Natl. Acad. Sci USA 81 : 5355-5359.

(4)   Pöhl, G., Källström, M., Bergsdorf, N., Wallén, P., and Jörnvall, H.
(1984)
Tissue plasminogen activator : peptide analyses confirm an indirectly
derived amino acid sequence, identify the active site serine residue,
establish glycosylation sites and localize variant differences.
Biochemistry 23 : 3701-3707.

(5)   Collen, D., Stassen, J.M., Marafino, B.J. Jr, Builder. S., De Cock, F.,
Ogez, I., Tajiri, D., Pennica, D., Bennett W.F., Salwa, J., and Hoyng C.F.
(1984).
Biological properties of human tissue type plasminogen activator obtained
by expression of recombinant DNA in animal cells.
J. Pharmacol. Exp. Therap. 231 : 146-152

(6)   Sarmientos P, Duchesne M, Denèfle P, Boiziau J, Fromage N, Delporte N,
Parker F, Lelièvre Y, Mayaux J.F., Cartwright T. (1989).
Synthesis and purification of active human tissue plasminogen activator
from E.coli.
Bio/technology 7 : 495-501.

(7)   Schimke, R. (1978)
Cene amplification in animal cells
Cell 37 : 705-713

(8)   Stark, G. and Wahl G. (1984)
Gene amplification
Ann. Rev. Biochem. 53 447-491

(9)   Duchesne M., Cartwright T, Crespo A, Boucher F and Fallourd A. (1984)
Localization of a Neutralization Epitope of Foot and Mouth Disease Virus

Using Neutralizing Monoclonal Antibodies.

J. Gen. Virol. __65__, : 1559-1566.

(10)   Harris, T.J.R., Patel, T., Marston, F.A.O, Little, S., Emtage S, Opendakker G, Volkaert G, Rombauts W, Billiau A and De Somer P. (1986).   —
Cloning of cDNA coding for human tPA and its expression in _E.coli_.
Mol.Biol.Med. __3__ : 279-292

(11)   Latta M, Knapp M, Sarmientos P, Brefort G, Becquart J, Guerrier L, Jung G and Mayaux J.F. (1987).
Synthesis and purification of native human serum albumin from _E.coli_.
Biol/Technology __5__ : 1309 - 1314

(12)   Graff R., lang K., Wrba A and Schmid F.X. (1986).
Folding mechanisms of porcine ribonuclease
J. Mol.Biol. __191__ : 281-293.

(13)   Points to consider in the production and testing of   new drugs and biologicals produced by recombinant DNA technology (1985)
Office of Biologics Research and Review, FDA.

(14)   Uzan A, Marin J, Mestre M, Imbault F, Lelièvre Y, Duchesne M, Fromage N, Cartwright T.
Umpublished results.

(15)   Milstone H, (1941)
J. Immunol __42__ : 109-116

(16)   Hansen L, Blue Y, Barone K, Collen D and Larsen G.R. (1988).
Functional effects of asparagine - linked oligosaccharide on natural and variant human tissue-type plasminogen activator.
J. Biol. Chem. __263__ : 15713 - 15719.

<u>**Paper of Cartwright**</u>

Kilburn: In your epitopes map did you consider what the
               immunogenicity would be like in humans rather than
               in mice?

Cartwright:

               It is difficult to do. It is always the question
               for any kind of testing of recombinant proteins.
               Animal testing, particularly immunogenicity, is of
               relatively limited value. In fact only a clinical
               study can tell you if there will be problems in
               humans.

Hentschel: There is a protein on the market from both E.coli
               and mammalian cells - namely HGH. The story is
               that the differences in fermentation are minor
               compared to all the other costs associated with
               getting something on the market. This is an easy
               protein to make with E.coli and there is clinical
               experience comparing the immunogenicity between
               mammalian and E.coli made material. There was
               evidence early on that the mammalian was better.

Cartwright:

               In each case the systems have got to be evaluated
               for the protein in question.

Sinacore: You showed the importance of the glycan structure
               of tPA in terms of its biological activity. Did
               you compare the glycan structure of the material
               from the CHO myeloma fusion cell line with the CHO
               cells?

Cartwright:
               No we haven't got that far.

Sinacore: What about the proportion of one chain to two chain
               tPA?

Cartwright:
               In all our preparations the proportion of two chain
               is 5% or less.

Tolbert: What was the stability of your CHO/myeloma fusion
               over long term culture?

Cartwright:

               Certainly stable for the 50-60 generations we have
               used it for.

ORAL POLIO VACCINE (SABIN) PRODUCED ON LARGE-SCALE VERO CELL CULTURE

Bernard MONTAGNON[1], Bernard FANGET[1], Roger VINAS[2], Lucien PEYRON[1], Jean-Claude VINCENT-FALQUET[1], and Pierre CAUDRELIER[1]

[1] : INSTITUT MERIEUX : 1541 Avenue Marcel Mérieux 69280 MARCY L'ETOILE - FRANCE
[2] : PASTEUR VACCINS : Parc Industriel d'Incarville 27100 VAL DE REUIL - FRANCE

Key Words : ORAL POLIO VACCINE, OPV, SABIN, VERO CONTINUOUS CELL LINE, LARGE-SCALE, MICROCARRIERS

ABSTRACT :

Due to the shortage of high quality primate sources for primary monkey kidney cells, Institut Mérieux moved towards Vero cells, grown on microcarrier, to prepare Oral Polio Vaccine (OPV) using Sabin strains. Series of 28 different monovalent have been produced equally distributed between the 3 serotypes : 9 for type 1, 10 for type 2 and 9 for type 3. The crude harvests were clarified and purified with combining chromatographic procedure and sucrose gradient zonal centrifugation. All the control tests of purity and potency (virus titration) were satisfactory. Particularly, the tests in monkeys for neurovirulence were all satisfactory, according to the WHO-test performed in comparison with WHO reference virus preparations. The clinical studies conducted in France and in Morocco showed efficacy as expected for OPV. After licensing, a post-marketing survey was performed in France, during distribution of more than 300,000 doses. In parallel, tests for the absence of neurovirulence in monkeys were applied by National Health Authorities. All tests were satisfactory and particularly the tests requested by the WHO/Biologicals to validate the new OPV for supplying to United Nations Agencies in addition to an international inspection of our facilities and procedures. The safety of the new OPV was confirmed for more than 50 million doses applied in the field, involving 33 different countries.

INTRODUCTION

Since 1959[1], Oral Polio Vaccine (OPV) prepared with Sabin strains was mainly produced by cultivation on primary monkey kidney cells (PMKC). But the quality of donor monkeys for PMKC was decreasing and rejection for latent contaminant viruses occurred with too high a frequency. On the other hand shortage of wild monkeys became an acute debate. In the same time, demand for OPV was growing. For all these reasons, we were incited to apply technology already developped for Inactivated Polio Vaccine (IPV)[2-3] to produce OPV on Vero cell line by large-scale cultivation on microcarriers.

MATERIAL AND METHODS

Cells and viruses

Vero cell line was received from American Type Culture Collection (ATCC) and developped through the Cell Banks system as previously[2-3] described. The Working Cell Banks (WCB) were at the 137th passage and the viruses were produced on cells developped at the 142nd passage. The microcarrier Cytodex-1[R] (PHARMACIA-Sweden) is prepared and sterilized as described in the booklet of the supplier[4].
The WCB was tested according to the WHO requirements when published[5]. The strains of Sabin Viruses were prepared in PMKC for virus seeds and for type 1 and 2, they were at SO + 3 (Sabin Original Seed + 3 passages) as production level. For type 3, we used the RNA-derived Pfizer strain, so called SOR, at SOR + 2 for production level.

Purification

When we started the production in 1985, we decided to apply a purification procedure in spite of the fact that OPV is an oral vaccine and all theoretical problems originated from a continuous cell line have no importance per oral route. However the experts thought that such a way could be an additional advantage to the new vaccine[6]. We apply routinely for each monovalent preparation lot of virus vaccine a chromatographic procedure based on an anion exchanger DEAE-Spherodex (IBF-France) combined with a sucrose gradient zonal centrifugation.

Controls

The crude harvests and monovalent lots are tested following the WHO Requirements as described for OPV produced in PMKC[7]. Particularly, the tests in monkeys for neurovirulence were performed following the WHO protocol, in comparison with reference virus preparations (homotypic). These Reference Virus preparations were the SO + 2 WHO Sabin Virus such as distributed by WHO. The lesions' score of histopathological sections of nervous tissues prepared from sacrificed inoculated valid monkeys was established by microscopic examination. The quantified scoring of the virus activity for each group of monkeys was obtained with a statistical evaluation comparing the mean score lesions of under test virus monovalent lot with the mean score value of Reference homotypic virus preparation.

Finished vaccines

Finished vaccines were prepared by dilution of monovalent virus vaccines in molar solution of magnesium chloride for stabilization of viruses. The virus titres and balanced formulations were made according to European Pharmacopœia Monograph at the starting studies. Later, the formulation has been adapted to every specific recommendations of United Nations' Agencies. For example, for each poliovirus type respectively 1, 2 and 3, the balanced formulations are : 3-1-3 (Europ. Pharm.), 10-1-3 (WHO) or 10-1-6 (PAHO and WHO recently).

Clinical studies

Immunogenicity of this new OPV was firstly studied in France[8]. A series of 118 children for primary vaccination and 116 children as booster immunization was studied for safety and efficacy. A complementary study of excretion/reversion[12] was conducted on two groups of children : one receiving OPV-Vero and another one OPV-PMKC-Stools samples for virus isolation were taken the same day but just before the first dose of vaccine and 1, 2, 3, 4, 6, 10, 20, 30 days after each one of 3 doses of vaccine. The isolated viruses were submitted to T-marker evaluation[7], sensitivity to monoclonal antibodies neutralization. Overmore, an assay to verify the sequence of RNA-genome of excreted viruses was undertaken especially in the 3'-non coding region of the genome[10].
A second set of clinical studies was applied in Morocco[9]. First part of study was concerning 200 children (mean age 3.2 months) for primary vaccination with 3 doses of OPV-Vero and 56 children (mean age 20.7 months) receiving the same vaccine as booster. The second part of the study was devoted to compare in newborns a schedule of 4 dose vaccines OPV-Vero versus OPV-PMKC.
The four doses were given at birth and 6, 10 and 14 weeks of age. Adsorbed DPT vaccine was also injected to all children on the same day as the OPV vaccine (last 3 OPV vaccine for newborns).

RESULTS

All the 28 monovalent lots were satisfactory as regarding all the classical tests for purity, identity and virus activity of OPV. Particularly the purity was examplified by residual Vero cell DNA determination[11]. The results of each lot were as low as less than 1 picogram per equivalent dose. All the rct/40 marker tests (table 1) and sensitivity to monoclonal antibodies neutralization showed that all virus lots were attenuated virus, Sabin-like. In addition, the sequencing of 3'-non coding region of the RNA viral genome of each of these 28 lots revealed the exact sequence comparable to the PMKC-produced virus and Sabin-like. By the neurovirulence test on monkeys the acceptability of all the 28 monovalent lots can be observed on the different tables 2, 3, 4 and fig. 1. All the mean lesions scores of the lots were lower than the scores of Reference Virus preparations.

Also interesting are the results of clinical studies. Immunogenicity of OPV-Vero in terms of primary vaccination was good enough to induce almost 100 % of seropositivity for all the 3 types of poliovirus after 3 doses as shown in table 5. The seroconversion rates were also of almost 100 % after 3 doses in seronegative children as described in table 6. These 2 tables were results of children studied in France. For Moroccan children, global figures are given in table 7. After 4 doses OPV-vaccine gave 95 %, 100 % and 90 % of seropositivity respectively for types 1, 2 and 3 of poliovirus comparing well with children having received OPV-PMKC. The immunogenicity was also assessed by a booster effect after administration to 77 children at 18 months and 39 as a 5 year booster. In Morocco 49 children at 18 months had also a booster effect for all 3 types as respectively 98 %, 100 % and 94 %.The safety of the vaccine was evaluated in France and in Morocco. Due to the concomitant administration of DT Pert. vaccine major side effects were fever and local reaction to DT Pert. injection. Diarrhea and vomiting were rare and always lower than 2 % and 1 % respectively. Furthermore, a post-marketing survey after licensing was assessed in France during 1989. After 10 months of marketing 350 000 doses have been sold in France. An effective epidemiological and virological surveillance as well a post-marketing surveillance did not show any paralytic poliomyelitis during this period.

DISCUSSION

When we decided to change the cell substrate for OPV production from PMKC to a continuous cell line such as Vero cell line, our aim was to produce an OPV identical to this one produced since 1961 and sold in France since 1966. All biological tests concerning purity, safety and efficacy the Vero-OPV were absolutely identical to PMKC-OPV. By cultivation on microcarrier system with a unique container such as fermentor (or Cytogenerator) cell growth and virus propagation can be regulated and maintained in more strict conditions of temperature, pH, pO_2 than in numerous units of glass or plastic bottles. The purification procedure could also have been selecting some more neurovirulent viral population, as sometimes discussed or evocated. In the reality, the series of 28 monovalent lots of OPV produced by Institut Mérieux affords an answer to this theoretical fear : all the series of respectively type 1, 2 and 3 have shown a regular consistency of results in "in vitro" marker (rct/40) or in neurovirulence tests performed in monkeys, compared with Reference virus preparations. The mean lesion scores evaluated by statistical methods were always lower than the scores obtained with Reference virus preparations. The study of excretion/reversion of virus after vaccination was undertaken. The immunological and virological markers in vitro are already known as Sabin-like strains. But the sequencing in the 3'-non coding region was much more delicate to perform. Untill now, they are not yet completed, but the preliminary results seem to show that Vero-OPV is giving the same profile of excretion/reversion than the PMKC-OPV.

The continuous cell line, particularly the Vero cell line used and certified for more than 10 year experience by Institut Mérieux, is a right alternative as substrate for preparing OPV at large-scale. This Vero OPV safe and efficaceous is now largely used in the Expanded Program of Immunization as more than 50 million doses have been already distributed through more 33 countries without complaint.

ACKNOWLEDGEMENTS

This study was carried out with the help of many contributors but more precisely : HILLION A.M., MENETRAT J.L., BAJARD A., BANDET R., BARGEL A., BEURLET J., CALLARD R., GENOUX P., GERDIL C., GIBELIN N., BEURLET J. and GOLDMAN C., HEIMENDINGER P., MOULIN J.Cl., PELLOQUIN F.,   SOUVRAS M., XUEREF C., GIRARD M., HORAUD F., CRAINIC R., AYMARD M., BRIGAUD M.
Please all receive our acknowledgements for their contribution.

REFERENCES

1   Sabin, A.B. Present position of immunization against poliomyelitis with live virus vaccines. Br Med. J. 1959, 663-680

2   Montagnon B.J. Polio and rabies vaccines produced in continuous cell lines : a reality for Vero cell line. Develop. biol. Standard. 1989, 70, 27-47

3   Montagnon B.J., Fanget B. and Nicolas A. The large scale cultivation of Vero cells in microcarrier culture for virus vaccine production. Preliminary results for killed poliovirus vaccine. Develop. biol. Standard. 1981, 47, 55-64

4   Pharmacia Fine chemicals. Microcarrier cell culture : principles and methods. Booklet of supplyier, Almqvist and Wiksell Tryckeri, Uppsala, 1981

5   World Health Organization (WHO). Requirements for continuous cell lines used for biological substances production. Requirements for biological substances n° 37. TRS 745 Annex 3, WHO, Geneva, 1987, 93-107

6   World Health Organization (WHO). Acceptability of cell substrates for production of biologicals. Report of a study group. TRS 747, WHO, Geneva, 1987, 16

7   World Health Organization (WHO). Requirements for Poliomyelitis Vaccine (Oral). Requirements for biological substances n° 7. Revised 1982. TRS-687 Annex 4, WHO, Geneva, 1983, 107-174

8   Guérin N. Clinical studies of OPV produced on Vero cells (in press)

9   Lahrech M.T. and Caudrelier P. Immunological response of Moroccan children and newborns to Oral Poliovirus Vaccine prepared on Vero cells. Vaccine 1990 (in press)

10   Minor P.D., John A., Ferguson M. and Icenogle J.P. Antigenic and molecular evolution of the vaccine strain of type 3 poliovirus during the period of excretion by a primary vaccinee. J. Gen. Virol. 1986, 67, 693-706

11   Montagnon B.J., Martin R., Bandet R., Fanget B., Paturel J. and   Mackowiak J.F. Residual Vero cell DNA and inactivated poliovaccine : detection by DNA-DNA molecular hybridization. In Vitro Cellular and Developmental Biology. Monograph number 6 (Hopps H.E. and Petricciani J.C. ed.) 82-89, OBRR/CDB/FDA, Bethesda, 1985

12   Brigaud M., Aymard M., Caudrelier P. Comparative study of poliovirus excretion after vaccination of infants with new OPV prepared on Vero cells or Monkey Kidney Cells (MK). In VI International Conference of Comparative and Applied Virology. BANFF, Alberta, Canada, October 15-21, 1989

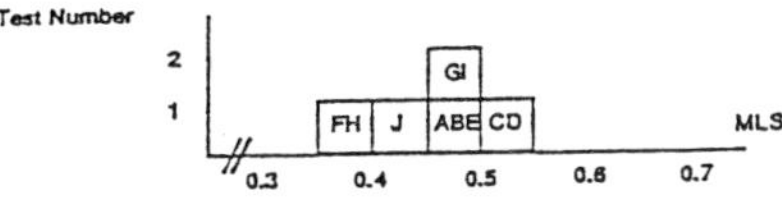

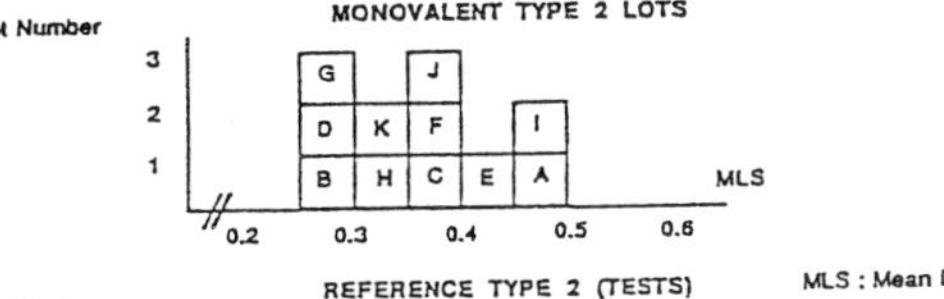

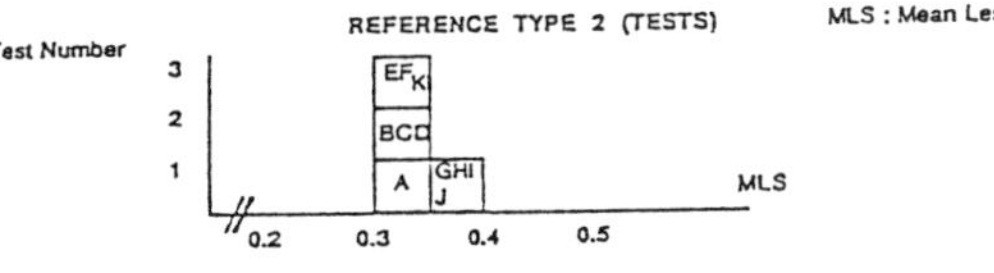

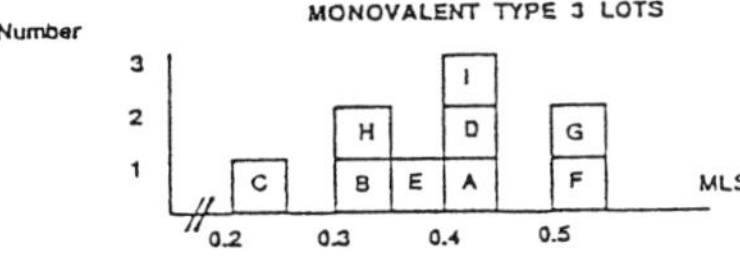

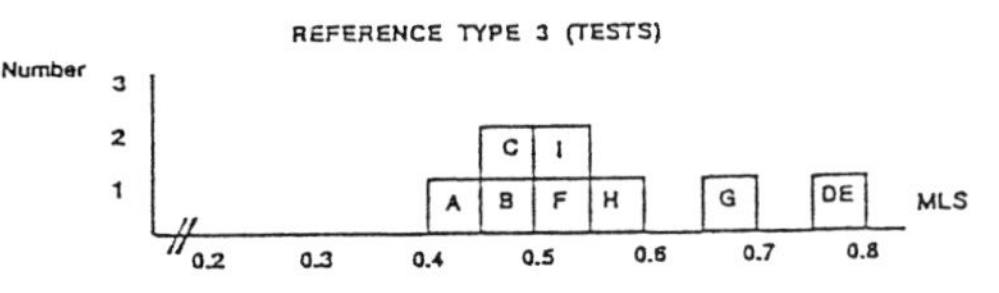

FIGURE 1

MEAN LESIONS SCORING OF HISTOPATHOLOGICAL
DATA FOR VALID MONKEYS OF OPV LOTS AND REFERENCE

TYPE 1

LOT NUMBER	DIFFERENCE OF TITER 34°C–40°C
016	$\frac{7.6}{10}$
017	$\frac{7.1}{10}$
018	$\frac{8}{10}$
019	$\frac{7.3}{10}$
020	$\frac{7.6}{10}$
021	$\frac{7.4}{10}$
022	$\frac{7.2}{10}$
023	$\frac{7.4}{10}$
024	$\frac{7.4}{10}$
SEED LOT TYPE 1	$\frac{7.4}{10}$

TYPE 2

LOT NUMBER	DIFFERENCE OF TITER 34°C–40°C
007	$\frac{7}{10}$
008	$\frac{6.9}{10}$
009	$\frac{7.5}{10}$
010	$\frac{7.1}{10}$
029	$\frac{8}{10}$
030	$\frac{8.3}{10}$
031	$\frac{8}{10}$
032	$\frac{8.2}{10}$
033	$\frac{8.4}{10}$
034	$\frac{8.2}{10}$
SEED LOT TYPE 2	$\frac{6.9}{10}$

TYPE 3

LOT NUMBER	DIFFERENCE OF TITER 34°C–40.3°C
011	$\frac{7.1}{10}$
012	$\frac{8.3}{10}$
013	$\frac{8.1}{10}$
014	$\frac{7.7}{10}$
015	$\frac{7.9}{10}$
025	$\frac{7.6}{10}$
026	$\frac{7.6}{10}$
027	$\frac{8}{10}$
028	$\frac{8}{10}$

TEST FOR CONSISTENCY OF VIRUS
CHARACTERISTICS rct/40 MARKER

Table 1

699

LOT NUMBER	PASSAGE LEVEL	PASSAGE IN VERO CELLS	MEAN LESION SCORE FOR REFERENCE $\bar{X}$ REF	MEAN LESION SCORE FOR THE VACCINE $\bar{X}$ TEST	C1	$\bar{X}$ TEST-$\bar{X}$ REF	ACTION
016	SO + 3	1	0.493	0.636	0.384	0.143	ACCEPTABLE
017	SO + 3	1	0.493	0.481	0.194	−0.012	ACCEPTABLE
018	SO + 3	1	0.511	0.674	0.439	0.163	ACCEPTABLE
019	SO + 3	1	0.511	0.323	0.333	−0.188	ACCEPTABLE
020	SO + 3	1	0.493	0.490	0.202	−0.003	ACCEPTABLE
021	SO + 3	1	0.370	0.500	0.266	0.130	ACCEPTABLE
022	SO + 4	1	0.478	0.340	0.284	−0.138	ACCEPTABLE
023	SO + 4	1	0.370	0.531	0.266	0.161	ACCEPTABLE
024	SO + 3	2	0.478	0.397	0.284	−0.081	ACCEPTABLE
SEED LOT TYPE 1	SO + 2	1	0.409	0.684	0.282	0.275	ACCEPTABLE

MONOVALENTS TYPE 1

TEST NUMBER	MEAN LESION SCORE	WITHIN TEST VARIANCE	WITHIN TEST DEVIATION	COEFFICIENT OF VARIATION
1	0.511	0.130461	0.361	0.707
2	0.493	0.047571	0.218	0.442
3	0.409	0.119853	0.346	0.846
4	0.370	0.056919	0.239	0.646
5	0.478	0.144725	0.360	0.795
ARITHMETIC MEAN	0.450	0.098852	0.314	0.698

WHO REFERENCE TYPE 1

"QUALIFYING" TESTS

Table 2   HISTOPATHOLOGICAL RESULTS - TYPE 1

LOT NUMBER	PASSAGE LEVEL	PASSAGE IN VERO CELLS	MEAN LESION SCORE FOR REFERENCE $\bar{X}$ REF	MEAN LESION SCORE FOR THE VACCINE $\bar{X}$ TEST	C1	$\bar{X}$ TEST–$\bar{X}$ REF	ACTION
007	S0 + 3	1	0.340	0.497	0.258	0.157	ACCEPTABLE
008	S0 + 3	1	0.311	0.288	0.181	−0.023	ACCEPTABLE
009	S0 + 3	1	0.311	0.370	0.182	0.059	ACCEPTABLE
010	S0 + 3	1	0.311	0.280	0.159	−0.031	ACCEPTABLE
029	S0 + 3	1	0.339	0.403	0.220	0.064	ACCEPTABLE
030	S0 + 3	1	0.339	0.378	0.191	0.039	ACCEPTABLE
031	S0 + 3	1	0.359	0.289	0.172	−0.070	ACCEPTABLE
032	S0 + 3	1	0.359	0.300	0.187	−0.059	ACCEPTABLE
033	S0 + 3	1	0.359	0.466	0.172	0.107	ACCEPTABLE
034	S0 + 3	1	0.359	0.368	0.172	0.009	ACCEPTABLE
SEED LOT TYPE 2	S0 + 2	1	0.339	0.324	0.181	−0.015	ACCEPTABLE

MONOVALENTS TYPE 2

TEST NUMBER	MEAN LESION SCORE	WITHIN TEST VARIANCE	WITHIN TEST DEVIATION	COEFFICIENT OF VARIATION
1	0.340	0.030626	0.174	0.513
2	0.311	0.030641	0.175	0.563
3	0.339	0.031535	0.178	0.525
4	0.359	0.051088	0.226	0.630
ARITHMETIC MEAN	0.338	0.036205	0.190	0.562

WHO REFERENCE TYPE 2

"QUALIFYING" TESTS

Table 3   HISTOPATHOLOGICAL RESULTS - TYPE 2

LOT NUMBER	PASSAGE LEVEL	PASSAGE IN VERO CELLS	MEAN LESION SCORE FOR REFERENCE $\bar{X}$ REF	MEAN LESION SCORE FOR THE VACCINE $\bar{X}$ TEST	C1	$\bar{X}$ TEST$-\bar{X}$ REF	ACTION
011	SOR + 2	1	0.440	0.449	0.406	0.009	ACCEPTABLE
012*	SOR + 2	1	0.486	0.335	0.309	−0.151	ACCEPTABLE
013*	SOR + 2	1	0.452	0.245	0.309	−0.207	ACCEPTABLE
014	SOR + 2	1	0.775	0.419	0.390	−0.356	ACCEPTABLE
015	SOR + 2	1	0.775	0.387	0.390	−0.388	ACCEPTABLE
025	SOR + 2	1	0.528	0.525	0.370	−0.003	ACCEPTABLE
026	SOR + 2	1	0.675	0.544	0.393	−0.131	ACCEPTABLE
027	SOR + 2	1	0.580	0.326	0.401	−0.254	ACCEPTABLE
028	SOR + 2	1	0.528	0.400	0.379	−0.128	ACCEPTABLE

<u>MONOVALENTS TYPE 3</u>

TEST NUMBER	MEAN LESION SCORE	WITHIN TEST VARIANCE	WITHIN TEST DEVIATION	COEFFICIENT OF VARIATION
1	0.595	0.217133	0.466	0.783
2	0.554	0.149865	0.387	0.699
3	1.028	0.328337	0.573	0.557
4	0.857	0.571499	0.756	0.882
5	0.775	0.280584	0.530	0.684
6	0.395	0.184462	0.430	1.089
7	0.440	0.173495	0.417	0.948
9	0.872	0.487329	0.698	0.801
10	0.580	0.174743	0.418	0.721
11	0.528	0.119224	0.345	0.653
12	0.675	0.339318	0.583	0.864
ARITHMETIC MEAN	0.670	0.277021	0.526	0.785

<u>WHO REFERENCE TYPE 3</u>

"QUALIFYING" LOTS

Table 4   HISTOPATHOLOGICAL RESULTS - TYPE 3

Number = 118	TYPE 1	TYPE 2	TYPE 3
Before vaccination % seropositivity	68/118 (57.6 %)	91/118 (77.1 %)	58/118 (49.2 %)
G.M.T. C.I. at 95 %	19.03 (15.2 - 23.9)	28.62 (23.1 - 35.5)	11.83 (9.7 - 14.4)
After 2 doses % seropositivity	106/115 (92.2 %)	114/115 (99.1 %)	105/115 (91.3 %)
G.M.T. C.I. at 95 %	125.39 (93.5 - 168.2)	816.70 (690.6 - 965.8)	168.15 (132.8 - 212.9)
% of titres x 4	83/115 (72.2 %)	110/115 (95.7 %)	96/115 (83.5 %)
After 3 doses % seropositivity	110/112 (98.2 %)	112/112 (100 %)	109/112 (97.3 %)
G.M.T. C.I. at 95 %	163.88 (127.0 - 211.5)	865.02 (724.2 - 1 033.2)	187.30 (151.7 - 231.3)
% of titres x 4	93/112 (83.0 %)	106/112 (94.6 %)	102/112 (91.1 %)

Table 5   <u>**IMMUNOGENICITY OF THE VERO SABIN VACCINE**</u>

<u>**AS PRIMARY VACCINATION**</u>

All children

	TYPE 1	TYPE 2	TYPE 3
After 2 doses % seroconversion	43/47 (91.5 %)	26/26 (100 %)	52/58 (89.7 %)
G.M.T. C.I. at 95 %	116.11 (76.0 - 177.3)	826.76 (532.5 - 1 283.7)	162.17 (118.8 - 221.3)
After 3 doses % seroconversion	45/45 (100 %)	26/26 (100 %)	54/55 (98.2 %)
G.M.T. C.I. at 95 %	130.84 (90.5 - 189.1)	903.75 (589.2 - 1 386.3)	186.20 (133.9 - 258.9)

Table 6   <u>**IMMUNOGENICITY OF THE VERO SABIN VACCINE**</u>

<u>**AS PRIMARY VACCINATION**</u>

Children seronegative before vaccination

	VERO OPV			PMK OPV		
	Type 1	Type 2	Type 3	Type 1	Type 2	Type 3
BEFORE						
Seropositivity rate *	93	88	81	90	83	64
AFTER 3 DOSES						
Seropositivity rate*	95	100	86	95	100	79
Seroconversion rate **	74	98	86	81	93	81
AFTER 4 DOSES						
Seropositivity rate *	95	100	90	86	100	89
Seroconversion rate **	92	100	95	86	97	94

* Percentage of titres ≥ 1:5

** Percentage of antibody titre multiplied at least by a factor of 4 compared to the titre theoretically observed if no vaccination was performed (calculated individually assuming a half-life of 4 weeks for maternal antibodies).

PMK : Primary Monkey Kidney Cell

OPV : Oral Polio Vaccine

<u>SEROPOSITIVITY AND SEROCONVERSION RATES IN BOTH</u>

Table 7 <u>VERO AND PMK CELL OPV GROUPS</u>

Velden de Groot:
I understand you used the same virus strains as for production from monkey kidney cells. Did you optimise again the culture conditions and the MOI in the Vero cells, and was there a change?

Montagnon: It was not necessary to optimise or adapt the cell conditions for the Sabin virus strain used in the monkey cells.

Velden de Groot:
Your main concern in purification is the cellular DNA I understand. Could you not have used an ion exchange step? Was it necessary to have a double purification step?

Montagnon: The purification procedure has been discussed by the WHO working group. It was not considered obligatory for the oral polio vaccine. Initially we thought it would be necessary to have two purification steps, and we maintained this process as the consistency of production was excellent.

STRATEGIES FOR IMPROVED PRODUCTION OF EPSTEIN-BARR VIRUS

Davies, A H[1][2]*, Huddelston, J[1], Evans, F J[3], Rickinson, A B[2] and Emery A N[1]

1.   Centre for Biochemical Engineering, University of Birmingham, U.K.
2.   Dept Cancer Studies, University of Birmingham, U.K.
3.   Dept of Pharmocognosy, London School of Pharmacy, London, U.K.
*   Present address: Institute of Virology, Mansfield Road, Oxford,

ABSTRACT

Epstein-Barr virus (EBV), a human herpesvirus endemic in all human populations, is the causal agent of infectious monoucleosis (IM), and is also linked to certain kinds of cancer. _In vitro_, EBV forms tightly latent infections of host cell lines: this lack of a simple permissive tissue culture system has made it difficult to obtain large quantities of virus for study.

The B95-8 cell line, established by infecting Marmoset B lymphocytes with EBV from an IM patient, is unusual in supporting a small proportion of cells which spontaneously release virus: enhancement of this population by adding the tumour promoter TPA, followed by a labour intensive, low yield ultracentrifugation step, is the standard method of preparing virus, and B95-8 the most studied source of EBV. Here we report the combined use of Sap A, a non-tumour-promoting analogue of TPA, large-scale mammalian cell culture and contained downstream processing by crossflow filtration, in a new strategy for EBV production. It has yielded virus preparations of unprecedented size, quality and infectious titre, making possible previously uncomtemplatable experiments and facilitating production of potential EBV vaccines.

KEYWORDS :
Cell culture; Epstein-Barr Virus; Induction; Membrane Filtration; Vaccine

INTRODUCTION

Interest in EBV stems from its cell growth transforming potential and from its clear linkage to several clinical conditions. Three principal problems have hindered large-scale virus production - 1) batch variability of virus preparations 2) the large scale use of tumour-promoting EBV inducers and 3) the poor efficiency of large scale recovery of biologically active vaccines and virus preparations. We submit here techniques and/or reagents which now offer the prospect of ameliorating these hindrances.

CULTURE OF EBV-INFECTED CELLS IN A BIOREACTOR

B95-8 cells were routinely cultured for our studies in a laboratory cell-culture reactor (SET 2CV - Setric Genie Industriel, Toulouse). Cultures were robust, insensitive to agitation speed over the 25-100 rpm

range and neither DOT nor pH control was needed - except for the latter
when serum-free low-protein media were used. Table 1 summarises results
for a range of conditions.

INDUCTION OF EBV IN MARMOSET B95-8 CELLS

The B95-8 cell line is unusual in supporting a small proportion of cells
which spontaneously release virus. Enhancement of this process by adding
TPA followed by a labour intensive low yield ultracentrifugation step has
become the generally accepted method of preparing virus. TPA is a
diterpene ester with profound short-term (irritancy) and long-term (tumour
promotion) toxic effects, and thus unsuitable for repeated use on a large
scale. We investigated a panel of tigliane analogues of TPA produced at
the London School of Pharmacy, finding one, designated Sap A, to be an
equipotent active analogue of TPA for EBV indution, but lacking the
latter's tumour promoting function. Structures for TPA and Sap A are
shown in figure 1.

PURIFICATION OF EBV USING TANGENTIAL FLOW FILTRATION

Conventional virus preparations use inefficient and labour intensive
processes which are not amenable to scale-up. We have demonstrated
contained separation of B95-8 cells from culture fluid using tangential
flow filtration with microporous membranes of pore size 0.45 μm, using the
'Minitan' flat membrane system (Millipore s.a., Molsheim). Concentration
of EBV particles, of average size 100nm in the resulting permeate, was
achieved with polysulphone ultrafiltration membranes in the same
equipment. Attempts to concentrate virus over a 100 kDa MWCO membrane
failed but the use of a 300 kDa NMWCO membrane was succesful and two
independent biological assays indicated the functional integrity of the
recovered virus.

CONTROL OF EPSTEIN-BARR VIRUS INFECTION

Current prospects for intervention in diseases in which EBV plays a role
include the development of prophylactic therapy based on the immune
response to a lytic viral antigen, gp350. gp350 has long been considered
as a potential anti-EBV vaccine. Despite the cloning and expression of
the gp350 gene in E.coli and mammalian cells however, little success has
been achieved in the maintenance of cultures with a significant proportion
of cells expressing gp350. Thus, pending significant advances in
recombinant vaccine design, the method of choice for preparation of the
immunogen remains FPLC purification from B95-8 cells. Small numbers of
Cottontop Tamarins were used in the animal trials of gp350: for the
currently projected human trials larger amounts of gp350 will be required.
As with production of the virus itself, this requires unprecedentedly
large quantities of B95-8 cells: these recent advances in cytotechnology
have facilitated such preparations.

ACKNOWLEDGMENTS :

The authors gratefully acknowledge the loan of equipment by Setric Genie
Industriel,Toulouse, and Millipore s.a., Molsheim.

Medium	pH	agitation (r.p.m)	μ_{max} (h.$^{-1}$)	MCD ($\times 10^{-6}$/ml)	$t_{\mu max}$ (h.)
RPM1/2% US	NR	25	0.029	1.19	58
		control	0.024	1.08	86
	NR	100	0.023	1.63	95
		control	0.023	1.77	32
RPM1/BIT	NR	25	0.010	0.64	84
		control	0.025	1.23	39
	7.2	25	0.023	1.14	39
		control	0.024	1.25	30
+Sap A (3×10^{-8}M)	7.2	25	0.022	1.35	60
		control	0.020	1.45	68

Table 1 : Growth of B95-8 cells in a stirred tank bioreactor (SGi)

Control cultures were grown in 10 ml. plastic tissue culture flasks
NR – not regulated

Virus dilution	original supernatant	permeate	retentate	washings
10^{0}	–	6/6	–	–
10^{-1}	–	5/6	–	–
10^{-2}	5/5	0/6	–	–
10^{-3}	6/6	0/6	–	4/6
10^{-4}	3/5	0/6	6/6	4/6
10^{-5}	2/6	0/6	6/6	5/6
10^{-6}	0/6	0/6	6/6	3/6
10^{-7}	–	–	6/6	1/6
10^{-8}	–	–	2/6	0/6

Table 2 Transforming litre of EBV concentrated by crossflow filtration.
The fraction of wells in which transformation had occured after 6 weeks is
given for serial dilutions of virus. The sources of virus assayed were
the original supernatant before concentration, and the permeate, retentate
and washings after concentration using a 300kDa membrane.

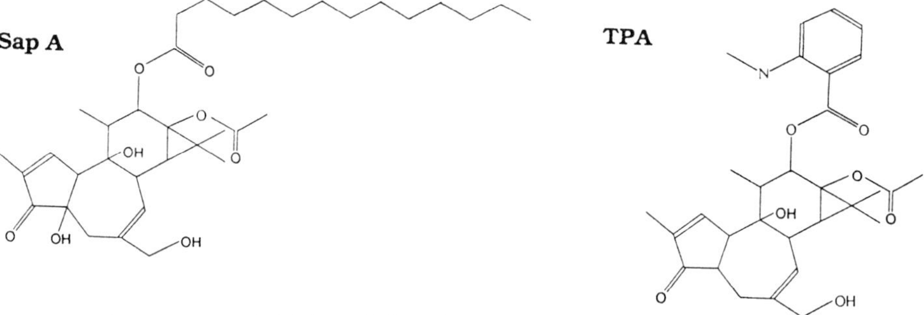

Figure 1. Structures of TPA and Sap A.

OPTIMAL CONDITIONS FOR THE GROWTH OF PIG KIDNEY ENDOTHELIAL CELLS (SK)
PROLIFERATED ON MICROCARRIERS AND PRODUCTION OF PIG PARVOVIRUS (PPV)
VACCINE

L. PORQUET, M. VAYREDA, C. AULINAS AND J. PLANA DURAN
LABORATORIOS SOBRINO, S.A. Vall de Bianya, Girona (Spain)

ABSTRACT

The goal is the utilization of cell growth technology on microcarriers in
order to determine Porcine Parvovirus (PPV) replication. Cell culture and
viral infection parameters have been studied. We also verified that virus,
obtained on SK cells grown on microcarriers, produces the same protection
levels than the classical vaccines obtained in roller bottles.

INTRODUCTION

PPV is one of the chief agents involved in reproductive problems of sows.
The different symptoms of the disease are: return to estrus, small lit-
ters, mummification and stillbirths. For this reason, our intention has
been to develop an effective vaccine against PPV.

MATERIAL AND METHODS

All the experiments were carried out with spinner flasks of 250 and 250 ml.
The culture medium was Glasgow M.E.M. with clex serum.
The conditions for culture were 37ºC and 5% of CO_2.
Cell counts by nuclear extrusion with crystal violet and citric acid.
The virus is titrated because of its capability for hemagglutinating gui
nea-pig red blood cells.
To use the viral antigen as vaccine, we inactivate it with binary ethyle-
nimine (B.E.I.) and manufacture a w/o/w type emulsion. One dose of the
vaccine contains 5120 HA units. The antibody titer is expressed in hemag-
glutination inhibition units.

RESULTS

Type of microcarrier: Cytodex 3.
Microcarrier concentration: 1 g / 1 l.
Cell inocula: For cell growth and future scale-up $1-2.10^5$ cells/ml
(Figure 1). For viral infection, $4-5.10^5$ cells/ml.
Stirring is at 20-25 r.p.m.
Infection at the same time that cells are put in suspension.
Number of virus/cell: from 5.10^{-5} to 5.10^{-4} HAu/ml (as verified by Figure 2
and Table 1).
Time of viral antigen collection: depending in every case on microscopic
observation (Figure 3) and titration per hemagglutination. Generally, the
supernatant is collected at least three times.
Serological response in rabbits is good, as shown in Figure 4 and Table 2.

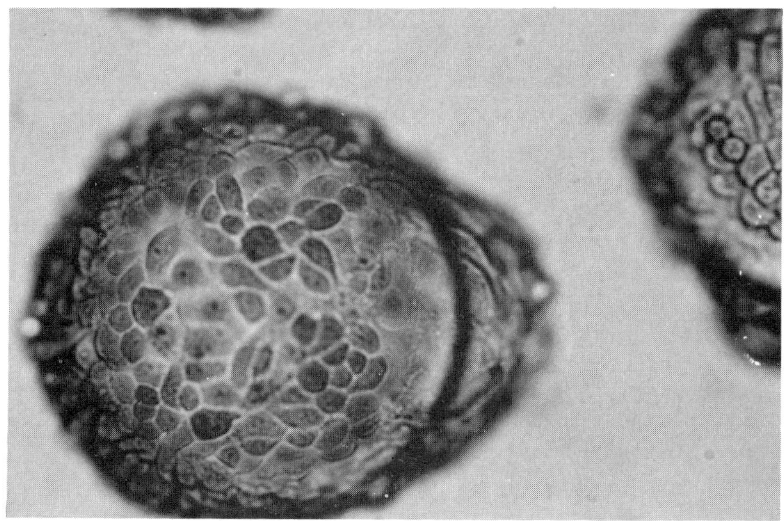

Figure 1

Cell Growth Curves

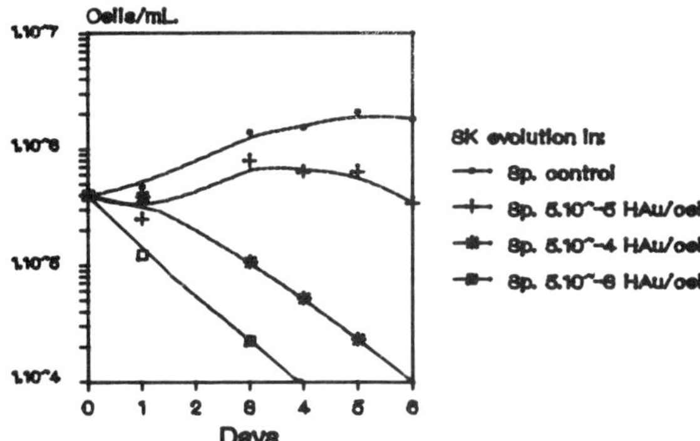

Figure 2. Pig Parvovirus infection, at the same time that cells are put in suspension, with three different virus Inocula:

5.10^{-3} HAu/cell
5.10^{-4} HAu/cell
5.10^{-5} HAu/cell

SK cells (cell/mL.) and PPV (total HA produced) evolution during 6 days.

Virus Production

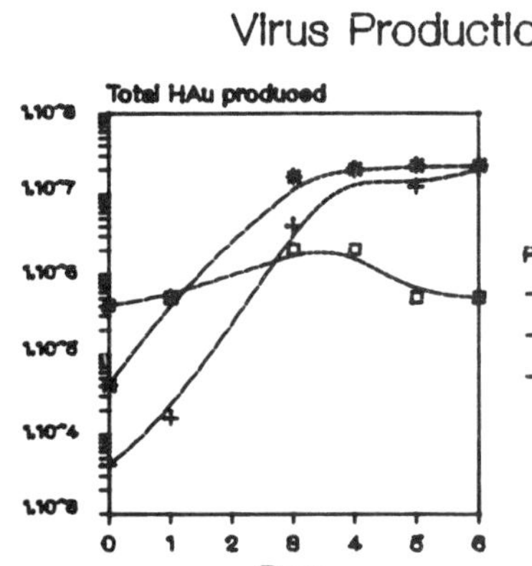

Days	Sp. 5.10^{-3}	Sp. 5.10^{-4}	Sp. 5.10^{-5}
0	$4.1.10^5$	$4.1.10^4$	$4.1.10^3$
1	$5.1.10^5$	$5.1.10^5$	$1.6.10^4$
3	$2.2.10^6$	$16.4.10^6$	$4.1.10^6$
4	$2.1.10^6$	$20.5.10^6$	$20.8.10^6$
5	$5.1.10^5$	$22.5.10^6$	$12.8.10^6$
6	$5.1.10^5$	$22.5.10^6$	$20.5.10^6$

Table 1. PPV evolution in the three different spinners.

710

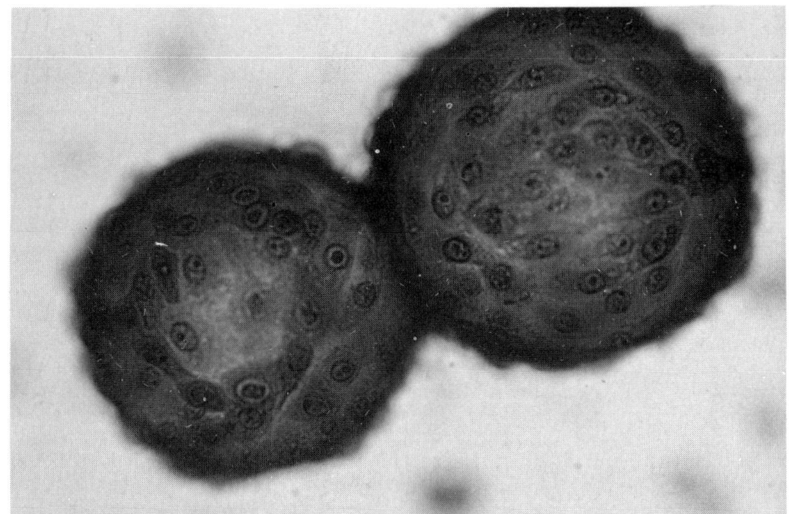

Figure 3

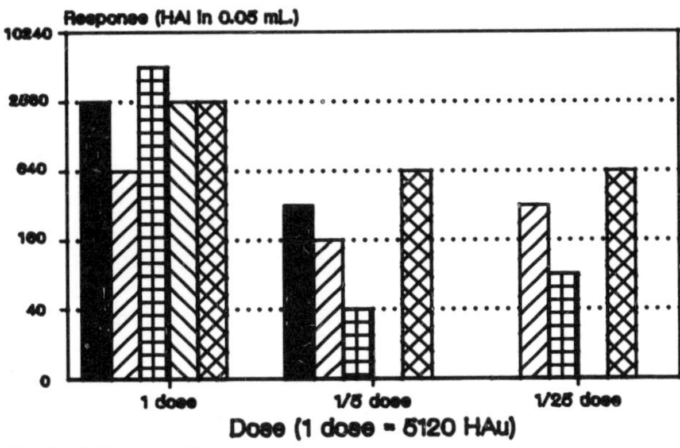

Figure 4. Serological response in rabbits 21 days after PPV vaccination.

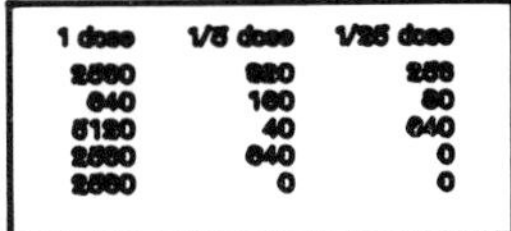

1 dose	1/5 dose	1/25 dose
2560	2560	2560
640	160	80
5120	40	640
2560	640	0
2560	0	0

Table 2

DISCUSSION

- SK cells grow very well on Cytodex microcarriers. Their cell multiplication rate is higher than in static culture or roller bottle.
- With extremely low quantities of virus/cell the viral yields obtained are good. The yield for PPV vaccine production is increased with micro carrier technology.
- This technology enables us to follow with accuracy viral infection by means of optical microscopy.
- We believe that the PPV vaccine obtained with this technology of micro carriers ensures the same level of protection in sows as with the classical roller-bottle vaccines.

CONTINUOUS PRODUCTION OF A NOVEL THROMBOLYTIC FROM 50/100 LITRE PERFUSED
MICROCARRIER CULTURES

Mannix, C.J., Pettman, G.R., Southwick, W.A.

Cell Products Unit, Biotechnology Department, SmithKline Beecham,
Biosciences Research Centre, Great Burgh, Epsom, Surrey, England KT18 5XQ.

ABSTRACT

Microcarrier cultures were evaluated as a means to scale-up production of
novel thrombolytic proteins from recombinant Chinese hamster ovary cells.
Conditions for growth of cells and production of the protein were
determined from small-scale cultures initially, and then applied to 50 or
100 litre perfused cultures.   Larger cultures were grown in serum-
containing medium, washed, and maintained in protein-free medium for
periods of up to ten weeks.   After an initial lag phase, the cultures
produced the recombinant product at an approximately constant rate, and
allowed recovery of gram quantities of material for evaluation.

KEYWORDS : recombinant cells, microcarriers, perfusion, protein-free
           medium, thrombolytic agents (t-PA).

INTRODUCTION

Within SmithKline Beecham, a series of novel thrombolytics, such as the
modified t-PA species described previously[1,2], have been required for
evaluation.   Small quantities of such proteins have been produced and
purified from mammalian cells grown in tissue culture flasks.   The object
of the present study was to evaluate the use of 50-100 litre microcarrier
cultures for production of gram quantities of product.

MATERIALS AND METHODS

A recombinant Chinese hamster ovary (CHO) cell line expressing the novel
thrombolytic was supplied by Dr. M.J. Browne (SB).   The cell line was
negative for mycoplasma contamination by both Hoechst stain (Calbiochem)
and Genprobe assays.   All culture reagents were supplied by Gibco unless
otherwise stated.   Growth medium was α-MEM supplemented with 10% dialysed
foetal bovine serum (dFBS).   Production medium was DMEM:Ham's F-12, 1:1.
Antibiotics are not used within the Cell Products Unit.   Cultures were
incubated at 37°C in an atmosphere of 5-10% CO_2 in air.   Stock cultures
were grown in 175 cm^2 flasks (Nunc) in the presence of 5 µM methotrexate
(Sigma), and were passaged as necessary by trypsinisation (0.25% trypsin
in Dulbecco's PBS 'A' (Oxoid).   Suspension cultures were grown in spinner
flasks (Techne MCS) stirred at 20-30 rpm, inoculated at approx. 2-4 x 10^4
cells per ml and grown to a maximum concentration of 6 x 10^5 cells per ml.
Cytodex 2 and 3 microcarriers (Pharmacia) for small scale cultures were
prepared according to the manufacturers instructions.   For reactor use,
microcarriers were swollen and washed in PBS (Dulbecco 'A'), washed with

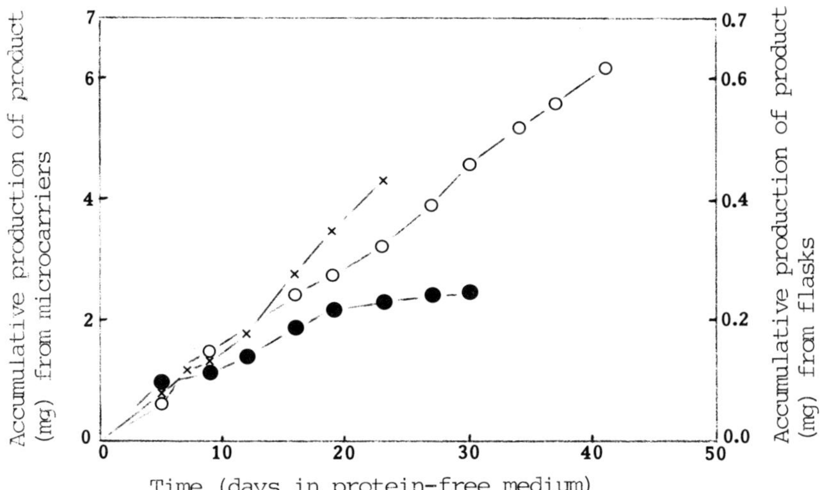

Duplicate cultures of CHO cells were grown on Cytodex 2 (●) and Cytodex 3 (○), in 200 ml cultures containing 0.6 g of microcarrier and the product produced in protein-free medium as described in Materials and Methods. Replicate flask cultures (80 cm^2, ×) were treated in parallel as a comparison.

Fig. 1   Production of thrombolytic protein by small-scale microcarrier cultures

deionised water to reduce the PBS to approx. 25%, and autoclaved. Concentrated (10 x) DMEM, glutamine and sodium bicarbonate were added aseptically to give a final composition of DMEM:PBS, 0.75:0.25 approx. The suspension was supplemented with 1-2 litres of dFBS, mixed and prewarmed to 37°C before transfer to reactors. Microcarrier cultures were initiated by addition of 2-5 g of Cytodex per litre of culture to vessels containing cells in suspension. Growth of microcarrier cultures was monitored by microscopic examination and by counting cells recovered by trypsinisation. Confluent microcarriers were washed three times with production medium, and incubated in the same medium. Spent medium containing product was recovered at 2-4 day intervals, and replaced with fresh production medium, or (reactors only) was continuously withdrawn and replaced with fresh medium. Product concentration was monitored by fibrin plate assay as described previously[3].

50 and 100 litre (working volume) stirred tank reactors were obtained from LH Engineering (Slough). An anular 75 μm filter was mounted on the top-driven agitator shaft, with access for pipework through the open top of the filter, above the level of liquid. Microcarriers were excluded from the inside of the filter, allowing recovery of spent culture medium free of microcarriers. Dissolved oxygen concentration and pH were controlled by sparging oxygen or carbon dioxide respectively into the inside of the filter. Medium could be supplied on demand using a level sensor. Media for reactor cultures was as for smaller cultures, except that they were prepared from powdered concentrate and sterilised by filtration (0.1 μm Ultipor, Pall) and the growth medium contained 0.005% DC 1520 antifoam (Dow-Corning).

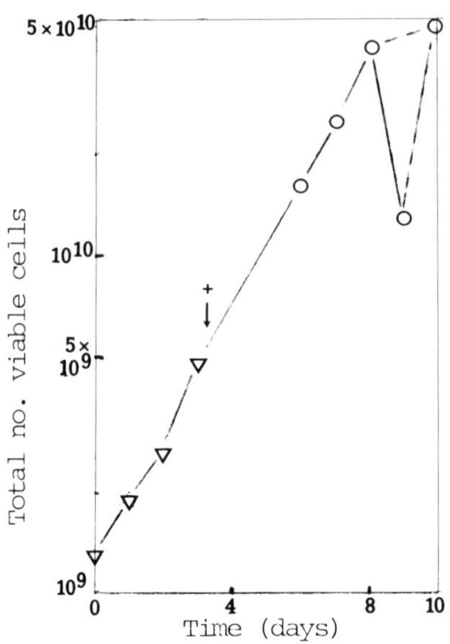

Fig 2 Growth of CHO cells
in 50 l reactor as suspension
(∇) and as microcarrier (+)
culture (o)
(see Materials and Methods)

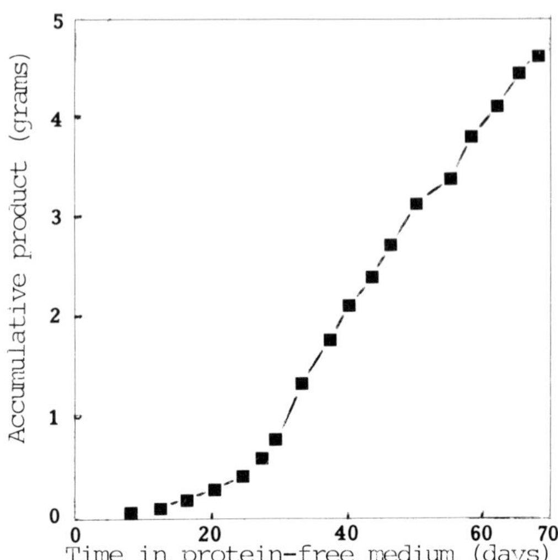

Fig 3 Production of thrombolytic
from 100 litre microcarrier culture
of CHO cells (see Materials and
Methods)

RESULTS AND DISCUSSION

Small-scale microcarrier cultures previously grown in the presence of
serum continued to produce the recombinant product in protein-free medium
for many weeks (fig. 1). The collagen-coated Cytodex 3 appeared to be
superior to Cytodex 2. Preparation of large-scale microcarrier cultures
was facilitated by initial growth of cells in suspension culture (fig. 2).
The 100 litre microcarrier culture produced only low levels of product
initially in the protein-free medium, which may have been caused by the
too rapid replacement of medium. Between 20 days and 70 days in protein-
free medium, the culture produced the product at an approximately linear
rate, and 5 g of recombinant protein was produced in approximately 2000
litres of medium (fig. 3). The use of protein-free medium facilitates
product purification and reduces production costs. However, the major
benefit of these cultures is the long productive period (months).

REFERENCES

1 Browne, M.J. et al, A tissue-type plasminogen activator mutant with
   prolonged clearance in vivo. J. Biol. Chem. 1988, 263, 1599-1602

2 Browne, M.J. et al, The role of tissue-type plasminogen activator
   A-chain domains in plasma clearance. Fibrinolysis 1989, 3, 207-214

3 Dodd, I., et al, Large-scale rapid purification of recombinant
   tissue-type plasminogen activator. Febs Lett 1986, 209, 13-17

PRODUCTION OF RECOMBINANT HUMAN THYROTROPIN AND ITS INCOMPLETE PROCESSING IN CHO CELLS

Sachihiko Watanabe, Yoshinori Nishitani, Machiko Hirono, and Hikaru Sonoda

Shionogi Research Laboratories, Shionogi & Co., Ltd., Osaka 553, Japan

ABSTRACT

Human thyrotropin(hTSH) β cDNA was expressed with α subunit cDNA in CHO cells. The production of recombinant hTSH increased efficiently with exposure to increasing concentrations of methotrexate and in a perfusion cell culture system with microcarrier. Recently we have, however, suggested that additional 6 amino acids at the C-terminus of β subunits are not completely removed in CHO cells, and that the hTSH cDNA without the 6 codons for C-terminal extension is also expressed in CHO cells to direct the synthesis of functional product. Thus, it may be advantageous to use β cDNA without the 6 codons instead of complete cDNA in the production of completely processed hTSH in CHO cells.

INTRODUCTON

Thyrotropin(thyroid-stimulating hormone, TSH) is a member of glycoprotein hormones. It consists of the two non-covalently associated subunits: a hormone-specific β subunit and an α subunit common to other glycoprotein hormones (1). The cDNAs and genes for the human TSH (hTSH) α and β subunits were isolated and sequenced (2,3), and we succeeded in its expression in CHO cells using cDNAs for the common α and hTSH β subunit(4). Here, we describe the efficient production of hTSH using gene amplification and high cell density cell culture techniques, although we suggested that the processing of recombinant β subunit is not complete in CHO cells(5).

MATERIALS AND METHODS

Construction of expression plasmids, cell cultures, and radioimmuno- and biological assays were described elsewhere (4,5).
Southern hybridization analysis. Chromosomal DNA was prepared from CHO cells, digested to completion with Hind III, electrophoresed on a 1.0% agarose gel, and blotted on nitrocellulose filter. Hybridization was carried out using nick-translated hTSH cDNA probe which had been obtained from pSV-TSH β with Bal I digestion.

RESULTS AND DISCUSSION

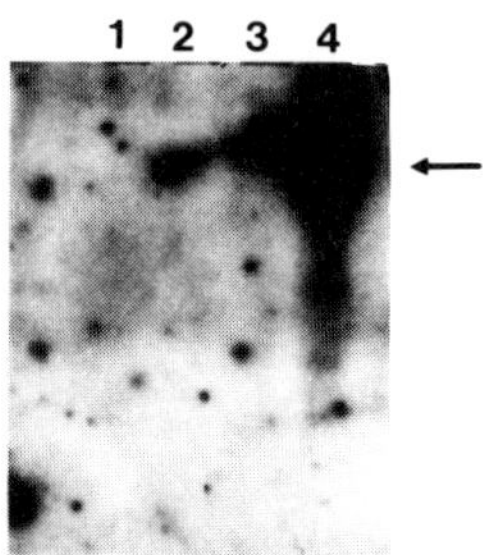

Figure 1 Southern blot analysis of dhfr⁺ MTX resistant hTSH secreting CHO cells. Genomic DNAs (5 μg each) from human placenta (lane 1), CHO dhfr⁻ cells (parental cell line, lane 2), CHO dhfr⁺ (CP43D20, lane 3) and CHO dfhr⁺ MTX resistant cells (CP43D20-10MTX500, lane 4) were analyzed as described in Materials and Methods.

Amplification of the dhfr gene by methotrexate(MTX) resistance led to enhanced expression of certain unselective marker genes (4). The yield of hTSH was 217 μU/ml in the hTSH-producing CHO cell line (CP43D 20) which is resistant to 100 nM of MTX. This cell line was exposed stepwise to higher concentrations of MTX to increase hTSH production, and we could obtain a CP43D20 derivative clone resistant to 500 nM MTX which produces more than 2000 μU/ml of hTSH. The production continued stably during more than 9 months. DNA copy number during MTX increases was analysized by Southern blotting (Fig.1). The 500 nM MTX-resistant cells contained at least 44 copies of the transfected plasmid.

Furthermore, CHO cells were cultured during 25 days on microcarriers in a perfusion cell culture system containing 1 L of culture medium (Fig.2), and we could find 1.6×10^7 μU (3,2 mg) of hTSH in resultant culture medium.

We purified recombinant hTSH using the following column chromatographies: S-Sepharose, DEAE-Sepharose, Concanavalin A-Sepharose, S-Sepharose, TSK-G2000SW and finally Bio-Gel P-30. Analysis of SDS-polyacrylamide gel electrophoresis and Western blot revealed that recombinant hTSH gives the same size pattern as that of the natural hTSH with a broad band. Two polypetides with approximately 24 Kd and 18 Kd corresponding to α and β subunits,respectively, appeared in the treatment of recombinant heterodimer hTSH with SH-reagent as already reported(5).

We have recently shown that additional 6 amino acids at the C-terminus of β subunits were not completely removed in CHO cells(5). Furthermore, both hTSHβ subunits without C-terminal extension and with incomplte extesion were functional as normal β-subunit in glycosylation, association with α-subunit, secretion and bioactivity(5). Thus, for the

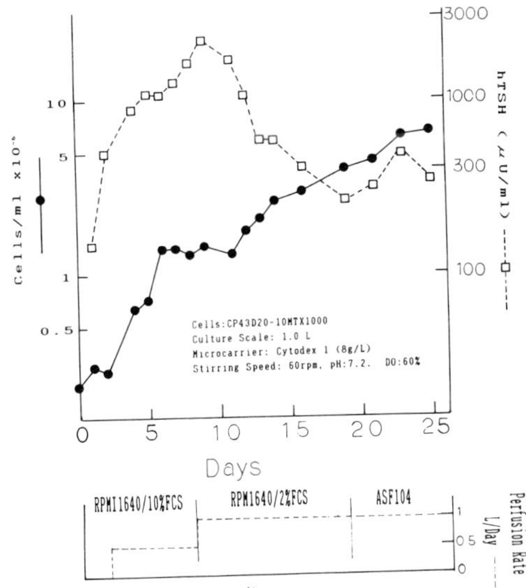

Figure 2 CHO cell growth and hTSH production with a cell culture system(6). The hTSH-producing CHO cells resistant to 1000 nM MTX (CP43D20-10MTX1000) were attached to 8 gr of microcarriers (Cytodex 1, Pharmacia) in 1l of RPMI1640 medium/10% FCS and then cultured in CL15 of a Celligen cell culture system (New Brunswick) at perfusion rates of 500 ml/day. The medium and perfusion rates were changed on day 8 and day 18 as indicated in Figure.

production of recombinant hTSH whose primary structure is completly identical with natural one it may be advantageous to use hTSH β cDNA without 6 codons for C-terminal extension.

ACKNOWLEDGMENTS

We thank Drs. N. Yoshida and T. Ono for their interest and help in TSH purification.

REFERENCES

1. Pierce, J. G. and Parsons, T. F. Annu. Rev. Biochem. 1981, 50, 465-495.
2. Fiddes, J. C. and Goodman, H. M. Nature 1980, 286, 684-687.
3. Hayashizaki, Y., Kato, Y., Miyai, K. and Matsubara, K. FEBS Lett. 1985, 188, 394-400.
4. Watanabe, S., Hayashizaki, Y., Endo, Y., Hirono, M., Takimoto, N., Tamaki, M., Teraoka, H., Miyai, K. and Matsubara, K. Biochem. Biophys. Res. Commun. 1987, 149, 1149-1155.
5. Takata, K., Watanabe, S., Hirono, M., Tamaki, M., Teraoka, H. and Hayashizaki, Y. Biochem. Biophys. Res. Commun. 1989, 165, 1035-1042.
6. Sonoda, H., Mori, H., Kikutani, H., Nishitani, Y., Hirono, M., Taniguchi, T. and Watanabe, S. J. Biotech. 1988, 9, 61-70.

Production of a monoklonal antibody against gelsolin

D.Lütkemeyer, H. Büntemeyer and J. Lehmann
Institute of Cell Culture Technique, University of Bielefeld, D-4800 Bielefeld 1, FRG

Introduction

Since Köhler and Milstein (1) have developed the technique to produce monoclonal antibodies, this technique is widely used for diagnostical and therapeutical purposes. For the technical production of monoclonal antibodies it is very important to work with high cell density and product concentration. Therefore, we use a high cell density perfusion system (2) with a medium especially optimized for each cell line. With this medium it is possible to perfuse with a low rate and use the whole medium more economically.

Materials and methods

The cells were cultivated in a 2 l perfusion bioreactor (Biostat MD, B. Braun, Melsungen, FRG). The reactor was equipped with a membrane basket with 2 m silicone tubing per litre for aeration and 2 m hydrophilized polypropylene hollow fibre membrane tubing per litre for medium exchange. The microfiltration membrane (0,3 μm) was connected at the input side via a peristaltic pump (Watson-Marlow 501-UR) with the medium reservoir and at the output side via another pump with the harvest tank (3). These two perfusion pumps controlled by a system creating a process cycle of harvesting and feeding depending on reactor volume and pump speed run alternatively. While running this cycle perfusion was carried out. Additionally, a third pump was connected to the reactor directly for cell harvest. Cells had to be remove from the reactor to reach steady state conditions. Temperature was set to 37 °C, pH to 7.2 and pO$_2$ to 40% air saturation.

The cell line used in this study were a mouse-mouse hybridoma (Mouse myeloma P3X63-Ag8.653 subclone / BALB/c) secreting a monoclonal antibody against gelsolin. Gelsolin, a 90 kdal protein, is an aktin modulator and plays a role in cytoskeleton of mammalian cells. The monoclonal antibody against gelsolin is of specific interest, because this antibody can tell the secreted gelsolin from the intracellular. The cell line was kindly supplied by Prof. Dr. B.M. Jockusch, Department of Biology, University of Bielefeld. Cell numbers were determined microscopically by trypan blue exclusion.

The serum free medium was a 1:1 mixture of IMDM and Ham's F12 supplemented with 2mM L-glutamine, 2mM pyruvate, 20 μM ethanolamine, 1 g/l bovine serum albumine complexed with 4 mg oleic acid, 10 mg/l human transferrin (Fe saturated), 10 mg/l bovine insulin. The medium and the supplements were sterilized by membrane filtration (0.2 μm).

The free amino acids in the samples of the fermentations were analysed using an automated reversed phase high performance liquid chromatographic system (RP-HPLC) with precolumn derivatization using the OPA method (4).

Glucose and lactic acid concentrations were analysed using an automatic analyzer system based on enzymatic and electrochemical reactions (YSI 2000, Yellow Springs Instruments, OH, USA).

In the supernatant the Antibody concentrations were analyzed by a kinetic sandwich ELISA method. The enzyme linked to the antibody (goat-anti-mouse antibody) was peroxidase converting o-phenylendiamine as substrate. For the kinetic analysis in each microplate well (standards and samples) an experimental point was taken every 3 minutes to control the complete enzyme reaction. In the linear part of this conversion curve (extinction versus time) the slope was calculated and correlated to the content of the standard solution. From this calibration function sample concentrations of several dilution steps were calculated.

Results

The fermentation of the hybridoma cell line (Figure 1) was subdivided into two parts: first part - batch; second part - perfusion with cell harvest. In the first part, when the rates of consumption of all nutrients were calculated (Figure 2), the cells grew up to a density of $1{,}8 \cdot 10^6$ cells/ml. Then the cells died, because of the limitation of amino acids (glutamine, methionine) (Figure 3); glucose concentration was not important during this period. Half of the volume of the fermenter was drained off, filled up again with fresh medium to start part two of the fermentation. The cells grew again and in this second part of the fermentation the fermenter was fed with fresh medium as described above (perfusion procedure). The feeding rate was raised from $D_P = 0.8$ d^{-1} at the beginning up to a maximum of $D_P = 1.7$ $^{-1}$; then cell harvest was started. Further changes of D_P were necessary to stabilize the steady state. The medium used in this part was optimized by supplementation of the limiting amino acids (Figure 2). The concentrations of asparagine, tryptophan, valine, isoleucine, leucine and phenylalanine were double, methionine and glutamine were triple and histidine was one and a half the time in respect to the basal medium, respectively. With this medium it was possible to supply $1 \cdot 10^7$ cells/ml (5,6,7). At $1 \cdot 10^7$ cells/ml cell harvest started to reach a steady state. During the rest of the fermentation 0.5-0.7 l·d^{-1} culture suspension was removed to keep the steady state constant. For a period of 20 days this steady state was

substrate	basal.	perfusion.	consumption rate
	μmol/l	μmol/l	nmol/10^6cells·d
ASP	162,7	162,7	21,8
GLU	304,9	304,9	38,3
ASN	144,6	289,2	33,4
SER	249,7	249,7	40,1
GLN	2500	7500	920,4
GLY	499,3	499,3	25,6
THR	448,8	448,8	70,9
ARG	700	700	100,2
ALA	190,2	190,2	-1475,5
TYR	309	309	45,5
TRP	44,2	88,4	9,7
MET	115,5	346,5	26,9
VAL	450,9	901,8	89,5
ILE	415,2	830,4	90,2
LEU	450,1	900,2	116,3
LYS	499,5	499,5	21,1
HIS	150,2	225,3	22,8
PHE	218,7	437,4	47,6
Glucose	17500	17500	1176,1
Lactat	-	-	-469,9
O_2			3012,2

Figure 2: Consumption rates in batch culture and amino acid concentrations in basal- and perfusion medium

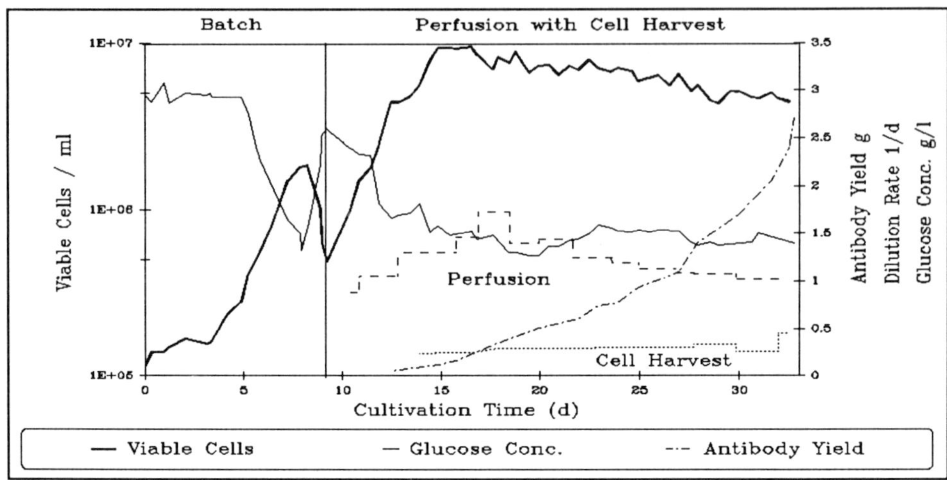

Figure 1: Perfusion fermentation in a 2 l bioreactor

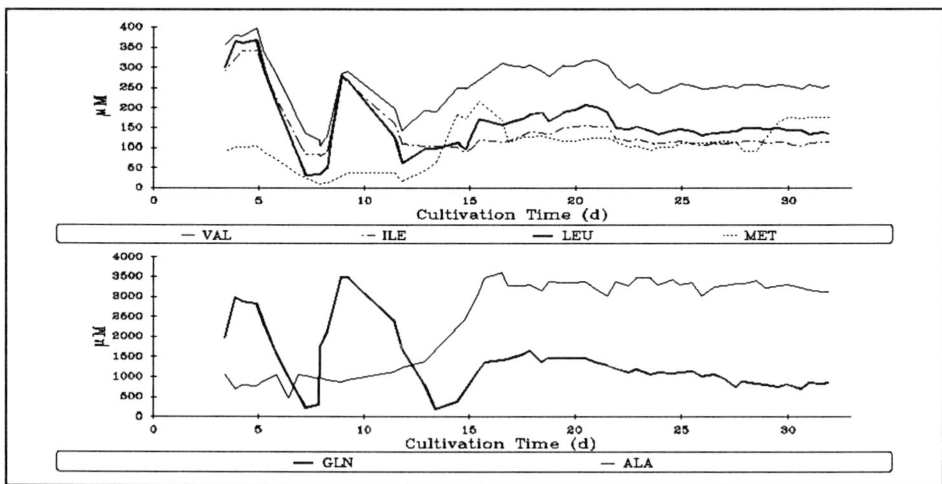

Figure 3: Amino acid concentrations in the perfusion fermentation

kept at a viable cell density of approx. $7 \cdot 10^6$ cells/ml. The amino acid concentrations in this period were constant, also indicating that a steady state point really was reached. These steady state conditions of optimal supply led to an antibody production of 8 μg $\cdot 10^{-6}$ cells $\cdot$ d^{-1} (8,9). This was remarkable higher than the productivity of 5 μg $\cdot 10^{-6}$ cells $\cdot$ d^{-1} observed in batch culture during exponential growth. The fermentation broth was concentrated by ultrafiltration (SP 20 Ultrafiltration System, Amicon). After precipitation (50 % $(NH_4)_2SO_4$) the antibody was purified by chromatographic techniques. First, the ammonium sulfate was removed by gelfiltration. After that step the antibody was purified by ion exchange chromatography. The purification success was controlled by SDS-PAGE electrophoresis on a PhastSystem (Pharmacia).

Discussion

From the data of the fermentation it is obvious that amino acid concentrations in serum-free medium are of tremendous importance for growth and production in animal cell cultures (10). The glucose concentration is not as interesting as some selected amino acid concentrations. Glutamine and especially methionine were of high importance. The calculation of amino acid consumption rates make it possible to optimize the medium for the perfusion fermentation, which was the premise for the high density cultivation of these cells and the higher productivity.

Literature:

1. Köhler G and Milstein C <u>Nature</u> 1975 <u>256</u>: 495-497
2. Lehmann J, Vorlop J and Büntemeyer H In: <u>Spier RE and Griffiths JB (eds) Animal Cell Biotechnology 3</u> 1988 (pp 221-237) Academic Press
3. Büntemeyer H, Bödeker BGD and Lehmann J In: <u>Spier RE, Griffiths JB (eds) Modern Approaches to Animal Cell Technology</u> 1987 (pp 411-419) Butterworths
4. Büntemeyer H Ph.D. Thesis. 1988, University of Hannover, FRG
5. Eagle H (1959) <u>Science</u> 1959 <u>130</u>: 432-437
6. Duval D, Geahel I, Dufau AF and Hache J In: <u>Spier RE, Griffiths JB, Stephenne J, Crooy PJ (eds) Advances in animal cell biology and technology for bioprocesses</u> 1989 (pp 257-259) Butterworths
7. Jäger V, Lehmann J and Friedl P <u>Cytotechnology</u> 1989 <u>1</u>:319-329
8. Geaugey V, Duval D, Geahel I, Marc A and Engasser JM <u>Cytotechnology</u> 1989 <u>2</u>:119-129
9. Wagner R, Ryll T, Krafft H and Lehmann J <u>Cytotechnology</u> 1988 <u>1</u>: 145-150
10. Zielke HR, Sumbilla CM, Zielke CL, Tildon JT and Ozand PT In: <u>Häussinger, Sies H (eds)</u> 1984 (pp 247-254) Springer

APPEARANCE OF NONSPECIFIC AMOUNTS OF MONOCLONAL ANTIBODY DURING FERMENTATION CAUSED BY DECREASED CELL VIABILITY

U. Marx[1], V. Jäger[2], S.T. Kiessig[1], R. Grunow[1], R.v. Baehr[1]

[1]Humboldt Univ. Berlin, Department of Med. Immunologie, GDR
[2]Gesellschaft für Biotechnol. Forschung, Braunschweig, FRG

ABSTRACT

A monoclonal anti-HIV-1 antibody (ab) from a murine hybridoma cell line was produced by repeated batch fermentation to compare the product quality in respect of its antigen (ag) binding specificity during cultivation. Cells are cultivated in a 1.2l stirred suspension reactor in a repeated batch mode. Cultivation was finished after cell viability dropped below 30%. Absolute amounts of specific reactive ab were detected by ag nonspecific and ag specific ELISA-techniques, respectively. It could be shown that the concentration of released specific non-reactive abs correlated with the decreased cell viability. Simultaneous immunoblots showed that this release could not be explained by the appearance of cytoplasmatic unlinked heavy and light immunoglobulin chains only.

INTRODUCTION

Additional amounts of abs appear in the culture fluid when cell viability is decreasing at the end of a batch culture process (1). This phenomenon can be used for the production of abs in batch, fed batch and repeated batch fermentation procedures, if the specific activity of the product does not change. Such changes may be caused by proteolytic degra-dation, deamidation, oxidation and other processes after considerable cell death in culture.

MATERIALS AND METHODS

Cells and media:
The abs were produced using the murine monoclonal hybridoma cell line CB-map24-4-1 (2). It belongs to the IgG2a sub-class, and recognizes the gag-coded protein p24 of HIV-1. Cells were grown in a modification of an earlier described serum-free medium (3). In this medium BSA/oleic acid comp-lexes are replaced by human serum albumin.

Reactor system:
Cells were propagated in a 1.2 liter reactor with bubble-free aeration through microporous moving membranes described previously (4).

Cultivation mode:
A repeated batch cultivation was performed. On day seven 900 ml of suspension were harvested and fresh medium was added. At that time density of living cells reached 10^7 cells/ml.

Viability decreased up to 70% (Fig. 1a).

Analysis of fermentation samples:
1. Cell numbers were determined by trypan blue exclusion.
2. Glucose and lactate concentrations of supernatants were
determined using glucose or lactate analyzers.
3. Amino acids were analyzed using HPLC (after derivatization
by orthophthaldialdehyde) (5).
4. Antibody concentration was determined in an anti-Fc mouse
IgG sandwich ELISA, ag specific reactivity was analyzed by ag
specific ELISA technique as described previously (6).
5. Ab molecules and fragments were detected by immunoblots
using a peroxidase-conjugated monospecific polyclonal anti-Fc
mouse IgG antiserum, for staining diaminobenzidin was used.

RESULTS AND DISCUSSION

A repeated batch fermentation procedure in a 1.2 liter
stirred reactor was performed over 12 days. On day seven
900ml of culture suspension were repleaced by fresh medium.
In the first and the second batch cycles IgG concentration
continuously increased (Fig. 1b). In contrast to ab concentration, viability decreased in the first batch growth cycle
as from day 5 and in the second cycle viability decreased
drastically away from day 9. The loss of viability correlates
with the limitation of GLU, MET and ASP in the medium (Fig.
1a). Other amino acids as well as glucose were never limited
during the whole procedure (data not shown). The specific
activity of produced abs is reduced by about 50% on day 6, in
correlation with the described amino acid limitation in
medium. During the second batch procedure (day 8 to 12)
specific activity is generally reduced by about 60%. Moreover, in contrast to increasing ab concentration, specific
activity decreased on day 12 (Fig. 1b). At the end of both
batches, as shown in anti-Fc mouse IgG HRP stained immunoblots, IgG fragments appeared (Fig. 2). Nevertheless,
especially over the second batch cycle, IgG fragment quantity
did not seem to correlate with the amounts of specific non-
reactive ab. On day 8 and 9, in contrast to the low specific
activity no fragments could be detected. Summarizing the
results, the partial loss of specific reactivity of the abs
could not be explained by the release of unlinked heavy and
light immunoglobulin chains out of dead cells alone. Amounts
of complete but specific non-reactive abs seemed to appear in
culture supernatant after limitation of medium components.
For our particular ab, posttranscriptional modifications,
such as deamidation of amino acids involved in the ag binding
site, may be a possible explanation. Similar effects are
discussed for ab molecules in serum-free media (7). In conclusion, for large scale production of this ab growth conditions guaranteeing high rates of viability must be
observed.

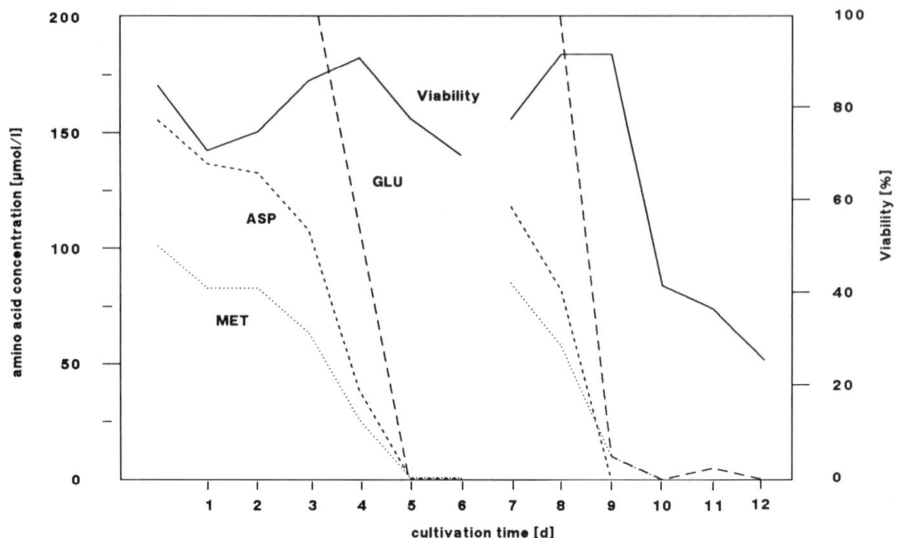

Fig. 1a: Viability and amino acid consumtion

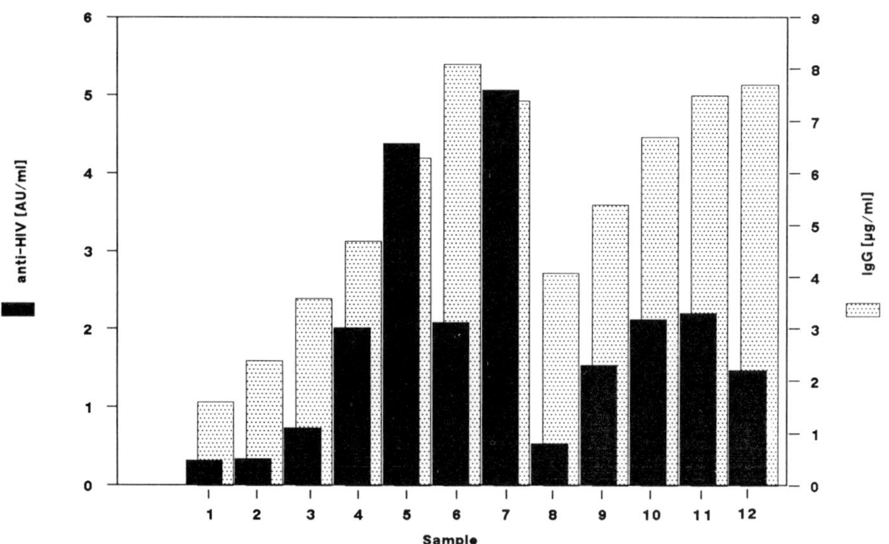

Fig. 1b: Amounts of specific reactive and specific non-reactive IgG

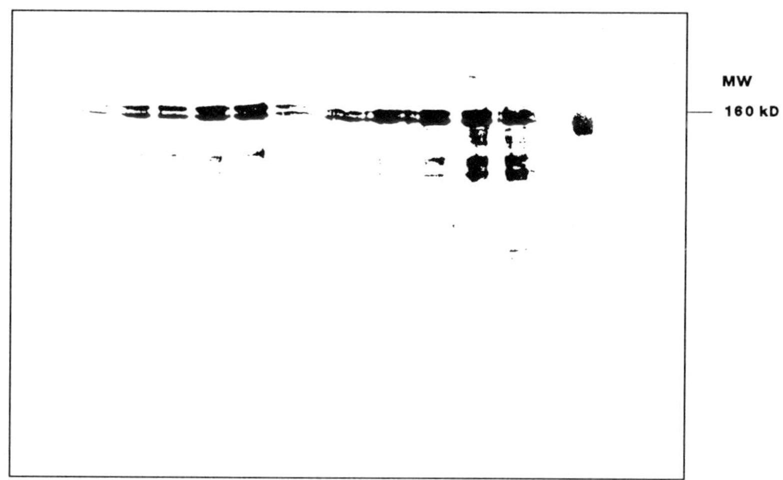

Fig.2: Detection of immuoglobulin fragments by western blot

REFERENCES

1 Katinger, H. <u>Massenproduktion monoklonaler Antikörper</u> in:
Monoklonale Antikörper: Anwendung in der Medizin.
Springer-Verlag Wien New York, 1989, pp.3-19

2 Grunow, R.; Giese, R.; Porstmann, T.; Doepel, H.; Haensel,
K. and Baehr, R.v. Development and biological testing of
human and murine monoclonal antibodies against HIV antigens. <u>Z.Klin.Med.</u>, 1990, <u>45</u>, Heft 4, 367-370

3 Jaeger, V.; Lehmann, J.; Friedl, P. Serum-free growth
medium for the cultivation of a wide 'spectrum of mammalian
cells in stirred bioreactors. <u>Cytotechnology</u>, 1988, <u>1</u>, 319-
329

4 Lehmann, J.; Piehl, GW.; Schulz, R. Bubble-free cell culture aeration with porous moving membranes. <u>Dev Biol.
Standart</u>, 1987, <u>66</u>, 227-240

5 Büntemeyer, H. Entwicklung eines Perfusionssystems zur
Kultivierung tierischer Zellen in Suspension. <u>Thesis</u>,
University of Hannover, FRG, 1987

6 Porstmann, T.; Porstmann, B.; Kießig, S.T.; Nugel, E.;
Scholz, D.; Grunow, R.; Volk, H.-D.; Ladhoff, A. and
v.Baehr, R. Diagnostik und Verlaufskontrolle von Infek-
tionen mit dem humanen Immundefizienzvirus (HIV). <u>Med.
aktuell</u> 1987, <u>13</u>, 448-450

7 Moellering, B.J.; Tedesco, J.L.; Townsend, R.R.; Hardy,
M.R.; Scott, R.W.; Prior, Ch.P. Electrophoretic differences
in a mab expressed in three media. <u>BioPharm 3(2)</u>,1990, 30-
38

PRODUCTION OF BIOLOGICALLY ACTIVE INSULIN-LIKE GROWTH FACTOR BY CELLS TRANSFECTED WITH A RECOMBINANT RETROVIRAL VECTOR ENCODING IGF-1

Patricia Looby Watts and Caroline MacDonald

Dept of Bioscience and Biotechnology, University of Strathclyde, Todd Centre, Glasgow G4 0NR.

ABSTRACT

Quiescent, serum-starved NIH 3T3 cells can be stimulated to incorporate ^{3}H-TdR by the addition of IGF-1 or EGF. However, when the two growth factors are added together a synergistic effect is achieved: the level of ^{3}H-TdR incorporation being more than two-fold greater than additive stimulation. We transfected a derivative of the NIH 3T3 cell line (a modified Y2 retrovirus packaging cell line) with a recombinant retroviral genome containing human IGF-1. Secreted IGF-1 was detected in the culture medium by radioimmunoassay and its biological activity has been demonstrated by measuring the synergistic response with exogenous EGF in 3T3 cells.

INTRODUCTION

The proliferation of normal diploid cells in culture is controlled by exogenous serum growth factors. In the absence of these factors, 3T3 cells leave the cell cycle and become reversibly arrested in the G_1/G_0 phase. Studies by Stiles *et al* (1) showed that in the presence of platelet-derived growth factor quiescent Balb/c3T3 cells become "competent" to replicate their DNA, but do not "progress" into S phase unless incubated with growth factors contained in platelet-poor plasma. More recently, Phillips and Cristofalo (2) have proposed a division of growth factors into three classes: class 1 or competence factors which include epidermal growth factor (EGF), fibroblast growth factor (FGF), platelet-derived growth factor (PDGF) and thrombin; class 2 or progressive factors such as insulin-like growth factor 1 (IGF-1), insulin-like growth factor 2 (IGF-2), multiplication-stimulating activity (MSA) and insulin; and class 3 factors such as dexamethasone and hydrocortisone. Different cell lines require different combinations of growth factors for proliferation in the absence of serum. In the normal human embryonic lung fibroblast cell line WI-38 all three classes of growth factor must be present to achieve maximum stimulation of DNA synthesis: the combination of EGF and IGF-1 is no better than either alone (2). In Swiss 3T3 cells, in contrast, these growth factors act synergistically and induce a 20-50 fold stimulation of ^{3}H-thymidine uptake over basal levels (3). In this paper we confirm this observation using NIH 3T3 cells, and show that the synergy between IGF-1 and EGF also occurs when the IGF-1 is supplied by conditioned medium obtained from the YspC5-5 cell line (C5-5) which expresses human IGF-1 from a retroviral vector.

MATERIALS AND METHODS

Cell culture and genetic engineering

Cells were grown in DMEM supplemented with 10% FCS (Gibco-BRL) and subcultured by 1:10 dilution twice weekly. Recombinant human IGF-1 and IGF-2 were obtained from Kabi-Gen; mouse sub-maxillary gland EGF (tissue culture grade) and human transferrin were obtained from Sigma. Conditioned medium was obtained from cells which were seeded at 2 x10^{5} cells per 25cm^{2} flask in DMEM + 10% FCS and grown to confluence (usually 3 days). After 3 rinses in DMEM without FCS, the cultures were re-incubated in serum-free DMEM. Samples of conditioned medium were harvested after a further 3 days growth. The vector p105-IGF1 contains the bacterial *neo* gene expressed from the MoMLV retroviral 5' LTR promoter, and the IGF-1 coding sequence expressed from the HSV-1 *tk* promoter in the reverse orientation with respect to viral transcription and terminated by an internal polyadenylation signal. This DNA was introduced into the ecotropic packaging cell line Y2sp1-4 (a modified Y2 line) by calcium phosphate-mediated DNA transformation (4). Colonies of G418-resistant cells were isolated by growth in 1 mg/ml Geneticin (Gibco-BRL). The Y2 line contains an integrated provirus sequence which lacks the retroviral packaging signal. After transfection with a retroviral vector containing the viral long terminal repeat sequences (LTRs) and the packaging signal this cell line will produce infectious virions which contain the transfected sequence. The Ysp1-4 line is similar, but contains additional mutations in the inserted provirus which reduce the likelihood of recombination between the endogenous and vector sequences to yield wild type virus. The titre of virus produced from the packaging cells was measured in samples of culture medium harvested during logarithmic growth, filtered through a 0.45µm filter and diluted. 3T3 cell cultures were infected with 2ml of this medium in the presence of 8µg/ml Polybrene (Sigma) for 2 hours and selected in 600µg/ml Geneticin. Colonies were counted after 2 weeks and the titre expressed as colony forming units/ml of culture medium. This work was done according to ACGM category 1 guidelines.

Analysis of RNA

RNA was isolated from cells using the single-step acid guanidinium thiocyanate-phenol-chloroform extraction method (5). Samples were spotted onto nitrocellulose (Millipore HAHY) filters and hybridisations carried out as described by Wahl *et al* (6). Probes were labelled with ^{32}P by nick translation to specific activities of 9×10^{7} dpm/μg, added at concentrations of 2-4 ng/ml, and incubated at 42°C for 3-5 hours. The probes used were the IGF-1 coding sequence excised from the vector and the whole plasmid sequence.

IGF-1 assays

Samples of conditioned serum-free medium were harvested after 3 days from confluent cultures and assayed using a radioimmunoassay kit obtained from Amersham. Cultures were deemed to be positive if the levels assayed were at least double the background levels in controls. The biological activity of the IGF was assessed by the ability of the conditioned culture medium to produce an synergistic effect with EGF on ^{3}H-thymidine uptake by NIH 3T3 cells. NIH 3T3 cells were seeded at 2×10^{5} cells per well in a 24 well plate in DMEM + 10% FCS for up to 24 hours to allow the cells to adhere. The cells were then washed three times in DMEM without FCS, and reincubated in DMEM without FCS for 24 hours. After a medium change the stimulant(s) and 1μCi/ml ^{3}H-TdR (83Ci/mmol, Amersham) were added to each well and the cells re-incubated for a further 24 hours. Cells were extracted with TCA, rinsed with ethanol, air-dried, then dissolved in 0.5ml 0.1M NaOH. The alkali-soluble portion was mixed with 4ml of Optiphase Safe (Pharmacia) for liquid scintillation counting. Proteins were separated on a Tricine-SDS-polyacrylamide gel and stained with Coomassie Blue (7).

RESULTS AND DISCUSSION

Characterisation of virus from the C5-5 packaging cell line

Expression of the retroviral vector in the C5-5 cell line has been demonstrated in two ways. Firstly, the cells have been shown to secrete infectious virus particles which confer G418 resistance to host cells and thus demonstrate the expression of the *neo* gene. The titre of virus produced by the C5-5 cell line was 10^{5} cfu/ml. Secondly, dot-blot hybridisation of viral RNA to ^{32}P-labelled IGF coding sequence and whole plasmid sequence has shown that IGF-1 is also present in the packaged viral genome.

Growth factor stimulation.

The incorporation of ^{3}H-thymidine by quiescent NIH 3T3 cells which had been serum-starved for 24 hours then incubated with medium to which combinations of growth factors had been added is shown in Fig 1. Cells incubated in the presence of one of the three growth factors (IGF-1, EGF or transferrin) alone showed at most a two-fold stimulation of incorporation of thymidine over the base level of incorporation in DMEM without serum. Cells incubated in IGF-1 plus transferrin show a two to three fold stimulation, the sum of the individual responses. In contrast, IGF-1 and EGF act synergistically on 3T3 cells, resulting in levels of thymidine incorporation over four times the individual responses, more than double the additive response.

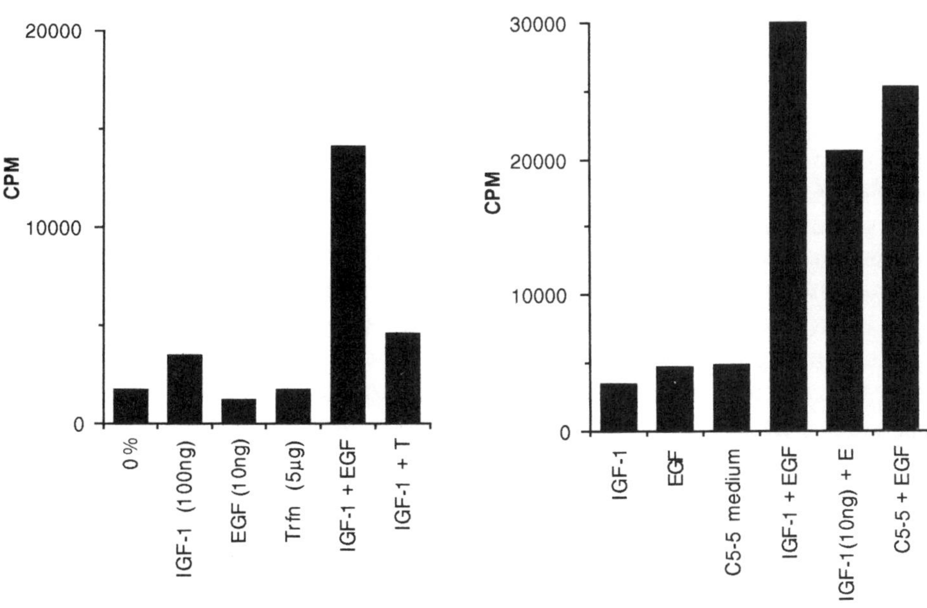

Fig. 1 Incorporation of ^{3}H-thymidine by serum-starved 3T3 cells incubated with growth factors.

Fig. 2 Incorporation of ^{3}H-thymidine by serum-starved 3T3 cells incubated with growth factors or C5-5 conditioned medium.

Expression of transfected IGF-1.

Five of seven clones of cells which had been transfected with the vector p105
secreted IGF-1 at levels between 300ng/ml and 1000ng/ml. Also, IGF-1 has
been visualised as a faint Coomassie Blue stained band in polyacrylamide gels
of medium from the C5-5 clone. Finally, biological activity has been
demonstrated by the synergistic response of C5-5 medium with EGF on
thymidine incorporation by 3T3 cells. When added on its own, the C5-5
conditioned medium produced an increase in ^{3}H-TdR incorporation similar to
that observed with the addition of IGF-1 (100ng/ml) or EGF (100ng/ml). C5-5
conditioned medium plus EGF (100ng/ml) stimulated an increase in thymidine
incorporation more than two-fold higher than the additive levels (Fig 2).

We have attempted to show that stimulation can also occur in an autocrine
fashion, ie that the transfected clone C5-5 can be rescued from quiescence by
the addition of EGF. Unfortunately, however, although C5-5 is a derivative of
the 3T3 cell line, confluent C5-5 cells do not become quiescent following 24
hour (or even 72 hour) serum-starvation. This may be due to the fact that the
IGF-1 gene is being expressed in a constitutive fashion and therefore the cells
are still being stimulated.

SUMMARY

In these experiments we have expressed a recombinant gene from a retroviral
vector in an ecotropic packaging cell line. This line not only expresses IGF-1
which is secreted into the culture medium, but also produces infectious virus
particles which contain the IGF-1 coding sequence and can be used to infect
target cells and thus introduce the growth factor gene into them. The ultimate
goal of this work is to show that genes for growth factors which have been
inserted into cells through genetic engineering techniques can allow sufficient
autocrine stimulation to enable the cultures to become self-perpetuating,
freed from serum dependence. The isolation of a packaging cell line such as
C5-5 means that growth factor genes can be rapidly introduced into different
cells.

ACKNOWLEDGEMENTS

The vector p105 was constructed by Dr Simon Hettle and provided by Professor

D Onions, and the modified Y2 packaging cell line, Ysp1-4 was a generous gift of Dr R Jarrett (Dept of Veterinary Pathology, University of Glasgow). This work was supported by grant no. GR/D 98525 from the SERC Biotechnology Directorate Animal Cell Biotechnology Club.

REFERENCES

1 Stiles, C. D., Capone, G. T., Scher, C. D., Antoniades, H. N., van Wyk, J. J. and Pledger, W. J., Dual control of cell growth by somatomedins and platelet-derived growth factor, <u>Proc. Natl. Acad. Sci. USA</u> 1979, <u>76</u>, 1279

2 Phillips, P. D. and Cristofalo, V. J., Classification system based on the functional equivalency of mitogens that regulate WI-38 cell proliferation, <u>Exp. Cell Res.</u> 1988, <u>175</u>, 396

3 Corps, A. N. and Brown, K. D., Ligand-receptor interactions involved in the stimulation of Swiss 3T3 fibroblasts by insulin-like growth factors and insulin, <u>Biochem. J.</u> 1988, <u>252</u>, 119

4 Gorman, C., High efficiency gene transfer into mammalian cells, in <u>DNA cloning, vol II</u>, (Ed. Glover, D. M.), IRL Press Ltd. <u>1985</u>, pp 143-190.

5 Chomczynski, P. and Sacchi, N., Single-step method of RNA isolation by acid guanidinium thiocyanate-phenol-chloroform extraction, <u>Anal. Biochem.</u> 1987, <u>162</u>, 156

6 Wahl, G. M., Stern, M. and Stark, G. R., Efficient transfer of large DNA fragments from agarose gels to diazobenzloxymethyl paper and rapid hybridisation by using dextran sulfate, <u>Proc. Natl. Acad. Sci. USA</u> 1979, <u>76</u>, 3683

7 Schagger, H. and von Jagow, G., Tricine-Sodium Dodecyl Sulfate-Polyacrylamide Gel Electrophoresis for the separation of proteins in the range from 1-100 kDa, <u>Anal. Biochem.</u> 1987, <u>166</u>, 368

8 Rechler, M. M. and Nissley, S. P., The nature and regulation of the receptors for insulin-like growth factors, <u>Ann. Rev. Physiol.</u>, 1985, <u>47</u>, 425

IN VITRO PRODUCTION OF GROWTH REGULATORS FOR HUMAN EPITHELIAL CELLS

Martin Clynes, Margaret Dooley, Breda Carey, Anne Godfrey, Angela O'Toole, Bernard Gregory and Eunan McGlinchey

National Cell & Tissue Culture Centre, (BioResearch Ireland), School of Biological Sciences, Dublin City University, Glasnevin, Dublin 9, Ireland.

ABSTRACT

The human carcinoma line RPMI 2650 produces at least 3 distinct growth factors including an autocrine stimulator. Growth factor production is a general characteristic of the cell population, since 8 independently-derived clones of RPMI 2650 all produced comparable levels of all of the 3 activities. Low levels of mycoplasma contamination may cause artifacts in screening cells for production of negative regulators of cell growth. Production of growth factors may play an important role in regulation of cell growth and productivity in vitro.

KEYWORDS: AUTOCRINE AND TRANSFORMING GROWTH FACTORS: HUMAN CARCINOMA LINES: CLONAL VARIATION: MYCOPLASMA.

INTRODUCTION

Cells in vitro can produce a variety of growth regulatory molecules, including transforming growth factors and autostimulatory or autocrine growth factors (1, 2). In some instances autocrine stimulation can occur intracellularly without the necessity for secretion of the autocrine factor (3). It appears likely that many cell populations in culture may simultaneously secrete several different growth regulatory molecules into culture medium (4), but the significance which this may have for regulation of growth of cells in culture is not clear. It is also unclear from the literature whether significant clonal variation in growth factor productivity exists within cell populations in vitro. The work described here aims to investigate growth factor diversity and clonal variation in growth factor production by the human carcinoma line RPMI 2650.

MATERIALS AND METHODS

Cell Lines and Growth Factor Assays

Details of all cell lines used are available in the ATCC catalogue. Details of TGF and autocrine assays are cited in refs. 1-4.

Isolation of clones of RPMI 2650

100 cells per dish were plated in 100 mm culture dishes. When clones had grown, they were trypsinized using a stainless-steel cloning ring sealed with autoclaved silicone grease. The cells were sequentially subcultured into 96-well, 24-well and 8-well plates, and finally to 25 cm^2 flasks before freezing.

RESULTS AND DISCUSSION

Table 1 shows that RPMI 2650 cell-conditioned medium (CM) contains an autostimulatory activity which can be concentrated by ultrafiltration through an Amicon YM2 1,000 M.W. cut off membrane.

TABLE 1

EFFECT OF RPMI 2650 CONDITIONED MEDIUM (CM) IN TGF AND AUTOCRINE BIOASSAYS

	TGF	TGF-B	AUTOCRINE
CM (10X Retentate)	7.45 ± 0.9	1.92 ± 0.3	2.14 ± 0.13
CM (Unconcentrated)	0.58 ± 0.5	0.23 ± 0.06	0.31 ± 0.08
Control Medium	0	0.02 ± 0.04	0.15 ± 0.02

(Data presented is colony forming efficiency (CFE) i.e. Colonies formed/Cells Plated)

It is also concentrated in the retentate a of 10,000 M.W. cutoff ultrafiltration membrane, so the autocrine factor(s) is probably of high molecular weight, although we cannot absolutely exclude the possibility that it is a low M.W. species which associates with large proteins.

Table 1 also shows that RPMI 2650 cells produce growth factors which are active in the TGF α plus β (NRK), and TGF-β (NRK-49F) assays, as well as in the autocrine assay. Concentrated RPMI 2650 CM competes with ^{125}I-EGF in a radioreceptor binding assay using A431 cells, confirming the presence in the CM of TGF-α-like molecules. Fractionation and stability studies suggest that the TGF-α-like, TGF-β-like and autocrine activities are attributable to at least 3 distinct molecular species. The fact that mammalian cells _in vitro_ may simultaneously produce several different growth regulatory (including autoregulatory) molecules may be of significance in understanding and controlling the regulation of growth and productivity in these systems, and warrants more intensive investigation. RPMI 2650 CM has also been shown to stimulate growth in monolayer at low density of other human carcinoma cells including Hep-2.

In attempting to characterize growth regulatory molecules produced by cells _in vitro_, it would be useful to obtain high-producer variant populations. It is unclear from the literature whether growth factor production is a general property of the producer cell population, or whether such populations contain a mixture of high- and low-level producers. Nister _et al_., (5) reported higher level production of PDGF by clones derived from later passages of a human malignant glioma line, but the general situation in cell culture populations remains unclear. In order to determine the situation in RPMI 2650 cells, we prepared a number of independent clones from this cell line.

TABLE 2

PRODUCTION OF GROWTH FACTORS BY CLONES OF RPMI 2650

	TGF-α		TGF-β		AUTOCRINE	
RPMI 2650	100 ± 16[*]		100 ± 15		100 ± 12	
Clone A	112 ± 28		106	2	72	20
Clone B	42	4	150	11	76	9
Clone C	86	24	134	9	47	9
Clone D	48	18	105	15	103	21
Clone E	83	14	108	11	70	7
Clone F	155	41	139	10	96	10
Clone G	73	28	164	18	82	10
Clone H	83	6	68	11	97	15

[*] To facilitate comparison, CFE supported by uncloned RPMI 2650 CM has been given a value of 100, for each assay type, and other CFEs are expressed relative to this.

The data presented in Table 2 shows that each of the 8 independently-derived clones of RPMI 2650 cells examined here produced comparable amounts of all three activities (TGF-α-like, TGF-β-like and autocrine). The considerable level of variation inherent in these assays makes it difficult to ascertain with certainty whether the differences observed between different clones are significant. It is clear, however, that growth factor production is a general property of the cells, rather than being a property of a few high-level producers. This again points to the importance of understanding the role of autologously-produced growth factors in cell culture production systems.

Finally, we are currently examining _in vitro_ production of growth inhibitors for human epithelial lines. In one instance, a potent high-molecular weight inhibitory activity produced by apparently healthy mouse cells proved to be an artifact due to mycoplasma contamination.

REFERENCES

1. Bascom, C., Sipes, N., Coffey, R. and Moses, H. (1989). Regulation of Epithelial Cell Proliferation by Transforming Growth Factors.
    J. Cell. Biochem. **39**, 25-32.
2. Heldin, C., & Westermark, B. (1989). Growth Factors as Transforming Proteins.
    Eur. J. Biochem. **184**, 487-496.
3. Browder, T., Dunbar, C. and Nienhuis, A. (1989).
    Private and Public Autocrine Loops in Neoplastic Cells.
    Cancer Cells **1**, 9-17.
4. McDonnell, S., Dooley, M. and Clynes, M. Growth Factors produced by human carcinoma cells in culture.
    Biochem Soc. Brans. **17**, 594-595.
5. Nister, M., Heldin, C. & Westermark, B. (1986). Clonal variation in the production of a PDGF-like protein and expression of corresponding receptors in a human malignant glioma.
    Cancer Res. **46**, 332-340.

PURIFICATION AND CHARACTERIZATION OF IMMUNOGLOBULIN PRODUCTION STIMULATING FACTOR IIα DERIVED FROM NAMALWA CELLS

Hiroki Murakami[1], Takuya Sugahara[2], Sanetaka Shirahata[1] and Koji Yamada[2]

[1]Graduate School of Genetic Resources Technology, [2]Department of Food Science and Technology, Faculty of Agriculture, Kyushu University, 6-10-1 Hakozaki, Fukuoka 812, Japan

ABSTRACT

Immunoglobulin production stimulating factor (IPSF) IIα was purified from Namalwa cell lyzate by ammonium sulfate precipitation, hydrophobic interaction chromatography and gel filtration.   The purified IPSF was estimated a 106 KD protein which was composed of a polypeptide of 40 KD and two polypeptides of 33KD by gel filtration and SDS polyacrylamide gel electro-phoresis.   The 33KD protein extracted from SDS polyacrylamide gel showed IPSF activity, but not the 40 KD protein.   The IPSF activity was fairly stable in alkaline but unstable in acidic solution.   In a serum-free medium, the IPSF-IIα stimulated IgM production of human-human and mouse-mouse hybridomas 4-15 and 2-fold, respectively. However, IgG production of neither human nor mouse was stimulated by the factor in the same serum-free medium.

INTRODUCTION

Monoclonal antibodies (MAbs), especially human MAbs, are desirable for not only diagnostics but also therapeutic uses. However, MAbs are now commercially expensive.   If a large amount of MAbs can be produced cheaper, MAbs will become more applicable to various areas.   Although a plasma cell (a matured B cell) in lymph nodes secrete 1.7×10^{14} immunoglobulin molecules/day *in vivo*[1,] immunoglobulin productivity of human-human hybridomas *in vitro* is now below a percent of that *in vivo*[2]. Thus it is required to enhance the immunoglobulin productivity of hybridomas for its mass production.

An IPSF was finally purified from Namalwa cells, and enhanced immunoglobulin productivity of human-human hybridomas in serum-free medium. We report here the purification and characterization of the IPSF.

MATERIALS AND METHODS

Cells and cell culture

Namalwa cells derived from human Burkitt lymphocytoma were cultured by the use of a high density culture system (Shimadzu, SHC-1 type). IgM-producing human-human hybridomas tested here were H15F1 which was a fusion product with a fusion partner HO-323 cells, and HB4C5 and HF10B4 fused with NAT-30, another fusion partner. IgG-producing human-human hybridomas K-1-5 obtained by fusion with HO-323, and HB731 and HB732 derived from HK-128, a fusion partner which was recently established for making IgG producing hybridomas[3] were also in the testing panels. F5 and D1 cells were mouse-mouse hybridomas producing IgM and 4F12 and 4C10B6 were mouse-mouse hybridomas producing IgG. All mouse-mouse hybridomas used here were derived from a fusion partner, P3-X63-Ag8 (P3U1) cells. These cells were cultured in ERDF (Kyokuto Seiyaku Co.) supplemented with 5% fetal bovine serum or ITES (10 µg/ml insulin, 20 µg/ml transferrin, 20 µM ethanolamine and 25 nM sodium selenite). Hybridomas for determining IPSF activity were cultured at 37 C under humidified 5% CO_2:95% air.

Namalwa cells were cultured to prepare IPSF in such a high density as 2×10^7 cells/ml in ERDF medium supplemented with 2% FBS or ITES.

Purification of IPSF-IIα from Namalwa cell lyzate

All procedures were described in the RESULTS section.

Polyacrylamide gel electrophoresis of IPSF-IIα

The IPSF-IIα was electrophoresed and silver-stained using a 3.3% stacking/5% running polyacrylamide gel in non-denaturation condition as described previously[4]. IPSF-IIα was also electrophoresed with SDS-polyacrylamide gel containing 12% acrylamide.

Assay of IPSF activity

IPSF activity was examined by measuring amounts of antibodies secreted by hybridoma cells to the medium during 6 h culture.

RESULTS

Namalwa cells (10^9 cells) were ultrasonically homogenized in 10 mM sodium phosphate buffer (pH 7.4). The IPSF activity in the lyzate was concentrated in the supernatant by 50% ammonium sulfate saturation, though most of the activity appeared in the supernatant after the treatment with 80% ammonium sulfate saturation. Further purification was performed after removal of ammonium sulfate.

Hydrophobic interaction chromatography

A hydrophobic interaction column (Butyl Toyopeal 650M, 22mm x 25 cm) was equilibrated with 2 M ammonium sulfate-10 mM sodium phosphate buffer (pH 7.4). The supernatant fraction obtained by a 50% ammonium sulfate saturation was applied to the column. IPSF activities were shown in the protein fractions eluted broadly at the concentration of ammonium sulfate less than 1 M (Fig. 1). Since the IPSF activities were broadly distributed, active fractions were grouped into A, B and C.

Fraction A obtained by hydrophobic interaction column chromatography was further gel-filtrated with TSK gel G3000SW (7.5 mm I.D. x 60 cm; TOSOH). After equilibration with 200 mM sodium phosphate buffer (pH 6.0), IPSF fraction A was applied to the column. The fractionated solution was dialyzed against 10 mM sodium phosphate buffer (pH 7.4) and IPSF activity was assayed. Strong IPSF activity was shown in a sharp single peak (data not shown). From the standard curve of molecular weight the IPSF was estimated about 110 KD. The IPSF was named IPSF-IIα, since we had already reported IPSF-I obtained from HO-323[4].

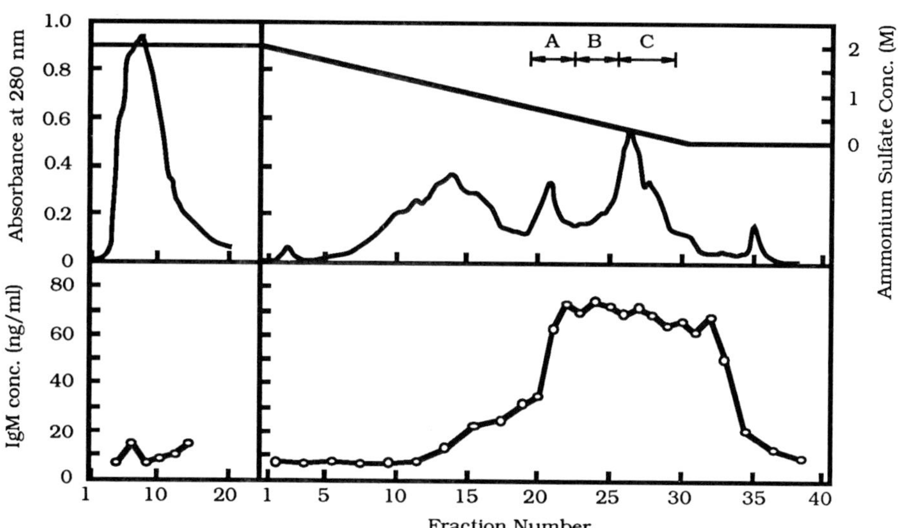

Fig. 1. Purification of IPSF-II from cell lyzate using hybrophobic interaction column (BUTYL TOYOPEARL 650M). A 50% ammonium sulfate saturated supernatant from Namalwa cell lyzate was applied to the column as described in the RESULTS section.

Polyacrylamide gel electrophoresis

The IPSF-IIα purified by gel filtration was electrophoresed
on a polyacrylamide gel. As shown in Fig. 2(A), a single band
was detected in non-denaturation condition, showing that the
protein was highly purified. The SDS polyacrylamide gel
electrophoresis of the IPSF-IIα revealed two bands of 44KD and
33KD (Fig. 2(B)). It was shown by densitometry that the
ratio of amount of the 44KD to 33KD bands was 1 to 2, taking
the molecular size of IPSF-IIα ca. 110 KD into the account.
These results suggests that IPSF-IIα is a 106 KD protein which
has a subunit structure composed of a 40 KD polypeptide chain
and two 33 KD polypeptide chains.
After SDS gel electrophoresis, proteins in each band were
extracted. The 33 KD subunit exclusively showed IPSF
activity. The 40 KD protein showed neither IPSF activity nor
the synergistic effect for IPSF activity of 33 KD subunit.
Thus, 33 KD subunit protein was responsible for IPSF activity
of IPSF-IIα. Though the role of the 40KD subunit is not known
yet, it may contribute to stabilize and transport 33 KD
subunit *in vivo*.

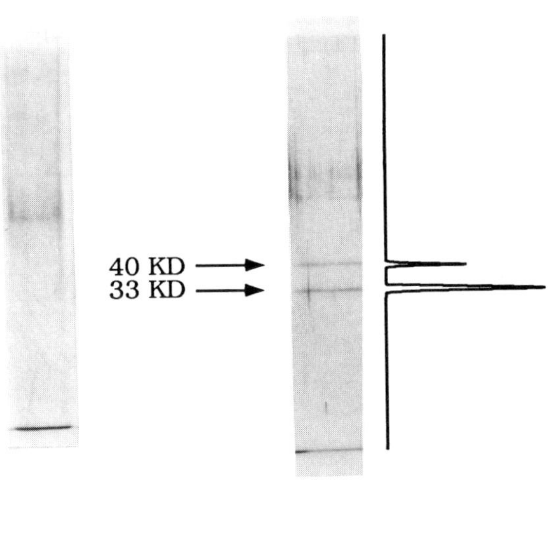

Fig. 2. Polyacrylamide
gel electrophoresis of
IPSF-IIα. Purified
IPSF-IIα was electro-
phoresed on (A) a 5%
polyacrylamide gel in
non-denaturation
condition; (B) a SDS-
polyacrylamide gel
containing 12%
acrylamide.

Analyses of pH and heat stability of IPSF-IIα

IPSF-IIα was stable in alkaline solution, especially at pH
9 (data not shown). It was unstable in acidic solution and
the activity was completely lost below pH 4. Heat stability

was also examined. IPSF-IIα rapidly lost its activity above
40 C (data not shown).

Specific activation of IgM producing hybridomas by IPSF-IIα in
serum-free medium.

IPSF-IIα purified from Namalwa cell lyzate enhanced IgM
productivity of hybridomas derived from both human and mouse
cells (Table 1).   H15F1 cells, a human-human hybridoma
derived HO-323 cells showed a 15 fold-enhanced IgM productivity by addition of 5 μg/ml IPSF-IIα. IgM productivities of
HB4C5 and HF10B4 cells were enhanced 4-and 8-fold by the IPSF-
IIα.   The IPSF-IIα enhanced IgM productivity of mouse-mouse
hybridomas ca.2 fold.   IPSF-IIα enhanced the IgG productivity
of neither human nor mouse hybridoma.

Hybridoma	Parent Cells	Isotype	Ig Conc. (ng/ml)		Relative Productivity
			IPSF	None	IPSF/None
Human					
HB731	HK-128	IgG	14.5	17.6	0.8
HB732	HK-128	IgG	10.7	11.9	0.9
K-1-5	HO-323	IgG	8.3	7.9	1.1
H15F1	HO-323	IgM	21.4	1.4	15.3
HB4C5	NAT-30	IgM	205	55.3	3.7
HF10B4	NAT-30	IgM	823	103	8.0
Mouse					
4F12	P3U1	IgG	454	474	1.0
4C10B6	P3U1	IgG	503	515	1.0
F5	P3U1	IgM	6270	3950	1.6
D2	P3U1	IgM	6810	3730	1.8

Table 1.   Specific activation of IgM producing hybridomas by
IPSF-IIα in serum-free medium.

DISCUSSION

IPSF was first found and partially purified from human lung
adenocarcinoma PC-8 cells[5]. A fusion partner cell line, HO-
323 cells also produced IPSF-I[4].   Although IPSF was partially
purified from Namalwa cell lyzate, it was difficult to purify
the IPSF because of the presence of a large amount of
irrelevant proteins[6].   Here we could effectively purify the
IPSF by using ammonium sulfate fractionation to remove
proteins before hydrophobic interaction column chromatography.   Since IPSF activities were detected in the fraction
which were eluted later from the hyrophobic interaction
column, IPSF may have high hydrophobicity or hydrophobic amino
acid residues on the surface.
IPSF-IIα stimulated IgM production but not IgG production
of hybridomas as well as IPSF-I derived from HO-323 cells.

Gene clonings of IPSFs are now undergoing.   Mass-production
of IPSF by recombinant bacteria or transfer of IPSF genes into
hybridomas will actualize enhancing IgM production of
hybridomas.
It can be expected by extensive survey to disclose active
substances which can stimulate the production of
immunoglobulins in other classes by corresponding hybridomas.

REFERENCES

1 Warner, NL. Membrane immunoglobulins and antigen receptors
on B and T lymphocytes. Adv. Immunol. 1974, 19, 67
2 Murakami, H. What should be focused in the study of cell
culture technology for production of bioactive proteins.
Cytotechnology 1990, 3, 3.
3 Kawahara, H., Yamada, K., Shirahata, S. and Murakami, H. A
new human fusion partner, HK-128, for making human-human
hybridomas producing monoclonal IgG antibodies.
Cytotechnology, in press
4 Toyoda, K., Sugahara, T., Inoue, K., Yamada, K., Shirahata,
S.and Murakami, H. Purification and characterization of the
immunoglobulin production stimulating factor derived from
human B lymphoblastoid cell HO-323. Cytotechnology 1990, 3,
189
5 Shinmoto, H., Murakami, H., Yamada, K., Dosako, S. and
Omura, H. Immunoglobulin production stimulating and
inhibiting factors derived from human lung adenocarcinoma
PC-8 cells. Cytotechnology 1988, 1, 295
6 Yamada, K., Akiyoshi, K., Murakami, H., Sugahara, T., Ikeda
I., Toyoda, K. and Omura, H. Partial purification and
characterization of immunoglobulin production stimulating
factor derived from Namalwa cells. In Vitro Cell. Develop.
Biol. 1989, 25, 243

<u>**Paper of Murakami**</u>

Sinacore: Were you able to ascertain whether or not your
immunoglobulin stimulating factor worked by
stimulating de novo synthesis, or by promoting
secretion of the immunoglobulin?

Murakami: We know that mRNA for Ig is enhanced so it works
by increasing copy numbers of mRNA.

Sinacore: You showed that the 33K proteins seemed to have a
3-fold stimulating action. In comparison you had
a 20-fold stimulation prior to fractionation on
polyacrylamide gel. Does this not suggest that
there was an additional sub-unit which was lost in
fractionation?

Murakami: I don't think so as we constructed that sub-unit
from the gel.

Schmidt: How did you establish 5 picogram/cell/min? Also
why can't you extrapolate this to standard
fermenter conditions?

Murakami: It was published 10 years ago in TC Reports. we
re-calculated the value from this paper in which
they used ratio-isotopes. There are other data eg
plasma cells produce 10^{11} Ig mols/day, which is
almost equivalent to that 5 pg. value.

PRODUCTION OF A CHIMERIC ANTIBODY FOR TUMOUR IMAGING AND THERAPY FROM CHINESE HAMSTER OVARY (CHO) AND MYELOMA CELLS

R.P. Field, H. Brand, G.L. Renner, H.A. Robertson & R. Boraston

Celltech Ltd., 216 Bath road, Slough, SL1 4EN, United Kingdom.

ABSTRACT

A human/murine chimeric antibody for tumour imaging and therapy has been made in a recombinant CHO cell line bearing a single copy of the antibody genes. A subclone of this line, chosen for its stability and authenticity and integrity of product, gave yields of 50 mg antibody/L in serum-free batch suspension culture; in fed-batch cultures yields were increased two fold. Using an alternative expression system, glutamine synthetase gene amplification in a myeloma host cell line, yields of this same antibody of up to 240 mg/L have been obtained in simple batch cultures.

INTRODUCTION

B72.3 is a murine monoclonal antibody directed against the tumour associated glycoprotein, TAG72, of breast and colon carcinoma cells. A humanised chimera of this antibody, cB72.3, consisting of murine variable region and human IgG4 constant region on both heavy and light chains has been made. This chimeric antibody, with suitable chemical modification such as attachment of a radiolabel, is currently in clinical trials for tumour imaging and therapy. Chinese hamster ovary (CHO-K1) cells and myeloma (NS0) cell lines have been used as hosts for expression of the chimeric antibody.

Antibody for clinical trials has been manufactured using the CHO-derived cell line. Process options for the culture of this cell line included scale up of attached cultures, either in multiple roller bottles or as large-scale microcarrier fermenter cultures, or as batch fermenter cultures in homogeneous suspension. Batch suspension culture was chosen by virtue of its relative simplicity and potential for rapid scale-up.

EXPRESSION OF CHIMERIC B72.3 ANTIBODY IN CHO CELLS

Cell Line

The CHO-derived cell line bears a single copy of each of the antibody light and heavy chain genes. The cell line was made by first transfecting with the light chain gene coupled to the *neo* gene for G418 resistance; G418 resistant cells were screened by ELISA for light chain production. Light chain transfectants were then retransfected with the heavy chain gene linked to the *gpt* gene for resistance to mycophenolic acid; resistant clones were screened by TAG72 antigen-binding ELISA. On the basis of antibody synthesis rate and authenticity and integrity of the product, clone F6G7 was chosen for manufacture of early batches of antibody. In batch suspension culture in a 100 litre airlift fermenter this cell line produced 40-50 mg antibody/L (Figure 1).

Recloning and Cell Line Stability

To ensure clonality of the cell line for manufacture of clinical trials material, the F6G7 line was recloned twice more by limiting dilution. Again, the criteria for selection of daughter clones were a high specific rate of antibody synthesis and integrity of the product; growth characteristics were of secondary importance since these could be optimized later by medium design. Following the second round of cloning, stability of product synthesis was also tested over approximately 100 generations (approximately 70 cell doublings are required for the establishment of master and working cell banks and for subsequent growth of cells to production generation in a 2000 litre manufacturing fermenter).

Of six candidate clones, 11G9 (clone 4 in Figure 2) exhibited the highest specific rate

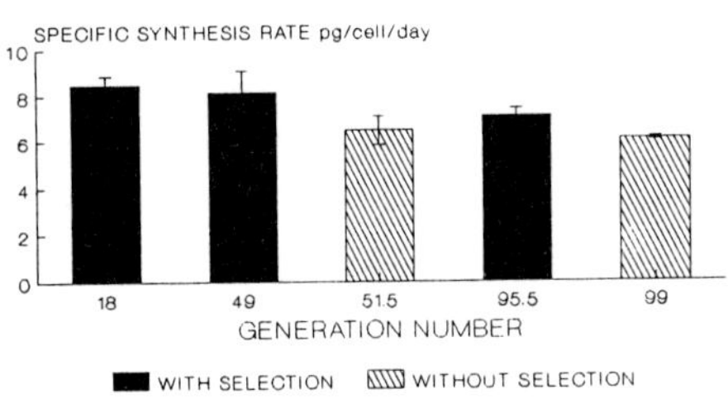

FIGURE 1

100L AIRLIFT FERMENTATION OF F6G7 CELLS MAKING cB72.3 ANTIBODY

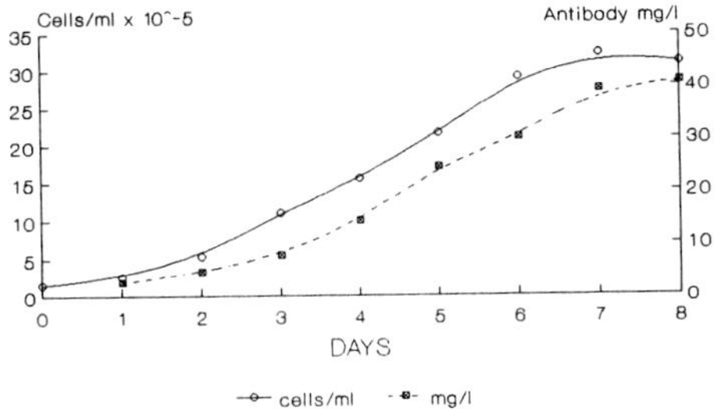

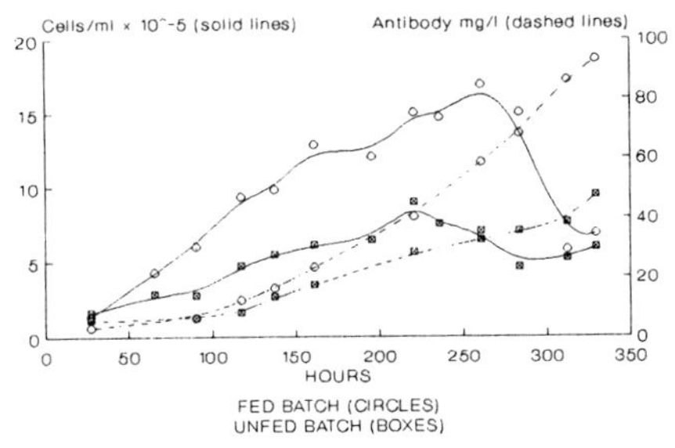

FIGURE 2

F6G7 SECOND ROUND RECLONES - GROWTH AND ANTIBODY SYNTHESIS

ANTIBODY SYNTHESIS RATE pg/cell/day
MAXIMUM CELL CONCENTRATION x10^-5/ml
HARVEST ANTIBODY CONCENTRATION mg/l

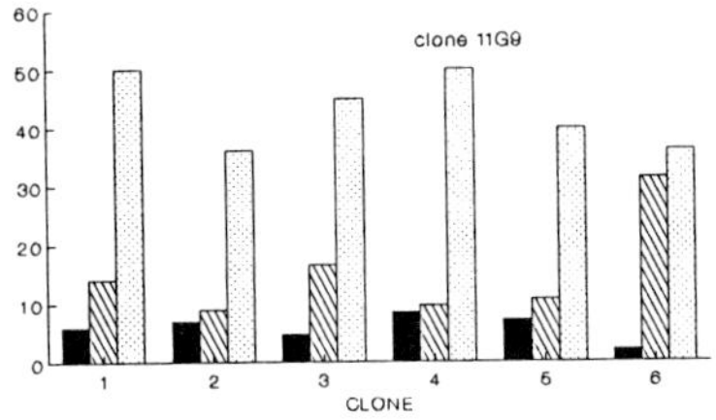

FIGURE 3

11G9- STABILITY OF ANTIBODY SYNTHESIS

WITH SELECTION   WITHOUT SELECTION

SELECTION SYSTEM IS GPT/NEO

*VALUES ARE MEANS +/- STANDARD ERROR.
*THE DIFFERENCE BETWEEN SAMPLE MEANS IS NOT SIGNIFICANT AT 5% LEVEL.

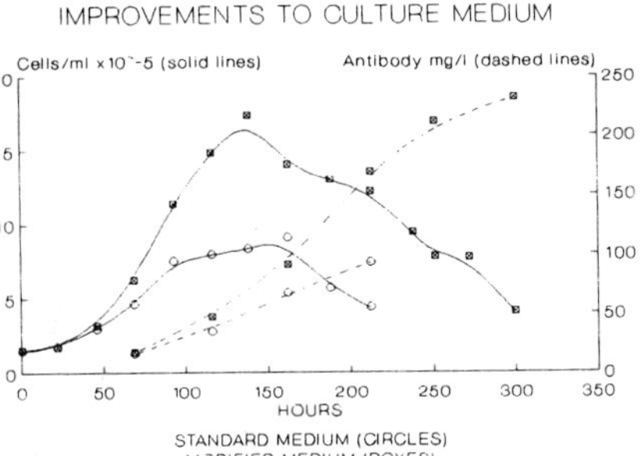

FIGURE 4

11G9 CELLS IN SERUM-FREE FERMENTER CULTURE- EFFECT OF NUTRIENT FEED

FED BATCH (CIRCLES)
UNFED BATCH (BOXES)

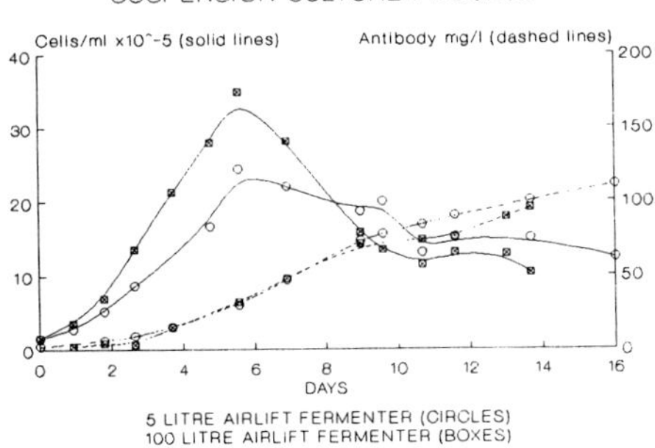

FIGURE 5

11G9 CELLS - SCALE UP OF FED-BATCH SUSPENSION CULTURE PROCESS

5 LITRE AIRLIFT FERMENTER (CIRCLES)
100 LITRE AIRLIFT FERMENTER (BOXES)

FIGURE 6

SERUM-FREE CULTURE OF GS-NSO (cB72.3) IMPROVEMENTS TO CULTURE MEDIUM

STANDARD MEDIUM (CIRCLES)
MODIFIED MEDIUM (BOXES)

of antibody synthesis and this rate was maintained over 99 generations, even in the absence of selection (Figure 3). This latter characteristic was considered particularly important since to maintain stability by continued use of cytotoxic drugs would be costly and require development and installation of quality control assays to demonstrate their clearance during product purification.

Medium Development and Scale-Up

While the cell line 11G9 exhibited high and stable rates of antibody synthesis, growth characteristics were poor compared to the other candidate clones. Thus optimization of growth offered scope to improve productivity. Serum-free adaptation and improvement in growth and antibody yield were achieved initially by supplementation of the production medium with an animal protein hydrolysate. Use of this supplement in a manufacturing medium was not favoured due to the presence of small (and potentially immunogenic) peptides, clearance of which could be difficult to demonstrate during product purification. Use of the protein hydrolysate supplement has been superceded by the use of nutrient feeds consisting of chemically defined components designed to accomodate the specific nutritional requirements of the 11G9 cell line. In small scale fermenter cultures this feed regime achieved a final product concentration of about 90 mg/L, a two-fold improvement over unfed cultures (Figure 4). That the process developed at small scale was reproducible in production scale fermenters is demonstrated by the profiles for growth and antibody accumulation in 5 and 100 litre airlift fermenters shown in Figure 5.

Product Quality

Samples taken through days 3-12 of the 100 litre fed-batch culture shown in Figure 5 were analysed by specific antigen-binding assays, PAGE and isoelectric focussing (IEF). The specific activity remained constant, light and heavy immunoglobulin chains migrated as single bands by PAGE, and the IEF banding pattern did not change over the duration of the culture.

EXPRESSION OF CHIMERIC B72.3 IN MYELOMA CELLS

The c.B72.3 antibody has more recently been expressed in NS0 myeloma cells using glutamine synthetase (GS) as a selectable marker. Cultivation of transfectants in the presence of methionine sulphoxamine (MSX) allows coamplification of the GS gene and the antibody gene to obtain high levels of expression. In simple batch culture using a standard serum-free medium this cell line produced 90 mg antibody/litre. Following extensive modifications to the medium final volumetric titres of 240 mg/L have been obtained in unfed batch cultures (Figure 6). An additional benefit of GS transfection is that cells will grow in media where glutamine is replaced by glutamic acid, a substrate that is both more stable than glutamine and metabolism of which does not generate the potentially cytotoxic concentrations of ammonia associated with glutamine metabolism. To date the stability of antibody synthesis by this cell line has been tested up to fifty generations; no decline in synthesis rate has been detected even in the absence of MSX selection.

CONCLUSIONS

Chimeric B72.3 antibody has been expressed in CHO cells. The recloned cell line is stable in the absence of drug-selection. Production of antibody has been scaled up in batch suspension culture in airlift fermenters; nutrient feeds are used to enhance product yield. Integrity and biological activity of the antibody are maintained throughout the culture process.

An alternative expression system for synthesis of the same antibody, consisting of GS amplification in a myeloma host cell line, has been developed. After medium optimization this cell line is 2-3 fold more productive than the CHO line.

OPTIMIZATION OF tPA PRODUCTION IN A 3 L
CONTINUOUS PERFUSION BIOREACTOR

U.Källström, <u>N.Chatzisavido</u>, F.Buzsáky, E.Lindner-Olsson
KabiGen AB, S-112 87 STOCKHOLM, SWEDEN

SUMMARY

We have used a 3L stirred tank bioreactor for the continuous
production of a tPA like trombolytic from CHO cells.
Recycling of cells, using a tangential flow filtration unit,
resulted in viable celldentisities between 5 to 10 million
cells per mL, at medium perfusion rates of 2 to 4 reactor
volumes per day. Volumetric productivity of the tPA variant
increased 15 to 18 fold using high persusion rates.

INTRODUCTION

The principles of continuous cultures have been known for 20
years but it is not until recently the technique has been
applied in large scale mammalian tissue culture. (1,2). With
the expanding demand for production of a number of proteins
of human therapeutic and diagnostic value the search for the
optimal production systems has become of outmost importance.
It ideally should be a homogeneous system allowing
optimization of the culture environment, eg admitting easy
control of physical parameters and cellstatus, facilitating
longterm cultures with lot to lot consistency and finally,
providing a high product yield. This can be achieved using a
stirred tank reactor with a continuously perfused culture.
Addition of critical nutrients and removal of waste products
result in high celldensity and product titers in the reactor.
Furthermore, proteins vulnerable to biodegradation can be
gradually removed to a gentler environment for subsequent
purification.

MATERIALS AND METHODS

Cells and cellculture conditions

Chinese hamster ovary (CHO) cells (line DG44 NY, obtained
from Dr L. Chasin, Sloan Cattering University New York, USA)
were transfected with a modified human tPA gene and amplified
with aminopterin using a standard protocol. (3) Cells were
routinely grown in 150 cm^2 T-flasks (Costar) and in 500 to
1000 ml spinner flasks at 30 RPM, (Techne UK). The reactor
was seeded at 7X10E5 cells/ml and the cells grew as monocell
suspension or in smaller aggregates of 5-10 cells.

Medium

The cells were grown in Dulbecco's modified Eagle's medium, DMEM and F12 (1:1), containing 3 g/L glucose (Gibco UK), supplemented with 100 U/mL penicillin, 100 μg/mL streptomycin (Sigma), 5 mg/L ascorbic acid, 7,8 μg/mL sodium selenite (Na_2SeO_3), 55 mg/L Sodium pyruvate (Merck) and 5 % FCS (Gibco UK). Between day 14 to 18, the medium was diluted 1:1 with PBS.

Assays

Cellviability and celldensity were determined by the Trypan-Blue exclusion method. Glucose and lactic acid levels were assayed with an YSI 2000 analyser (Yellow Springs Ohio, USA). For rapid product analysis of active tPA variant a fibrinolytic assay was used. For quantification of product in the reactor and in the harvest we used an ELISA.

RESULTS AND DISCUSSION

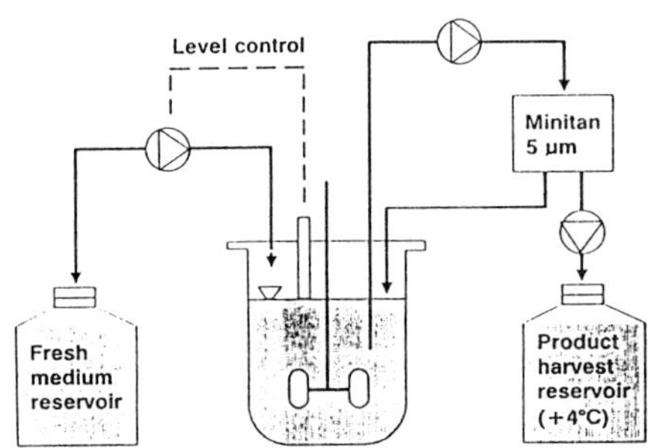

Fig 1   BIOREACTOR

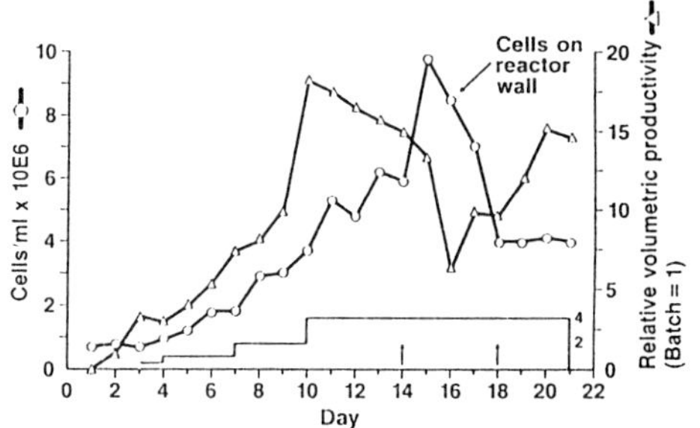

Fig 2 PRODUCTION AS FUNCTION OF
CELLDENSITY AND MEDIAFLOW

A 3 L stirred tank (Belach Sweden) was used for this perfusion culture. A schematic chart is shown in Fig 1. Working level was 2L in the reactor, pH was kept at 7,1, Dissolved Oxygen Tension (DOT) at 40 % and agitation rate at 90 RPM. A cross flow filtraiton unit, Minitan (Millipore), with 5μ poresize DVLP membrane and total surface area of 0,24 m^2 was used to separate cells from the culture medium for recirculation into the reactor. Culture fluid was pumped through the channel plate and over the membrane surface forcing cell-free fluid through the membrane, which could be collected in the harvest reservoir. Cellrecirculationrate was 6L/h at start with a gradual increase to 13 L/h the last days of the culture. Tree different flowrates (1,2 and 4 reactor volumes/day) were tested.

Cellviability never decreased below 95 %. The drop in celldensity between day 14-18 is a combination effect of the mediumdilution (1:1 with PBS) and the fact that, due to

746

frequent sparging to keep the set levels of DO, cells were
accumulating around the headspace of the reactor walls.
Typical glucose levels in the fermenter varied between 1,5-
2,0 g/L. Lactic acid did not exceed 1,1 g/L at any time (Data
not shown)
There was a constant raise in relative production of tPA with
increased flowrates. Optimal production occured at
celldensities of approximately 5x10E6 cells/mL. (Day 10-12).
Relative volumetric productivity compared to a batch culture,
run in the same reactor with the same cell inoculum,
increased 15 to 18 fold at perfusionrates of 4 rv/d.
At high celldensities, eg >7X10E6 cells/mL, perfusionrates of
4 rv/d were not sufficient to hold the productivity at the
highest levels already reached and there was a gradual
decrease in relative production starting at day 12. Diluting
the medium with PBS (1:1), resulted in a further drop in
productivity to a 10 fold increase compared to the control.
This could be explained as a result of the decrease in
nutrient and energy supply. Production levels decreased to
the levels previously achieved with perfusionrates of 2 rv/d,
(same energy supply) but a lower celldensities, at days 7 to
10. Finally, shifting back to the original medium with a
high perfusionrate, did not improve celldensity, but the
relative production was raised to a 15 fold increase compared
to the control (Fig 2).

CONCLUSIONS

We could increase celldensities in the continuously perfused
culture, from 2X10E6 cells/mL normally reached in a batch
culture, to 10X10E6 cells/mL by altering the medium
flowrates. We got a good production of a variant form of tPA
using a flow rate of 4 reactor volumes per day with moderate
celldensities, eg 4X10E6 cells/mL. Production potential was
determined by the availability of nutrients and of energy
source and did not seem to be an effect of inhibitor dilution
or "wash out". High celldensities, eg >7X10E6 cells/mL, in
combination with high perfusion rates but low nutrient supply
gave a production of tPA similar to the amounts produced when
having lower celldensities supplied with the same nutrient
and glucose concentration.

REFERENCES

1   Himmelfarb, P.,Thayer, P.S. and Martin, H.E. 1969
      SCIENCE 164: 555-557

2   McMichael, G.J 1988
      Amer. Biotech. Labor. 6: 34

3   Kaufman, R. and Sharp P. 1982
      J.Mol. Biol. 159: 601-621

THE PRODUCTION AND ASSAY OF tPA FROM MAMMALIAN CELLS

A.W. Grierson, C. Darnbrough and C. MacDonald

Department of Bioscience and Biotechnology, University of Strathclyde, The Todd Centre, 31 Taylor Street, Glasgow G4 ONR, Scotland.

ABSTRACT

A comparative study of a spectrophotometric assay and a fibrin-plate assay for the detection of human tissue-type plasminogen activator (tPA) showed differences in sensitivity and accuracy between the methods. The assays were used to detect transient levels of production of tPA in the serum from mammalian cell lines (CHO, PQXB). The tPA gene was introduced into the cell lines in a range of plasmid vectors, using both calcium phosphate- and lipofectin-mediated transfection. Each vector contained a cDNA copy of tPA under the control of different 5' and 3' regulatory elements. The transfection and subsequent assay therefore provide a system for estimating how different regulatory elements can affect the production of proteins, in this case tPA, from mammalian cells.

INTRODUCTION

tPA plays an important part in the human fibrinolytic system: it converts plasminogen into plasmin which in turn proteolytically degrades the fibrin network associated with blood clots (1). Optimisation of tPA, in its active form, is therefore of great commercial important. for this reason, both assays used directly measure the activity of tPA produced from the cell lines transfected with the range of vectors. Both assays were based on the following reaction:

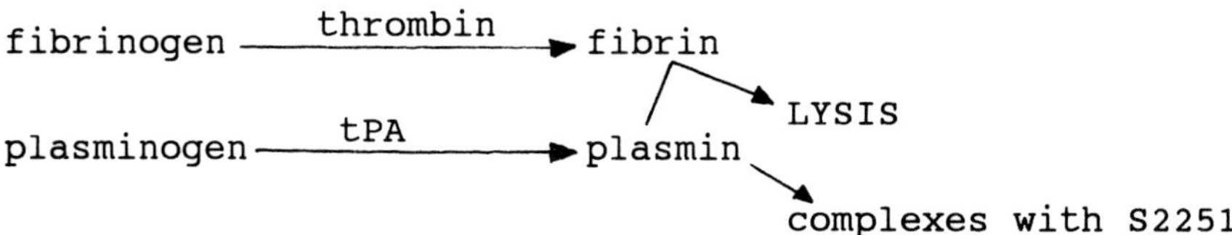

METHODS

Cell culture and vector construction

tPA was expressed in CHO cells, and the murine hybridoma cell lines PQXB2/2 and a derivative line (sf PQXB) adapted to grow in serum-free conditions. Both PQXB cell lines were supplied by ICI. Transfections were carried out using either the calcium phosphate mediated method (2), or the lipid-mediated method (3). Liposomes were supplied by GIBCO BRL.

pTR315 contains RSV LTR, tPA cDNA sequence and the SV40 poly A signal/small t intron. Standard manipulations produced vectors in which the tPA gene was under the control of different regulatory elements:

pKT40KPA:	tk promoter and SV40 poly A/small t intron
pKT40:	tk promoter and tk poly A
pHCMV-tPA-SV40:	HCMV promoter/enhancer and SV40 poly A/small t intron.

tPA assays

Two types of assays were compared. The plate assay (4) involved casting agarose gels containing fibrinogen, plasminogen and thrombin in immunodiffusion plates. tPA samples were then added to wells in the gel and the subsequent area of lysis was measured after incubation at 37°C. In the spectrophotometric assay (5), any plasmin produced from plasminogen due to the action of tPA on the surface of fibrinogen fragments was detected due to the presence of the plasmin-specific chromogenic substrate S-2251. The absorbance change at 405 mins directly related to the amount of tPA in the sample.

RESULTS

Assays (see Figs. 1 and 2)

The plate assay is more sensitive, reliably detecting 0.01ng/ul tPA; this is tenfold more sensitive than the spectrophotometric assay. The plate assay is also more discriminating: there is a greater degree of change in the diameter of lysis between standards in Fig.1 than there is between absorbance changes in Fig. 2. Altering the pH of the assay reaction mixture had no effect between pH 3-11 on the standard curve in Fig. 1 (data not shown).

Transfections

CHO cells have a background level of tPA production equivalent to approximately 1.5pg/cell/24 hrs. PQXB 2/2 and sf PQXB produce levels of tPA too low to be detected by either assay system. Transfection of sf PQXB and CHO (in serum-free conditions) with pTR315 and pKT40KPA increased the level of production of tPA to approximately 2pg/cell/24 hrs. This value was consistently less for pTR315 suggesting that the tk promoter is stronger than the RSV LTR in these cell lines. No data is yet available for pHCMV-tPA-SV40.

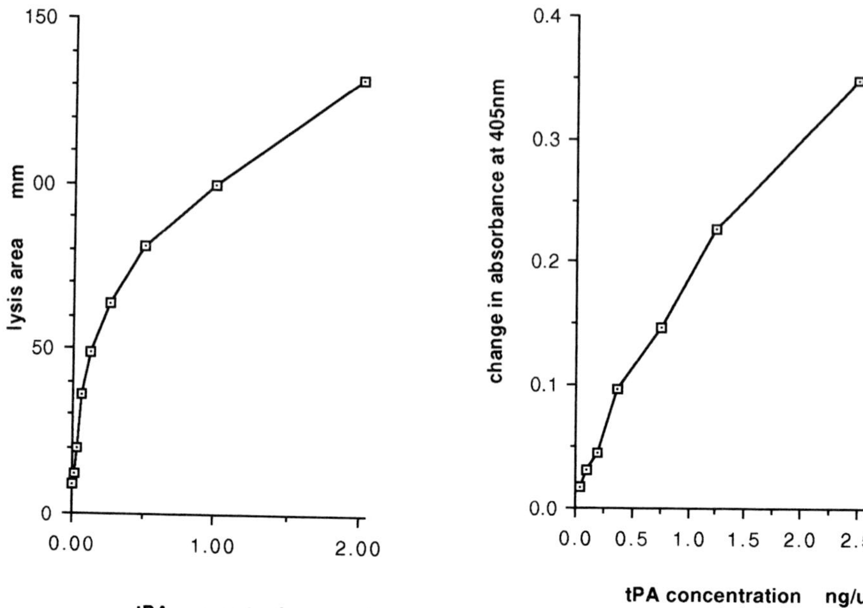

Fig. 1   Standard Curve   Fig. 2   Standard Curve for
          for Plate Assay   Spectrophotometric
                                            Assay

ACKNOWLEDGEMENTS

We would like to thank Dr. C. Bebbington (Celltech) for providing pEe6hCMV-BglII, which contains the promoter/enhancer sequences from the human cytomegalovirus, and Dr. M. Brown (SmithKline Beecham) for providing pTR315 which contains the tPA cDNA sequence.

REFERENCES

1   Kadouri, A. and Bohak, Z. (1983) _Biotechnology_ _1_, 1983, 354

2   Gorman, C. in _DNA_ _Cloning_ _Vol_ _II_, (Ed. Glover, D.M.), IRL Press, 1985, p143-190

3   Felgner, P.E., Cradek, T.R., Holm, M., Roman, R., Chan, H.W., Wenz, M., Northrop, J.P., Ringold, G.M. and Danielsen, M. _Proc._ _Natl._ _Acad._ _Sci._ _USA.,_ 1987, _84_, 7413.

4   Schumacher, G.F.B. _Anal._ _Biochem._, 1972, _48_, 9

5   Mahmoud, M. and Gaffnay, P.J. _Thomb._ _Haemostas.,_ 1985, _53_, 356

CONSTITUTIVE SECRETION OF SOLUBLE CD23 RECEPTORS IN HOLLOW FIBER REACTORS.

A. Bernard, C. Cavegn, T. Jomotte, P. Graber , J.Y. Bonnefoy

GLAXO IMB , 46 Route des Acacias, CH 1211, Geneva , Switzerland

ABSTRACT

A hollow fiber reactor was used for immobilizing the EBV-transformed B cell line RPMI8866. It constitutively expresses membrane CD23 receptors which are subsequently cleaved into several soluble fragments, ranging from 14 to 37 kDa. We report here on the large scale preparation of the 37 kDa moiety. The titer of the 37 kDa can be increased to 80000 U/ml but the molecule is highly aggregated and can not be recovered in its native conformation.

INTRODUCTION

CD23 is a 45 kDa cell membrane antigen which seems to be implicated in several B cell activities such as proliferation (1), differentiation (2), IgE production (3), and inhibition of macrophage migration (4). Some of these activities may be mediated by the soluble forms of the molecule with an apparent MW of 37, 33, 25 and 14 kDa. We report here on the production and purification of the soluble 37 kDa receptor. We chose to use a hollow fiber cartridge which would allow high cell densities together with product retention.

MATERIALS AND METHODS

Cell line

We use the EBV-transformed B cell line RPMI8866 (5) which is a natural CD23 secretor.

Media

RMPI 1640 supplemented with 2 mM L-Glutamine, 10 mM Hepes, 50 ppm Gentamycin and 0.01% Pluronic F68 is used in the reactor and the extracapillary space (ECS) of the hollow fiber cartridge is supplemented with a mixture of FCS, Ultroser HY (USHY), and RPMI 1640.

Hollow fiber reactor

We assembled the hollow fiber cartridge (Disscap 140E) as described by Klerx et al. (7). It is connected to a conventional Chemap stirred reactor (15 l) for medium conditioning. 2.10^8 cells are inoculated into the 200 ml ECS. The fermenter medium is renewed as soon as glucose concentration falls below 0.2 g/l. At the same time, the ECS is harvested and then reinjected with the mixture FCS/USHY/RPMI 1640. (Table 1).

Analytical methods

Glucose is measured by a glucose analyzer 2000 (YSI, USA). Western Blot analysis is used to follow purification. The 37 kDa titer is determined by an ELISA method in which 100 units (U) represent the amount of sCd23 released overnight by 10^6 RPMI 8866 cells/ml that yields a half-maximal absorbance.

Purification method

Purification of material was performed by selective ammonium sulfate precipitations, followed by gel filtration (ACA 44 column).

RESULTS

Each addition of nutrients (Table 1), after 250 hrs, corresponds to an ECS harvest operation, for which the harvested volume and the product titer are plotted in Figure 1. At c.a. 900 hours, the titer increased from 1000 U/ml to 80000 U/ml for an unexplained reason. The harvested volume decreased steadily from 100 ml initially to almost 20 ml after 2 months. This decrease is explained by a corresponding increase of cell mass and debris in the ECS.

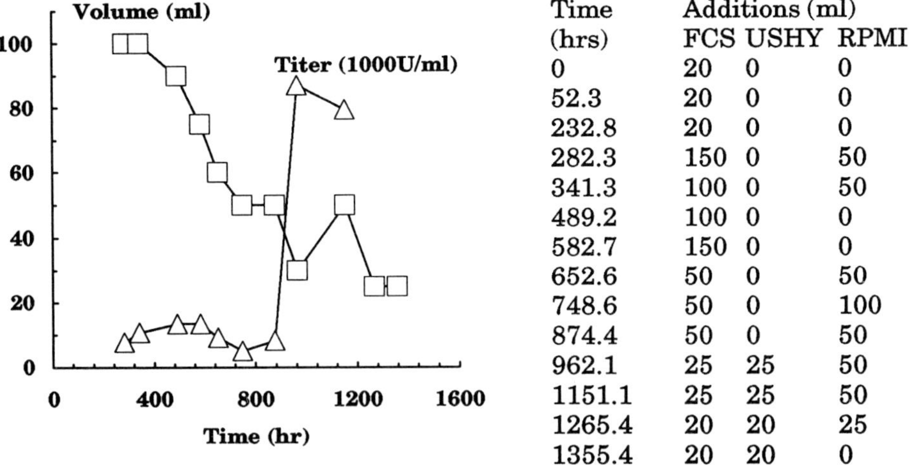

Time (hrs)	Additions (ml)		
	FCS	USHY	RPMI
0	20	0	0
52.3	20	0	0
232.8	20	0	0
282.3	150	0	50
341.3	100	0	50
489.2	100	0	0
582.7	150	0	0
652.6	50	0	50
748.6	50	0	100
874.4	50	0	50
962.1	25	25	50
1151.1	25	25	50
1265.4	20	20	25
1355.4	20	20	0

Figure 1 Titer and volume harvested

Table 1 ECS additions

During purification (Figure 2), the 37kDa form is found in greatest proportion in the 36-41% ammonium sulfate cut (Lane 2). Unfortunately this fraction contains highly aggregated 37kDa as evidenced by gel filtration (data not shown). Because of this, it was impossible to purify it in the native form.

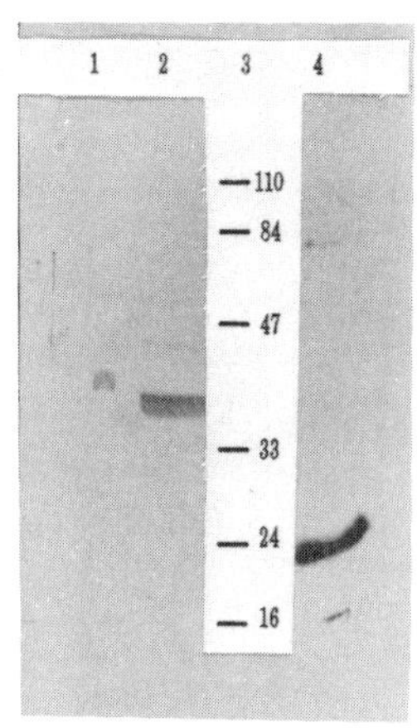

Figure 2   Western Blot of purified fractions.

1 $(NH_4)_2SO_4$ cut 41-46 %
2 $(NH_4)_2SO_4$ cut 36-41 %
3 Prestained MW standards
4 Pure recombinant 25kDa

CONCLUSIONS

The hollow fiber technology appears suitable for producing large quantities of the CD23 soluble forms. The maximum titer achieved represents a 200 fold difference versus suspension culture titers. However, the molecule is highly aggregated and not easily recoverable.

REFERENCES

1 Swendeman, S. and Thorley-Lawson, D.A. <u>EMBO J</u>. 1987, <u>6</u>, 137
2 Brieva, J.A., Kagan, J.M., Saxon, A. and Stevens, R.H. submitted for publication
3 Sarfati, M., Bron, D., Lagneaux, L., Fonteyn, C., Frost, H. and Delespesse, G. <u>Blood</u>. 1988, <u>71</u>, 94
4 Flores-Romo, L., Cairns, J., Millsum, M.J. and Gordon J. <u>Immunology</u> 1989, <u>67</u>, 547
5 Gonzalez-Molina, A. and Spiegelberg, H.L. <u>J.Clin. Invest.</u> 1977, <u>59</u>, 116
6 Klerx, J.P.A.M., Jansen Verplanke, C., Blonk, C.J. and Twaalfhoven, L.C. <u>J. Immunol. Methods</u> 1988, <u>111</u>, 179

PRODUCTION OF PROTEINS FROM CELL NUCLEI BY CYCLIC CONTINUOUS FERMENTATION

B. Röder[1], G.-W. Piehl[1], J. Lehmann[2]

1) GBF-Gesellschaft für Biotechnologische Forschung mbH, FRG
2) University of Bielefeld, FRG

Introduction

Product concentrations in mammalian cell cultivations are usually very low. For economic production advanced fermentation techniques are required. Normally, desired compounds are excreted into the culture broth. For production of these compounds different fermentation techniques have been developed.
If the desired compound is cellbound or part of the cell nucleus, high cell concentration will be the key parameter. In this study, production of a cell nucleus protein, required for transcription studies, from HeLa cells is demonstrated. This protein can only be obtained from the cell nucleus if the cells were harvested in the exponential growth phase (1). For production, a combination of repeated batch and perfusion is used. Fermentations were carried out in 1.4 and 21.5 liter volume.

Experimental

<u>Cell-line:</u> HeLa (obtained from P. Gruss, ZMBH-Heidelberg, FRG).
<u>Medium:</u> serumfree composition (2) with following modifications: IMDM without Hepes, sodium bicarbonate 2.8 g/l, no additional glutamine, no ethanolamine.
<u>Fermentor:</u> Membrane stirred reactor (3) with polypropylene membrane for aeration and filtration (perfusion).
<u>Fermentation conditions:</u> dO: 50 % air saturation, pH: 6.8 - 7.1, culture volumes: 1.4 l and 21.5 l, feed rates: 0.053 l/h (1.4 l) and 0.810 l/h (21.5 l), temperature: 37°C, stirrer speed: 20 rpm.
<u>Cell counting:</u> cells were counted by trypan blue dye exclusion method in a haemocytometer.

Results

Two aspects have to be considered for fermentation: first, cells must grow exponentially up to the harvesting and second, a high cell concentration should be obtained in the reactor for economical production. Using a conventional batch process, maximum concentration of 1×10^6 cells/ml can be obtained during the exponential growth phase. For higher cell concentrations, fed batch or continuous operation with cell retainment can be used. Previous experiments have shown that continuous operation with total cell retainment results in higher cell concentrations than fed batch and therefore has been used in the process described here.

In fig. 1, the time course of the fermentaion in a 1.4 l reactor is shown. After inocculation cells grow exponentially. At a cell concentration of 1 x 10⁶ viable cells/ml continuous operation was started using a dilution rate of 0.038 1/h. Cells continue to grow exponentially up to a cell concentration of 7 x 10⁶ viable cells/ml, the maximum value which could be obtained in the exponential growth phase. At that concentration the main part of the cells was harvested and continuous fermentation restarted after addition of new medium at a cell concentration of 1 x 10⁶ cells/ml. This procedure could be performed for several cycles without any change in cell growth rate, maximum cell concentration and productivity as shown in fig. 1.

The process was scaled up from 1.4 to 21.5 liters. As shown in fig. 2, the growth rate, the productivity and maximum cell concentration in the 21.5 l reactor were identical compared to the 1.4 l reactor. After a fermen-tation time of 195 h (2 cycles) in the 21.5 l reactor a total amount of 2.8 x 10¹¹ cells was obtained.

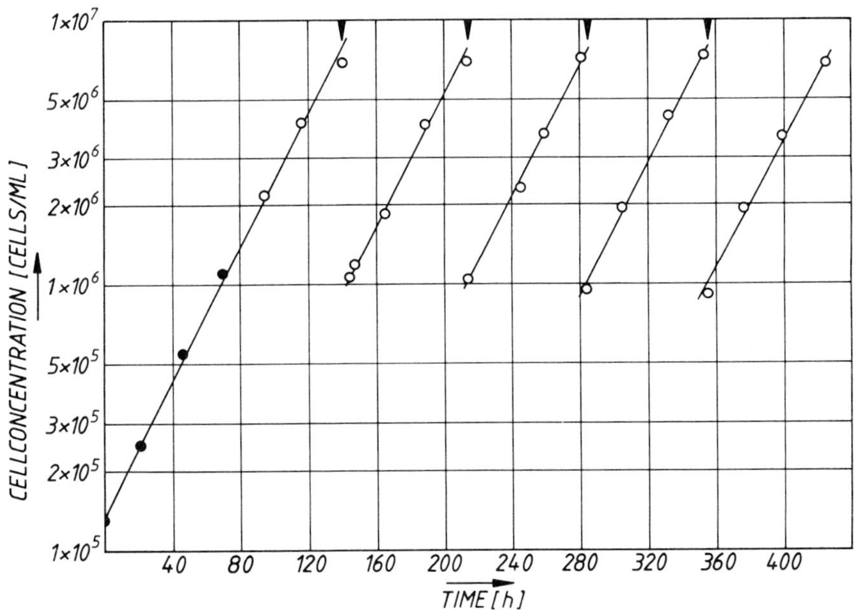

Fig. 1: Scale 1.4 l: Cyclic continuous fermentation of HeLa cells. Cell concentration (viable cells) as a function of time. Black dots: batch operation, open dots: continuous operation, black arrows: cyclic cell harvest.

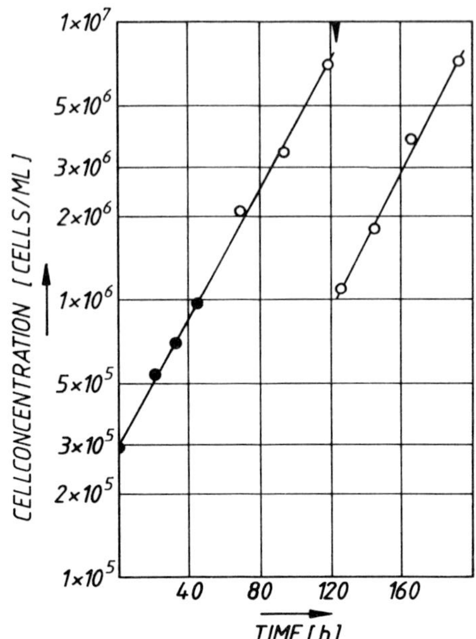

Fig. 2: Scale 21.5 l: Cyclic continuous fermentation of HeLa cells. Cell concentration (viable cells) as a function of time. Black dots: batch operation, open dots: continuous operation, black arrows: cyclic cell harvest.

References

(1) Schlokat, U. Immunoglobluin Enhancer Bindende Faktoren: Identification, Charakterisierung, Reinigung und Wechselwirkung mit anderen Enhancer Elementen; PhD Thesis, University of Heidelberg, 1987

(2) Jäger, V.; Lehmann, J. and Friedl, P. Serum-free growth medium for the cultivation of a wide spectrum of mammalian cells in stirred bioreactors; Cytotechnology, 1988, 1, 319

(3) Büntemeyer, H., Bödeker, B. G. D., Lehmann, J. In: Modern Approaches To Animal Cell Technology (eds. Spier, R. E. and Griffith, J. B.) Butterworth, Borough Green, Sevenoaks, UK, 1987, 221

Section 11
Regulatory issues

BIOLOGICALS AND REGULATORY ASPECTS IN THE E.E.C.

Florian HORAUD

Institut Pasteur - Virologie Médicale

75724 PARIS CEDEX 15, France

In order to ensure the free circulation of biological products among member countries of the E.E.C., the Council of Ministers of the E.E.C. adopted, in 1986, four directives aimed at harmonizing the manufacture, quality control and registration of biological products. (E.E.C. official form No. L15 of 17.01.1987). A Committee for Proprietary Medicinal Products (CPMP) was created (Directive 87/22/EEC) to authorize, refuse or withdraw products derived from biotechnology or high technology procedures. The CPMP is assisted in its activity by a group of experts forming a Biotechnology/Pharmacy working party. Created in 1985, this team plays two main roles: 1) it gives an opinion to the CPMP on individual applications in agreement with E.E.C. biotechnology consultation, and 2) it drafts specific recommendations on the production and quality control of different categories of biologicals. This second task is particularly important, because it should create the scientific basis on which products issuing from biotechnology are regulated. Because the E.E.C. is a federation of independent countries, and because each member of this community will maintain its regulatory organisations, the recommendations drafted by the Biotechnology/Pharmacy group are the main factor in the harmonization coordination of the requirements necessary for the licensing of biologicals in Europe.

The Biotechnology/Pharmacy working party in Brussels, chaired by G. Schild (NBSB/U.K.), drafted several recommendations, shown in Table I. Among the documents listed in Table I, special attention should be given to the draft entitled "Validation of virus removal and inactivation procedures" that was already sent by CPMP to the EPI for comments. This guideline is unique because it is the first time when the problem of validation of the purification method to remove viruses and the validation of viral inactivation is discussed in a regulatory document. In the past, viral inactivation has been considered only from the point of view of killed viral vaccine, while the removal of viruses contaminating the cell substrate used to prepare biologicals has never been discussed. The reason was simple, because in the past the presence of a virus in a cell culture used to produce a biological disqualified the cells. However, in the last ten years, this concept was revised because the new developments in biotechnology have made it possible to exploit new animal cell substrates, mainly continuous cell lines. It is well known that animal cell lines commonly used in rDNA technology, like the CHO cells, contain endogenous retroviruses. The same holds true for murine hybridoma producing monoclonal antibodies.

In order to understand the necessary approach for the acceptability of such cells, some data have to be evoked concerning the use of biologicals. Historically, viral vaccines were the first biological products recognized to be capable of causing severe accidents. The following examples are illustrative.

In the time just following the introduction of rabies vaccination by Pasteur, severe accidents were generated by the incomplete inactivation

of rabies virus in the vaccine. Rabies vaccine prepared in the CNS of
animals was also the cause of an allergic encephalitis generated by an
immunological reaction against myelin present in the vaccine. Allergic
encephalitis was the first post-vaccine clinical accident in which a
component of the cell substrate used to amplify the immunogenic virus was
identified as a source of adverse effect.

In the year 1940, some yellow fever vaccine, prepared in embryonated
eggs and lyophilized, was contaminated with hepatitis B virus contained
in the human sera used as a stabilizer. This accident is significant
because it showed that a reagent used as additive can introduce in a
"clean" vaccine a contaminant highly pathogenic for humans. But there is
no doubt that the SV40 incident was the most dramatic accident in which
vaccine was contaminated by an adventitious virus present in the cell
substrate, in this case, primary cell culture of rhesus kydney.[5] In the
1950s, SV40 contaminated killed poliovaccine because this agent is very
resistant to formaldehyde, live poliovaccine and adenovirus vaccine.
Contaminated killed poliovaccine was administered in the U.S.A. and in
Europe to 100 million subjects, while in Eastern Europe, more than 200
million children received oral poliovaccine containing high quantities of
SV40. Fortunately, this incident had a happy outcome because simian SV40
replicates poorly in humans, but its importance remained an illustrative
event for the evaluation of viral safety of biologicals.

The E.E.C. Biotech draft concerning viral validation of removal and/or
inactivation covers not only products derived from tissue culture but
also blood and plasma derivatives or other pharmaceuticals prepared from
animal or human tissues. Here again, viruses like HIV or hepatitis B
present in blood were at the origin of the world-wide spread of these
infections to humans. Recently the administration to haemophiliac

patients of some batches of Factor VIII or Factor IX containing residual active HIV induced AIDS in these patients. The particular aspects of the inactivation of viruses in the plasma derivatives will be drafted in greater detail by the E.E.C. Biotech group in the recommendations concerning medicinal products derived from human blood and plasma (see Table I).

If we have a look back to the biologicals that were contaminated with viruses, we can realize that the identification of the contaminating agent was possible only many years after the product had been introduced onto the market.

The E.E.C. Biotech document discussed first the sources of viral contamination, making clear that this problem is very complex, because of the new methodology used to prepare biologicals. In connection with the origin of virus contamination of products, the document considers afterward the concept of validation for viruses. In principle, three approaches can be used to check for potential contamination of a biological product: 1) testing source material; 2) testing the capacity of the manufacturing procedure to remove and/or inactivate viruses; and 3) testing the product at appropriate stages of manufacture, including concentrated final bulk. However, the document recognized that no single approach will necessarily establish the safety of the product, for two main reasons: 1) the inherent limits of virus assays that are not able to detect virus at low concentrations; and 2) the hazardous nature of many potential contaminants. The validation of the purification and/or inactivation, in spite of its limitations, can provide essential information on the safety of biologicals. This concept is particularly important in the case of blood and plasma derivatives, in which the characterization of source material is complicated by its diversity and by its

762

potential contamination with hazardous viruses like HIV or hepatitis B.

The criteria that should be considered in the choice of viruses for validation are discussed in detail, together with the design of viral validation assays, and a table of viruses useful in such studies is given (see Table II). The document recommends that a number of 3-4 viruses should be enough to be used in validation procedures by using specific viruses that can occur in some source material like HIV in blood derivatives, murine retroviruses in hybridoma cells, etc. and model viruses representing a range of viruses having physico-chemical structures as SV40, Sabin-type poliovirus, etc. Finally, the document is accompanied by two appendices analyzing the sensitivity of virus assays and calculating the reduction factor that is a major issue of validation experiments.

The Biotech group recommendations for the validation of virus removal and inactivation procedures is a document considering that, in order to testify to the virological safety of biologicals, the particular characteristics of each product must be evaluated. The tests performed for viral safety studies should be considered in their totality. Actually, biologicals manufactured in animal cells have a risk that is not different from those obtained from bacteria and yeast. This is the main reason that the guidelines do not go into details and consider that only case-by-case analysis allows regulatory policy to be decided for every product. Since understanding the document produced by the Biotech group in Brussels requires a minimum knowledge of virology, the correct design of viral validation assays is asking for the cooperation of professional virologists. Producers should be aware of the important role their collaboration with virologists can play in assuming the virus safety of biologicals.

Table 1

REGULATORY DOCUMENTS DRAFTED BY THE EEC-BIOTECHNOLOGY/PHARMACY WORKING PARTY

- Guidelines on the production and quality control of medicinal products derived by recombinant DNA technology. (1)

- Guidelines on the production and quality control of monoclonal antibodies of murine origin intended for use in man. (2)

- Guidelines on the preclinical biological safety testing of medicinal products derived from biotechnology. (3)

- Guidelines on the production and quality control of cytokine products derived by modern biotechnological processes. (4)

- Production and quality control of human monoclonal antibodies intented for use in man. (released).

- Validation of virus removal and inactivation procedures. (Sent to CPMP)

- Medicinal products derived from human blood and plasma. (in preparation)

Table II.   Examples of Viruses which have been used in Virus Validation Studies
according to the E.E.C. Biotech Working Party

Virus	Family	Natural Host	Genome	Env	Size	Shape	Resistance to Physicochemical Reagents
HIV	Retro	Man	RNA	Yes	80-100nm	Spherical	Low
Murine Leukemia virus (MuLV)	Retro	Mouse	RNA	Yes	80-110nm	Spherical	v. Low
Reovirus 3	Reo	Various	RNA	No	60-80nm	Spherical	High
Parainfluenza virus	Paramyxo	Various	RNA	Yes	150-300nm	Pleo-Spher	Low
Influenza virus, PR8	Orthomyxo	Man	RNA	Yes	80-120nm	Pleo-Spher	Low
Poliovirus, Sabin type 1	Picorna	Man	RNA	No	25-30nm	Icosahedral	Med
SV40	Papova	Monkey	DNA	No	45nm	Icosahedral	High
Pseudorabies virus	Herpes	Swine	DNA	Yes	120-200nm	Spherical	Med
Vesicular Stomatitis Virus	Rhabdo	Bovine	RNA	Yes	80-90nm	Bullet shaped	Low
Vaccinia virus	Pox	?	DNA	Yes	500-700nm	Brick shaped	High

REFERENCES

1. TIBTECH, December 1987, Vol. 5. or J. Biol. Standard. (1989), <u>17</u>, 223-231.

2. TIBTECH, January 1988, Vol. 6 or J. Biol. Standard. (1989), <u>17</u>, 213-222.

3. TIBTECH, February 1989, Vol. 7. or J. Biol. Standard. (1989), <u>17</u>, 203-212.

4. TIBTECH, October 1988, Vol. 6. (released)

5. Shah, K. and Nathanson, N.: Human Exposure to SV40: Review and Comment. Am. J. of Epidemiology (1976), <u>103</u>, 1-12.

Onions: I would like to endorse Florian's comments about
contamination.   In the UK the HSE has been engaged in
an exercise to quantitate those instances when virus
transmission has occurred.   We now know of 7 incidents
which have occurred in the last 20 years of
transspecies transmission and these have occurred
primarily in vaccines but not exclusively so.   On each
occasion a species jump has occurred and has caused
disease. The latest example of that in Britain is BSE
and I think we should be concerned about 2 new viruses
HHV6 has been demonstrated in 90% of people and we are
picking it up in 10^5 cells from everybody and a new
murine gamma Herpes virus which we are all going to be
concerned about because it is unknown to everybody here
so far and this now exists in mouse populations and
could turn up in hybridomas.   I re-emphasise the
transspecies jump and we know herpes viruses can cross
species barriers.   We need to be very concerned about
this.

Horaud: This confirms that we are exposed to new and unknown
dangers and this is the reason that regulatory agencies
are so cautious.   While some producers are aware of the
problems those Companies which are dominated by the
biochemical engineering aspects are not as cautious.
So everything should be validated so the examples of
David Onions are heuristic.   What now happens to sera
which could be derived from animals infected with the
BSE agent is a real problem as this agent comes from
Sheep Scrapie and it could relate to Creutzfelds Jacobs
disease in humans.   We are always operating at the
limits of safety; I encourage people to work with
animal cells but do your best to ensure safety.

<u>**Workshop of Regulatory Matters**</u>

Geyer:

It is obvious from the talk of Dr Horaud that the licensing of drugs in the USA is different from what happens in Europe at the moment. As I have worked for a European Company recently I have had to deal with the regulatory concerns in both places, so when I think about the harmonization of regulatory practices I think of the potential advantages leading to a streamline registration process for new products. For example there should be a concerted response to the emergence of a new viral contaminant as alluded to by Dr. Onions earlier as well as the more rapid assimilation and dissemination of technical advances such as DNA fingerprinting for the efficient introduction of new clinical entities on a world-wide basis as soon as possible. The situation in the USA is much simpler and there is a consistency to the regulatory process which those in US companies are getting used to. Where we have a similar situation which is akin to Europe is in the deliberate release of genetically modified organisms which is still a field of controversy and debate between the EPA and USDA as to which agency has precedence over making and enforcing regulations in this area.

Spier:

There should be concern about questions of regulation, for each $1 of work to achieve the demonstration of the feasibility of a product it takes a further $10 to obtain a licence to sell that product on the market. The tail is wagging the dog. Can this be reversed? How much do we charge society by the time it takes to get a product into the market place and the on-cost of the drugs which have to recover the costs of going through the regulatory process particularly in the developing world as well as the developed world.

Specifically can I ask Florian that while, you have recognised that you can put in an application to any one of 33 European countries (12 of them in the EEC) new legislation dealing with the release of genetically modified organisms is based on a one-stop shopping approach to obtaining a licence is this a possibility in the area of licensing therapeutics and prophylactic biologicals.

Horaud:

Brussels is saying that it is responsible for licences whereas the Council for Europe (which represents all the European countries including those is the Community) can make recommendations. If you reside in a member state of the EEC and you want a licence you get in touch with the national authority or you can initiate a file in Brussels. It is important to realise that both national and EEC authorities are open

to hear verbal submissions before a document file is
submitted. This helps in getting the approach for the
submission for the licence in the appropriate form.
You should get in touch with the Agencies as soon as
possible before the official registration application
is done. If you are outside the EEC, and from the USA
you need to go to Brussels as do the other non-EEC
European Countries. Since June 1989 you need a licence
from Brussels. In January 1992 after the market is
opened up a Brussels licence will entitle the holder to
market products in any of the EEC countries
automatically.

Also as the regulatory committee meets every two months
it is important to prevent delays to get the dossier
representing the product as correct as possible as
early as possible and this could mean assembling a pile
of papers 1-2 metres high. The scientific quality of
the material in the file is the most significant
feature of the submission leading to its acceptance.

Spier: We also need to mention the OECD who have made
recommendations about the release of GMO's. Members of
our society should be aware of these papers.

Horaud   There are also groups in Brussels working on this
problem but communication between the various parts of
the Brussels organizations is not very good so often
work is duplicated and contradictions ensue.

Spier: One of the factors which limits progress in this area
is the number of regulators or the people who process
these metre high packages of paper, would we like a
recommendation to go forward from this Society for a 10
fold increase in the number of such people. Because
the biggest delays in getting approval occurs between
the submission of papers and the receipt of answers-
it could be 6 months, for one interaction.

Onions: I sit on the new Committee on the genetically
manipulated organisms release, I think that for new
regulatory systems we go for a one stop shopping stage
system. In the UK we provide people with a flow chart
of what the steps are so that we can be fairly rapid in
our processing of applications. I also agree heartily
with Professor Spier because we do need more people
processing paper because this is where things are
clogging up and having to look at some of the stuff
myself I understand why.

Arathoon: Are there proposals with the CPMP or the EEC
regulations that would permit the more rapid clearing
or approval of a submission which has already been
cleared by the FDA or the Japanese authorities.

Horaud: It is not a single procedure as there are 12 autonomous
               units in the EEC which makes a difference with the USA.
               But after 1st. Jan 1992 there could be a new, single
               and more rapid decision making process which will
               depend on the quality of the dossier. A good dossier
               can take 6 months but a poor one 2 years but Companies
               will get to be good at making dossiers.

Arathoon: But if the USA can approve a dossier why should it be a
               problem at the EEC.

Horaud: We have good relations with the FDA but we have our own
               responsibilities in Europe. It is a good point to have
               FDA approval but an American dossier would be
               reexamined in the light of European Philosophy.

Estefanell: The regulatory problems are not only technical but they
               also have a commercial aspect.   The individual
               countries in Europe have started out from the point of
               protecting their own industry.   Europe is trying to
               break down these barriers. There is a similar problem
               between the USA, Europe and Canada which is mindful of
               the commercial aspects of market penetration.

Draper: In a lot of areas the regulatory agencies have not got
               their act together. We heard Norman Finter talk about
               a Solera process for interferon which he is allowed to
               operate without changing the cell for a whole year
               while for veterinary viral vaccines this would not be
               allowed even when you are selling to a Third World
               country.

Spier: Don't you think it is now more practical to obtain
               licences for products from transformed cell lines now
               that some such products have been licensed you should
               be able to run a Solera process for an FMD vaccine for
               a year.

Spier: The feature which is dominating the relationships
               between the manufacturers and the regulatory agencies
               is the science of the product under investigation.
               Jack Obijeski impressed me with the observation that
               until 5 or so years ago the regulatory agencies were
               dominated by thoughts of the conjectural possibilities
               of damage which was influenced by a hyperactive press
               which seized on this as a new issue.   This type of
               hype has died down now that we have genetically
               modified organisms released into the environment-
               pseudomona syringiae. Also the pioneering situations
               like lymphoblastoid interferon and genetically
               engineered tPA and insulin where we are injecting a
               genetically engineered product into people. We are now
               left with a great body of work to validate our

production systems. Are people satisfied that such an
amount of work is necessary? or how do people respond
to the monopolistic situation engendered by the cost of
obtaining a product licence which can only be afforded
by the large companies who have already had past
successes viz a vis the SME's (small and medium
enterprise) who have yet to obtain a produce licence
the cost of which could be so high as to keep them out
of this market place. You need $100 million in the
bank for any one product or to be practical a company
needs $500 million to counter the 1 in 5 chance of
arriving at a commercially successfully product. Thus
the SME's don't stand a chance in spite of having much
of the innovation going on in them. Of course when an
SME has something which looks as if it will succeed the
SME tends to be purchased by one of the large
established companies. Is this a healthy situation.?

Spier: Let's return to the scientific and technical issue of
the unknown virus lurking in cells for which we do not
have a diagnostic method or even a detection method.
Using our present knowledge and the new techniques can
we look at our own, normal human cells and determine
how many viral genomes are lingering there. Would we
find many Herpes viruses and Retroviruses?

Onions: If it was that simple we would have done it. There are
viruses we have not yet even discovered the two clear
examples are HHV6 which we only knew of 2 years ago and
the new gamma Herpes virus of murines which has only
been characterised in the last year. There will be
others.

Spier: From your experience in identifying these two new
viruses is there now a protocol which would search out
further new viruses?

Onions: Some of those come from HIV, we are now finding many
new viruses in people who have been immunosuppressed by
their HIV infections. This is how HHV6 was discovered,
but first we must look for the viruses we know about
and also design processes which are effective in
removing a wide range of viruses - a belt and braces
philosophy to clear out the ones we know about and
inactivate the ones we don't know about.

Horaud: I agree with Prof. Onions. As a virologist I feel
frustrated in not being able to answer Ray's question.
An example of a difficult problem in BSE; we do not
know how to search for this agent in bovine sera.
There is another papovavirus like virus found in bovine
sera that was described 25 years ago by Dr Sha as a
virus of new world monkeys but it is not a virus of new
world monkeys it is a contaminant of sera which becomes

Spier:
apparent after replication in cells. We cannot rule out, whatever we do, the possibility that there will be a self-replicating agent in the final product.
Talking of BSE the review by Prusinier in Ann. Rev. Microbiol, 1989., indicates that the 30KD glycoprotein does not of itself replicate but takes advantage of the existence of the gene for the protein backbone of the molecule being present in at least all mammals. The properties of the infectious material is different from the native material. What we could be looking for is possibly an aberrant glycosylation of a native protein (see an article on this expected in the Oxoid Review, Autumn 1990 by Spier).

Onions:
In the UK we no longer use bovine serum of UK origin for manufacture and it is proclaimed that BSE is not present elsewhere. In a recent meeting (3 weeks ago) representatives of the USA reported that it looks as though an agent resembling BSE was present in US cattle in Wisconsin where an outbreak of Mink encephalopathy has been attributed to the bovine carcass material fed to the mink. So it looks as if the BSE type infection is more widespread and that indeed cattle may have their own indigenous agent. We have to be aware of this. The only way we can detect these agents is in mice or hamsters but the assays take a long time.

Spier:
Can the DNA fingerprinting technique be more defined to be able to identify mutants within a cell type.

Stacey:
In looking at the mini satellite sequence we are looking at a basket work of DNA around genes and not specific mutations within the functional genes. If you want to look at single mutations you may need a single locus probe; the present technique is based on a multilocus probe. This latter method thus will not pick up the small differences.

Seefried:
In Canada we have had 4 or 5 outbreaks of Scrapie in sheep and these animals were eradicated. All animals which are suspected as having contracted Rabies are now automatically examined for spongiform encephalopathy and so far they have not found any BSE in Canada.

Handa-Corrigan:
While most of the regulatory issues are focused at the manufacturers of products does there not need to be a separate set of rules which operate at the laboratory scale where we, for example, produce gramme quantities of material for testing by clinicians in named patient trial experiments.

Wisher:
Peter Greenblott at the National Center Institute in USA has suggested a minimal testing procedure for monoclonals to be used in cancer therapy. As many of

the trials are in terminally ill cancer patients the
problem of inducing an infection is not crucial.   In
the situation where the clinical trial expands to many,
non-terminally ill patients an investigation of
possible infection by possible retroviruses etc is
required. contaminations.

Pietrowski: In possible opposition to what has been said so far I
hold that the regulatory requirements of the FDA are
quite reasonable. Both the FDA and the EEC authorities
are asking us to understand our starting materials and
the capabilities of our processes and with the
exception of the limit which has been put on the DNA in
the final product, I do not feel that what we are being
asked to do is too onerous.

Spier: It's the complaint of the manufacturers that in order
to get a product licence you have to generate such a
mass of paper that you can barely get it into a small
sized office. We are thinking of the forests as much
as anything.

Pietrowski: I agree, I think that much of what is submitted is not
what the authorities wish to see.   It is unfortunate
that different authorities wish to see the same data in
different formats. Delays tend to be caused by the
applicants not complying to the requirements.

Spier: Maybe we need clearer and tighter guidelines to find
out what the authorities want sooner rather than find
out what they thought they wanted later.

Pietrowski: The vast majority of the required information is
available.

Omstead: I also think the requirements are not undue although
they take a lot of paper to write down. There are many
steps which take time.   Having obtained approval for
two products in my country the requirements are not
unreasonable. How is the beginning of 1992 going to
change the length of time taken to obtain approval for
a drug?   In our experience you have to go through the
rapporteur, then the working party to the CPMP then the
independent nation review. The only thing which would
be shortened would be the last step. There are a lot
of reasonable questions which will have to be
incorporated in the procedure which will have to
account for the different views of the different
countries.

Horaud: It depends on the product and the process. If you use
a CHO cell and a vector which has already been used the
examination would be much quicker than if you came with
a completely new system.   Companies who employ

excellent molecular biologists often come up with
something new but it is not easy to get through the
agency.

Omstead: I agree the review can't be more streamlined without
decreasing the scientific quality of the review.

MAPPING OF N-LINKED OLIGOSACCHARIDES FROM HUMAN RECOMBINANT GLYCOPROTEINS: QUALITY CONTROL OF GLYCOSYLATED THERAPEUTIC POLYPEPTIDES

Harald S. Conradt, Karin Schaper, Christiane Proppe and Manfred Nimtz

Department of Genetics and Cell Biology, GBF-Gesellschaft für Biotechnologische Forschung mbH, Mascheroder Weg 1, D-3300 Braunschweig

ABSTRACT

The demonstration of lot-to-lot consistency for biotechnologically prepared glycoproteins with respect to oligosaccharide structures is described and examplified by the mapping of N-glycosidically linked oligosaccharides from recombinant human EPO expressed in BHK-21 cells. By comparison with reference oligosaccharides of known structure, high-pH anion-exchange chromatography (HPAE-PAD) of N-glycans liberated by PNGase treatment of the glycoprotein or glycopeptides thereof generated by proteolytic degradation/peptide mapping, can be used to detect even subtle lot-to-lot deviations. The method enables the detection/quantification of the antennarity of glycoprotein oligosaccharides, NeuAc as well as lactosamine repeat content and the presence of proximal fucose. The simple chromatographic procedure is applicable *to routine batch analysis of biotechnologically prepared glycoproteins* (as we could show for AT III, t-PA and IFN-ß from several recombinant host cell lines), is highly reproducible, superior to conventional chromatographic techniques and does not need expensive instrumentation (GC-MS, FAB-MS, NMR), which is required for primary structural analysis of oligosaccharides derived from glycoproteins.

INTRODUCTION

The production of clinically important human glycoproteins in heterologous mammalian cell lines has attracted interest, since it has become increasingly clear, that the carbohydrate portion of these polypeptides play a significant role in their overall biological properties. Apart from the primary structural analysis of the carbohydrate portion of recombinant glycoproteins expressed in various mammalian host cell lines (1) which is required to clarify important biological properties of these products (carbohydrates may affect their : clearance in vivo (NeuAc content), antigenicity (e.g.Galα1-3Gal), susceptibility to proteolytic attack, physicochemical properties), there is a need to control the identity of different biotechnologically prepared glycoprotein batches destined for subsequent clinical trials. A method is required, which enables the rapid evaluation of the quality (with respect to carbohydrate status) of a biotechnological product. Furthermore, elucidation of glycan structures at individual glycosylation sites is desired.

MATERIALS AND METHODS

Purified Human Erythropoietin (EPO)
Human recombinant EPO is a product of Merckle GmbH (Ulm, FRG) and was produced by expression in Baby Hamster Kidney cells (BHK-21). The final product was 99% pure as checked by SDS-PAGE and tryptic mapping of the protein.

High-pH Anion-Exchange Chromatography (HPAE-PAD)
HPAE-PAD was performed using a Dionex BioLC system (Dionex, Sunnyvale, CA, USA) equipped with a CarboPac PA1 column and a pulsed amperometric detector (detection potentials of +0.05, +0,60 and -0.60 V were used). Elution of oligosaccharides was performed by using two gradient programs. Solvent A was 0.1 M NaOH and solvent B was 0.1 M NaOH containing 0.5 M Na-acetate; flow rate was 1ml/min (gradient I : a 30 min linear gradient from 0-10 % B was applied, then a 10 min gradient to 20% B followed by a 10 min isocratic run; gradient II : 20 min from 0-20% solvent B, a 5 min run to 30% B and a further 20 min run to 100% B.

Reference Oligosaccharides
Bi- and triantennary N-glycans bearing α2-3 linked NeuAc and containing proximally α1-6 linked fucose were prepared as described elsewhere (4,5). Bi-antennary N-glycans without proximal fucose, bearing α2-6 linked NeuAc were isolated from human serum antithrombin III (Behringwerke Marburg, FRG). Tetra- and tri-antennary N-glycans were isolated from recombinant EPO expressed in BHK cells (6). The structures of all reference oligosacccharides are established by GC-MS, FAB-MS and 600 MHZ spectroscopy as well as exoglycosidase digestion in combination with HPLC or gel filtration (6,7).

Enzymic treatments
Recombinant human EPO (50-100 micrograms) was incubated in 0.5 ml 100mM Na-phosphate buffer pH 7.7 containing 0.02% Na-azide with 2-5 units of PNGase (Boehringer, Mannheim, FRG) at 37^0C. Complete liberation of N-glycans was checked by SDS-PAGE of the protein. Treatments with neuraminidase and α-fucosidase were performed as described (5,6,7) but pH for incubations with the latter enzyme was 6.5 to inhibit the neuraminidase activity in the preparation used. Oligosaccharides were desalted using a Fast Desalting column (FPLC, Pharmacia) prior to HPAE-PAD analysis.

Carbohydrate structure analysis
GC-MS, FAB-MS and 600 MHZ ^{1}H-NMR spectroscopy were performed similar as described in (4,5,7,8) and will be completely detailed elsewhere (6).

RESULTS AND DISCUSSION

Detailed structural analysis of N-linked oligosaccharides by GC-MS (methylation and compositional analysis), FAB-MS and ^{1}H-NMR revealed the presence of bi- tri- and tetraantennary oligosaccharides (with and without lactosamine repeats) in recombinant human EPO from BHK-21 cells (6). Since the presence of NeuAc has been discussed to be prerequisite for the full biological activity of erythropoietin, we were interested to establish a procedure enabling the rapid analysis of the sialylation state of different batches of recombinant human EPO. In principle, FAB-MS of permethylated oligosaccharides (9), by evaluation of fragment ions derived from the non-reducing end allows important structural informations on N-glycans to be obtained from the presence/absence of the following characteristic ions as examplified in Fig.1 : NeuAc m/z=376(344,minus CH$_3$OH); NeuAc-Hex m/z=580; NeuAc-Hex-HexNAc m/z=825(793); NeuAc-Hex-HexNAc-Hex-HexNAc m/z=1274; Hex-HexNAc-Hex-HexNAc m/z=913(881); Hex-HexNAc m/z=464(432) or the potential human antigenic Galα1-3Galß1-4-GlcNAc structures (Hex-Hex-HexNAc m/z=668) as well as proximal Fucα1-6GlcNAc-OH (deoxyHex-HexNAc-ol m/z= 450). From the relative abundance of these fragment ions (see Fig.1) a high sialylation state of EPO-derived N-linked oligosaccharides can be inferred as well as the absence of Galα1-3Gal. The methodology, however, requires highly sophisticated instrumentation and comparatively high amounts of material (10-50 micrograms of N-glycan). Furthermore, chemical derivatization procedures (reduction and methylation) are required.

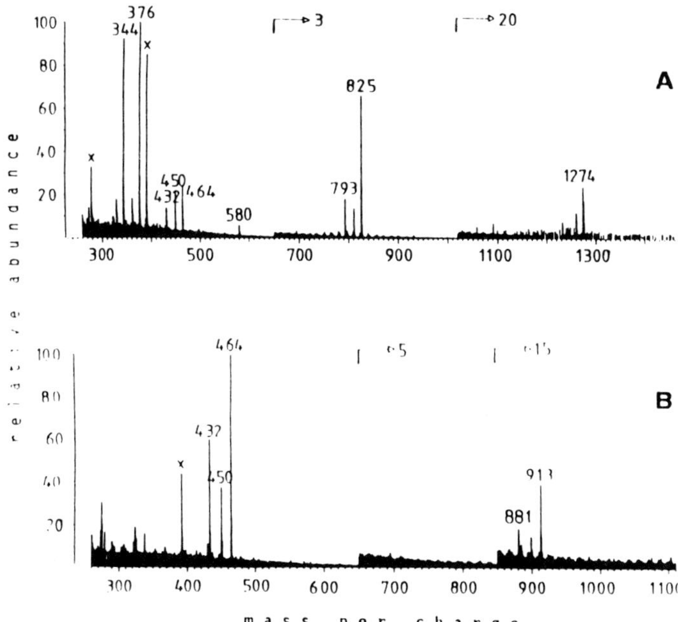

Fig.1.: FAB-MS spectra of reduced and permethylated total N-glycans from recombinant EPO from BHK cells before (A) and after (B) desialylation. Only fragment ions of the lower mass range were recorded in the positive ion mode.

Alternatively, the recently developed high-pH anion-exchange chromatography in conjunction with pulsed amperometric detection (2,3) permits carbohydrate separations and (by comparison with retention times of structurally defined reference oligosaccharides) the analysis of complex oligosaccharide mixtures to be carried out at the subnanomole level.

As shown in Fig. 2 oligosaccharides can be separated in 4 groups according to the number of NeuAc residues present. The monosialylated fraction contains 50% of biantennary structures, the remainder being triantennary structures with a branch at the 6-linked core-mannose and tetraantennary structures in equimolar ratios. The disialylated fraction contains 60% of tetraantennary oligosaccharides, 20% of biantennary chains, triantennary glycans as well as tetraantennary chains with 1 or 2 repeats. The trisialylated fraction contains both isomeric forms of triantennary structures, and 70% of tetraantennary oligosaccharides plus small amounts of 1+2 lactosamine repeats containing derivatives thereof. The tetrasialylated fraction is composed of about 70% of pure tetraantennary chains, 25 % of tetraantennary chains with 1 repeat and small amounts bearing 2 repeats (detailed analysis will be published elsewhere).

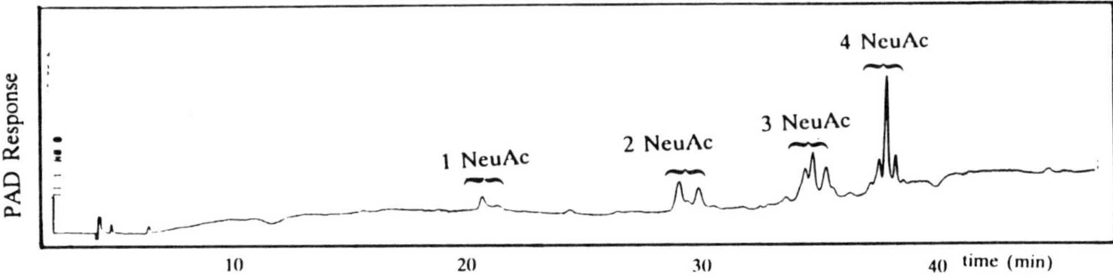

Fig.2 : HPAE-PAD of N-linked oligosaccharides from recombinant human EPO expressed in BHK-21 cells. 100 micrograms of recombinant EPO were digested with PNGase and (after desalting as described under M+M) 1/5 of the liberated oligosaccharides were analyzed by HPAE-PAD using gradient I.

The overall pattern of the neutral oligosaccharide structures after removal of NeuAc by V.cholerae neuraminidase is shown in Fig.3. Obviously, tetraantennary chains (peak 4 = tetrantennary, peak 5 = tetraantennary with 1 repeat (two isomeric forms!) and peaks 6 and 7 = teraantennary with two and three repeats, respectively make up about 90% of oligosaccharides present in the protein. Peak 1 represents the biantennary glycan, peaks 2 and 3 are the two triantennary isomeric glycans with Man-3 and Man-6 being substituted in position 4, or position 6, respectively. *HPAE-PAD of desialylated N-glycans, therefore, allows for detection of antennarity, presence of lactosamine repeats and, addionally, enables the dicrimination between isomeric triantennary forms.*

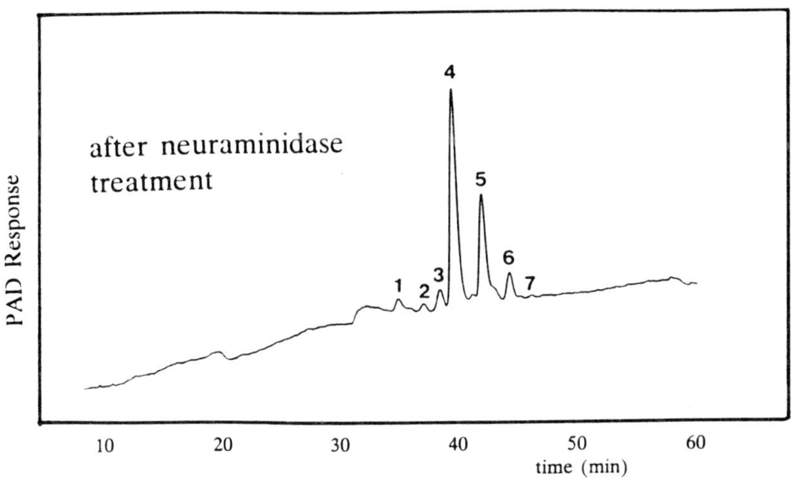

Fig.3 : HPAE-PAD of desialylated N-linked oligosaccharides from human recombinant EPO from BHK-21 cells. Gradient I was used. Structures of peaks 1-7 are explained in the text.

HPAE-PAD allows the detection of proximally linked α1-6 linked fucose in N-glycans. As depicted in Fig.4, after incubation with α-fucosidase , the retention times of tetrasialylated structures (isolated by ion-exchange FPLC using a Mono Q column, Pharmacia) peak a = tetraantennary + 4 NeuAc, b= tetraantennary with 1 repeat + 4 NeuAc as well as c= tetrantennary with 2 repeats + 4 NeuAc are increased significantly.

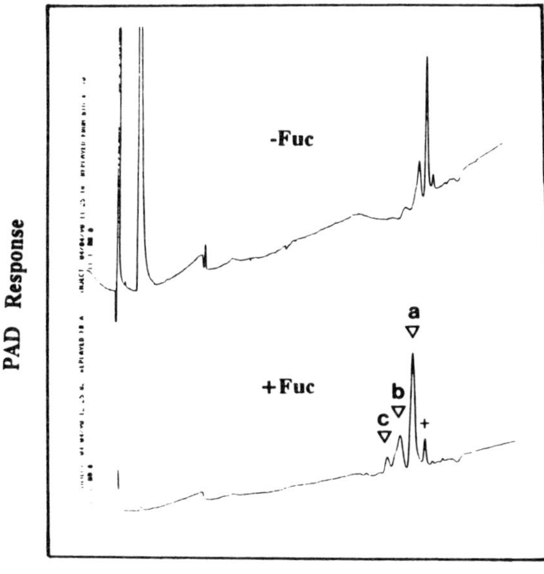

Fig. 4 : HPAE-PAD of tetra-sialylated N-linked oligosaccharides from human recombinant EPO from BHK-21 cells before (+Fuc) and after (-Fuc) treatment with α-fucosidase. Gradient II was used. Structures of peaks a-c as described in the text. The peak marked (+) presumably represents an epimeric form of the tetraantennary oligo-saccharide (a) which is generated under the alkaline conditions during HPAE-PAD.

The elution characteristics in HPAE-PAD of individual oligosaccharide chains bearing different substitutions (antennarity, number of NeuAc residues, linkage type of NeuAc (α2-6 vs. α2-3 to Galß1-4Gal-R), lactosamine repeat content, presence/absence of proximal fucose (see Fig's. 2-4) and Galα1-3Gal) permits the detection of novel oligosaccharides and changes in relative ratios of individual structures in different glycoprotein batches.

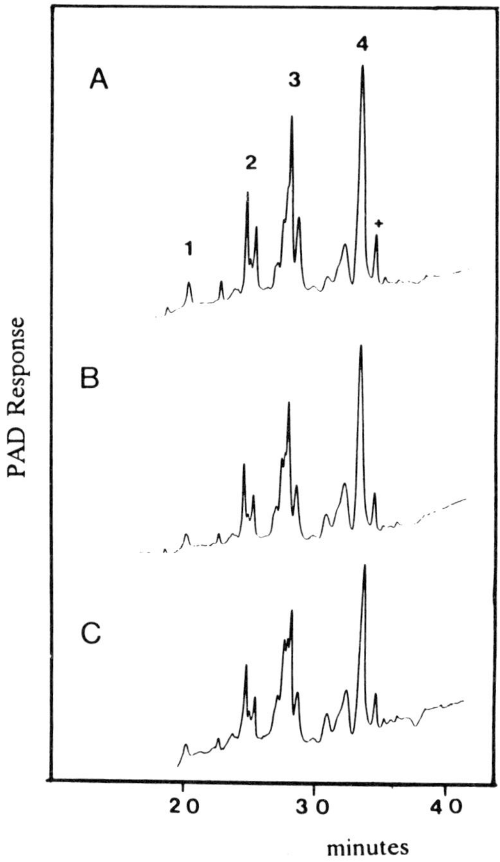

Fig.5 : Comparison of oligosaccharide elution profiles from three recombinant human EPO preparations after HPAE-PAD. 1-4 correspond to oligosaccharide fractions with 1-4 NeuAc residues (compare Fig.2).
Gradient II was used.

Fig.5 shows, that three batches of recombinant human EPO exhibit an almost identical carbohydrate profile; even small differences between batches can be detected (compare the trisialylated oligosaccharide group 3 in panel A+B, Fig.5). *HPAE-PAD represents a rapid and valuable tool for the control of lot-to-lot consistency of oligosaccharides from biotechnologically produced glycoproteins.*

Fig.6 shows the HPAE-PAD profile of oligosaccharides derived from human EPO glycosylation site III (Asn-83). The corresponding tryptic peptide was obtained after peptide-mapping on a Vydac C-18 HPLC-column. Clearly, the proportion of highly sialylated tetra- and triantennary glycans is more pronounced at Asn-83 when compared to the total oligosaccharides released from all N-glycosylation sites (see Fig.5 and Fig.6).

HPAE-PAD enables the detection of subtle differences in oligosaccharide structures of glycoproteins at the level of individual N-glycosylation sites.

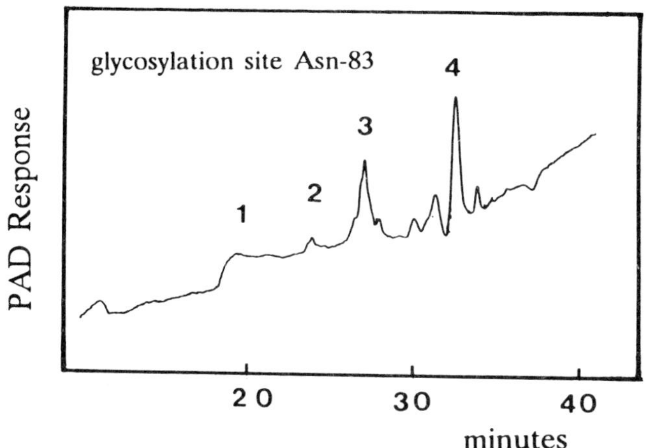

Fig.6 : HPAE-PAD of N-linked oligosaccharides from glycosylation site III (Asn-83) of human EPO from recombinant BHK-21 cells.

References :

1   H.S.Conradt, B.Hofer and H.Hauser, Trends in Glycosci.Glycotech. (1990) in press

3   L.-M.Chen, M.-G.Yet and M.-C.Shao, FASEB J., 2, 2819-2824 (1988)

2   M.R.Hardy and R.R.Townsend, Proc.Natl.Acad.Sci.U.S.A., 85, 3289-3293 (1988)

4   G.Zettlmeissl, H.S.Conradt, M.Nimtz and H.E.Karger
J.Biol.Chem, 264, 21153-21159 (1989)

5   H.S.Conradt, H.Egge, J.Peter-Katalinic, J.Reiser, T.Siklosi and K.Schaper
J.Biol.Chem. 262, 14600-14605 (1987)

6   M.Nimtz and H.S.Conradt (1990) in preparation

7   H.S.Conradt,M.Nimtz,K.E.J.Dittmar,W.Lindenmaier,J.Hoppe and H.Hauser
J.Biol.Chem. 264, 17368-17373 (1989)

8   H.S.Conradt and M.Nimtz
Proceedings of the Xth International Symposium on Glycoconjugates, Jerusalem, Sept.10-15 1989,N.Sharon ed.,pp.162-163

9   A.Dell, Adv.Carbohydr.Chem.Biochem., 45, 19-72 (1987)

Curling: When you look at the different forms of sialic acid
            did you find over prolonged culture that any are
            actually affected? De-sialated oligosaccharides
            do not have a long half-life.

Conradt: We have studied this. The sialation state does not
            matter if you have enough protein in your medium.
            Maybe if you have higher cell densities you will
            get problems with sialidases released. We have in
            all cases found the same amount of sialic acid
            under all culture conditions, except when we have
            introduced glucosamine or galactosamine into the
            medium. These reduced the glycosylation of all
            glycoproteins in all cultures.

Curling: Does it affect the _in vivo_ activity?

Conradt: If there is some sialic acid missing there is a
            decrease of _in vivo_ activity – the clearance rate
            is greatly enhanced.

VALIDATION OF DOWNSTREAM PROCESSING

Gillian Lees [1] and David Onions [2]

[1]Quality Biotech, 6.04 Kelvin Campus, West of Scotland Science Park, Glasgow G20 OSP Scotland.
[2]LRF Virus Centre, University of Glasgow, Glasgow G61 1QH.

ABSTRACT AND INTRODUCTION

Validation helps establish the safety of a product by determining whether unknown or undetected viruses would be removed by the purification process. The safety of a biological product depends on control and testing at several stages.

- . Testing the source material e.g. master working cell bank and extended bank.

- . Testing the bulk product and final product - to determine if latent or introduced viruses are present.

- . Validating the downstream process to remove or preferably inactivate viruses.

Testing the source material and product may fail to reveal mycoplasma or viral contaminants as these can be missed at low concentration unless many repeat samples are made. Similarly, unknown viruses may be present. There are several instances of human and veterinary vaccines being contaminated by viruses including the contamination of poliovirus vaccine by SV-40 present in the rhesus monkey cells used to prepare early vaccines. In the veterinary field such viral contaminants have resulted in transpecies transmission and disease induction on a wide scale as occurred in the transmission of adenovirus 76.

BASIC PRINCIPLES OF A VALIDATION DESIGN

The basic principles of a validation are shown in the accompanying diagram. A downscaled system is constructed and the size of the system is constrained by (1) a need to introduce a minimum virus spike of 10^8 infectious units in 10% or less of the load volume (2) a requirement to keep the retained output volume low to be able to titrate the virus (3) a requirement to keep transit times and protein concentrations as near as possible to the full scale system. The output buffers have to be tested for cytotoxicity. When buffers are cytotoxic,

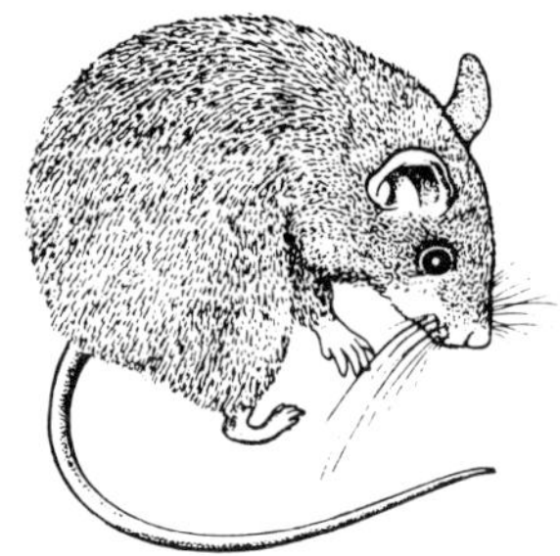

MURINE   HYBRIDOMAS

RETROVIRUS   MuLV
(ss RNA enveloped)

The retrovirus is present in all hybridomas
as DNA provirus which may be expressed

HERPESVIRUS   HSV
(ds DNA enveloped)

Herpesviruses may remain as latent infection
in lymphoid cells.   A new member of the
gamma-herpesviruses has recently been identified
in mice

PICORNOVIRUS   Poliovirus
(ss RNA unenveloped)

This small RNA virus displays high to medium
resistance to most physicochemical agents

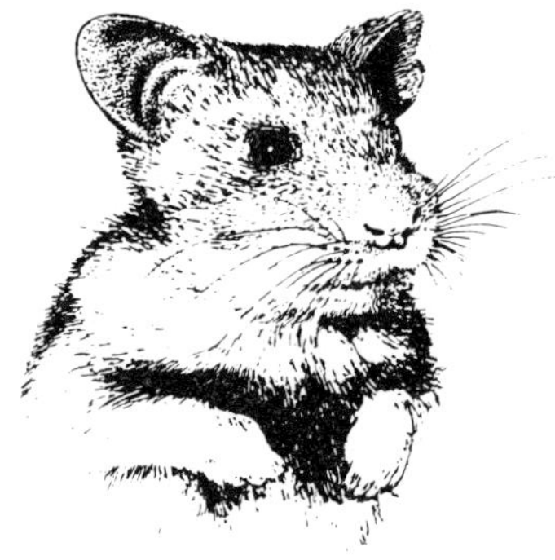

CHO   CELLS

Viruses   above but in addition one   may include:-

REOVIRUS 3
(ds RNA unenveloped)

This virus displays high resistance to physico-
chemical agents and can infect both man
and CHO cells

validated virus concentration and purification methods have to be used.

The volume of the retained output should be as low as possible. Note that if no virus is detected in small 1-2ml samples of the output a minimum titre is assumed from the Poisson distribution. For instance if the true titre is 1×10^3 iu/ml a 1 ml sample will be negative on 37% of occasions but at 5×10^3 iu/ml will be negative on only 0.67% of occasions. If 5 iu/ml is assumed in the retained output the total assumed titre is equal to the volume x 5.

In order to determine if inactivation or clearance is occurring it is necessary to conduct inactivation studies, but it is also useful to monitor the levels of virus in the non-retained fractions. A validation positive control is included to assess the effects of freeze-thawing and storage on the spike virus.

VIRUSES IN VALIDATIONS

Validations may be conducted for DNA, mycoplasma, viruses and agents like Scrapie or BSE. For virus validations a minimum of 3 viruses are chosen. One virus should be a retrovirus since these may be inherited in the germ line or remain as latent infections. For murine hybridomas and CHO cells MuLV is appropriate, but for human cells the Maedi-Visna virus is preferable as, like the human lentivirus HIV, it is more resistant to temperature and other physical parameters.

The other viruses are chosen to represent a range of physico-chemical properties and in general at least one virus should be resistant to many physical and chemical agents. In those cases where a virus is known to be present it should also be included in the validation. A herpesvirus like herpes simplex 1 should be included. In our experience they are more resistant than retroviruses and they may remain as latent viruses in lymphoid and other cell types. Poliovirus provides a severe test, being a small unenveloped virus resistant to many physical and chemical effects. However each validation has to be considered separately and viruses chosen with knowledge of the starting material and the types of risk associated with it.

PROBLEMS IN EVALUATING VALIDATIONS

Several factors affect the interpretation of the results of a validation. The overall clearance of a system is often regarded as the sum of the logarithm of the clearance at each stage (multiplicative clearance). However, several factors can lead to additive clearance. If, as shown in the diagram below, inactivation of one step in a stage is dependent on a specific buffer and this used as the input of a second stage, this can lead to an inactivation step being counted twice.

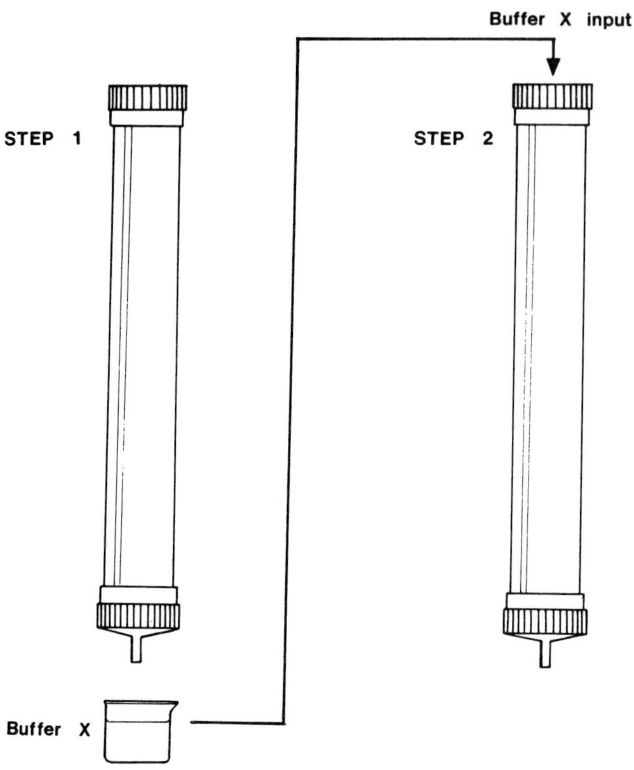

Input Buffer of STEP 2 is the same as output of STEP 1.   Inactivation of virus may be counted twice

CLEARANCE MAY BE ADDITIVE

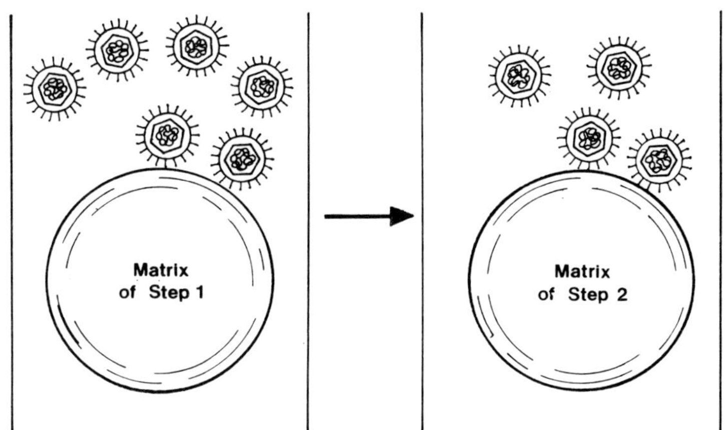

Clearance is dependent on binding of virus to matrix. Total clearance may therefore be dependent on total matrix volume and become additive not mutiplicative between stages

VIRUS BUILDS UP ON MATRIX

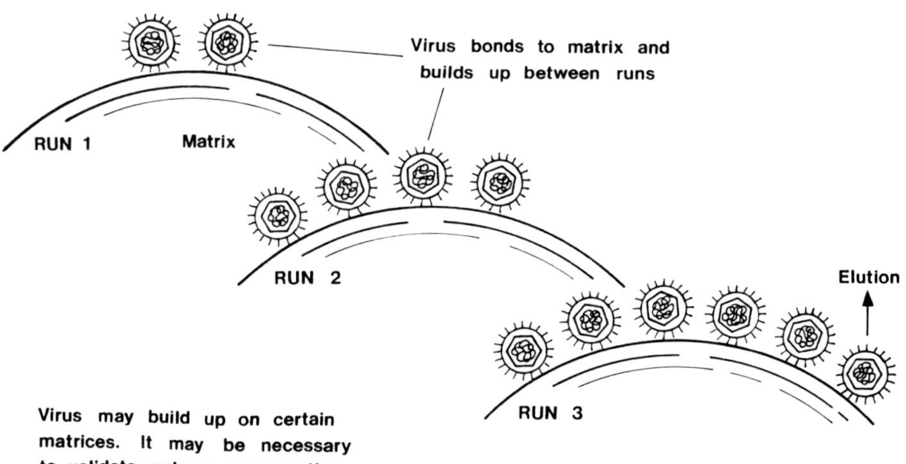

Virus may build up on certain
matrices. It may be necessary
to validate column regeneration

Virus prepared from tissue culture may aggregate and virus can escape inactivation by being present in the centre of clumps leading to a 'persistent fraction'. Similarly if virus clearance is dependent on adsorption to the column matrix, this can lead to additive rather than multiplicative clearance between stages.

<u>INACTIVATION VERSUS CLEARANCE</u>

Wherever possible inactivation steps are preferable to clearance steps and specific inactivation steps should be conducted. However our experience with the inactivation of the retrovirus feline leukaemia virus indicates that inactivation is often non-linear with a persistent fraction forming. Temperature and pH inactivation steps can be altered by protein and divalent cations and the levels of these should reflect the situation seen in the downstream process. Viruses also vary widely in their susceptibility to different inactivation processes as shown for the effects of UV irradiation and temperature on retroviruses.

	Heat	UV Inactivation
Retrovirus (FeLV)	t 1/2 6 hrs at 37°C	2nd Order kinetics
Poliovirus	t 1/2 Infectivity > 24 hrs at 37°C	1st Order kinetics

THE CULTURE ENVIRONMENT AFFECTS RECOMBINANT PROTEIN PROCESSING IN CHO
CELLS

P. Hayter, E. Curling, A. Baines, A. Bull, I. Salmon, P. Strange, and N.
Jenkins

Biological Laboratory, University of Kent, Canterbury, Kent, CT2 7NJ,
U.K.

ABSTRACT

The effect of the culture environment on the expression of recombinant
human interferon-gamma (IFN-γ) in Chinese hamster ovary cells (CHO) was
investigated. In typical batch cultures IFN-γ production appeared to be
growth-related, however it was possible to manipulate the environment
such that IFN-γ production continued in the absence of cell growth. This
suggests that IFN-γ production was influenced by the metabolic state of
the cell rather than the specific growth rate per se. The degree of IFN-γ
glycosylation also varied with the physiological state of the cell with a
gradual increase in the proportion of underglycosylated IFN-γ produced by
the cells towards the end of the growth phase.

INTRODUCTION

The efficacy of many therapeutic mammalian proteins is dependent upon the
accuracy of post translational modifications carried out during their
synthesis (1,2). It has therefore been considered that such proteins can
only be effectively expressed in mammalian cells which are able to carry
out the correct post translational modifications (3,4). The disadvantages
with mammalian cell production systems lie with the relatively low
product yields achieved and considerable attention has been given to the
improvement of cell and product yields by manipulation of the cell
environment. However there is less information on the effect of the cell
environment on the accuracy of protein expression.

In this study we have examined both the kinetics of recombinant
human interferon-γ production and the variation in product heterogeneity
in Chinese hamster ovary cells (CHO). IFN-γ consists of a single
polypeptide with two N-linked glycosylation sites at asparagine residues
28 and 100. Both natural and IFN-γ produced by CHO cells show
heterogeneity in the degree of glycosylation (5,6). Although
glycosylation of IFN-γ is not essential for its biological activity it is
nonetheless a useful model in which to study the effect of the culture
environment on the expression and heterogeneity of a recombinant protein.

MATERIALS AND METHODS

The cells used in this investigation were derived from a DHFR$^-$ mutant of
CHO-K1 cells. These cells were expressing human interferon-γ which was
co-amplified with DHFR by methotrexate selection.

The medium was a serum-free formulation based on RPMI 1640 supplemented with 5mg/ml bovine serum albumin (Miles Laboratories), 5μg/ml
insulin, 5μg/ml transferrin, 1mM pyruvic acid, 0.1mM alanine, 1μM
putrescine, 3μM $FeSO_4$, 3μM $ZnSO_4$, 10nM Na_2SeO_3 and 10nM $CuSO_4$ (Sigma).

Cells for fermenter studies were harvested from 500ml spinner cultures (Techne, Cambridge) and seeded at 1 x 10^5/ml in a 2 litre fermenter (Bioengineering AG, Wald, Switzerland). The pH was controlled at 7.2 by automatic CO_2 addition and the dissolved oxygen tension was controlled at 50% by the automatic sparging of air.

Shake flask cultures (100ml) were performed in 250ml Erlenmeyer flasks. The headspace of the flask was purged with a mixture of 5% CO_2 in air to maintain pH. The flasks were shaken at 100rpm in a shaking incubator at 37°C.

Glucose and lactate concentrations were determined using commercial assays (Sigma test no. 635 and 826-UV), ammonia concentrations were determined by the method of Fawcett and Scott (7) and IFN-γ concentrations were determined by sandwich ELISA using monoclonal antibodies supplied by Celltech. Ltd.

IFN-γ for SDS-polyacrylamide gel (PAGE) analysis was immunoprecipitated using a monoclonal antibody which recognises all IFN-γ variants and purified using protein A-Sepharose. Proteins were revealed by silver staining (8) and the relative intensity of the protein bands determined by scanning densitometry.

RESULTS AND DISCUSSION

CHO cells seeded at 1 x 10^5 cells/ml reached approximately 1 x 10^6 cells/ml after 100 hours after which there was a rapid decline in cell viability (Fig. 1). The maximum cell growth rate was 0.032h^{-1} but declined after about 50-60 hours. IFN-γ was produced during the growth phase with the highest production rate associated with the exponential phase of cell growth. The rate of IFN-γ production (q_{IFN}), declined in parallel with cell growth rate suggesting that there was a relationship between cell growth and IFN-γ production.

Glucose was consumed rapidly and was exhausted by the end of the growth phase (Fig. 2). Lactic acid and ammonia accumulated during growth reaching concentrations of 12mM and 2mM respectively. The rate of glucose uptake (q_{glc}) and the rates of lactate and ammonia production (q_{lac}, q_{amm}) also declined during the growth phase. The changes in cell growth rate and metabolism could not be attributed to pH changes or oxygen starvation since both these parameters were maintained at a constant level.

IFN-γ produced by CHO cells in batch culture was immunoprecipitated and analysed by SDS-PAGE. Using this technique several molecular weight variants could be discerned (Fig. 3). The bands formed three clusters at molecular weights of 23-27kDa, 19-21 and 15-17kDa. It has been confirmed by N-glycanase and tunicamycin treatment that the clusters of bands at 19-21kDa and 23-27 represent glycosylated variants of the protein whereas the bands at 15-17kDa represent the non-glycosylated form (data not shown). The presence of multiple bands within each glycosylation variant is probably due to proteolytic processing at the carboxyl terminal of the IFN-γ polypeptide (9).

Analysis of samples taken during a batch culture of CHO cells showed that the proportions of each glycosylation variant changed as the culture progressed (Fig. 3). There was a gradual decline in the proportion of the doubly glycosylated variants from 60% to 30% and an increase in the proportion of non-glycosylated variants from undetectable levels to 30% of the total IFN-γ by the end of the culture. These changes were not observed in metabolically labelled IFN-γ which was added to CHO cell cultures suggesting that the changes in protein heterogeneity occurred

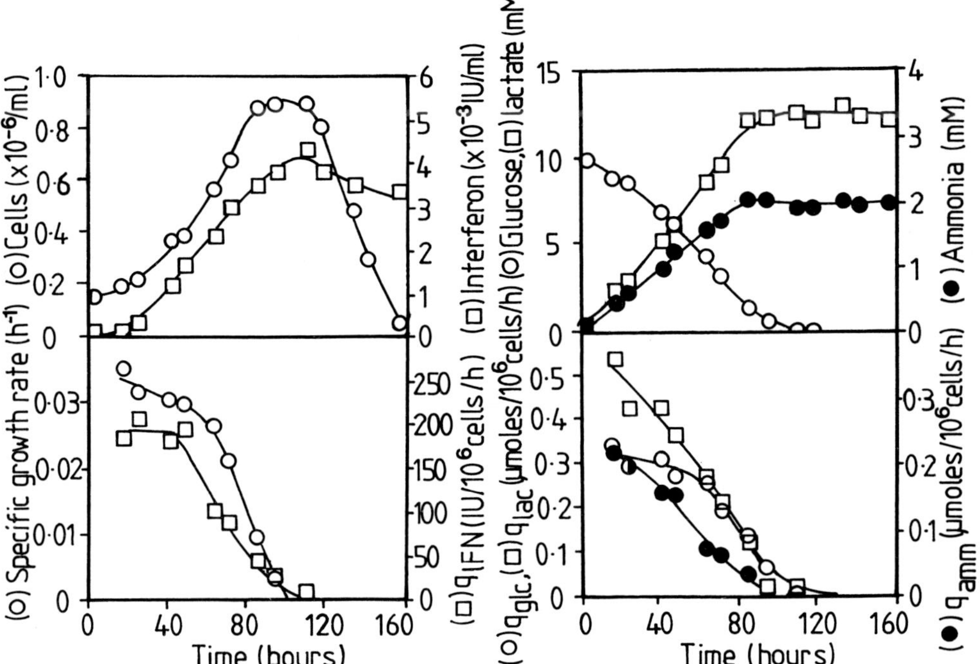

Figure 1. Cell growth and IFN-γ production in stirred batch culture

Figure 2. Cell metabolism in stirred batch culture

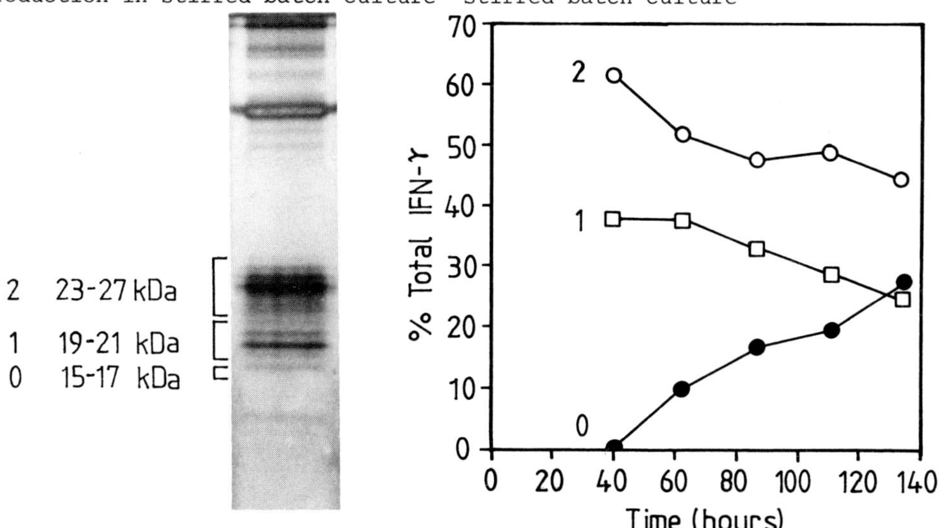

Figure 3. Interferon heterogeneity in stirred batch culture. The groups of bands resolved by SDS-PAGE represent 0, non-glycosylated IFN-γ, 15-17kD (●); 1, glycosylation at one Asn residue, 19-21kD (□) and 2, glycosylation at both Asn residues 23-27kD (O).

during IFN-γ biosynthesis and were not due to degradation of the product in the medium. Thus it appears that alterations in IFN-γ heterogeneity are likely to be a reflection of the changes in cell metabolic activity during the course of a batch culture.

It was considered possible that the increase in the proportion of under glycosylated variants could be due to glucose starvation since glucose was exhausted by the end of the growth phase. It has been shown that factors which perturb carbohydrate metabolism such as glucose starvation can cause defects in protein glycosylation (10).

To determine whether the depletion of glucose was responsible for the changes in IFN-γ glycosylation, batch cultures were initiated at a higher initial glucose concentration (22mM as opposed to 10mM in previous cultures). No significant differences in either cell growth or IFN-γ production were observed at the higher initial glucose concentration (Fig. 4). Glucose was not exhausted in these cultures but the glucose uptake rate was considerably higher during the growth phase and continued at a high rate during the decline phase. Despite the high rate of glucose metabolism, the proportion of fully glycosylated IFN-γ variants declined during the latter half of the growth phase. By the end of the growth phase there were similar proportions of each variant as were seen in batch cultures with lower glucose concentrations (Fig. 5). This suggests that there is no simple relationship between glycolytic flux and protein glycosylation in these cells.

Analysis of amino acid metabolism by CHO cells showed that glutamine was the most rapidly depleted amino acid and it was exhausted by the end of the growth phase in batch cultures (data not shown). For this reason the effect of varying the glutamine concentration on CHO cell growth and IFN-γ production was investigated. To ensure that glucose was not limiting at higher glutamine concentrations the experiments were carried out at both normal (10mM) and high glucose concentrations (20mM) in 100ml shake flask cultures.

No difference in either cell growth or IFN-γ production was observed when the glutamine concentration was increased from 2mM to 4mM (Table 1). However there was a reduction in cell growth at 1mM glutamine and no growth in the absence of glutamine although cell viability remained high for 240 hours. It is notable that IFN-γ production continued in the glutamine-starved cells and the rate of Ifn-γ production was similar for proliferating and non-proliferating cells. The maintenance of high cell viability and continued protein synthesis in the absence of cell growth indicates that the rate of IFN-γ production in these cells is affected more by the physiological state of the cell than the cell growth rate per se.

Together these findings suggest that both the rate of production and the accuracy of protein processing in CHO cells are influenced by the physiological state of the cell. This in turn is influenced by changes in the cell's environment which may result from nutrient depletion or metabolite accumulation. Identification of those factors which affect not only the kinetics but also the fidelity of protein expression will facilitate the monitoring and control of protein production by mammalian cell cultures.

ACKNOWLEDGEMENTS

We thank Richard Willson for expert technical assistance; Wellcome Biotechnology Ltd. for the CHO cell line; Celltech Ltd. for the monoclonal antibodies and the SERC Biotechnology Directorate, Celltech,

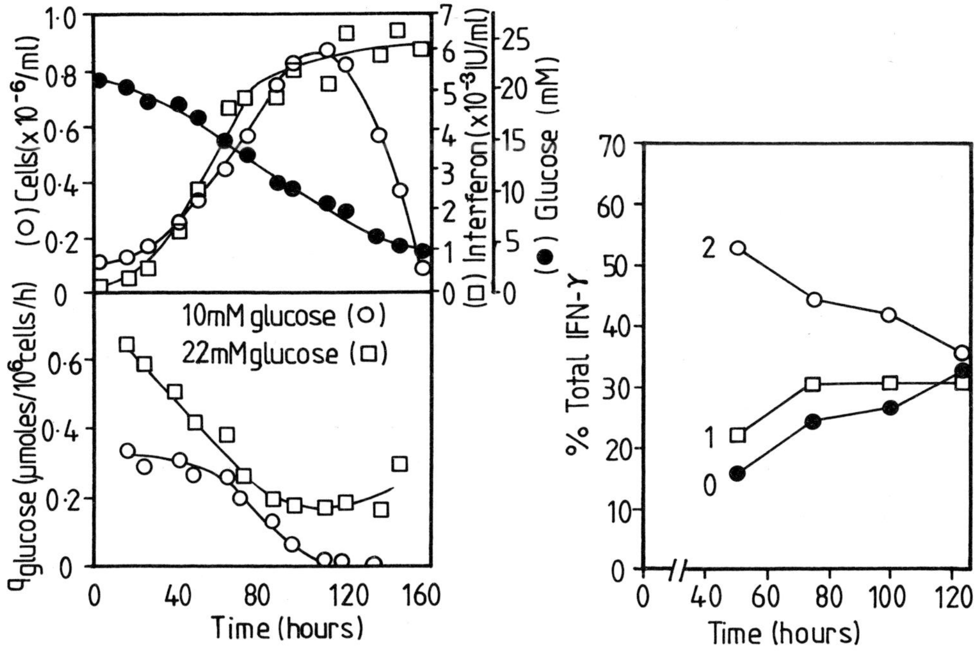

Figure 4. Effect of glucose on cell growth and IFN-γ production.

Figure 5. Effect of glucose on IFN-γ heterogeneity.

10mM glucose Glutamine (mM)	Cell number (x10⁶/ml)	Specific growth rate (h⁻¹)	Interferon concentration (IU/ml)	q_{IFN} (IU/10⁶ cells/h)
0	0.17	0.001	1350	74
1	1.07	0.021	3000	54
2	1.31	0.027	3650	68
4	1.36	0.026	3500	59

20mM glucose Glutamine (mM)				
0	0.18	0.001	1150	44
1	1.09	0.021	3000	54
2	1.31	0.026	3500	51
4	1.34	0.027	3800	53

Table 1. Effect of glutamine on cell growth and IFN-γ production.

Glaxo, Porton Internatinal, Smith-Kline Beecham and Wellcome Biotechnology for support of the research program of which the work described here was part.

REFERENCES

1. Busby, S., Kumar, A., Jospeh, M., Halfpap, L., Insley, M., Berkner, K., Kurachi, K. and Woodbury, R. Expression of active human factor IX in transfected cells. Nature 1985, 316, 271
2. Dube, S., Fisher, J.W. and Powell, J.S. Glycosylation at specific sites of erythropoietin is essential for biosynthesis, secretion and biological function. J. Biol. Chem. 1988, 263, 17516
3. Bebbington, C. and Hentschel, C. The expression of recombinant DNA products in mammalian cells. Trends Biotechnol. 1985, 3, 314
4. Lubiniecki, A.S. Pharmaceutical applications of recombinant DNA-modified mammalian cells. Develop. Industrial Microbiol. 1987, 28, 133
5. Rinderknecht, E., O'Connor, B.H. and Rodriguez, H. Natural human interferon-γ. Complete aminoa cid sequence and determination of sites of glycosylation. J. Biol. Chem. 1984, 259, 6790
6. Mutsaers, J.H.G.M., Kammerling, J.P., Devos, R., Guisez, Y., Friers, W. and Vliegenthart, J.F.G. Structural studies of the carbohydrate chains of human γ-interferon. Eur. J. Biochem. 1986, 156, 651
7. Fawcett, J.K. and Scott, J.E. A rapid and precise method for the determination of urea. J. Clin. Pathol. 1960, 13, 156
8. Johnson, A. and Thorpe, R. Immunochemistry in Practice. 2nd ed. Blackwells, U.K. 1987, pp. 150-151
9. Arakawa, T., Hsu, Y.R., Parker, C.G. and Lai, P.H. Role of polycationic C-terminal portion in the structure and activity of recombinant human interferon-γ. J. Biol. Chem. 1986, 261, 8534
10. Chapman, A.E. and Calhoun, J.C. Effects of glucose starvation and puromycin treatment on lipid-linked oligosaccharide precursors and biosynthetic enzymes in Chinese hamster ovary cells in vivo and in vitro. Arch. Biochem. Biophys. 1988, 260, 320

Gerbert: Do you know whether the sugars on your molecule changed with serum and serum-free growth?

Hayter: We get the same pattern.

Gerbert: Do you see any change if you grow your cells with different types of sugars, or with lipid supplements?

Hayter: We have tried supplementing mannose, N-acetyl glucosamine and several other sugars and we saw no effect at all.

Gerbert: Did you see any de-sialation of your molecules upon standing of the media at 4°C?

Hayter: I don't know if this occurs.

THE Medi-Cult® HYBRITEST - A NEW TEST FOR *IN VITRO* TOXICOLOGY

Hans Ingolf Nielsen[1] and Kjell Bertheussen[2]

[1]Medi-Cult a/s, Kanalholmen 12, DK-2650 Hvidovre, Denmark, and
[2]Dept. of Clinical Medicine, University of Tromsø, Norway.

ABSTRACT

The Medi-Cult® Hybritest is based on the proliferation of a
sensitive, but rapidly growing murine hybridoma cell line (1E6)
in the protein-free RPMI-SR3 medium. Due to the fact that this
medium is protein-free, the system becomes very sensitive,
since there are no possibilities for toxins to be bound and
neutralized by binding proteins like albumin, transferrin and
antibodies, etc.
Keywords: In vitro toxicology, Toxicity, Bioassay, Serum-free
media, Defined media, Cell culture, Quality control.

INTRODUCTION

Many bioassays for cytotoxicity testing and based upon cultures
cells or mouse embryos present problems due to either the
medium or the cells or simply the complexity of the measurements. Often the sensitivity is poor due to the high concentrations of detoxifying, binding proteins in the medium -
such as albumin, transferrin, antibodies, etc. For anchorage
dependent cells, adherence problems caused by e.g. the
substrata may also interfere with the results. A way of
avoiding these problems would be to use a sensitive and
anchorage independent cell line, which proliferates rapidly in
a protein-free medium.

MATERIALS AND METHODS

In the method described here, the practically protein-free
medium RPMI-SR3 Medi-Cult a/s, Denmark) was used (1,2). This
medium contains insulin as the only peptide (0.5 mg/l). As test
cells were chosen the murine hybridoma cell line 1E6. This cell
line combines a high sensitivity to toxins with a rapid
proliferation. The cells are seeded at a density of 1-2 x 10^4
cells/ml and within 7-8 days reach a maximum density of around
10^6 cells/ml in case of no toxicity.

The Hybritest is simply based on the proliferation rate. In
order to count the cells in the middle of the exponential
growth, they are harvested after 4 days, and - in case of no
toxicity - typically yield around 2 x 10^5 cells/ml. The
Hybritest is presently being used for testing basal cell
culture media, water, cell separation media, drugs, chemicals,
plastics, glassware etc.

Hybritest procedure for fluid media.
1. Test medium and RPMI-SR3 is mixed 1:1, and possible deviations in pH and osmolality compensated for
2. 1 ml medium is pipetted into each 1.9 cm^2 culture well (quadruplicate)
3. 2 x10^4 cells are added per well
4. Incubation for 4 days
5. Cells are counted
6. Growth inhibition is calculated relative to a control culture in a known batch of RPMI-SR3. A minimum of 10 times increase in cell number is normally required.

Hybritest procedure for water.
1. RPMI-SR3 is made up using the test water
2 - 6. as above.

Hybritest procedure for powdered media.
1. Test medium is made up with a known batch of water, and mixed 1:1 with RPMI-SR3
2 - 6. as above.

Hybritest procedure for chemicals and drugs.
1. Chemical or drug is added to RPMI-SR3 in the required concentrations
2 - 6. as above.

Hybritest procedure for plastics, glassware, paraffin etc.
1. Extraction in RPMI-SR3 in darkness with specified temperature, time and shaking
2 - 6. as above.

RESULTS AND DISCUSSION

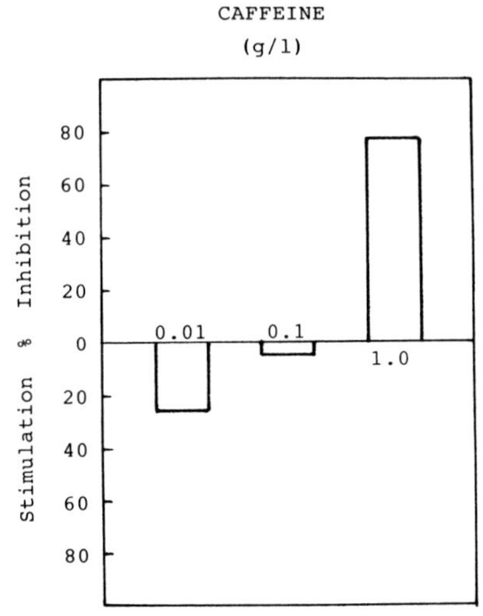

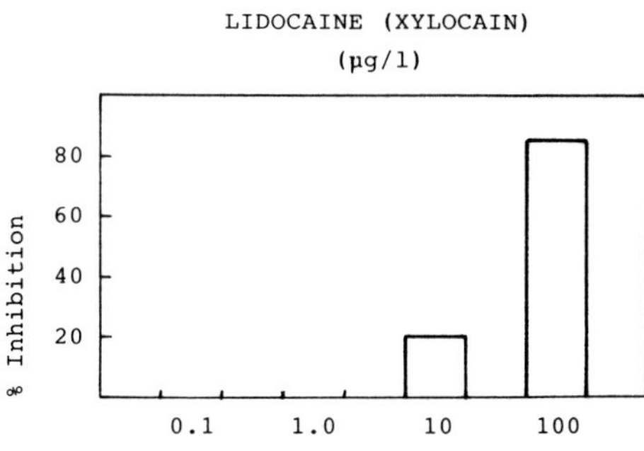

Figures 1 - 2. Examples of Hybritests of chemicals

It is a well-known fact that fluid media degrade relatively rapidly and become cytotoxic (3). This is particularly critical if such media are used in serum-free culture. A Hybritest study at the University of Tromsø using ready-made fluid media from three producers showed as an example a cytotoxicity of 0 - 92% for EBSS (5 batches) and 61 - 100% for Ham's F10 (3 batches). Studies on powdered media from the same producers gave the encouraging result of no toxicity at all. This shows the importance of using a freshly made-up medium. It is, however, of great importance to use water of a high quality. In a Hybritest study of 11 brands of commercially available, sterile water, 9 were found to be toxin-free, whereas the remaining two had toxicities of 11% and 88%, respectively.

Figures 1 - 2 show examples of Hybritests of chemicals. Note that the Hybritest is not only able to show growth inhibition, but may indicate growth stimulation, as well.

ACKNOWLEDGEMENTS

The skilful assistance of Anna-Lise Poulsen and Susanne Rasmussen is gratefully acknowledged.

REFERENCES

1. Bertheussen, K., N.Holst, F.Forsdahl and K.E.Høie. A new cell culture assay for quality control in IVF. _Human Reproduction_, 1989, _4_, 531-535.
2. Nielsen, H.I. and K.Bertheussen. The Medi-Cult® Hybritest for _in vitro_ toxicology and quality control. _ATLA_, 1990, _17_, 199-202.
3. Nielsen, H.I. and K.Bertheussen. Degrading effect of light on cell culture media. _This volume_.

List of exhibitors

Alfa-Laval Centritech AB
Amicon
Applikon
B. Braun Sciencetec
Bio/Technology
Bocknek Ltd
Cellon Sarl
Celltech Ltd
Chemap Groupe Alfa-Laval
Cytolab
ECACC
Gibco
Hyclone
IBF
Immuno-Chemical Products
Ingold France
Institut Jacques Boy

Intermed SA
In Vitron Corporation
LH Fermentation Ltd
LSL Biolaffitte
MBR Bio Reactor AG
Medical and Veterinary Supplies Ltd
Microbiological Associates Ltd
Miles
Millipore
New Brunswick Scientific
PAA-Labor-und Forschungs
Quality Biotech Ltd
Sera-Lab
SGI
Sigma Chimie
Sorebio
Verax Corporation

List of Participants

ADAMSON S. ROBERT
GENETICS INSTITUTE INC.
ONE BURTT ROAD
01810　　ANDOVER MA
ETATS UNIS

AGUILON FRANCOIS
SANOFI ELF BIO-RECHERCHES
LABEGE -INNOPOLE - VOIE NO 1
B.P 137
31328　　LABEGE CEDEX
FRANCE

AKAI KUNIHISA
SNOW BRAND MILK PRODUCTS CO LT
519 SHIMO-ISHIBASHI
ISHIBASHI-MACHI
329-05　　SHIMOTSUGA-GUN
JAPON

AL-RUBEAI MOHAMED
SCHOOL OF CHEMICAL ENGINEERING
UNIVERSITY OF BIRMINGHAM
B15 2TT　BIRMINGHAM
GRANDE BRETAGNE

ALBAHN HENRIK
DEPT. OF BIOTECHNOLOGY
BLOCK 223, THE TECHNICAL
UNIVERSITY OF DENMARK
DK-2800　LYNGBY
DANEMARK

ALMGREN JOAKIM K.G.
HYCLONE AB
SOLVEG 41
S-22370　LUND
SUEDE

ANDERSON KEVIN PATRICK
GENENTECH, INC.
460 POINT SAN BRUNO BLVD.
94080　　SOUTH SAN FRANCISCO CA
ETATS UNIS

APELMAN STIG
ALFA-LAVAL CENTRITECH AB
S-147 80 TUMBA
SUEDE

ARATHOON ROBERT
460 PT. SAN BRUNO BLVD.
M.S. #32
94080　　SOUTH SAN FRANCISCO, CA
ETATS UNIS

ARCHINARD PH.
BIOMERIEUX
69280　　MARCY L'ETOILE
FRANCE

AVIGNON JEAN-LOUIS
B.P 19
69780　　ST PIERRE DE CHAUDIEU
FRANCE

BAIJOT BRUNO
SMITH KLINE BIOLOGICALS
RUE DE L'INSTITUT 89
1330　　RIXENSART
BELGIQUE

BAILLET PASCALE
INSTITUT MERIEUX
1541 AVENUE MARCEL MERIEUX
69280　　MARCY L'ETOILE
FRANCE

BARBER ALAN
LH FERMENTATION LTD
PORTON HOUSE, VANWALL ROAD
SL6 40B　MAIDENHEAD
GRANDE BRETAGNE

BECHSTEDT WOLFGANG
CHEMIEANLAGENBAU
LEIPZIG-GRIMMA
PF 674 LEIPZIG
7010　　LEIPZIG
REPUB. DEMOCRAT. ALLEMANDE

BEHRENDT ULRICH
BOEHRINGER MANNHEIM GMBH
NONNENWALD 2
D-8122　PENZBERG
ALLEMAGNE FEDERALE

BELL SARAH LORAINE
DEPARTMENT OF MICROBIOLOGY
SURREY UNIVERSITY
GU2 5XH　GUILDFORD
GRANDE BRETAGNE

BELLANGER LAURENT
CIS BIOINDUSTRIES
B.P 171
30205　　BAGNOLS SUR CEZE CEDEX
FRANCE

BENAROYA ANDRE
FLOBIO
15 RUE ARMAND SYLVESTRE
92400　　COURBEVOIE
FRANCE

BENAROYA LAURENT
FLOBIO
15 RUE ARMAND SYLVESTRE
92400　　COURBEVOIE
FRANCE

BENET GERARD
RHONE MERIEUX LABORATORY
254 RUE MARCEL MERIEUX
B.P 7009
69342　　LYON CEDEX 07
FRANCE

BERNARD ALAIN
GLAXO-IMB
46 ROUTE DES ACACIAS
CH-1211　GENEVE
CONFEDERATION HELVETIQUE

BERTHOLD WOLFGANG
DR. KARL THOMAE GMBH
ABT. BIOTECHNISCHE PRODUKTION
BIRKENDORFER STRABE 65
D-7950　　BIBERACH/RIB
ALLEMAGNE FEDERALE

BEY ELKE
P.O BOX 488
KELVIN
2054　　SANDTON
AFRIQUE DU SUD

BILL EBERHARD
BIOFERON BIOCHEMISCHE SUSTANZ.
GMBH&CO
ERWIN-RENTSCHLER-STR 21
D-7958　　LAUPHEIM
ALLEMAGNE FEDERALE

BILLIG DAVID
POLYDEX BIOLOGICALS LTD
415 COMSTOCK ROAD
M1L 2H4　SCARBOROUGH, ONTARIO
CANADA

BISELLI MANFRED
INSTITUT FUR BIOTECHNOLOGIE
KFA JULICH POSTFACH 1913
5170　　JULICH
ALLEMAGNE FEDERALE

BJOERLING TORSTEN
ALFA-LAVAL CENTRITECH AB
S-147 80 TUMBA
SUEDE

BLAKE KAREN
ECACC, PHLS - CAMR
PORTON DOWN
SP4 0JG　SALISBURY, WILTS
GRANDE BRETAGNE

BLASEY HORST
GLAXO
INSTITUTE FOR MOLECULAR
BIOLOGY SA
CH-1211　GENEVA
CONFEDERATION HELVETIQUE

BLIEM RUDOLF
BRISTOL-MYERS COMPANY
PO BOX 4755
NY13221-4755
　　　　SYRACUSE
ETATS UNIS

BLUML GERALD
INSTITUTE OF APPLIED MICROBIOL
UNIVERSITY OF AGRICULTURE
PETER JORDANSTR 82
A-1180　WIEN
AUTRICHE

BOCKNEK GAIL
165 BETHRIDGE ROAD
M9W 1N4　TORONTO, ONTARIO
CANADA

BODY MARIELLE
DEVINEAU SA
42 RUE DE PARADIS
75010   PARIS
FRANCE

BOEDEKER BERTHOLD
CUTTER LABS
4th. & PARKER STREETS
94701   BERKELEY
ETATS UNIS

BOGOSSIAN EVELYNE
CRBA - PROCIDA RU
B.P 1
13367   MARSEILLE
FRANCE

BOLLO ENRICO
SORIN BIOMEDICA SPA
VIA CRESCENTINO
13040   SALUGGIA (VC)
ITALIE

BOLTON BRYAN JOHN
ECACC, PHLS - CAMR
PORTON DOWN
SP4 OJG SALISBURY, WILTSHIRE
GRANDE BRETAGNE

BORASTON ROBERT CHARLES
CELLTECH LTD.
216 BATH ROAD
SLI 4EN SLOUGH, BERKSHIRE
GRANDE BRETAGNE

BOSCHETTI EGISTO
I.B.F.
35 AVENUE JEAN JAURES
92390   VILLENEUVE LA GARENNE
FRANCE

BOUSICAUX ALAIN
BIOVIRUS
BP 86
69280   MARCY L'ETOILE
FRANCE

BRATTLE MALCOLM
QUALITY BIOTECH LTD
WEST OF SCOTLAND SCIENCE PARK,
KELVIN CAMPUS
           GLASGOW
GRANDE BRETAGNE

BROLY HERVE
CENTRE REGIONAL DE TRANSFUSION
SANGUINE
21 RUE CAMILLE GUERIN
59012   LILLE CEDEX
FRANCE

BROWN PETER C.
CHIRON CORPORATION
4560 HORTON ST.
CA 94608 EMERYVILLE
ETATS UNIS

BUNTEMEYER HEINO
UNIVERSITAT BIELEFELD, TECHN.
FAKULTAT, ZELLKULTURTECHNIK
P.O BOX 8640
4800   BIELEFELD
ALLEMAGNE FEDERALE

BURNS ROBERT B.
ICN FLOW
P.O BOX 17
KA12 8NB IRVINE
GRANDE BRETAGNE

BUSHELL MICHAEL EDWARD
DEPT. OF MICROBIOLOGY
UNIVERSITY OF SURREY
GU2 5XH GUILDFORD
GRANDE BRETAGNE

BUTLER MICHAEL
DEPT BIOLOGICAL SCIENCES
MANCHESTER POLYTECHNIC
CHESTER STREET
M1 5GD   MANCHESTER
GRANDE BRETAGNE

CAMERON DONALD ROSS
ECACC, PHLS CAMR
PORTON DOWN
SP4 OJG SALISBURY
GRANDE BRETAGNE

CARBONELL DELPHINE
SDFMA/SEATN
BAT 352
CEN CADARACHE
13108 ST PAUL LEZ DURANCE CEDEX
FRANCE

CARTWRIGHT TERENCE
CENTRE DE RECHERCHES RHONE
POULENC
13 QUAI JULES GUESDE
94400   VITRY SUR SEINE
FRANCE

CAULCOTT CELIA ANN
ICI PHARMACEUTICALS
BIOTECHNOLOGY DEPARTMENT
MERESIDE, ALDERLEY PARK
SK10 4TG MACCLESFIELD, CHESHIRE
GRANDE BRETAGNE

CHABERT PHILIPPE
BIO MERIEUX
CHEMIN DE L'ORME
69280   MARCY L'ETOILE
FRANCE

CHARLIER GERARD J.W
NATIONAL INST. FOR VETERINARY
RESEARCH
GROESELENBERG 99
1180   BRUSSELS'
BELGIQUE

CHATZISAVIDO NATHALIE
KABIGEN AB
S-112 87 STOCKHOLM
SUEDE

CHOTTEAU VERONIQUE, MARIE
UNIVERSITE LIBRE DE BRUXELLES
SERVICE CHIMIE GENERALE 1
CP 160 - 50 AV. F.D ROOSEVELT
1050   BRUSSEL
BELGIQUE

CLARK T.J.
CELLON SARL
22 RUE DERNIER SOL
L-2543   LUXEMBOURG
LUXEMBOURG

CLARK STUART AIRDRIE
PHLS, CAMR
PORTON DOWN
SP4 OJF SALISBURY
GRANDE BRETAGNE

CLARKE JOHN BRIAN
P.H.L.S. CENTRE FOR APPLIED
MICROBIOLOGY & RESEARCH
PORTON DOWN
SP4 OJG SALISBURY, WILTS
GRANDE BRETAGNE

CLYNES MARTIN
NAT. CELL&TISSUE CULTURE CENTR
SCHOOL OF BIO. SCI
DUBLIN CITY UNIVERSITY
9   DUBLIN, GLASNEVIN
REPUBLIQUE D'IRLANDE

COGAN DIANE
BUTTERWORTHS
PO BOX 63
WESTBURY HOUSE, BURY STREET
GU2 5BH GUILDFORD, SURREY
GRANDE BRETAGNE

COLINET GERARD
SMITHKLINE BIOLOGICALS
89 RUE DE L'INSTITUT
1330   RIXENSART
BELGIQUE

COMER MICHAEL JAMES
BOEHRINGER MANNHEIM GMBH
NONNEWALD GMBH
D-8122   PENZBERG/OBB
ALLEMAGNE FEDERALE

CONRADT HARALD S.
GBF - DEPT. OF GENETICS
MASCHERODER WEG 1
D-3300   BRAUNSCHWEIG
ALLEMAGNE FEDERALE

COSSONS NANDINI HEATHER
BIOLOGICAL LABORATORY
UNIVERSITY OF KENT
CT2 7NJ CANTERBURY
GRANDE BRETAGNE

COUDERC RENE
SANOFI ELF BIO-RECHERCHES
LABEGE - INNOPOLE - VOIE 1
B.P 137
31328   LABEGE CEDEX
FRANCE

COURTIADE BERNADETTE
CRBA - PROCIDA RU
BP 1
13367   MARSEILLE
FRANCE

COUSINS RODERICK BRUCE
BIOTECHNOLOGY UNIT
STRATHCLYDE UNIVERSITY
131 ALBION STREET
G1 1SD   GLASGOW
GRANDE BRETAGNE

CROOY P.
SMITHKLINE BIOLOGICALS
RUE DE L'INSTITUT,89
B-1330   RIXENSART
BELGIQUE

CRUZ DAVID
NEW BRUNSWICK SCIENTIFIC
P.O BOX 6826
6503   NIJMEGEN
PAYS BAS

CURLING ELISABETH MARY ANN
BIOLOGY DEPARTMENT
UNIVERSITY OF KENT
CT2 7NJ CANTERBURY
GRANDE BRETAGNE

CYMBALISTA SAMUEL
LABORATOIRES SERONO SA
ZI DE L'OURIETTAZ
1170   AUBONNE
CONFEDERATION HELVETIQUE

D'HONDT ERIK
SMITH KLINE BIOLOGICALS
RUE DE L'INSTITUT 89
1330   RIXENSART
BELGIQUE

D'OULTREMONT PHILIPPE
SOLVAY & CIE S.A
CENTRAL DIRECTION OF RESEARCH
RUE DE RANSBECK 310
1120   BRUXELLES
BELGIQUE

DACHS FRANZ
PAA-LABORATORY
WIENERSTRASSE 131
A-4020   LINZ
AUTRICHE

DAVIS JOHN MICHAEL
R & D DEPARTMENT
BLOOD PRODUCTS LAB
DAGGER LANE - ELSTREE
WD6 3BX   BOREHAMWOOD, HERTS
GRANDE BRETAGNE

DE BOER EIZE
DUPHAR B.V.
ANIMAL HEALTH DIVISION
P.O BOX 900
1380 DA   WEESP
PAYS BAS

DELAPLACE BRIGITTE
IBF BIOTECHNICS
35 AVENUE JEAN JAURES
92390   VILLENEUVE LA GARENNE
FRANCE

DEMANGEL CAROLINE
BERTIN ET CIE
B.P 3
78373   PLAISIR CEDEX
FRANCE

DENY CORALIE
DEVINEAU SA
42 RUE DE PARADIS
75010   PARIS
FRANCE

DERAMOUDT FRANCOIS-XAVIER
Z.A. DE COURTABOEUF
3 AVENUE DES TROPIQUES
91943   LES ULIS
FRANCE

DESCAMPS ERIC
INSTITUT JACQUES BOY
45 RUE COGNACQ JAY
51100   REIMS
FRANCE

DEVINE JOAN
BRITISH BIOTECHNOLOGY LTD
BROOK HOUSE
WATLINGTON ROAD, COWLEY
OX4SLY   OXFORD
GRANDE BRETAGNE

DEYGAS
SOCIETE INTERMED
Z.I DES RICHARDETS
24 RUE DU BALLON
93160   NOISY LE GRAND
FRANCE

DIAZ ISABELLE
PASTEUR VACCINS
PARC INDUSTRIEL D'INCARVILLE
27100   VAL DE REUIL
FRANCE

DIDELEZ JEAN
SMITHKLINE BIOLOGICALS
RUE DE L'INSTITUT 89
1330   RIXENSART
BELGIQUE

DIENER FREDERICO
CHEMAP AG
HOLZLIKIESENSTR. 5
8604   VOLKESUIL
CONFEDERATION HELVETIQUE

DIEZ IBANEZ MIGUEL
PLATE FORME DE PREDEVELOPEMENT
EN BIOTECHNOLOGIE
INRA DIJON
21034   DIJON
FRANCE

DINKA STEPHEN K.
P.O BOX 567
R.D #1
SANATORIUM ROAD
10963   OTISVILLE, NEW YORK
ETATS UNIS

DOCHERTY ROBERT
LIFE TECHNOLOGIES LTD
P.O BOX 35
TRIDENT HOUSE, RENFREW ROAD
PA34EP   PAISLEY
GRANDE BRETAGNE

DOUSSAU GUY
PALL INDUSTRIE
B.P 253
3 RUE DES GAUDINES
78104   ST GERMAIN EN LAYE
FRANCE

DOYLE ALAN
ECACC, PHLS, CAMR
PORTON DOWN
SP4 0JG   SALISBURY
GRANDE BRETAGNE

DRAPER MARIAN ELAINE
THE PIRBRIGHT LABORATORY
PITMAN-MOORE ASH ROAD
PIRBRIGHT
GU24 ONQ WOKING, SURREY
GRANDE BRETAGNE

DUNKER REINHARD
E. MERCK
DEPT. BIOTECHNOLOGY
P.O BOX 41 19
6100   DARMSTADT
ALLEMAGNE FEDERALE

DUNN IRVING
CHEMICAL ENGINEERING
ETH
8092   ZURICH
ALLEMAGNE FEDERALE

DUVAL DOMINIQUE
BERTIN ET CIE
B.P 3
78373   PLAISIR CEDEX
FRANCE

EBERHARD ULRICH
BEHRINGWERKE AG
P.O BOX 11 40
D-3550   MARBURG
ALLEMAGNE FEDERALE

ELLUARD MARIE-PAULE
SDFMA/SEATN
BAT 352
CEN CADARACHE
13108   ST PAUL LEZ DURANCE
FRANCE

EMBORG CLAUS
DEPT OF BIOLOGICAL, BLOCK 223
THE TECHNICAL UNIVERSITY OF
DENMARK
DK-2800 LYNGBY
DANEMARK

EMERY NICK
SCHOOL OF CHEMICAL ENGINEERING
UNIVERSITY OF BIRMINGHAM
B15 2TT BIRMINGHAM
GRANDE BRETAGNE

ENGASSER J.M
ENSALA
54500   VANDOEUVRE-LES-NANCY
FRANCE

ERNST WOLFGANG
INSTITUTE OF APPLIED MICROBIOL
UNIVERSITY OF AGRICULTURE
PETER JORDANSTR 82
A-1190   WIEN
AUTRICHE

ESPUNA MASSO ENRIC
LES PRADES S/A
LABORATORIOS HIPPRA
17170   AMER (GIRONA)
ESPAGNE

ESTEFANELL DE MARIA JORGE ANDRES
PRODUCTION DIRECTOR
COOPER-ZELTIA S.A.
APARTADO 16
36400   PORRINO (PONTEVEDRA)
ESPAGNE

EWART KRISTINA
ORION CORPORATION
ORION DIAGNOSTICA
P.O BOX 83
02101   ESPOO
FINLANDE

EYER KURT
CHEMICAL ENGINEERING DEPT.
ETH ZENTRUM
CH-8092 ZURICH
CONFEDERATION HELVETIQUE

FABRY LUC
SMITH KLINE BIOLOGICALS
RUE DE L'INSTITUT, 89
1330   RIXENSART
BELGIQUE

FALASH ZVY
C/O INTERPHARM LABORATORIES LT
KYRYAT WEIZMANN
76110   NESS-ZIONA
ISRAEL

FANGET BERNARD
INSTITUT MERIEUX
1541 AVENUE MARCEL MERIEUX
69280   MARCY L'ETOILE
FRANCE

FEDER JOSEPH
INVITRON CORPORATION
4649 LE BOURGET DRIVE
63134   ST. LOUIS, MISSOURI
ETATS UNIS

FENGE CHRISTEL
C/O B.BRAUN DIESSEL BIOTECH
SCHWARZENBERGER WEG 73 - 79
D-3508   MELSUNGEN
ALLEMAGNE FEDERALE

FERNANDEZ PEREZ ALBERTO
MILES ESPANA S.A.
PLAZA DE ESPANA 10
28008   MADRID
ESPAGNE

FERTIG GEORG
TECHNICAL UNIVERSITY
INSTITUTE OF ZOOLOGY
SCHNITTSPAHNSTR. 3
6100   DARMSTADT
ALLEMAGNE FEDERALE

FIGUEROA CARLOS
MILES, INC.
4TH PARKER STREETS
94701   BERKELEY, CA
ETATS UNIS

FINTER
WELLCOME BIOTECHNOLOGY LTD
LANGLEY COURT
BECKENHAM
BR3 3BS KENT
GRANDE BRETAGNE

FIORENTINI DAVID
BIOLOGICAL INDUSTRIES
25115   KIBBUTZ BET HAEMEK
ISRAEL

FISCHER DINA
C/O INTERPHARM LABORATORIES LT
KYRIAT WEIZMANN
76110   NESS-ZIONA
ISRAEL

FITZPATRICK LORNA HILLARY
BIOTECHNOLOGY LABORATORIES
MANCHESTER POLYTECHNIC
CHESTER STREET
M1 5GD   MANCHESTER
GRANDE BRETAGNE

FOSTER ROSEMARY
MACMILLAN PRESS
1 MELBOURNE PLACE
WC2B 4LF LONDON
GRANDE BRETAGNE

FRAUNE ELISABETH
B.BRAUN DIESSEL BIOTECH GMBH
SCHWARZENBERGER WEG 73 - 79
D-3508   MELSUNGEN
ALLEMAGNE FEDERALE

FRECHE JEAN-PAUL
BIOTEC CENTRE S.A.
12 AVENUE DE CONCYR
45100   ORLEANS
FRANCE

FRESHNEY ROBERT IAN
CRC DEPT. MEDICAL ONCOLOGY
ALEXANDER STONE BUILDING
GARSCUBE ESTATE, BEARSOEN
G61 1BD GLASGOW
GRANDE BRETAGNE

FRETTA ANTONELLA
FARMITALIA CARLO ERBA
VIA DEI GRACCHI 35
20146   MILANO
ITALIE

FRIEBERG HANS
S.V.A.
DEPT OF CELL CULTURE
BOX 585 BMC
S-75123 UPPSALA
SUEDE

FRIELING KLAUS H.
C/O PAUL EHRLICH INSTITUT
PAUL EHRLICHSTRASSE 51-59
D-6070   LANGEN
ALLEMAGNE FEDERALE

FROUD STEPHEN JAMES
CELLTECH LTD
216 BATH ROAD
SL1 4EN SLOUGH, BERKSHIRE
GRANDE BRETAGNE

FUJIYOSHI NOBUO
KYOWA HAKKO KOGYO CO. LTD.
6-1, OHTEMACHI,
1-CHOME, CHIYODAKU
100   TOKYO
JAPON

GALLILI GILAD
B.L.T.
P.O BOX 27047
         JERUSALEM
ISRAEL

GANNE VINCENT
CNTS
3 AVENUE DES TROPIQUES
BP 100
91943   LES ULIS CEDEX
FRANCE

GANNON FRANK
NATIONAL DIAGNOSTICS CENTRE
BIORESEARCH IRELAND
UNIVERSITY COLLEGE GALWAY
         GALWAY
REPUBLIQUE D'IRLANDE

GARDNER CATHERINE ANNE
MEDICAL & VETERINARY SUPPLIES
LTD,
BOTOLPH CLAYDON
MK18 2LR BUCKINGHAM
GRANDE BRETAGNE

GATINEAU ERIC
CNTS -
AVENUE DES TROPIQUES
BP 100
91940   LES ULIS
FRANCE

GEAHEL ISABELLE
BERTIN ET CIE
B.P 3
78373   PLAISIR CEDEX
FRANCE

GEAUGEY VALERY
BERTIN ET CIE
59 RUE PIERRE CURIE
ZI DES GATINES
78393   PLAISIR CEDEX
FRANCE

GEBERT CAROL
THE UNIVERSITY OF NEW SOUTH
WALES
PO BOX 1
2033   KENSINGTON
AUSTRALIE

GEISSE SABINE
SANDOZ PHARMA LTD.
PRECLINICAL RESEARCH, BIOTEC.
BLDG. 506/304
CH-4002 BALE
CONFEDERATION HELVETIQUE

GENGENBACH RALF
BASH-AG ZET/ZH- A15
6700   LUDWIGSHAFEN
ALLEMAGNE FEDERALE

GERARD JEAN-PHILIPPE
C.N.T.S. INNOVATION ATR
AVENUE DES TROPIQUES
91943   LES ULIS
FRANCE

GEYER SCOTT
ARES-SERONO
100 LONGWATER CIRCLE
02061   NORWELL, MASSACHUSSETES
ETATS UNIS

GHEYSEN DIRK RICHARD
SMITHKLINE BIOLOGICALS
LAB MOL & CELL BIOLOGY
B-1330   RIXENSART
BELGIQUE

GLAD MAGNUS
PERSTORP BIOLYTICA AB
S-22370 LUND
SUEDE

GOERGEN JEAN-LOUIS
LSGC - CNRS - INPL
1 RUE GRANDVILLE
BP 451
54001   NANCY
FRANCE

GOETGHEBEUR STEPHANE PAUL
45 AVENUE DE FLANDRE
59491   VILLENEUVE D'ASCQ
FRANCE

GORIS AGNES
N.V. ECO BIO
WOUDSTRAAT 25
B-3600   GENK
BELGIQUE

GOTOH TATSUO
1239 SHINZAIRE, ABOSHI-KU
HIMEJI, HYOGO
671-12   HIMEJI
JAPON

GRAHAM HENRY A.
74 SAND HILL ROAD
08801   ANNANDALE, NY
ETATS UNIS

GRATION K.A.F.
ANIMAL HEALTH BIOLOGY
PFIZER CENTRAL RESEARCH
         SANDWICH, KENT
GRANDE BRETAGNE

GRAY PETER PHILIP
UNIVERS. OF NEW SOUTH WALES
DEPARTMENT OF BIOTECHNOLOGY
P.O BOX 1
2033   SYDNEY
AUSTRALIE

GRIERSON ALASTAIR
DEPT OF BIOSCIENCE & BIOTECH.
UNIVERSITY OF STRATHLLYDE
TODD CENTRE
G4 ONR   GLASGOW
GRANDE BRETAGNE

GRIFFITHS BRYAN
DIVISION OF BIOLOGICS
PHLS CAMR PORTON DOWN
SP4 0JG SALISBURY, WILTS
GRANDE BRETAGNE

HAFFENDEN PAUL
165 BETHRIDGE ROAD
M9W 1N44 TORONTO, ONTARIO
CANADA

HAGGSTROM LENA
DEPT. OF BIOCHEMISTRY AND
BIOTECHNOLOGY
INSTITUTE OF TECHNOLOGY
S-100 44 STOCKHOLM
SUEDE

HAMILTON ALLISTER
LIFE TECHNOLOGIES LTD
PO BOX 35
TRIDENT HOUSE RENFREW ROAD
PA 3 4EP PAISLEY
GRANDE BRETAGNE

HAMPSON BRIAN S.
CHARLES RIVER U.K. LTD
MANSTON ROAD
CT9 4LT MARGATE, KENT
GRANDE BRETAGNE

HANDA-CORRIGAN ANITA
DEPT. MICROBIOLOGY
UNIVERSITY OF SURREY
GU2 5XH GUILDFORD, SURREY
GRANDE BRETAGNE

HARBOUR COLIN
DEPART. OF INFECTIONS DISEASES
THE UNIVERSITY OF SYDNEY
NSW 2006 SYDNEY
AUSTRALIE

HARDY E.
MEDICAL & VETERINARY SUPPLIES
BOTOLPH CLAYDON
MK18 2LR BUCKINGHAM
GRANDE BRETAGNE

HASSA ECKHARD D.
MBR
WERKSTR. 4
8620   WETEIKON
CONFEDERATION HELVETIQUE

HAUSER HANSJORG
GBF
MASCHERODE WEG 1
D-3300   RAUNSCHWEIG
ALLEMAGNE FEDERALE

HAYTER PAUL
BIOLOGICAL LABORATORY
UNIVERSITY OF KENT
CT2 7NJ CANTERBURY
GRANDE BRETAGNE

HEIRWECH KRISTIEN
INDUSTRIEPARK ZWIJNAARDE 7
BUS 4
9710   GENT
BELGIQUE

HEIRWEGH KRISTIEN
N.V. INNOGENETICS S.A
INDUSTRIEPARK ZWIJNAARDE
7 BOX 4
B-9710   GHENT
BELGIQUE

HENNO PATRICK
BIOSYS SA
21 QUAI DU CLOS DES ROSES
60200   COMPIEGNE
FRANCE

HENTSCHEL CHRIS
MRC COLLABORATIVE CENTER
1-3 BURTON HOLE LANE
MILL HILL
W71 AD   LONDON
GRANDE BRETAGNE

HERBST DETLEV
BYK GULDEN ITALIA
VIA GIOTTO 1
20032   CORMANO (MILANO)
ITALIE

HEWLETT GUY
BAYER AG - INST. FUR VIROLOGIE
PHARMA-FORSCHUNGSZNTRUM
5600   WUPPERTAL 1
ALLEMAGNE FEDERALE

HIRATA TERUAKI
MINISTRY OF HEALTH AND WELFARE
HEALTH SCIENCES DIV.
1-2-2 KASUMIGASEKI-CHIYODA-KU
100-45   TOKYO
JAPON

HIROSE YOSHIO
JAPAN HEALTH SCIENCES FOUNDAT.
I,K BLDG - 3-6-9 NIKONGASHI,
HENCHO, CHUOKU
103   TOKYO
JAPON

HODGES GISELE M.
IMPERIAL CANCER RESEARCH FUND
2ND FLOOR AFRICA HOUSE
64-78 KINGSWAY
WC2B 6BG LONDON
GRANDE BRETAGNE

HOFMANN FRIEDER
BIOTECHNETICS
4116 SORRENTO VALLEY BLVD.
92121   SAN DIEGO
ETATS UNIS

HOLMBERG ANN
PERSTORP BIOLYTICA
S-22370 LUND
SUEDE

HOLTORF ANKE-PEGGY
K681.1.02
CIBA GEIGY
DEPT BIOTECHNOLOGY
CH-4002 BASLE
CONFEDERATION HELVETIQUE

HOPE SANDRA
MICROBIOLOGICAL ASS. INTERNAT.
STIRLING UNIVERSITY INNOVATION
PARK
FK9 4LA STIRLING
GRANDE BRETAGNE

HOPPE HENRY
GENZYME
1 MOUNTAIN ROAD
FRAMINGHAM
01720   FRAMINGHAM
ETATS UNIS

HORAUD FLORIAN
INSTITUT PASTEUR
28 RUE DU DOCTEUR ROUX
75724   PARIS CEDEX 15
FRANCE

HU   WEI-SHOU
UNIVERSITY OF MINNESOTA
421 WASHINGTON AVE S.E
55455   MINNEAPOLIS, M.N
ETATS UNIS

HUBER-WEGMANN GABRIELA
SANDOZ AG, BIOTECHNOLOGIE
506/304
4002   BASEL
CONFEDERATION HELVETIQUE

HUXFORD ROSIE
SERA-LAB
HOPHURST LANE
CRAWLEY DOWN
RH10 4FF SUSSEX
GRANDE BRETAGNE

HWANG CHRIS
DEPARTMENT OF BIOLOGY
M.I.T.
ROOM 56-125

ETATS UNIS

JACOBS MARITTA
PFEIFER & LANGEN
FRANKENSTR 25
P.O 100 320
D-4047   DORMAGEN
ALLEMAGNE FEDERALE

JAEGER VOLKER
GESELLSCHAFT FUER BIOTECHNOLOG
FORSCHUNG
MASCHERODER WEG 1
D-3300   BRAUNSCHWEIG
ALLEMAGNE FEDERALE

JAIN DEEPAK
MERCK & CO. INC.
P.O BOX 2000
R 30Y
07065   RAHWAY
ETATS UNIS

JAKUBEK EVA-BRITT
SVA DEPT. OF CELL CULTURE
BOX 585 BMC
S-75123 UPPSALA
SUEDE

JALANKO ANU
ORION CORPORATION,
BIOTECHNOLOGY
VALIMOTIE 7
00380   HELSINKI
FINLANDE

JENKINS NIGEL
BIOLOGICAL LABORATORY
UNIVERSITY OF KENT
CT2 7NJ CANTERBURY
GRANDE BRETAGNE

JOHANSSON KERSTIN M.
PHARMACIA DIAGNOSTICS AB
F51-1
751 82   UPPSALA
SUEDE

JOHNSON BRIAN
PITNAN-MOORE EUROPE
BERKHAMSTEAD HILL
HP4 2QE BERKHAMSTEAD
GRANDE BRETAGNE

JONES ELISABETH EIRIAN
DEPARTMENT OF BIOLOGICAL
SCIENCES
MANCHESTER POLYTECHNIC
M1 5GD   MANCHESTER
GRANDE BRETAGNE

JORDAN MARTIN
INSTITUT FUR ZELLBIOLOGIE
HPM F27
ETH - HONGGERBERG
8093   ZURICH
CONFEDERATION HELVETIQUE

KAKES ERIK
PO BOX 149
3100 AC SCHIEDAM
PAYS BAS

KANZLER OTTO
BENDER & CO.GES MBH
DR BOEHRINGERGASSE 5-11
A-1121   VIENNA
AUTRICHE

KARES ERIK
APPLIKON
PO BOX 149
3100 AC SCHIEDAM
PAYS BAS

KASPI LEA
BIOLOGICAL INDUSTRIES
25115   KIBBUTZ BET HAEMEK
ISRAEL

KATINGER HERMANN
INSTITUTE OF APPLIED MICROBIOL
PETER JORDAN STR. 82
A-1190   VIENNA
AUTRICHE

KELLER INGRID
PFEIFER & LANGEN
ABT. PHARMA
POSTFACH 100 320
D-4047   DORMAGEN
ALLEMAGNE FEDERALE

KELLER JURG
CHEMICAL ENGINEERING DEPT.
ETH ZENTRUM
CH-8092 ZURICH
CONFEDERATION HELVETIQUE

KIERULFF JESPER V.
DEPT OF BIOTECHNOLOGY
BLOCK 223 - THE TECHNICAL
UNIVERSITY OF DENMARK
DK-2800 LYNGBY
DANEMARK

KILBURN DOUGLAS
BIOTECHNOLOGY LAB
UNIVERSITY OF BRITISH COLUMBIA
V6T IW5 VANCOUVER
CANADA

KLEMENT GERHARD
CENTOCOR EUROPE BV
PO BOX 251
2300 AG LEIDEN
PAYS BAS

KLEUSER BEATE
SANDOZ PHARMA AG
BAU 316 / 514
POSTFACH
4002   BASEL
CONFEDERATION HELVETIQUE

KLOFT MICHAEL
BIOTEST PHARMA GMBH
LANDSTEINERSTRABE 5
D-6072   DREIEICH
ALLEMAGNE FEDERALE

KLOPPINGER MARTINA
TECHNICAL UNIVERSITY
INSTITUTE OF ZOOLOGY
SCHNITTSPAHNSTR. 3
6100   DARMSTADT
ALLEMAGNE FEDERALE

KNUDSEN IDA MOELGAARD
NOVO NORDISK A/S
BUILDING 3B
DK-2880 BAGSVAERD
DANEMARK

KOCH STEFAN
BOEHRINGER MANNHEIM GMBH
NONNENWALD 2
D-8122   PENZBERG
ALLEMAGNE FEDERALE

KOEHL MICHEL
TRANSGENE
11 RUE DE MOLSHEIM
67000   STRASBOURG
FRANCE

KONGERSLEV LEIF
NIELS STEENSENSVEJ 1
DK-2820 GENTOFTE
DANEMARK

KONOPITZKY KURT
BENDER & CO.GESMBH
DR BOEHRINGERGASSE 5-11
A-1121   VIENNA
AUTRICHE

KRATJE RICARDO
GBF - GESELLSCHAFT FUR BIOTECH
FORSHUNG
MASCHERODER WEG 1
D-3300   BRAUNSCHWEIG
ALLEMAGNE FEDERALE

KRETZMER GERLINDE
INSTITUT FUER TECHNISCHE CHEMI
CALLINSTRASSE 3
D-3000   HANNOVER 1
ALLEMAGNE FEDERALE

KREUZBURG UTE
DEPT OF BIOSCIENCE & BIOTECH.
UNIVESITY OF STRATHLLYDE
TODD CENTRE
G4 ONR   GLASGOW
GRANDE BRETAGNE

LANGUET BERNARD
RHONE MERIEUX
LABORATOIRE IFFA
254 RUE MARCEL MERIEUX
69007   LYON
FRANCE

LATRILLE FRANCK
SOREBIO
BORDEAUX TECHNOPOLIS
SITE MONTESQUIEU
33650   MARTILLAC-LA BREDE
FRANCE

LE BOUTEILLER CHRISTINE
SANOFI ELF BIO-RECHERCHES
LABEGE - INNOPOLE - VOIE NO 1
B.P 137
31328   LABEGE CEDEX
FRANCE

LEHMANN JURGEN
INST. OF CELL CULTURE TECHNOL.
UNIVERSITY OF BIELEFELD
D-4800   BIELEFELD
ALLEMAGNE FEDERALE

LEHUU BERTRAND
INSTITUT PASTEUR TEXCELL
28 RUE DU DOCTEUR ROUX
75724   PARIS CEDEX 15
FRANCE

LEITNER ORITH
CHEMICAL IMMUNOLOGY
WEIZMANN INSTITUTE OF SCIENCE
P.O.B 26
76100   REHOVOT
ISRAEL

LENO MICHEL
LAB. DE TECHNOLOGIE CELLULAIRE
INSTITUT PASTEUR
28 RUE DU DOCTEUR ROUX
75724   PARIS CEDEX 15
FRANCE

LESSART PIERRE
SDFMA/SEATN
BT 352
CEN CADARACHE
13108 ST PAUL LEZ DURANCE CEDEX
FRANCE

LEVERING PIET R.
ORGANON INTERNATIONAL B.V
POSTBUS 20
5340 BH OSS
PAYS BAS

LI SHU-YING
GBF
MASCHRODER WEG 1
3300   BRAUNSCHWEIG
ALLEMAGNE FEDERALE

LIND WALDEMAR
GBF, ARBEITSGRUPPE ZELLKULTUR-
TECHNIK
MASCHERODER 1
D-3300   BRAUNSCHWEIG
ALLEMAGNE FEDERALE

LINDNER-OLSSON ELISABETH
KABIGEN AB
S-112 87 STOCKHOLM
SUEDE

LITWIN JACK
STATE BACTERIOLOGY LAB.
10521   STOCKHOLM
SUEDE

LIZEN ETIENNE
SMITH KLINE BIOLOGICALS
RUE DE L'INSTITUT 89
1330   RIXENSART
BELGIQUE

LOBMANN MICHELE
SMITHKLINE BECKMAN
ANIMAL HEALTH PRODUCTS
89 RUE DE L'INSTITUT
1330   RIXENSART
BELGIQUE

LOOBY DENIS
PHLS CAMR
PORTON DOWN
SP4 0JG SALISBURY, WILTSHIRE
GRANDE BRETAGNE

LOOKER T.
MANCHESTER POLYTECHNIC
CHESTER STREET
M1 5GD   MANCHESTER
GRANDE BRETAGNE

LOVE RICHARD
SERONO LAB.
100 LONGWATER CIRCLE
02061   NORWELL, MA
ETATS UNIS

LUBINIECKI ANTHONY S.
VP BIOPHARMACEUTICAL
P.O BOX 1539 - L-28
PA 19406-0939
              KING OF PRUSSIA
ETATS UNIS

LUCKI-LANGE MONA
GBF, ARBEITSGRUPPE ZELLKULTUR-
TECHNIK
MASCHERODER WEG 1
D-3300   BRAUNSCHWEIG
ALLEMAGNE FEDERALE

LUNDGREN BJORN
PHARMACIA DIAGNOSTICS AB
F51-1
751-82   UPPSALA
SUEDE

LUPKER JAN
SANOFI ELF BIO-RECHERCHES
LABEGE-INNOPOLE - VOIE NO 1
B.P 137
31328   LABEGE CEDEX FRANCE

LUTKEMEYER DIRK
UNIVERSITAT BIELEFELD
INSTITUTE OF CELL CULTURE
TECHNIQUE
4800   BIELEFELD
ALLEMAGNE FEDERALE

MACDONALD CAROLINE
DEPT OF BIOSCIENCE & BIOTECH.
UNIVERSITY OF STRAHLLYDE
TODD CENTRE
G4 ONR   GLASGOW
GRANDE BRETAGNE

MADDALO FRANCIS
SERONO LABORATORIES
100 LONGWATER CIRCLE
02061   NORWELL, MASSACHUSSETTES
ETATS UNIS

MAILLY EMMANUEL
LSGC - CNRS - INPL
1 RUE GRANDVILLE
B.P 451
54001   NANCY
FRANCE

MALARME DANIEL
SOLVAY & CIE S.A
310 RUE DE RANSBEEK
1120   BRUXELLES
BELGIQUE

MALMSTROEM ULF
ALFA-LAVAL CENTRITECH AB
S-147 80 TUMBA
SUEDE

MANLEY QUENTIN JOHN
CELLTECH
216 BATH ROAD
SL1 4EN SLOUGH
GRANDE BRETAGNE

MANNIX CHRIS
BEECHAM PHARMACEUTICALS RES.
1 YEW TREE BOTTOM ROAD
KT18 5XQ EPSOM, SURREY
GRANDE BRETAGNE

MARC ANNIE
LSGC - CNRS - INPL
1 RUE GRANDVILLE
B.P 451
54001   NANCY
FRANCE

MARCUS DINO
ISRAEL INSTITUTE FOR
BIOLOGICAL RESEARCH
70450   NESS-ZIONA
ISRAEL

MARTIAL ADELE
LSGC - CNRS - INPL
1 RUE GRANDVILLE
B.P 451
54001   NANCY
FRANCE

MARTIN CHRISTIAN-MONIQUE
DIAGNOSTICS TRANSFUSION - RECH
& DEVELOP. LAB CULTURE CELLUL.
3 BD RAYMOND POINCARE - BP 20
92430   MARNES LA COQUETTE
FRANCE

MARX UWE
HU ZU BERLIN, CHARITE
INST. OF MED. IMMUNOLOGIE
SCHUMANNSTR. 20/21
1040   BERLIN
ALLEMAGNE FEDERALE

MASCARELLA FONT RICART
LABORATORIOS SOBRINO S.A.
CRTA. CAMPRODON S/N
17813   VALL DE BRIANYA
ESPAGNE

MASTRODICASA MARCO
LEPETIT RESEARCH CENTER
VIA R. LEPETIT 34
21040   GERENZANO (VARESE)
ITALIE

MC GLYNN ELAINE
CIBA-GEIGY
K125 4 12
4002   BASEL
CONFEDERATION HELVETIQUE

MCLEAN JOHN STEPHEN
ICI BIOTECHNOLOGY
ALDERLEY PARK
SL6 8QR MACCLESFIELD, CHESHIRE
GRANDE BRETAGNE

MCLEOD ALEXANDER
PROTEIN FRACTIONATION CENTRE
21 ELLEN'S GLEN ROAD
EH17 7QT EDINBURGH
GRANDE BRETAGNE

MCSWEENEY BARRY
BIORESEARCH IRELAND, EOLAS
GLASNEVIN
9   DUBLIN
REPUBLIQUE D'IRLANDE

MEIGNIER BERNARD
INTITUT MERIEUX
1541 AV. MARCEL MERIEUX
69280   MARCY L'ETOILE
FRANCE

MELLANO DIEGO
IZO
VIA BIANCHI 7
25124   BRESCIA
ITALIE

MELLSTROM KARIN
KABIGEN AB
STRANDBERGSGATAN 49
S-11287 STOCKHOLM
SUEDE

MERTEN OTTO-WILHELM
INSTITUT PASTEUR
LAB. DE TECHNOLOGIE CELLULAIRE
25 RUE DU DOCTEUR ROUX
75724   PARIS CEDEX 15
FRANCE

MILES
PLAZA DE ESPANA, 10
28008   MADRID
ESPAGNE

MIZRAHI A.
ISRAEL RESEARCH
BIOLOGICAL RESEARCH
70450   NESS ZIONA
ISRAEL

MONTAGNON BERNARD JEAN
INSTITUT MERIEUX
DIRECTOR OF VIROLOGY UNIT.
1541 AVENUE MARCEL MERIEUX
69280   MARCY L'ETOILE
FRANCE

MONTALTO JOSEPH
195 W BIRCH
60901   KANKAKEE
ETATS UNIS

MORANDI MAURIZIO
SCLAVO SPA
VIA FIORENTINA 1
53100   SIENA
ITALIE

MOREIRA JOSE LUIS
INSTITUTO DE BIOLOGIA EXPERIM.
E TECHNOLOGICA (IBET)
APARTADO 12
2780   OEIRAS
PORTUGAL

MORIMOTO YUUKI
MITSUBISHI KASEI CORP.
1000 KAMOSHDA, MIDORI-KU
227   YOKOHAMA
JAPON

MOUSCADET JEAN-PIERRE
DEVINEAU SA
42 RUE DE PARADIS
75010   PARIS
FRANCE

MOWLES JON MARTIN
ECACC, PHLS, CAMR
PORTON DOWN
SP4 0JG SALISBURY
GRANDE BRETAGNE

MUNDT WOLFGANG
BIOMEDICAL RESEARCH CENTER
UFERSTRABE 15
A-2304   ORTH DONAU
AUTRICHE

MUNSTER MICHAEL J.
R.W JOHNSON PHARMACEUTICAL
RESEARCH INSTITUTE
ROUTE 202, PO BOX 300
008869   RARITAN, NEW JERSEY
ETATS UNIS

MURAKAMI HIROKI
GRADUATE SCHOOL OF GENETIC
RESOURCES AND TECHNOLOGY
KYUSHU UNIVERSITY
812   FUKUOKA
JAPON

MURNANE AMY
P.O BOX 1539
MAIL CODE L-36
19406-0939
          KING OF PRUSSIA, PA
ETATS UNIS

MURPHY MARIE
CHIROPRACTIC CLINIC
KILWORTH VILLAGE
          CO.CORK
REPUBLIQUE D'IRLANDE

MUSGRAVE STEPHEN CHRISTOPHER
WELLCOME BIOTECH
FERMENTATION DEPT.
LANGLEY COURT
BR33BS   BECKENHAM
GRANDE BRETAGNE

NAGAMINE KENICHI
HIGASHIMUTAYAMA CITY
KUMEGANOCHO 1-52-14
NICHIREI RESEARCH INSTITUTE
189   HIGASHIMURAYAMA
JAPON

NARENDRA-NATHAN TINA J.
WELLCOME BIOTECH
FERMENTATION DEPT.
LANGLEY COURT
BR33BS   BECKENHAM
GRANDE BRETAGNE

NEWELL DIANE
PHLS - DIVISION OF BIOLOGICS
PORTON DOWN
SALISBURY
SP4 0JG WILTSHIRE
GRANDE BRETAGNE

NIELSEN VILLY
A/S NUNC
KAMSTRUPVEJ 90
KAMSTRUP
4000   ROSKILDE
DANEMARK

NIELSEN HANS INGOLF
MEDI-CULT A/S
KANALHOLMEN 12
DK-2650 HVIDOVRE
DANEMARK

NIELSEN LARS KELD
DALSO PARK 11B
3500   VAERLOSE
DANEMARK

NIKOLAY SIMON DIETER PHILLIP
WOLFSON CYZOZECHNOLOTY LAB.
DEPT. OF MICROBIOLOGY
UNIVERSITY OF SURREY
GU2 5XH GUILDFORD, SURREY
GRANDE BRETAGNE

NILSSON KJELL
PERCELL BIOLYTICA
S-22370 LUND
SUEDE

NILSSON LOTTA
FLOBIO
15 RUE ARMAND SYLVESTRE
92400   COURBEVOIE
FRANCE

NOE WOLFGANG
DR. KARL THOMAE GMBH.
ABT. BIOTECHNISCHE PRODUKTION
BIRKENDORFER STRABE 65
D-7950   BIBERACH/RIB
ALLEMAGNE FEDERALE

NORDLANDER EVA KRISTINA
PHARMACIA AB
BJORKGATAN 30
75122   UPPSALA
SUEDE

OHASHI HIDEYA
PHARMACEUTICAL LABORATORY
KIVIN BRAWERY CO. LTD
22 SOUJA-MACHI ICHOME
371   MAEBASHI GUNMA
JAPON

OHMAN MARIE
PHARMACIA DIAGNOSTICS AB
F51-1
75182   UPPSALA
SUEDE

OKA MELVIN S.
SMITHLINE & FRENCH LABORATORIE
P.O BOX 1539, L-39
19406-0939
           KING OF PRUSSIA, PA
ETATS UNIS

OLIVER ALAN SPENCER
PORTON PRODUCTS
PORTON DOWN
SP4 OJG SALISBURY
GRANDE BRETAGNE

OLOFSSON MATS
KABIGEN AB
S-112 87 STOCKHOLM
SUEDE

OMSTEAD DANIEL
RW JOHNSON PHARMACEUTICAL
RESEARCH INSTITUTE
ROUTE 202, P.O BOX 300
08869   RARITAN, NEW JERSEY
ETATS UNIS

ONIONS DAVID
L.R.F. VIRUS CENTRE
UNIVERSITY OF GLASGOW
G61 1QH GLASGOW
GRANDE BRETAGNE

OUDOT CATHERINE
GIBCO BRL SARL
BP 7050
95051   CERGY PONTOISE CEDEX
FRANCE

PAGE KEITH
SERA-LAB LTD.
HOPHURST LANE
CRAWLEY DOWN
RH10 4FF SUSSEX
GRANDE BRETAGNE

PANINA GIANFRANCO
ISTIT. ZOOPROFILATTICO SPERIM.
DELLA LOMBARDIA E DELL'EMILIA
VIA A. BRANCHI NO. 7
25125   BRESCIA
ITALIE

PAPOUTSAKIS E. TERRY
DEPT. CHEM. ENGINEERING
NORTHWESTERN UNIVERSITY
2145 SHERIDAN ROAD
60208   EVANSTON, ILLINOIS
ETATS UNIS

PARODI BARBARA
I.S.T.
VIALE BENEDETTO XV 10
I-16132 GENOVA
ITALIE

PERSSON LENA
SVA DEPT OF CELL CULTURE
BOX 585 BMC
S-75123 UPPSALA
SUEDE

PERSSON BO
DEPT. OF BIOTECHNOLOGY
BLOCK 223 - THE TECHNICAL
UNIVERSITY OF DENMARK
DK-2800 LYNGBY
DANEMARK

PETRI THOMAS
SCHERING AG
MUELLERSTR. 170/178
D-1000   BERLIN 65
ALLEMAGNE FEDERALE

PIETROWSKI ROBERT ANDREW
EVANS BIOLOGICALS LTD
GASKILL ROAD SPEKE
L24 9GR LIVERPOOL
GRANDE BRETAGNE

PINGEON BERNARD
DIAGNOSTICS PASTEUR
CULTURE CELLULAIRE
ROUTE DE GISSEL
69114   STEENVOORDE
FRANCE

PINTON HERVE
SETRIC GENIE INDUSTRIEL (SGI)
15 ALLEES DE BELLEFONTAINE
31100   TOULOUSE
FRANCE

PIRET JAMES
BIOTECHNOLOGY LAB
#237-6174 UNIVERSITY BLVD.
V6T 1W5 VANCOUVER
CANADA

PLANA DURAN JUAN
LABORATORIOS SORRINO S.A.
CRTA. CAMPRODON S/N
17813   VALL DE BIANYA
ESPAGNE

POINSARD A.
CELLON SARL
22 RUE DERNIER SOL
L-2543   LUXEMBOURG
FRANCE

PORQUET GARANTO LOURDES
LABORATORIOS SOBRINO S.A.
CRTA. CAMPRODON S/N
17813   VALL DE BIANYA
ESPAGNE

POURADIER DUTEIL XAVIER
IMEDEX
Z.I LES TRAQUES
B.P 38
69630   CHAPONOST
FRANCE

POUZET AGNES
DIAGNOSTICS TRANSFUSION
3 BLD RAYMOND POINCARE
92430   MARNES LA COQUETTE
FRANCE

PRESTON ALAN ELEY
MEDICAL & VETERINARY SUPPLIES
LTD,
BOTOLPH CLAYDON
MK18 2LR BUCKINGHAM
GRANDE BRETAGNE

PUENTE GONZALEZ JOSE ANTONIO
P.C.S. PROD. MANAGER
COOPER-ZELTIA S.A.
APARTADO 16
36400   PORRINO (PONTEVEDRA)
ESPAGNE

RABAUD JEAN-NOEL
SETRIC GENIE INDUSTRIEL (SGI)
15 ALLEES DE BELLEFONTAINE
31100   TOULOUSE
FRANCE

RACHER ANDREW JOHN
PHLS CAMR
DIVISION OF BIOLOGICS
PORTON DOWN
SP4 OJG SALISBURY
GRANDE BRETAGNE

RASMUSSEN BENTE
HYBRIDOMALABORATORY
STATENS SERUMINSTITUT
ARTELLERIVEJ 5
2300   COPENHAGEN S.
DANEMARK

REARDON PAUL CHARLES
GRACE INDUSTRIAL CHEMICALS
AVENUE MONTCHOISI 35
1001   LAUSANNE
CONFEDERATION HELVETIQUE

REUSCHENBACH PETER
BASF ZHBIF A30
ZH/ZT - B 9
D-6700   LUDWIGSHAFEN
ALLEMAGNE FEDERALE

REUVENY SHAUL
ISRAEL INST. BIOLOGICAL RES.
DEPARTMENT BIOTECH
P.O BOX 19
70450   NESS-ZIONA
ISRAEL

REY SPEND LOVE
FLOBIO
15 RUE ARMAND SYLVESTRE
92400   COURBEVOIE
FRANCE

RIEMANN HOLGER
GENETIC ENGINEERING GROUP
LUNDTOFTEVEJ 100
BUILD 227
2800   LYNGBY
DANEMARK

RIMMELE DOMINIQUE
INSTITUT JACQUES BOY SA
45 RUE COGNACQ JAY
51100   REIMS
FRANCE

RODER BETTINA
MASCHERODER WEG 1
D-3300   BRAUNSCHWEIG
ALLEMAGNE FEDERALE

ROMETTE JEAN-LOUIS
CHEMAP AG
HOLZLIWISENSTRASSE 5
CH-8604 VOLKETSWIL
CONFEDERATION HELVETIQUE

RONFARD VINCENT
CENTRE REGIONAL DE TRANSFUSION
SANGUINE
59012   LILLE CEDEX
FRANCE

RONNING OYSTEIN W.
CENTER FOR INDUSTRIAL RESEARCH
P.O BOX 124 - BLINDERN
0314   OSLO 3
NORVEGE

RUPP HEIKE
GBF, ARBEITSGRUPPE ZELLKULTUR-
TECHNIK
MASCHERODER WEG 1
D-3300   BRAUNSCHWEIG
ALLEMAGNE FEDERALE

RYLL THOMAS
GBF, ARBEITSGRUPPE ZELLKULTUR-
TECHNIK
MASCHERODER WEG 1
D-3300   BRAUNSCHWEIG
ALLEMAGNE FEDERALE

SAMARUT JACQUES
ECOLE NORMALE SUP. DE LYON
LAB. DE BIOLOGIE MOLECULAIRE &
CELLULAIRE - 46 ALL. D'ITALIE
69364   LYON
FRANCE

SANDERS PETER GEORGE
MICROBIOLOGY DEPT.
SURREY UNIVERSITY
GU2 5XH GUILDFORD
GRANDE BRETAGNE

SCHEIRER WINFRIED
SANDOZ FORSCHUNGSINSTITUT GMBH
BRUNNERSTRASSE 59
A-2235   VIENNA
AUTRICHE

SCHLAEGER ERNSZT-JURGEN
HOFFMANN - LA ROCHE LTD
BAU 66/108 GRENZACHERSTR. 124
4002   BASEL
CONFEDERATION HELVETIQUE

SCHMID GEORG
HOFFMANN-LA ROCHE LTD
BAU 66/302
GRENZACHERSTR. 124
4002   BASEL
CONFEDERATION HELVETIQUE

SCHONHERR OTTO THOMAS
DIOSYNTH BV
P.O BOX 20
5340 BH   OSS
PAYS BAS

SCHREIBER REGINE
RHONE MERIEUX LABORATOIRE IFFA
254 RUE MARCEL MERIEUX
69007   LYON
FRANCE

SCHURCH ULRICH HANS ANDREAS
SCHWEIZERISCHES SERUM + IMPF
INSTITUT
REHAGSTR 79
3001   BERN
CONFEDERATION HELVETIQUE

SCHUTZ CLAUDIA
GBF, ARBEITSGRUPPE ZELLKULTUR-
TECHNIK
MASCHERODER WEG 1
D-3300   BRAUNSCHWEIG
ALLEMAGNE FEDERALE

SCHWARZBARD ZIVIA
LABORATOIRES SERONO SA
ZI DE L'OURIETTAZ
1170   AUBONNE
CONFEDERATION HELVETIQUE

SCOTT MICHELLE
DEPARTMENT OF MICROBIOLOGY
UNIVERSITY OF SURREY
GU2 5XH   GUILDFORD
GRANDE BRETAGNE

SEAR CHRISTOPHER H.J.
CHARLES RIVER UK LTD
MANSTON ROAD
CT9 4LT   MARGATE, KENT
GRANDE BRETAGNE

SHARPIN ROSEMARY
IMMUNO-CHEMICAL PRODUCTS LTD
P.O BOX 1607
          AUCKLAND 1
NOUVELLE ZELANDE

SHIRAGAMI MAKOTO
MINISTRY OF HEALTH AND WELFARE
PHARCENTICALS CHEM. SAFETY DIV
1-2-2 KASUMIGASEKI, CHIYODA-KU
100-45   TOKYO
JAPON

SIEWERT DETLEF
INVITRON CORPORATION
4649 LE BOURGET DRIVE
63134   ST LOUIS, MISSOURI
ETATS UNIS

SILLEKENS
EUROCLONE B.V.
PLESMANLAAN 125
1066 CX   AMSTERDAM
PAYS BAS

SINACORE MARTIN S.
GENETICS INSTITUTE, INC
ONE BURTT ROAD
01810   ANDOVER, MA
ETATS UNIS

SINSKEY ANTHONY J.
DEPART. OF BIOLOGY
MIT ROOM ROOM 56-121
MA 02139 CAMBRIDGE
ETATS UNIS

SJOEBERG MIKAEL
ALFA-LAVAL CENTRITECH AB
S-147 80 TUMBA
SUEDE

SOUVRAS MICHEL
INSTITUT MERIEUX
1541 AVENUE MARCEL MERIEUX
69280   MARCY L'ETOILE
FRANCE

SPIELMANN
SOCIETE NUNC - C/O INTERMED
Z.I DES RICHARDETS
24 RUE DU BALLON
93160   NOISY LE GRAND
FRANCE

SPIER R.
UNIVERSITY OF SURREY
GU2 5XH   GUILFORD
GRANDE BRETAGNE

STACEY GLYN
ECACC, PHLS-CAMR
PORTON DOWN
SP4 OJG   WILTSHIRE
GRANDE BRETAGNE

STADLER PETER
BAYER AG, PH-P VE BIOCHEMIE
BLDG 46
P.O BOX 10 17 09
D-5600   WUPPERTAL 1
ALLEMAGNE FEDERALE

STEIN PETER
INVITRON CORPORATION
4649 LE BOURGET DRIVE
63134   ST LOUIS - MISSOURI
ETATS UNIS

STEINER ULRICH
BAYER AG
VE BIOCHEMIE, GEB 50
D-5600   WUPPERTAL 1
ALLEMAGNE FEDERALE

STEPHENNE J.
SMITHKLINE BIOLOGICALS
RUE DE L'INSTITUT, 89
B-1330   RIXENSART
BELGIQUE

SUGIMURA KEIJIRO
2716-1, IKAZA-AKATWA
AZA-KARAKAKE
CHIYODA-MACHI
370-05   OHRA-GUN, GUNMA
JAPON

SUMEGHY ZOLTAN
SANDOZ PHAMA AG
LOICHTSTR.
4002   BASEL
CONFEDERATION HELVETIQUE

TAKADA HIROSHI
KASUGADE NAKA 3-1-98
KONOHANAKU
554   OSAKA
JAPON

TAKAHARA YOSHIYUKI
AJINOMOTORO, INC
1-1 SUZUKI-CHO, KAWASAKI-KU.
KAWASAKI
210   KAWASAKI
JAPON

TAKASHINA MAKOTO
SHIMAYA 1-14-3
KONOHANA-KU. OSAKA
SUMITOMO ELECTRIC INDUSTRIES
554   OSAKA
JAPON

TAKEBE HIDEHI
PHARMACEUTICAL RESEARCH CENTER
HEIJI SEIKA KAISHA LTD
788 KAYAMA, ODAWAYA, KANAGARA
          ODAWARA
JAPON

TAKEUCHI MASAO
INSTITUTE FOR FERMENTATION
OSAKA,TAKEDA CHEMICAL INDUSTR.
LTD . 2-17-85 JUSO-HONCHO
532   OSAKA
JAPON

TALLMAN BONITA M.
RD #4
BOX 85
17756   MUNCY, PA
ETATS UNIS

TANI SHOSHANA
C/O INTERPHARM LABORATORIES LT
KIRYAT WEIZMANN
76110   NESS-ZIONA
ISRAEL

TENTE WILLIAM E.
ARES ADVANCED TECHNOLOGIES
SERONO LABORATORIES
100 LONGWATER CIRCLE
02061   NORWELL, MASSACHUSSETS
ETATS UNIS

TETTEROO P.A.T.
CENTOCOR EUROPE B.V.
P.O BOX 251
2300 AG   LEIDEN
PAYS BAS

THALER THOMAS F.
MBR BIO REACTOR AG
WERKSTRASSE 4
CH-8620   WETZIKON
CONFEDERATION HELVETIQUE

THALMANN ERNST
CHEMAP AG
HOLZLIWISENSTR. 5
8604   VOLKETSWIL
CONFEDERATION HELVETIQUE

THIERY JEAN-PAUL
ECOLE NORMALE SUPERIEURE
PHYSIO-PATHOLOGIE DU DEVELOP.
46 RUE D'ULM
75230   PARIS CEDEX 15
FRANCE

THOMAS RUTH HELEN
BIOTECHNOLOGY LABORATORIES
MANCHESTER POLYTECHNIC
CHESTER STREET
MI 5GD   MANCHESTER
GRANDE BRETAGNE

THOMPSON KEITH JOHN
BIOSCOT LTD
KINGS BUILDINGS
WEST MAINS ROAD
EH9 3JF   EDINBURGH
GRANDE BRETAGNE

THORPE JANE
STERILIN LTD
CULDROSE HOUSE -
1, FREDERICK STREET - ALDERSHO
GU11 ILQ HAMPSHIRE
GRANDE BRETAGNE

TOKASHIKI MICHIYUKI
TEIJIN TOKYO RESEARCH CENTER
4-3-2 ASAHIGAOKA, HINO
191   TOKYO
JAPON

TOLBERT WILLIAM R.
INVITRON CORPORATION
4649 LE BOURGET DRIVE
63134   ST LOUIS MO.
ETATS UNIS

TOMLINSON NICOLA JANE
BIOLOGICFAL LABORATORY
UNIVERSITY OF KENT
CT2 7NJ CANTERBURY
GRANDE BRETAGNE

TONDON JOEL
IBF BIOTECHNICS
35 AVENUE JEAN JAURES
92390   VILLENEUVE LA GARENNE
FRANCE

TONG JEREMY MICHAEL
BIOLOGICAL LABORATORY
UNIVERSITY OF KENT
CT2 7NJ CANTERBURY
GRANDE BRETAGNE

TROTEMANN PIERRE
INSTITUT MERIEUX
1541 AV. MARCEL MERIEUX
69280   MARCY L'ETOILE
FRANCE

VAN DER VELDEN-DE GROOT TINY
RIVM - LAB. INACTIV.VIRAL VACC
P.O BOX 1
3720 BA BILTHOVEN
PAYS BAS

VAN GELDER PIETER, T.J.A.
INTERVET INTERNATIONAL B.V.
POSTBOX 31
5830 AA BOXMEER
PAYS BAS

VAN MEEL FRANCK C.M.
ORGANON INTERNATIONAL B.V.
POSTBUS 20
5340 BH OSS
PAYS BAS

VAN WEPEREN J.
TURFTORENSTR. 12
9712 BP GRONINGEN
PAYS BAS

VENAK J.
MBR BIO REACTOR AG
WERKSTRASSE 4
CH-8620 WETZIKON
CONFEDERATION HELVETIQUE

VICAN CHARLIE
MILLIPORE S.A
BP 307
78054 ST QUENTIN YVELINES CEDEX
FRANCE

VICKROY T. BRUCE
709 SWEDELAND ROAD
19406   KING OF PRUSSIA, PA
ETATS UNIS

VINAS ROGER
PASTEUR - VACCINS
PARC INDUSTRIEL D'INCARVILLE
27100   VAL DE REUIL
FRANCE

VON SEEFRIED ADOLF
165 BETHRIDGE ROAD
M9W 1N4 TORONTO, ONTARIO
CANADA

VOURNAKIS JOHN N.
VERAX CORPORATION
ETNA ROAD
NH 03766 LEBANON
ETATS UNIS

WAGNER ROLAND
G.B.F.
BIOVERFAHRENSTECHNIK
MASCHERODER WEG 1
D-3300   BRAUNSCHWEIG
ALLEMAGNE FEDERALE

WAHL JURGEN
BOEHRINGER MANNHEIM GMBH
NONNENWALD 2
D-8122   PENEBERG
ALLEMAGNE FEDERALE

WALLBERG CHRISTER
MONOCARB AB
S-223 70 LUND
SUEDE

WALZ FRANZ
DR. KARL THOMAE GMBH
BIRKENDORFER STR. 65
7950   BIBERACH
ALLEMAGNE FEDERALE

WARDELL JOHN NOEL
DEPT. OF MICROBIOLOGY
UNIVERSITY OF SURREY
GU2 5XH GUILDFORD
GRANDE BRETAGNE

WATANABE SACHIHIKO
SHIONOGI RESEARCH LABORATORIES
SHIONOGI & CO. LTD.
FUKUSHIMAKU
553   OSAKA
JAPON

WATANABE KAZUO
2-1-3-9 KATATA
OTSU - CITY
              OTSU
JAPON

WATTS PATRICIA
DEPT OF BIOSCIENCE & BIOTECH.
UNIVERSITY OF STRATHLLYDE
TODD CENTRE
G4 ONR   GLASGOW
GRANDE BRETAGNE

WEGGLER ROBERT
VOGELBUSCH GES MBH
ZWEIGNIEDERLASSUNG SCHWEIZ
BUCHGRINDELSTRASSE 13
CH-8621 WETZIKON 4
CONFEDERATION HELVETIQUE

WERENNE J.
FACULTY OF SCIENCES CP 160
UNIVERSITE LIBRE DE BRUXELLES
50 AV D.D. ROOSEVELT
B-1050   BRUXELLES
BELGIQUE

WHITE MICHAEL
BIOTECHNETICS
4116 SORRENTO VALLEY BLVD.
92121   SAN DIEGO, CALIFORNIA
ETATS UNIS

WHITESIDE JONATHAN PETER
MICROBIOZOGY DEPT
UNIVERSITY OF SURREY
GU2 5XH GUILDORD, SURREY
GRANDE BRETAGNE

WHITFIELD ALAN
SERA-LAB LTD
HOPHURST LANE
CRAWLEY DOWN
RH10 4FF SUSSEX
GRANDE BRETAGNE

WIRTH MANFRED
G.B.F
MASCHERODER WEG 1
D-3300   BRAUNSCHWEIG
ALLEMAGNE FEDERALE

WISHER MARTIN
MICROBIOLOGICAL ASSOCIATES INT
STIRLING UNIVERSITY INNOVATION
PARK
FK9 4LA STIRLING
GRANDE BRETAGNE

WURM FLORIAN MARIA
GENENTECH INC. CELL CULTURE
RES. + DEVELOP.
460 POINT SAN BRUNO BLVD.
94080   SOUTH SAN-FRANCISCO,CALIFORNIE
ETATS UNIS

WYATT DIANNE
SERA-LAB LTD
HOPHURST LANE
CRAWLEY DOWN
RH10 4FF SUSSEX
GRANDE BRETAGNE

YOUNG MICHAEL
VERAX CORPORATION
HC61, BOX 6 ETNA ROAD
03766   LEBANON, NEW HAMPSHIRE
ETATS UNIS

ZILIOTTO PAUL
FARMITALIA CARLO ERBA
VIA DEI GRACCHI 35
20146   MILANO
ITALIE

ZOLETTO RENZO
ISTITUTO ZOOPROFILATTICO DELLE
VIA G. ORUS 2
35100   PADOVA
ITALIE

Subject index

Baby hamster kidney cells (*cont.*)
human recombinant glycoproteins, 144, 775
influence of shear stress, 244
interleukin-2 production, 180
LDH-release, 244
morphology, 244
PCFIA measurement, 597
porous ceramic matrix, 400
protease activity, 196
reference cell line, 46
serum-free medium, suspended aggregates, 429
size distribution, 244
viability, 244
Bacterial fermentors, growth of mammalian cells, 381
Baculovirus,
expression vector system, 345
insect pathogens, 470
Basal nutrient, chemically defined, 190
Batch cultures,
kinetic model, 634
LDH release, 569
production of anti-HIV–a antibody, 722
production of antibodies, 390
protein free medium, 625
Bioassays, cytotoxicity, 796
Biological products,
quality control,
EEC directives, 759
and registration, 759
safety and testing, 783
Biomass estimation, VERO cells, 580
Bioreactor system,
airlift system, monoclonal antibodies, 390
antithrombin III-producing BHK cells, 445
bioreactor system *vs* low-tech system, 381
bleeding-out dead cells, 394
comparative studies, 517–540
contained, scale-up, 519
continuous cell lines, flow cytometric analysis, 576
continuous cultures,
antithrombin III production, 445
continuous suspension, dilution rates compared, 616
high density, absence of insulin, 606
on-line removal of cells, 416
production of antibodies, 390
sedimentation chambers, CHO cells, 416
control parameters, 363
double membrane perfusion, antithrombin III-producing BHK cells, 445
entrapment bioreactor, monitoring of monoclonal antibody, 149
fixed bed, 519
fixed membrane *vs* microporous membrane, 537
flask system, 519
fluidized-bed, 502, 513, 528
hardware, 385–420
high density perfusion culture, 262, 370

Bioreactor system (*cont.*)
kinetics and modelling, 601–636
large scale polymodal 225 dm^3 plant, 387
LDH release, 569
membrane aeration, 498
membrane *vs* stirred-tank reactor, oxygen availability, 454
monitoring and assay of animal cell parameters, 541–600
optimization via metabolism, 477–516
overview, 361–384
oxygen supply and glucose concentration, effect on lymphoblastoid cells, 247
particles, 421–442
production of antibodies, 390
productivity, 363
protein-free medium, development, 170
rotating wire cage, 370
stirred tank, 533, 745
stirred tank *vs* fluidized-bed, 528
suspension cultures, 110, 180, 429, 519, 722
see also Perfusion bioreactor
Blood fractionation process, development, 95
Bovine anti-testosterone monoclonal antibodies, cloning and expression, 335
Bovine serum albumin (BSA), as additive to serum-free medium, 148
Branched-chain amino acids, as substrates, 73
Bubble-free aeration,
in fixed membrane reactors, 537
in microporous membrane reactors, 537
oxygen transfer characteristics, 451
in perfused fluidized bed reactor, 528
stirred tank perfusion, 460
suspension culture, 180
Butyrate, effect on Factor VIII, CHO cells, 104
By-products *see* Secondary metabolites

C-type retrovirus, density characteristic, 39
Calcium phosphate precipitation, plasmid sequences, 15
Carcinoma cells,
adhesion and motility factors, 52
growth factors, 732
metastasis, and FGF, 52
Carrier proteins, in downstream processing, 155
CD4, production from recombinant proteins, 90
CD4 chimaeric molecules, production by mouse myeloma cell lines, 18
CD23 receptors, constitutive secretion, 751
Cell adhesion molecules, morphogenesis, 52
Cell banks, characterization by DNA fingerprinting, 28
Cell culture media,
components,
estimation technique, 603
optimisation of protein production, 76
composition, estimation procedures, 603
defined, 796
dialysed, 67

Cell culture media (*cont.*)
  gradients, scale-up difficulties, 407
  and light sensitivity, 82
  protein and serum-free, 131–204
  recycle flow, measurement of downstream
      concentrations, 457
  reference cell lines, 46
  requirements, growth and antibody production,
      625
  safety of medium supplements, 117
  special supplements, 59–130
  see also Large-scale cell culture; Serum-free
      media; Protein-free media
Cell culture process, optimization, 76, 110, 180,
    718
Cell cycle,
  laser flow cytometry, 587
  stages, transferrin receptor levels, 125
Cell death,
  lactate dehydrogenase as an indicator, 569
  laser flow cytometry, 587
Cell density, estimation, 603
Cell density, high, 363, 460, 486, 514
  advantages of fluidized bed reactor, 754
  bioreactor development, 370
  maintenance of cultures, 606
Cell fragility, 381
Cell function modulators (CFM), 95
Cell growth,
  FBS substitutes, evaluation, 95
  role of dissolved oxygen, 256
Cell growth activators (CGA), effect on cell
    replication and protein expression, 95
Cell Line Data Base (CLDB), 48, 49
Cell lines,
  characterization, 13–58
  lipoprotein requirements, 67
Cell longevity, 137
Cell manufacturing processes, development, 363
Cell nucleus protein, from HeLa cells, 754
Cell physiology, 205–284
  adaptation to glutamine-free medium, 276
  ATP and other nucleotides, 236
  critical shear stress level, BHK cells, 244
  cytoskeletal filament network, 229
  effect of by-products, 226
  effect of oxygen and glucose, 247, 256
  factors affecting cell attachment, 266
  investigations, 262
  oligoadenylate synthetase, multienzyme
      system, 279
  osmolarity, 259
  parameters, flask and macroporous glass sphere
      cultures, 479
  pulse experiments, 609
  removal of inhibitory factors, 218
  secondary metabolites, 207
Cell replication, effect of CFM and CGA, 95
Cell stocks, quality control, DNA fingerprinting,
    28
Cell viability, anti-HIV-1 production, 722

Cell-specific productivity, 363
Cellular storage lipids, mammalian cells, fatty
    acid composition, 61
Cell–virus interaction, 519
Centrifuge, continuous, bleeding out dead cells,
    394
Chemostat, antibody cultivation, 247
Chimeric antibody, subclone CHO cells, stability,
    742
Chinese hamster ovary cells,
  defective endogenous retrovirus-like particles,
      39
  evaluation of genetic stability, 576
  expressing FSH, 76
  Factor VIII production, semicontinuous *vs*
      perfusion culture, 523
  FISH (Fluorescence *in situ* hybridization), 316
  human thyrotropin beta cDNA expression, 715
  human/murine recombinant antibody for
      tumour imaging, 742
  IFN-γ, effect of culture environment, 309, 789
  increased expression of Factor VIII, 104
  media supplements, screening experiment, 76
  microcarriers, Dormacell, 439
  microsphere-induced aggregate culture, 416,
      423
  polyamine-enhanced product expression, 107
  producing Factor VIII, 523
  production of antithrombin, III, 498
  productivity enhanced by pluronic F-68, 502
  reference cell line, 46
  release of trypsin-like serine protease, 110
  serum-free media, suspended aggregates, 429
  staining for rapid visualization, 543
  thrombolytic proteins, novel, 712
  tPA production, 669
  transfection with tPA gene, 745
Cholesterol,
  in cell cultivation, 170
  Ex-Cyte as source, 67
Chromatography,
  affinity, MAb purification, 662
  cleaning in place, 639
  high performance liquid affinity
      chromatography, 594
  HPAE-PAD, N-glycans, 775
  ion exchange, MAb purification, 658
  ion exchange chromatography,
      composite high flow rate, 651
      hybridoma cells, 236
      interference of purification, 658
      MAb purification, 658
      sanitization, 651
  leachables, toxicology, 639
Chromatography supports, serum-free, serum
    substitutes, behaviour, 658
Chromosome studies, stability of amplified DNA,
    CHO studies, 309
Cleaning, separation techniques, 637
Clonal variation, 732
Clone, protein-free, transformation, 190

Colchicine, treatment of hybridoma cells, 229
Collagen microspheres, in fluidized-bed
    bioreactors, 502
Collagen types, epithelial cell line reponse, 52
Collagenase, SV40 virus-containing plasmids, 15
Computer simulation, hybridoma cell growth, 631
Conditioned medium, 85
Contamination, separation techniques, 637
Continuous cultures, *see* Bioreactor system
Continuous-flow ultracentrifugation, 39, 394
Couette viscometer, 229
Crossflow filtration, downstream processing, 706
Cytochalasin E, treatment of hybridoma cells, 229
Cytoskeletal microfilament network, resistance to
    shear injury, 229
Cytotoxicity testing, bioassays, and *in vitro*
    techniques, 796

Data banks, cell culture, 48, 49
Data filtering procedure, estimation techniques,
    603
DEAE resin, behaviour of 'serum free' cell
    supernatants, 658
Death phase, hybridoma cultures, 609
Death rates, as function of dilution rate, 616
Deep-end filtration system, hybridoma cell lines,
    454
Defined media *see* Cell culture media; Protein-
    free media; Serum-free media
Desferrioxamine, effect on transferrin receptor
    expression, 125
'Designer proteins', synthesis, 287
Dexamethasone, cell cultivation, 170
DHFR, 309
Dialysed media,
    culture of hybridoma cell lines, 85
    dialysis cartridge, 85
Dicistronic transcription units, correlated dual
    gene expression, 338
Dihydrofolate reductase, co-amplification with
    IFN-Γ gene, 309
Dilution rate, 616
Direct sparging, oxygen transfer characteristics,
    451
DNA,
    amplified, stability in CHO cells, 309
    demethylation, butyrate effect on factor VIII
        expression, 104
    fingerprints, European Collection of Animal
        Cell Cultures, 28
    minisatellite, 28
    Southern analysis, 104
    synthesis, 70
DNA-index determination, evaluation of cell
    stability, 576
'Donor Bovine Serum', as 'safe' supplement, 117
Double membrane stirrer, in fluidized bed
    bioreactor, 528
Downstream concentration measurement,
    medium recycle flow reactors, 457

Downstream processing,
    affinity processing for purification of MAbs,
        662
    composite high flow rate ion exchangers,
        economic scale-up, 651
    isolation of biologicals, 639
    productivity of mammalian cell culture, 363
    protein-free medium, 180
    serum-free media and serum substitutes, 658
    validation, 783
Drosophila melanogaster, insect cell lines, 460

E1A gene, induction of immortalization, 55
E7 oncogene, human papillomavirus, induction of
    immortalization, 55
ECACC *see* European Collection of Animal Cell
    Cultures
Ecotropic viruses, 34
Electrophoresis, purification, monitoring, 662
ELISA, kinetic techniques, purification success,
    662
Embryonic cells,
    adhesion and motility, 52
    human, SV40 virus-containing plasmids, 15
Encapsulation, 548
Endogenous and exogenous retroviruses, safety
    evaluation, 39
Energetics, glutaminolysis, 79
Energy metabolism, growth and antibody
    production, 625
Environment, manipulation, IFN-γ production,
    789
Enzymes, iso-enzyme analysis, evaluation of
    genetic stability of cells, 576
Epidermal growth factor, 726
Epithelial cells,
    in vitro production of growth regulators, 732
    induction of immortalization, 55
EPO-linked oligosaccharide mapping, 775
Epstein–Barr virus,
    B95-8 cell line, marmaset lymphocytes, 706
    transformed B cell line RPM18866,
        hollow fibre reactors, 751
        polyamine-enhanced product expression, 107
Erythrocytes, immunoglobulin-coated,
    phagocytosis, 15
Escherichia coli, tPA production, 669
Esterase, SV40 virus-containing plasmids, 15
European Collection of Animal Cell Cultures,
    DNA fingerprints, 28
European Community,
    biologicals and regulatory aspects, 759
    'BRIDGE' programme, 48
European Database, animal cell lines, 48
Ex-Cyte lipoprotein, 67
Exogenous retroviruses, latent infection, 34

Factor VIII production,
    Chinese hamster ovary cells, 104, 523
        semicontinuous *vs* perfusion culture, 523

Purification process, validation of downstream
    processing, 783
Purine–pyrimidine ratio, ion-pair HPLC, 236
Purity testing, VERO cell culture, 695
Putrescine, polyamine-enhanced product
    expression, 107

Quality control,
    biological products, 759
    EEC directives, 796

Rb protein, anti-oncogene, inactivating cellular
    protein, 55
Recombinant cell lines, HIV gp120 production,
    110
Recombinant CHO cells *see* Chinese hamster
    ovary cells
Recombinant proteins, production,
    CD4, 90
    large-scale, baculovirus expression vector
        system, 345
Recombinant retroviruses, transfection, 55
Redox state, monitoring growth of mammal cells,
    548
Reference cell lines, 46
Registration, biological products, EC directives,
    759
Regulatory issues, 757–798
Respiration, inhibition by KCN treatment, 229
Retinoblasts, human embryo, SV40-containing
    plasmids, 15
Retrovirus-like particles, defective, Chinese
    hamster ovary cells, 39
Retroviruses,
    C-type, 39
    exogenous, 34
    safety evaluation, 34
Reverse transcriptase, 39
RNA, Northern analysis, 104
Roller bottle,
    cultivation of e-RDF medium, 167
    vaccine production, 709
Rotating sieve, oxygen transfer characteristics,
    451

Safety,
    biological product, 783
    safe medium supplements, 117
Sanitization, of ion exchangers, 651
Scale-up,
    bioreactor system, 519
    PBRs, difficulties, 407
    porous ceramic matrix, 400
    see also Large scale production
Schneider-2 cells, protein testing, ultrafiltration
    unit, 460
Screening systems, 338
Secondary metabolites,
    effect on cell cultures, 207, 226
    production rates, growth rate μ function, 616

Sedimentation chambers, continuous culture,
    Chinese hamster ovary cells, 416
Selenous acid, enhancement of Ex-Cyte, 67
Separation methods, diversity, 637
Serine proteases, 196
Serum albumin, 658
Serum replacement concentrate, in serum-free
    culture, 429
Serum substitutes, downstream considerations,
    658
Serum supplements, high density perfusion, 262
Serum-free culture, 187, 196, 247, 345
    anchorage-dependent cells, 137
    antibody cultivation, 247
    cell adaptation, 18
    cell development, 133
    cell growth activators, 95
    cells as suspended aggregates, 429
    chimeric antibody production, 742
    Chinese hamster ovary cell line, 309
    fibronectin production, 167
    in hollow fibre technology, 495
    hybridoma cultures, 133, 140, 149, 606
        kinetic effects, 606
    IPSF purification, 735
    large-scale continuous growth, hybridoma cell
        line, 148
    and light degradation, 82
    and lipid preparations, 67
    mammalian cells, various lines, 140
    NIH 3T3 cells,
        addition of IGF-1, 726
        synergism of IGF-1 and EGF, 726
    pluronic F-68 addition, 502
    protein expression levels, 76
    and protein preparations, 445
    recombinant cell cultures, 502
    RPMI–SR3 medium, Hybritest, 796
    serum substitutes, downstream considerations,
        658
    supplements, 155
    upstream and downstream processing, 155
    von Willebrand factor, 525
Serum-free media, 131–204
    hybridoma cell lines, 259
    sf-9 cells, 46
Shear injury, resistance of cytoskeletal
    microfilament network, 229
Shear-sensitivity, mammalian cells, 381
Sparging, direct, 498
    oxygen transfer rates, 451
Specific growth rate μ,
    cultured cells, 61, 616
    as function of dilution rate, 616
Specific production rate, specialized bioreactors,
    381
Spectrophotometric assay, tPA detection, 748
Spermidine, polyamine-enhanced product
    expression, 107
SSR *see* Protein-free medium, synthetic serum-
    free

Draper, 770
Driesel, A. J., 460
Drouet, X., 247
Duband, J. L., 52
Dufour, S., 52
Dunn, I. J., 513
Duval, D., 256, 454

Eberhard, U., 26, 498
Egly, J. M., 658
Emborg, C., 133, 307, 381
Emery, A. H., 706
Emery, A. N., 70, 379, 398, 414, 589
Engasser, J. M., 454, 486, 569, 575, 603, 606, 634
Estefanell, 568, 650, 770
Evans, F. J., 706

Fabry, L., 580
Fanget, B., 695
Faure, T., 104, 525
Favre, E., 370
Fenge, C., 262
Fertig, G., 470, 576
Field, R. P., 742
Figueroa, 414, 428
Finter, N. B., 3, 568
Fiorentini, D., 137
Fonteix, 603
Fraune, E., 262, 470
Freeman, A., 266
Freshney, 56, 57, 324
Frieberg, H., 622
Fritchmann, K., 190
Froud, S. J., 107, 110, 116, 325
Fung, V., 316

Ganne, V., 104
Gannon, 32
Garcia de Castro, A., 533
Gariepy, P., 95
Gaspard, V., 525
Gavrilovic, J., 52
Geahel, I., 256
Geaugey, V., 454, 569
Gebert, C. A., 66, 76, 129, 274, 308, 795
Geyer, 768
Glad, M., 651, 657
Gleave, S., 226
Godfrey, A., 732
Goergen, J. L., 569, 634
Goetghebeur, S., 423
Gould, S., 345
Graber, P., 751
Grace, J. R., 400
Graf, H., 658
Gray, P. P., 76
Greenfield, P. F., 625
Gregory, B., 732
Grierson, A. W., 748
Griffiths, B., 387
Griffiths, J. B., 46, 48, 65, 149, 308, 398, 479, 519

Gronvik, K. O., 622
Grunow, R., 722
Guerin, P., 104
Gummich, G., 439

Hache, J., 352
Haffenden, P., 117
Haggstrom, L., 79, 622
Hambleton, P., 387
Handa-Corrigan, A., 224, 398, 415, 489, 494, 533, 650, 772
Harbour, C., 307, 631
Harris, E. L. V., 110
Hassell, T., 226
Hauser, H., 338
Hayter, P. M., 309, 789, 795
Heirwegh, K., 148
Heinzle, E., 513
Henno, P., 85
Hentschel, C. C., 26, 27, 287, 302, 303, 325, 694
Herrera, A., 279
Hewlett, G., 67
Hirono, M., 715
Hjertstedt, M., 523
Hofmann, F., 26, 165, 186, 190, 274, 275, 324, 369, 379, 414, 494, 568, 657
Holmberg, A., 594
Holtorf, 274, 307
Hope, J., 363
Hoppe, 32
Horaud, F., 31, 32, 56, 325, 767, 768, 769, 770, 771, 773, 759
Hu, W.-S., 379, 380, 423, 428
Huddleston, J., 706
Hunt, G., 345
Hwang, C., 275, 379, 548, 568

Iannotta, B., 49

Jackson, T., 335
Jacobs, M., 439
Jager, V., 155, 165, 166, 196, 236, 460, 528, 722
Jain, D., 345, 351
Jannin, J., 525
Jenkins, H. A., 203, 276, 512
Jenkins, N., 309, 789
Jennings, P., 226
Jervis, E., 597
Johanssen, R., 144, 498
Johnson, A., 316
Jomotte, T., 75
Jouanneau, J., 52
Junker, B., 345

Kallstrom, U., 745
Kanzler, O., 390
Kaplan, Y., 266
Kaspi, L., 137
Katinger, 57
Keller, G., 39
Keller, H., 170, 609